S0-AWP-687

SYSTEMS ANALYSIS & DESIGN METHODS

The Whitten-Bentley-Ho System of Instruction

- Instructor's Guide with Transparency Masters
- Projects and Cases
- Test Items
- QUESTBANK Computerized Testing Package (for IBM PC or Apple Computers)

All of these supplements were written by Jeffrey L. Whitten and Lonnie D. Bentley. When combined with the *Systems Analysis and Design Methods* text, they provide a complete system of instruction for teaching systems analysis and design. For more information see the *Preface* in this text or call Times Mirror/ Mosby College Publishing at 800-325-4177.

SYSTEMS ANALYSIS & DESIGN METHODS

Jeffrey L. Whitten, MS, CDP
Associate Professor

Lonnie D. Bentley, MS, CDP
Assistant Professor

Thomas I.M. Ho, PhD
Professor

All at Purdue University

Times Mirror/Mosby College Publishing
St. Louis   Toronto   Santa Clara   1986

Dedication

To my Mother and Father, who have always been my source of inspiration.—Jeff

To my lovely wife Cheryl and son Robert.—Lonnie

To Jeff and Lonnie, who are accomplishing what we believe.—Tom

To the students of the Computer Technology Department. May all your experiences be successes.—Jeff, Lonnie, and Tom

Editor	Susan Newman Solomon
Editorial Assistants	Lisa Donohoe and Pam Lanam
Text and Cover Designer	Nancy Benedict
Production Coordinator	Mary Forkner, Publication Alternatives
Illustrators	Reese Thornton and Deborah Thornton

FIRST EDITION

A division of The C.V. Mosby Company
11830 Westline Industrial Drive, St. Louis, MO 63146

Printed in the United States of America

Library of Congress Cataloging in Publication Data

Whitten, Jeffrey L.
Systems analysis and design methods.

Includes index.
1. Systems designs. 2. Systems analysis. I. Bentley, Lonnie D. II. Ho, Thomas I. M., 1948– . III. Title
QA76.9.S88W48 1986 003 85–28535
ISBN 0–8016–5464–5

PR/VH/VH 9 8 7 6 5 4 3 2 1 03/D/317

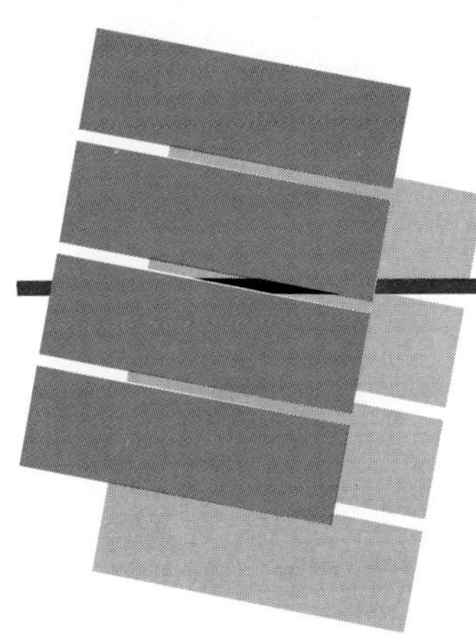

Contents in Brief

Part Three
Systems Design and Implementation: Tools and Techniques 356

Part Four
Skills that Overlap Systems Analysis, Design, and Implementation 708

Contents in Detail

Each chapter begins with What Will You Learn in this Chapter? *and concludes with* Problems and Exercises *and* Annotated References and Suggested Readings.

15 *Designing Computer-Based Methods and Procedures* *568*

16 *Designing Programs and Packaging Program Specifications* *613*

17 *How to Perform Systems Implementation* *656*

Module B Fact-Finding Techniques 733

Module C Communications Skills for the Systems Analyst 756

Module D Feasibility and Cost-Benefit Analysis Techniques 781

Module E Database: The Alternative to Files 806

Index 835

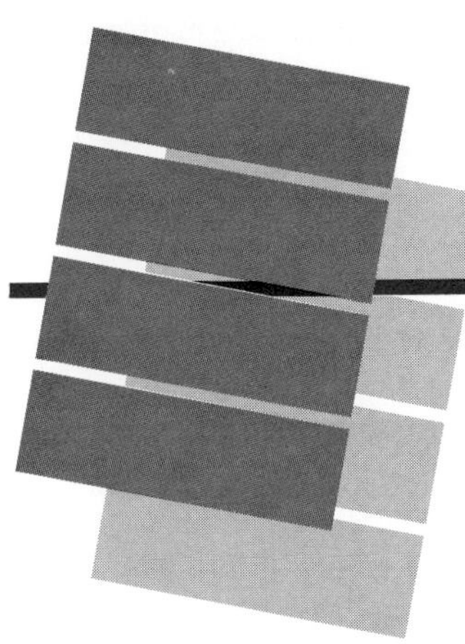

Preface

The Intended Audience for this Book

Systems Analysis and Design Methods is intended to support a practical first course in computer information systems development. This course is normally taught at the sophomore or junior level in two and four year colleges and trade schools. We recommend that students have taken an introductory data processing or computer concepts course and at least one computer programming course before using this book. The book can be used for any introductory systems course in either the DPMA, ACM, or independent computer science or computer information systems curriculum.

Why We Wrote This Book

Today's students have become ''consumer-oriented''—they want their money's worth for every course. They expect to walk away from a course with more than just a grade and the promise that someday they'll appreciate the concepts and knowledge. They want to leave a course having practiced and mastered career-oriented skills. Thus, like most instructors, we require practical projects for our systems analysis and design course. Our enthusiasm for teaching this subject, however, has been tempered by student and instructor dissatisfaction with the available textbooks. We wrote this book to solve the problems we found in other books. Specifically, we note the following:

- *Many books are too conceptual.* Students perceive concepts as "fillers." Actually most books do reinforce the concepts, but this reinforcement is not immediately apparent to the naive and inexperienced student.
- *Other books are very practical, but too mechanical.* These books leave students with the impression that systems analysis is only tools and techniques, and they do not get a sense of the "people side" of systems analysis and design — working with users, resolving conflicts, facing frustrations, fulfilling responsibilities to users.
- *Most books perpetuate the myth that classical and structured tools are mutually exclusive.* To the practitioner, nothing could be further from the truth. Both classical and structured tools and techniques offer advantages and disadvantages. Furthermore, they can and should be applied in a complementary strategy to build more effective information systems.
- *Virtually all books lack sufficient examples to demonstrate the practical requirements of projects.* Students consistently complain that examples are too few, too simple, not interrelated, etc. This problem places tremendous office and classtime burdens on faculty, who feel compelled to "fill in the holes."
- *Most books do not offer a glimpse into the future of systems work.* The next generation of systems analysis and design will be very different from the current generation. Students know this because they read trade journals regularly; but they find correlating the trends with specific jobs and career options difficult, as the trade journals are written to a more experienced audience.

Why We Think You Should Consider This Book

Like most authors, we are excited about our book. We really believe that it is different and that you should consider adopting this textbook for your course because:

- *Instructors provided market research for this book.* Before we began writing our publisher solicited more than 1500 detailed questionnaires from systems analysis and design instructors all over the country. Their responses helped us appreciate the variety in systems analysis and design courses and significantly influenced the structure and content of our work. This book reflects what instructors want.

- *This book is more complete than other texts.* We cover several subjects that receive no coverage or only partial coverage in many other books. For example, we provide *entire* chapters on:
  - Terminal dialogue design for on-line systems
  - Data dictionaries and codes
  - Data flow diagrams
  - On-line systems design
  - Interpersonal skills
- *We present both concepts and tools as important to systems analysis and design.* The book's organization provides a solid learning path from concepts and trends to tools and techniques. Concepts are reinforced throughout the book via a visual model (the pyramid) and via the systems development life cycle orientation.
- *Our book is skills oriented and practical, but not mechanical.* We emphasize the role of the analyst, as well as people skills, human engineering considerations and user interaction—so necessary throughout the systems development life cycle.
- *We integrate the use of classical and structured tools and techniques.* Students are not likely to graduate into the pure structured shop, pure classical shop, or any other strict advocate of a single methodology. So, unlike any other book, we show how to make the transition from the newer structured tools of systems analysis to the tried-and-true tools of classical systems design. Further, this is the only book that demonstrates the packaging of classical design specifications around the tools and techniques of structured design.
- *We have included many more examples than other systems texts.* Reviewers have consistently noted the abundance of practical examples provided by this text. Students learn by doing; any good manager will tell you (and every instructor knows) that employees (and students) can't master something that hasn't been adequately demonstrated.
- *This book is up to date and points to the future of systems analysis and design.* We cover (not just mention) all the latest tools and topics. Through our *Next Generation* box feature we give valuable insight into future applications, methods, tools and

techniques — such as prototyping, productivity tools and information systems issues. The *Next Generation* is intended to be more thought-provoking than informative and to sensitize students to the need to "keep current" in this rapidly changing field.

- *This book offers flexibility of topic coverage.* Specialized skills that overlap multiple phases of systems development (such as fact finding, cost-benefit analysis, interpersonal communications and so on) or that are not included in all first courses are presented as "modules" in a separate unit that may be taught any time after Chapter 5.

- *Our in-text learning aids have been carefully developed to maximize student learning:*
  1. *Minicases.* Most chapters begin with a minicase and discussion questions to sensitize the reader to the chapter's issues. Some cases demonstrate successes and others demonstrate failures. A few cases issue challenges that intentionally present a problem to students — a problem that can be solved by reading the chapter.
  2. *What Will You Learn in This Chapter?* Each chapter includes behavioral objectives toward which the student can strive. These objectives are specifically tested via the problems and exercises at the end of the chapters and modules. The correspondence between the objectives and the problems and exercises is documented in the Instructor's Guide.
  3. *Problems and Exercises.* Each chapter includes problems and exercises that are specifically patterned after the behavioral objectives for that chapter. Most problems and exercises are designed so they won't burn themselves out — that is, so their effectiveness is not diminished by the buildup of students' files containing answers. This is accomplished by having the student draw upon previous or current work experience, or research and interviews. Several problems offer no single, correct solution and call for some subjective analysis.
  4. *Annotated References and Suggested Readings.* This section is more than a bibliography. Many references are annotated with the authors' insights into their favorite books, some of them competitors.
  5. *A Running Case Study — Analysts in Action.* This case study features a typical project presented in eight episodes. A run-

ning case is not a unique concept, but "Analysts in Action" has two unique and noteworthy differences:

- The case emphasizes the people interaction of systems work, especially interaction between analysts and users. Tools and techniques are demonstrated, but not emphasized, in the episodes.
- The episodes introduce rather than reinforce chapter content to enhance student motivation. The student, having seen the tool in the context of the working environment, is more highly motivated to master that tool.

- *We have written the book using a lively, conversational tone.* Today's students often lose interest in textbooks because they are written in a dry, factual tone. We see no reason to tarnish an exciting subject by writing in a dull, academic style. Therefore, we wrote this text in a conversational, "talk with you, not at you" tone. By making the material more interesting as well as informative and instructional, we believe this text will maintain students' reading interest over a longer period of time.

We hope the reasons above will convince you to consider this book. We hope also that you will discover it to be the systems analysis and design book you've been waiting for.

How to Use This Book

Systems Analysis and Design Methods is divided into four parts. The first three parts are normally covered in sequence although some instructors may prefer to resequence some chapters. Part One, "Systems Anslysis and Design: Concepts, Philosophies, and Trends," presents the information systems development situation. These chapters introduce the systems analyst career option, modern information systems functions and capabilities, and the systems development life cycle. We take great comfort in the fact that the concepts underlying today's trends are not different from those we learned as students—that certainly says something for concepts. We add interest to the presentation of these concepts through the use of practical examples that demonstrate the current state-of-practice in the field. To reinforce concepts, two *visual* models are developed—the information system pyramid and the life cycle. These visual models are repeated throughout the text to reinforce the concepts as they are applied in the skill-oriented chapters.

Parts Two and Three present "Systems Analysis Tools and Techniques" and "Systems Design and Implementation Tools and Techniques." We organized the chapters around the proven roadpath to successful systems, the systems development life cycle. Each part begins with a chapter that takes a more detailed look at the appropriate phases of the life cycle. Subsequent chapters develop specific skills that the student can immediately apply to projects and problems. We place considerable emphasis on the business perspective and human engineering aspects of systems anslysis and design.

Part Four is quite unique! Market research indicated that a set of skills and topics is included in some introductory systems courses but not in others (such as data base, cost/benefit analysis and project management). Our research indicated further that because these skills and topics overlap the traditional analysis, design, and implementation phases, different instructors prefer to introduce the material at different points during the course. We organized these subjects, therefore, into self-contained modules, Part Four. Instructors may elect to cover none or all of the modules, may introduce them at their discretion, and may prefer to review any module at other appropriate times during the course. Any prerequisite chapters are mentioned at the beginning of the modules.

Additional course design alternatives and textbook use guidelines may be found in the *Instructor's Guide* that accompanies our text.

Supplements

It is our purpose to provide instructors with a course, not just a book. The large numbers of part-time instructors, teaching assistants, overworked researchers, and adjunct faculty motivated us to assemble a powerful supplements package.

Instructor's Guide

Not just your everyday combination of key terms, topical outline, problem answers, and transparency masters! Instead, we've written an instructor's guide with substance. Our guide includes:

- *Course planning, design, scheduling, and control suggestions* for both quarter and semester plans of study.
- *Textbook conversion aids* to help instructors convert from their current text to Whitten/Bentley/Ho.

- *Lesson planning guidelines* that offer numerous options for using classroom time. Lessons are designed around student behavioral objectives. For each objective, alternative classroom approaches (i.e., lecture, discussion, lab, workshop, demonstration) are directed to the objective. Evaluation mechanisms, other than those in the book and the *Projects and Cases* supplement, are offered. Instructors can build interesting and varied lessons around these guidelines.
- *Additional references* for the instructor's preparation.
- *Answers or answer guidelines* for textbook discussion questions, challenges, problems, and exercises.
- *Guidelines for using the Projects and Cases supplement.*
- *Chapter enhancements* for higher level classes or very motivated students.
- *Blank forms and charts* with duplication permission. (Permission to duplicate is contingent upon adoption of the textbook or the *Projects and Cases* supplement.)
- *100 transparency masters* of (1) key graphics that appear in the book, (2) of adaptations of textbook graphics, and (3) of totally new illustrations.

Projects and Cases

Not just a case book! The best designed casebooks are usually flawed. This is not the author's fault; it's a problem with the concept of a casebook itself. The author of a case is trying to distill the complexities of a realistic, practical situation and put them on paper using the English language, a tool that analysts have long since abandoned as ambiguous. As a result, cases often contain omissions and discrepancies that the instructor is forced to resolve. Perhaps it's realistic to leave holes in a case, but the instructor often pays the price.

We offer an alternative that has been class tested and proven for ten semesters! Our *Projects and Cases* offers the following distinctive features:

- *Build Your Own Case.* A controlled approach allows students to build a systems analysis and design project from their own work experience (which doesn't have to be in data processing). Students' familiarity with the business environment increases their interest and frees the instructor from case development.

Case development results from the direct application of the concepts and philosophies found in Part One of the text. Meanwhile, carefully conceived guidelines ensure that each student's case is equivalent in size and complexity. These guidelines permit both individual and team projects.

- *Adapt a Case.* Students are provided with an overview of traditional commercial systems applications. Through directed research, the student establishes an industry and business situation using the concepts in Part One of the textbook. Once again, the burden of case development is on the student, who takes an active role in the project's direction.
- *Programming Instruction Cases.* Computer programming instructors often spend as much time debugging their assignment specifications for the students as they do teaching the art of computer programming. This project option directs a small team of students to develop thorough programming assignment specifications using an instructor's course goals and objectives.
- *Milestones.* For each of the above options, this supplement is divided into project milestones that are cross-referenced to our textbook as well as selected other texts. Each milestone describes the assignment and provides a final checklist for common errors and omissions.
- *Forms and Charts.* Blank forms and charts with duplication permission are provided. (Permission to duplicate is contingent upon adoption of the textbook or the *Projects and Cases.*)

Test Bank

A written test bank includes 3000 items using the following formats:

- True/False
- Multiple Choice
- Matching
- Sentence Completion
- Essay

The test bank includes both correct answers and a unique feature — explanations or rationales for incorect answers. A computerized testing package, *QUESTBANK,* is available from our publisher for adopters.

Acknowledgements

We are indebted to many individuals who have contributed to the development of this textbook. We want to thank the reviewers and market research respondents whose feedback was both constructive and invaluable.

Reviewers

Joyce Abler
Central Michigan University

Maryam Alavi
University of Houston, Central

Sarah Baker
Miami University

Steven Baumgartner
California State University, Los Angeles

Lynn Bell
DeVry Institute of Technology, Phoenix

Charles Bilbrey
James Madison University

Seth Carmody
Illinois State University

Ronald Cerruti
City College of San Francisco

William Cotterman
Georgia State University

Kevin Duggan
Midlands Technical College

Lance B. Eliot
California State University, Long Beach

J. Patrick Fenton
West Valley Community College

Jack Gillman
Florida International University

Sallyann Hanson
Mercer County Community College

Claudia Harris
Tulsa Junior College

Don Harris
Lincoln Land Community College

C. Brian Honess
University of South Carolina, Columbia Campus

Jean-Margaret Hynes
University of Illinois, Chicago

Blake Ives
Dartmouth College

Wallace Jewell
Edinboro University of Pennsylvania

Carol Kaplan
Rockland Community College

Bob Keim
Arizona State University

Paul Maxwell
Bentley College

Marilyn Puchalski
Bucks County Community College

Lora Robinson
St. Cloud State University

Bruce Saulnier
Quinnipiac College

Craig Slinkman
University of Texas, Arlington

Alfred St. Onge
Springfield Technical Community College

Carole Timinskis
Ferris State College

Joyce Walton
Seneca College

Frank White
Catonsville Community College

John G. Williams
Indiana University/Purdue University, Indianapolis

Ronald Williams
Central Piedmont Community College

Market Research Respondents:

Alabama: J. Allen, Imao Chen, Patricia Cole, Roy Daigle, Betty Hinkson, John Pearson, K. Reilley, Fejinder Sara, John Willhardt, Kenneth Williams, F. H. Wood. **Arizona:** Carole Meeks, W. Pagnotta. **Arkansas:** Tim Baird, D. G. Barber, James Behel, Glenn Coleman, Carolyn Easley, H. H. Hartman, David Kratzer, Don Roberts. **California:** G. Michael Barnes, Stephen Baumgartner, Clifford Brown, Evan Brown, Jeff Buckwalter, Michael Capsuto, Ronald Cerruti, Carl DeWitt, Ed Dionne, Ronald Eaves, Ben Edmonson, Raymond Fanselau, Peter Freeman, Fred Friedman, Kenneth Gardner, Stanley Gryde, David Harris, William Key, Sidney Kitchel, Richard Meyer, D. Michelepoulos, Mary Pavlovich, C. V. Ramamoorthy, Lance Rand, John Randall, George Rice, Jesse Sacilana, Jeane Schildberg, John Sonquist, John Spagnoletti, John Stoob, Lavette Teague, Jim Vigen, Gerald Wagner, Joseph Waters, Robert Wilson. **Colorado:** Magnus Braunagel, Roberta Canter, Deane Carter, Ray Clarke, Ronald Dehn, Curtiss Mallory. **Connecticut:** Richard Close, F. Hilson, R. A. Kambertz, Earl McCoy, Bruce Saulnier. **District of Columbia:** Eugene Dolan, Nanette Levinson, H. Maisel, I. D. Welt. **Delaware:** Alan Buttles, Roxine MacDonald, Philip Mackey, Jack O'Day. **Florida:** Richard Earp, Fred Harold, Joseph King, Kathryn Kinsley, Gus Klebingot, Pete Kokoros, Keith Merwin, Joseph Moder, H. C. Munns, Jack Munyan, Richard Plate, Douglas Shaw, W. B. Wright. **Georgia:** Lucio Chiaraviglio, John Mitchell, Leonard Rodrigues, Erich Stocker, Reneva Vincent. **Hawaii:** Kay Hoke. **Idaho:** Byron Dangerfield, Ross Ruchti. **Illinois:** Jerome Banoss, William Burkhardt, Jack Caldwell, Mira Carlson, Don Distler, John Fendrich, Peg Goetz, Wanda Grabow, Dwight Graham, Donald Harris, Shankar Hedge, T. Hjelem, Paul Hrycewicz, David Kephart, J. Nadis, Norman Noerder, Alan Pfeifer, Samuel Pincus, Linda Salchenberger, Dean Sanders, Larry Vail, Russell Vernor, John Weir. **Indiana:** A. J. Adams, Leon Adkinson, R. A. Barrett, W. J. Brown, Jean Heinemann, Paul Hemmeter, Carl Hommer, David Hutchinson, Donald Kurtz, T. C. Lee, Robert Leiper, N. J. Smith, Ed Solinski, James Westfall. **Iowa:** Richard Chlopan, Raymond Hardy, Don Hansen, William Lee, Stephen Smith, Karen Sturm. **Kansas:** G. H. Anderson, Ricky Barker, H. R. Gentry, David Gustafson, Gary King, Jack Logan, Gretchen Ryan. **Kentucky:** Marvin Albin, Keith Arnold, John Crenshaw, Richard DiSilvestro, Tom Hughes, John McGregor, Paul Mulcahy, Rammohan Ragade, James Sherrard, Gladys Smith, William Toll. **Louisiana:** W. F. Denny, Brenda Erfurdt, Patricia Farer, Ruby Halliday, Walter Hollingsworth, W. H. Hyams, S. Sitharama Iyengar. **Massachusetts:** L. Clarke, W. Clarke, Robert Graham, John Hafferty, Pat Hagan, Maurice Halliday, D. Hastings, Jane Hill, Ernest Kallman, Paul Maxwell, David Russell, Gwendolyn Sams, Mark Schuh, Jean Smelewicz, J. MacGregor Smith, Alfred St. Onge, Sandra Stalker. **Maryland:** G. Balog, Dale Murray, Frank White. **Maine:** Thomas

Byther. **Michigan:** Joseph Adamski, Jack Burgess, T. S. Greff, Charlene Griffin, Richard Howell, Sandra Poindexter, David Rosteck, John Schneider, D. Stephen, Carole Timinskis, Lawrence Turner. **Minnesota:** Michael Bozonie, R. Christenson, R. Folz, Larry Grover, Ambrose Kodet, John Lehman, Roderick McMillan, J. David Naumann, David Weldon, Richard Weisgerber. **Mississippi:** Kirk Arnett, Ralph Bisland, Jr., C. D. Burgg, Elias Callahan, James Christine, Barbara Pettway, Brady Rimes, Donald Smith. **Missouri:** Wayne Bailey, Richard Batt, H. D. Byron, John Craigin, J. Steve Earney, Tom Franklin, Raymond Freese, Mike Martin, Owen Miller, Joe Otterson, S. V. Pollack, David Race, A. Wilson. **Montana:** Walter Briggs, John Rettenmayer. **North Carolina:** Bob Blackwelder, James Carland, Aubrey Claton, David Cooke, Gail Lee Elmore, Jim Finn, Stan Grady, Michael Hall, G. L. Hershey, Carol Jones, James Hunter, Robert Kinch, James Land, E. L. Morton, Robert Ralph, Steve Robertson, W. R. Spickerman, Fu Yao Wang, Bruno Wichnoski, Stan Wilkinson, Dianne Williams, Ronald Williams. **Nebraska:** Elizabeth Behrens; C. Vaughn Johnson, William Longley, Marilyn Mantel-Guss, Rene Mayo, Glenn Morey, Jim Scott. **New Hampshire:** Dick Bennett, Kurt Hyde, Blake Ives. **New Jersey:** Rene Asgari, David Bellin, Kevin Byron, Thomas Dunn, Tony Fini, George Gugel, Jim Lawaich, C. Mitchell, H. Terry Reid, Jerry Segal, Shirley Tainow, Jacqui Vail, W. Westphal, Ed Winchester, D. C. Winters. **New Mexico:** L. B. Keaty. **New York:** John Bockelman, Michael Breban, Richard Coll, Joan Danehy, Maryangela Gadikian, Harry Goldberg, Myron Goldberg, Ron Gwynn, Joseph Hoffman, W. S. Holmes, David Hopkins, Carol Kaplan, Keith LaBudde, Jim Leone, Lawrence Levine, Susan Luman, Krishna Moothy, Eta Nagle, Jane Peaslee, Edwin Reilly, E. H. Rogers, John Rooney, Kenneth Rule, Donald Stasiw, Daniel Sterns, Paul Szabo, Gilbert Traub, Joe Turner, J. S. Williams, C. Zamifirescu. **Ohio:** Beverly Atwell, Sarah Baker, G. D. Bouw, Richard Bialac, C. M. Brown, John Chappelear, Tom Critzer, Carl Crosswhite, W. S. Davis, Carl Evert, Donald Fairburn, George Field, R. A. Hovis, James Kriz, David Kroger, Richard Little, Carol Lobenhofer, Marianne Massi, John McKinney, Ronald Moreau, Sharon Morel, J. O'Loughlin, David Osborne, Karl Rieppel, Erwin Roster, Ravinderpahl Sandhu, Joseph Speier, T. Srager, Elaine Shillito, Douglas Troy, Gail Weisman. **Oklahoma:** Frank Chimente, Milford Chisum, Tom Ford, Ralph Foster, Claudia Harris, G. E. Hedrick, James Holland, Jacques La France, Robert Lanctot. **Oregon:** Mads Ledet, John Shaw, Ken Thomason. **Pennsylvania:** Fred Bierly, Mario Cecchetti, Angelo De Cesaris, William Doyle, Harold Frey, James Gardmen, Wallace Jewell, Jr., Frederick Kohun, Ralph Kuhn, John Lane, Robert Little, Melvin Mitchell, Myron Morford, Prashant Palvia, Dennis Pearson, King Perry, Marilyn Puchalski, H. Prywes, Paul Ross, Jeff Routh, Harold Schwartz, Edward Styborski, Charles Taylor, Stephen Tillman, Samuel Wiley. **Rhode Island:** D. Richard Allen, David Rolfe. **South Carolina:** Carter Bays, Kevin Duggan, W. Greg Huseth, E. L. Menes, Linda Metcalf. **South Dakota:** James Johnson. **Tennessee:** John Beckell, Wayne Brown, L. Edward Hart, C. Bruce Myers, Jerry Peters, Charles Pfluger, Clinton Smullen, Bill Truex, James Westmoreland. **Texas:** John Anderson, Ida Mae Baxter, James Beane, David Burris, C. M. Bush, Larry Crisp, G. Cunningham, Alton Dillaha, Arnold English,

Victor Fixe, William Harkrider, John Harrison, Paul Hewitt, Fred Homeyer, Roy Martin, Leonard McLaughlin, C. H. Nestman, Joseph Pennington, Camilla Rice, Theodore Robinson, Les Rydl, Fred Sheicklgruber, Craig Slinkman, Ron Tabor, Ken Veatch, Suriya Yadan. **Utah:** Russell Anderson, Larry Chaston, Greg Jones, Robert Lewis, Marshall Rowney. **Virginia:** David Ameen, Ben Bauman, Charles Bilbrey, E. E. Blanks, R. F. Brogan, Terri Burner, James Clements, Edward Cross, Gerald Engel, G. W. Gorsline, Berton Hodge, Willard Keeling, Paul Laski, J. Lee, Charles Reynolds, Daniel Reynolds, J. W. Riehl, Arline Sachs, Hilton Souther, Walter Strain, Howard Ward. **Washington:** Robert Ball, Bob Mathews, George Miller, Susan Solomon, W. N. Wittstruck. **Wisconsin:** Pierre Bettelli, David Dean, William Fieldbinder, Jacob Gerlach, Mohan Gill, Michael Meeker, Robert Morshew, Len Myers, Paul Pham, Allen Schmidt, Ralph Smieja, Janice Weinberg. **West Virginia:** Robert Marsburn, Robert Perry. **Wyoming:** Richard Cliver, Rod Southworth, Althea Stevens. **Puerto Rico:** Alvin Martinez. **Canada:** Peter Abel, Frank Allair, J. A. Anderson, E. Arojmandi, Tom Austin, Frank Brearton, David Daniels, William Davenport, Victor Dawson, Bob Fawcett, Diane Fletcher, K. Dale Fletcher, Grant Hamilton, D. J. Hanbury, E. Heither, Misbah Islam, Herbert Kempe, Gerry Kowalchuk, Rosa Lam, Alan Law, C. E. Law, A. P. B. Lissett, Jack Mathews, David May, L. L. McCurdy, J. Mitchell, R. J. Miller, R. A. Moss, Alan Moore, H. Mueller, J. F. Newman, David Nolting, Riley O'Connor, R. Smith, Gordon Veinot, Mike Webb, Georgette Weiss.

Special thanks is given to Dorothy Jane Miller, our secretary, who provided encouragement, overtime, and patience, especially during the weeks and evenings that preceded project deadlines.

We offer thanks to the students of the Computer Technology Department of Purdue University. You have been truly special and made teaching a rewarding experience. Your patience and understanding during early drafts of the textbook, handouts, and projects was much appreciated. This book is for you! We'd like to single out the following students who made special contributions to the project: Henry Yee, Daina Mathews, Karen Kincaid, Tammy Bullock Fisher, Mike and Jeannine Stoltz, Lorraine Demelio, and Judy Stork. Each of these individuals contributed through reviews, development, special materials, or ideas.

Finally, wc'd likc to thank our new family, the publishing staff of Times Mirror/Mosby. Special thanks is given to Susan Newman Solomon, our sponsoring editor and the best in the business. Prospective authors who appreciate the professionalism and style of this book would do well to contact Susan. Additional thanks is offered to Mary Forkner, Nancy Benedict, Sandra West, Reese and Deborah Thornton, Claudia Wilrodt, Dick Schiding, Sue Platts, Pam Lanam, and Lisa Donohoe.

We hope we haven't forgotten anyone. And we assume full responsibility for any inadequacies or errors in this text. Any comments, criticisms, suggestions, or improvements are welcome and appreciated. Write to us in care of Times Mirror/Mosby, 4633 Old Ironsides Drive, Suite 410, Santa Clara, CA 95054.

We think that if you compare *Systems Analysis and Design Methods* to other texts, you will truly "discover the difference." And now we must start the sequel, an exciting, unique approach to the structured systems analysis and design methodology. No rest for the weary. . . .

Jeff Whitten
Lonnie Bentley
Tom Ho

SYSTEMS ANALYSIS &
DESIGN METHODS

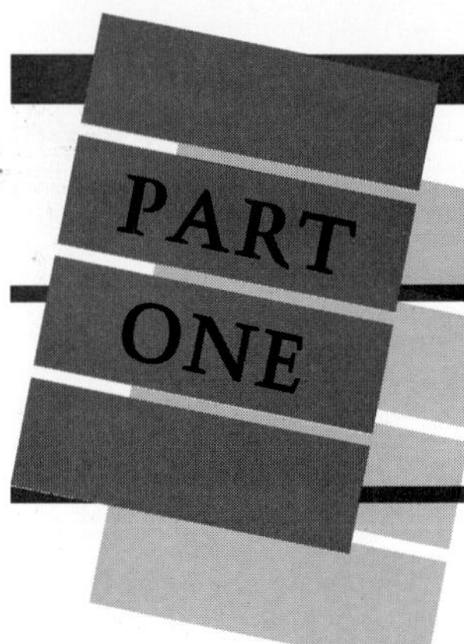

Systems Analysis and Design: Concepts, Philosophies, and Trends

We can almost read your mind: "Con'-cepts? Phi-los'-o-phies? Trends? (Well, that one's OK) . . . WAIT A MINUTE! I thought this was supposed to be a practical book." We worried about that title. Honest! So many concepts units seem only to fill space in textbooks. They have that "Because I told you so!" feel to them. So why should you study this unit? Well, titles can be very misleading. This is going to be the most applied, involving concepts unit you have ever read. We'll give you plenty of examples to sink your teeth into.

Systems analysis and design aren't mechanical activities. There are no magical methodologies for success (although there are many snake oil merchants who say there are); no perfect tools and techniques. Programming may be a skill, but systems analysis and design is also very much an art. Fortunately, many of us have the natural abilities we need to succeed in this art (although it is becoming somewhat of an engineering discipline in some respects). But we need to be schooled; we need to refine and extend our natural abilities. We start, here, with the basics.

Systems analysis and design are practical disciplines. Fortunately, the practice is governed by some basic concepts and philosophies. If you understand these concepts and philosophies, you will be able to apply, with confidence, the tools and techniques we present. Furthermore, you will find yourself better able to adapt to new situations and methods. In addition to concepts and philosophies, we will also discuss trends that will impact systems analysis and design.

Five chapters make up this unit. Chapter 1 introduces you to the systems analyst, the professional most likely to practice the methods presented in this book. Chapter 2 introduces the knowledge worker and the business as the benefactors of the computer-based information systems the systems analyst will analyze and design. The cast of characters having been established, Chapter 3 focuses on the information system itself. Because the information system is the product the systems analyst is developing, it is important for you to have a good understanding of that product. We describe the information system in terms of capabilities, inputs, outputs, and processing elements. In Chapter 4 we survey the problems typically encountered by systems analysts when developing modern information systems and establish some basic principles for successful system development. Finally, Chapter 5 introduces the system development life cycle, the process by which systems analysts build information systems. These five chapters are designed to give you a solid foundation upon which to build your study of the tools and techniques presented in Parts II, III, and IV of this book.

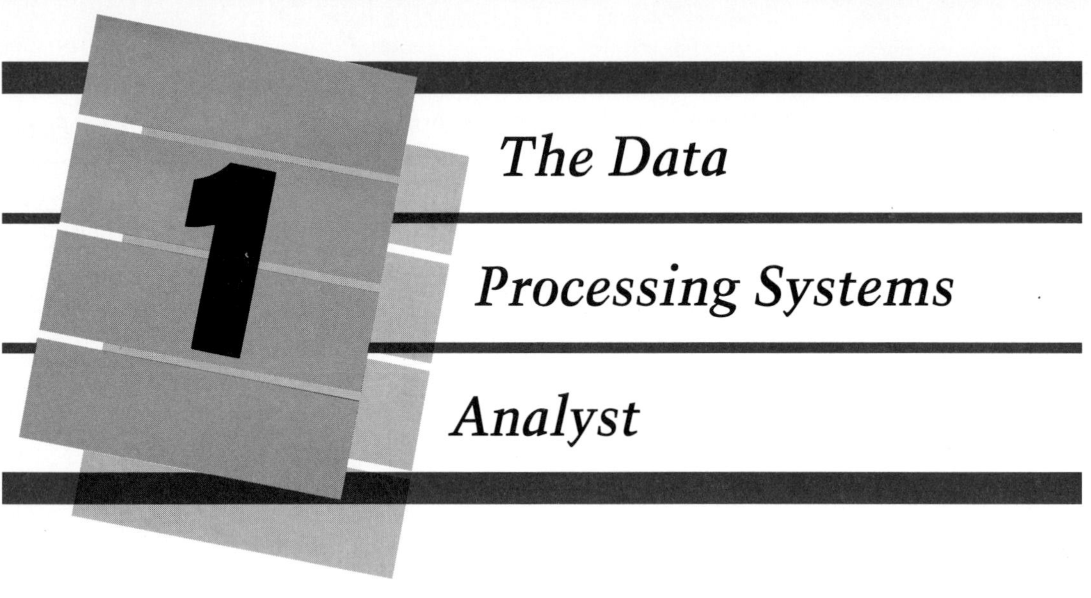

1 The Data Processing Systems Analyst

WHAT WILL YOU LEARN IN THIS CHAPTER?

This chapter introduces the systems analyst — the person this book is about. You will know that you understand the systems analyst function when you can

1. Define the systems analyst's role and responsibilities in a typical organization.
2. Define *systems analysis, systems design,* and *systems implementation* — the three principle activities performed by the analyst.
3. Differentiate between a *systems analyst,* a *programmer/analyst,* and an *information analyst.*
4. Differentiate between the types of work done by the systems analyst and the computer programmer.
5. Describe how the systems analyst fits into the data processing function.
6. Develop a plan of study for your education or continuing education that will prepare you for a career as a systems analyst.

WHO SHOULD READ THIS BOOK?

Why are you interested in systems analysis and design methods? Perhaps one of the following scenarios describes your interest:

- You have aspirations of becoming a data processing systems analyst or a programmer/analyst (hereafter referred to as an analyst).
- You have aspirations of becoming a computer programmer, and you realize that computer programmers must work closely with analysts.
- You have aspirations of becoming a business manager, consultant, or professional staff (for example, accountant, marketing specialist, or production manager), and you realize that you will work closely with analysts to define your computer support needs.
- You are a computer programmer (or programming student), and you find yourself doing — or redoing — work normally done by an analyst. (This situation is not unusual because programmers frequently encounter incomplete or inadequate programming specifications prepared by analysts.)
- You have been asked or assigned to write computer programs for a business application you know little or nothing about.
- You are an analyst (or student), and you have been introduced to the new structured methodologies; you are interested in integrating their use with the more classical tools and techniques.

If any of these situations describes you, you should read this book. The pertinent character in each of our scenarios is the analyst. But just what is a systems analyst and what does one do? The answers to these questions lie in this book.

WHERE DID THE SYSTEMS ANALYST COME FROM?

In the beginning, there was the computer — or so it seems! Truly, computers have become a way of life for today's high-tech society. Look around you. There are computers in many of your home appliances. There are computers in most new cars. Most of your bills are generated by computers. You receive junk mail because you are on everybody's computer list. You can get money from the bank at all hours if you have access to a computerized teller. Do you have any idea how much information a person could obtain about you if they gave a computer your social security number? The computer revolution has changed all our lives. But you haven't seen anything yet!

Why is all this happening? It may surprise you to discover that the computer technological revolution is firmly rooted in common sand and quartz. Silicon, an element that is second only to oxygen as the most abundant substance on Earth, is found in sand and quartz. And silicon is used to manufacture the tiny computer chips that contain thousands of microscopic electronic circuits. Today's microprocessor chips carry a hundred thousand or more electronic circuits and execute ten million or more instructions per second, and these chips are getting better every day! Furthermore, they are getting smaller and cheaper! As a result of this technological revolution, every business will soon be able to afford a computer. And businesses that have been using computers all along will be able to acquire greater numbers of computers that are more and more powerful.

Still, despite all of its current and future technological capabilities, the computer owes its power and usefulness to people. Business people define the applications and problems to be solved by the computer. Computer programmers and technicians apply the technology to well-defined applications and problems. Thus, we see that computers are only tools that offer the opportunity to collect and store enormous volumes of data, process business transactions with great speed and accuracy, and provide timely, relevant information for management. Unfortunately, this potential has not been fully or even adequately realized in most businesses. Business users do not fully understand the capabilities, limitations, and technology of the computer. Likewise, the computer programmers and technicians frequently do not understand the business applications, problems, and needs that they are trying to solve. Indeed, a communications gap has dcvcloped between those who need the computer and those who understand the technology.

The systems analyst was born during the Industrial Revolution when business was suddenly forced to study and design efficient production methods and procedures for people and machines. The data processing systems analyst evolved from the need to improve use of the computer resource for the information processing needs of business applications. We've already characterized the computer as a tool in a more complex entity—the business. Many of the failures and disappointments of business computing can be traced to our preoccupation with the computer and the failure of the computer professional to recognize the problems and needs of the business system. All too frequently, computer solutions are designed without regard for the people who will use them. The systems analyst is our answer to bridging the communications gap that has developed between the business user and computer programmer/technician.

Has this new breed of systems analyst truly bridged the communications gap between the business user and computer programmer/technician? Not really! We recognized the need for the data processing systems analyst long before we developed effective tools, techniques, and methodologies to build the bridge. Today, these methods exist! And new methods promise higher productivity and increased success for future systems analysts. This book is about some of those methods, current and future.

WHAT DOES THE SYSTEMS ANALYST DO?

Let's summarize the systems analyst's role and responsibilities:

> A **systems analyst** studies the problems and needs of an organization to determine how people, methods, tasks, and computer technology can best accomplish improvements for the business.
>
> When computer technology is used, the systems analyst is responsible for the efficient capture of data from its business source, the flow of that data to the computer, the processing and storage of that data by the computer, and the flow of useful and timely information back to business users.

Note that the systems analyst's first responsibility is to the business and its managers. If a computer is used, that responsibility is extended to include the efficient use of the computer resource.

Unfortunately, the title *systems analyst* is frequently misused in the industry. Organizations may assign this title to anyone from a computer programmer to a sophisticated designer of computer applications. What is even more confusing is that, in many organizations, computer programmers actually perform some or all of the duties of the systems analyst; and in other organizations, systems analysts perform the duties of the computer programmer. So how can you identify a true systems analyst? It is best to regard the title of systems analyst with some degree of skepticism until you see or hear a formal job description. A typical systems analyst job description is depicted in Figure 1.1.

Unfortunately, there are several legitimate variations on the title *systems analyst.* Two of the more common aliases are defined as follows:

Programmer/Analyst A person whose job includes the responsibilities of both the computer programmer (described later in this chapter) and the systems analyst.

Information Analyst A person whose job is limited to the study of a business problem or need and specification of the business requirements but does not extend to the design of the computer-based system.

Other titles for the systems analyst include business analyst, systems designer, systems consultant, and systems engineer. Because there is so much confusion in this area and because in practice there is such a wide range of duties assigned to the role, it should be evident that a job description is indeed necessary to identify a true systems analyst.

The Responsibilities of the Systems Analyst and Programmer: A Comparison

Essentially, the systems analyst performs systems analysis, systems design, and systems implementation for developing computer-based business applications. *Systems analysis* is the study of a current business system and its problems, the definition of business needs and requirements, and the evaluation of alternative solutions. *Systems design* is the general and detailed specification of a computer-based solution that was selected during systems analysis. Design specifications are typically forwarded to the computer programmers and technicians for systems implementation. During

Figure 1.1 ▶

Job description for a typical systems analyst. The job description for a systems analyst will vary from firm to firm. This description is representative of a systems analyst.

JOB TITLE: Systems Analyst   REPORTS TO: Manager of Systems and Procedures

NARRATIVE DESCRIPTION Gathers and analyzes data for developing information systems. A systems analyst shall be responsible for studying the problems and needs set forth by this organization to determine how computer equipment, business procedures, and people can best solve these problems and accomplish improvements. Designs and specifies systems and methods for installing computer-based information systems and guides their installation. Makes formal presentations of findings, recommendations, and specifications in formal reports and in oral presentations.

RESPONSIBILITIES

1. Defining requirements for improving or replacing systems.
2. Evaluating alternative solutions for feasibility.
3. Guiding all systems development activities.
4. Designing systems flow and procedures to ensure control.
5. Testing systems segments to ensure adequacy in meeting needs.

DUTIES

1. Estimate personnel requirements, cost and time for systems projects.
2. Review and approve proposed systems solutions.
3. Develop, implement, and enforce systems development standards.
4. Plan and direct acquisiton, training, and development of systems personnel.
5. Educate management and users in data processing capabilities and requirements.
6. Document current systems operations.
7. Perform interviews and other data gathering.
8. Apply current technology to business solutions.
9. Prepare specifications for systems improvements.
10. Define systems security and control features.
11. Develop systems testing and conversion plans.
12. Supervise other project personnel as required.
13. Design file structures, forms inputs, and outputs.
14. Design data collection, processing, and control features.
15. Guide programmers and procedure writers.
16. Document the results of analysis, design, and implementation.

EXTERNAL CONTACTS

1. User management and technical personnel
2. Managers
3. Other systems analysts
4. Operations personnel
5. Vendors of computer equipment and software
6. Programmers

QUALIFYING EXPERIENCE

1. Bachelor's or Master's degree in computing, business, or statistics is preferred.
2. Data processing experience as a programmer.
3. Training in business functions and in systems analysis and design.
4. Thorough familiarity with organizational information needs.
5. Good communications skills.

systems implementation, computer programs are written and tested, managers and users are trained to use the new system, and operations are converted from the old system to the new system. The analyst plays a pivotal role in all three phases.

The one assumption of this book is that you are familiar with the job of a computer programmer. With this in mind, we should compare the responsibilities and job characteristics of the systems analyst with those of the computer programmer. The jobs are certainly not similar. For the computer programmer, we note the following (adapted from Demarco, 1978):

1. The programmer's responsibility rarely extends beyond the actual computer program. The scope of the programmer's world includes the computer, the operating system and utilities, and the programming languages in use (for example, COBOL or BASIC).
2. The programmer's work is very *precise.* That is to say, a program instruction is right or wrong. The program's logic is correct or incorrect. Although you may not enjoy debugging a program, the task is relatively straightforward.
3. The programmer's job involves few interpersonal relationships. The programmer normally deals with other programmers and with the systems analysts who prepared the program specifications. Provided that the analyst has done the job correctly, the programmer should not have to visit the user or become familiar with the business problem.

How do the analyst's responsibilities and job characteristics differ from those of a programmer? We note the following job characteristics for the systems analyst [again, adapted from Demarco, 1978]:

1. The systems analyst must deal with more than just computer programs. The analyst is responsible for the computer equipment selected, the people who will use the system, the procedural aspects of the system (such as how data will be captured), and the files and databases of the system. These components must fit together like pieces of a puzzle if the system is to benefit the business.
2. The work cannot be considered precise. There are few right or wrong answers. System solutions are often compromise solu-

tions. Many solutions change so often that fulfilling requirements (which change frequently themselves) is like shooting at a moving target.

3. The interpersonal relationships are numerous and complex. The analyst must be able to deal with users (who are often hostile) as well as with programmers, managers, audit personnel, data processing operators, and data processing salespersons (all of whom have their own motivations and jargon).

So why would any sane person want to be a systems analyst? We have certainly painted a picture of a complex world, and therein lies the answer. The job of the systems analyst presents a fascinating challenge to many individuals. It is exciting! It offers opportunities for decision making and creativity. Today, organizations seek analysts who are smart enough to define problems in terms of causes and effects rather than settling for simple remedies that may only treat the symptoms of a problem. And they want analysts who can see the big picture, who can look beyond one business function (for example, marketing), to see the impact of an idea upon another business function (such as production or inventory control).

Systems analyst is a job in the organization that:

- Allows you to participate in middle- and high-level management decision making concerned with business methods, tasks, forms, and strategies
- Forces you to look at the big picture or *systems view* early in your career
- Requires you to learn problem-solving skills and exercise creativity in your solutions

Many organizations are beginning to recognize that a good, experienced systems analyst has the proper business perspective for promotion to positions of greater management responsibility.

The Analyst's Position and Role Within the Data Processing Function

The internal organization of the data processing (DP) function can be depicted by organization charts. Although the structure of the DP function varies from company to company, the structure pre-

The Next Generation

Applications Development Without Programmers: How Will the Analyst's Job Change?

For many years now, we have written computer programs in procedural languages, such as COBOL, FORTRAN, and BASIC. By *procedural,* we mean that the programmer uses instructions to describe, in considerable detail, exactly how to accomplish an intended task. Today, we are seeing the evolution of nonprocedural languages. Instead of specifying exactly how to perform a task, nonprocedural languages simply specify what is to be accomplished. Nonprocedural languages use a simpler, English-like syntax to update data bases, generate reports, create graphs, and answer inquiries. At the risk of oversimplifying the result, "the computer does the rest." Examples of nonprocedural languages include FOCUS, RAMIS, SAS, and DBASE. Many of these languages can now be used on microcomputers. And it is generally believed that end users, those with little or no data processing background, will soon be using such languages to write many of their own computer programs.

How will data processing jobs change? If you are a programmer, you may be wondering about job security. Fear not! Nonprocedural languages are still immature—occasionally awkward and sometimes limited in capability. Therefore, processing efficiency or complex requirements may dictate the use of more conventional languages, at least for the time being. We will still be needing programmers for many more years!

And what about the systems analyst? We will need analysts more than ever! Fourth-generation languages can greatly speed the design and implementation of computer applications. However, the analysis of those applications is still necessary. Why? Because nonprocedural languages, like any other tool, can be misused. End users, like analysts, may create incorrect, incomplete, and inflexible solutions to their own problems. Additionally, other tasks await systems analysts in the nonprocedural language environment.

Most nonprocedural languages are built around databases that must be carefully developed to fully exploit the language. Therefore, many systems analysts will become more involved in *database analysis* and *design* (see Part IV, Module E). Other analysts will become *techniques specialists,* who will help users determine whether or not specific problems are suited to nonprocedural languages. And still other analysts will become experts and consultants for end users, helping them learn and apply the nonprocedural languages to their problems. The roles will change, but the systems analyst will survive!

In the immediate future, you can expect analysts to use fourth-generation languages to prototype systems. What is prototyping? *Prototyping* is an engineering-inspired design approach where you quickly build a system or subsystem that works but that may not be complete. This prototype can be demonstrated to users and then easily modified. Prototypes can be more rapidly developed by using the nonprocedural languages. Sometimes the prototype even becomes the final system. Other times, the prototype must be rewritten in a procedural language to improve efficiency or add features. But in any event, design by prototyping accelerates the analyst's system development efforts.

Does this environment sound too futuristic to believe? If so, read James Martin's book, *Application Development Without Programmers* (Prentice-Hall, 1982). It's a real eye-opener!

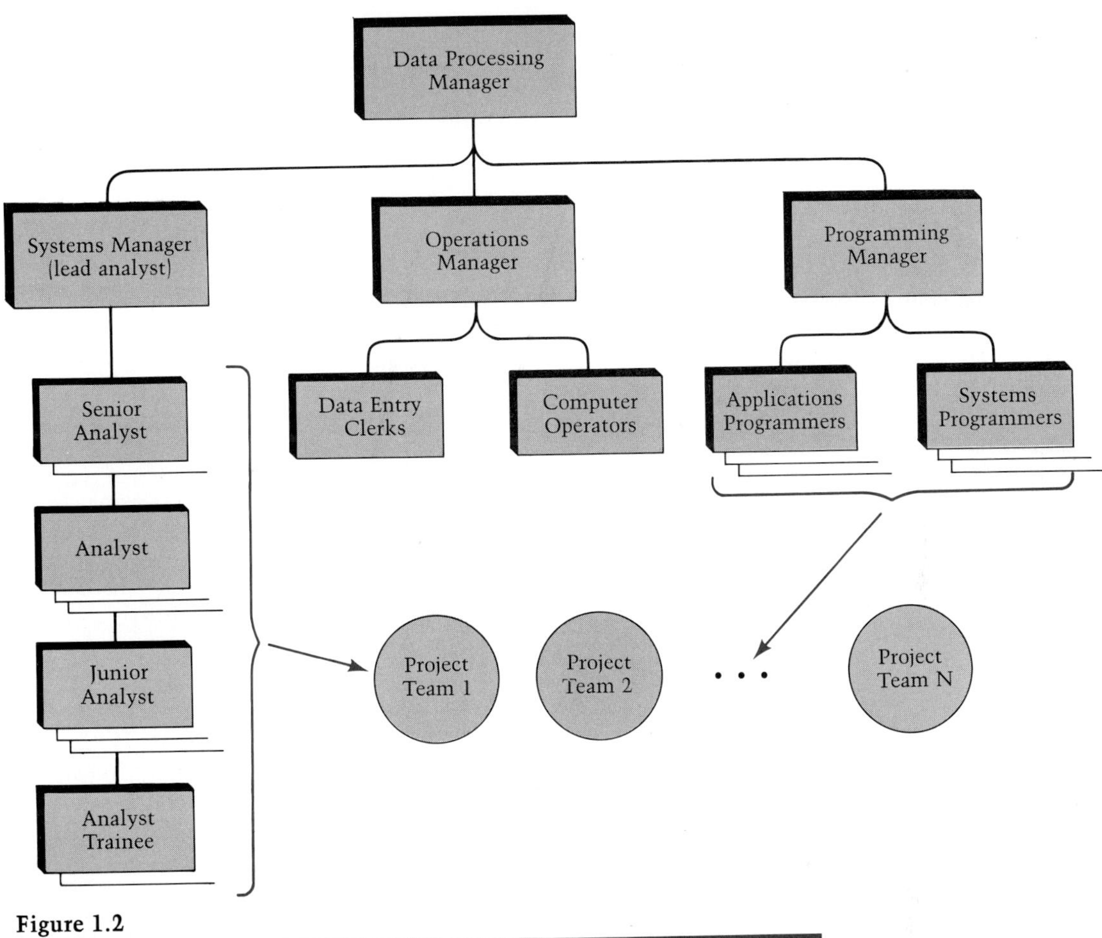

Figure 1.2

The organization of the data processing function. Every data processing shop develops its own unique structure; however, this structure is fairly typical. Notice how programmers and systems analysts are organized into project teams. These teams are created and disbanded as projects are started and completed or canceled.

sented in Figure 1.2 is fairly typical. Note that the lowest levels of the DP function are organized into project teams. These teams are formed and disbanded as projects come and go.

What is the analyst's role in the system project? We prefer to look at the analyst as a facilitator. The analyst acts as the interface among many different types of people and facilitates the development of computer applications through these people (see Figure

Figure 1.3

People with whom the analyst must work. As a facilitator of systems development, the analyst must work with many types of people, both technical and nontechnical. The joint efforts of these professionals, as coordinated by the analyst, will result in successful computer applications.

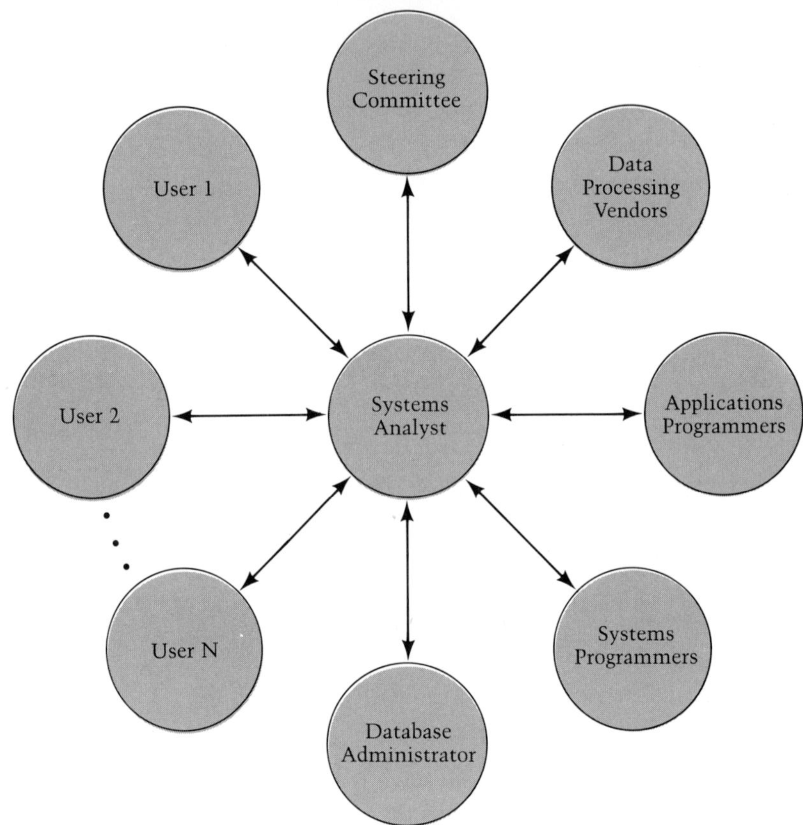

1.3). The analyst may very well be the only individual who sees the total picture of the system!

At this point, it becomes worth our while to take a careful look at the organization of the systems analysis professionals. Within the systems analyst job category, various levels of responsibility exist. Brief job descriptions for the various levels include:

- *Lead Analyst* A systems manager or high-level systems analyst who is probably in charge of all or many systems activities and projects in the department
- *Senior Analyst* An experienced systems analyst who may lead a project team or work independently on any or all phases of a system project; may be in charge of all projects within a specific business function

- *Analyst* A less experienced systems analyst who can generally work without supervision but may sometimes require assistance
- *Junior Analyst* An inexperienced systems analyst who generally works under direct supervision

Of course, each firm may have its own classifications, dividing up the range of responsibilities differently, or using different titles for the same categories.

PREPARING FOR A CAREER AS A SYSTEMS ANALYST

A book will not make you a competent systems analyst any more than your first programming book or course made you a competent computer programmer. You will, however, be able immediately to apply the skills and concepts you learn in this book to small computer applications, although you may need some supervision. Furthermore, you will have a solid foundation on which to base additional systems training.

What Does It Take to Become a Successful Systems Analyst?

We have suggested that the analyst is the principle link between business users and computer programmers. What does it take to become a successful systems analyst? First, we should look at two things that almost all systems analysts have in common:

1. Most analysts become analysts after obtaining experience as computer programmers. At a very minimum, the analyst has a programming education.
2. Most analysts lack any formal training or education in systems analysis and design. This situation is slowly changing.

Most organizations consider computer programming experience to be a prerequisite to systems analysis and design experience. The reasoning is sound. An analyst must be able to develop technically feasible solutions and precise program specifications. You should not, however, assume that a good programmer will become a good analyst or that a bad programmer could not become a good analyst. There is no such correlation. Unfortunately, many organizations insist on promoting good programmers who become poor or mediocre systems analysts. Worse still, poor programmers are often passed over in the belief that they cannot become good analysts.

That brings us back to our original question, *what does it take to become a successful systems analyst?* One writer suggests the following:

> I submit that systems analysts are people who communicate with management and users at the management/user level; document their experience; understand problems before proposing solutions; think before they speak; facilitate systems development, not originate it; are supportive of the organization in question and understand its goals and objectives; use good tools and approaches to help solve systems problems; and enjoy working with people [Wood, 1979. Copyright 1979 by CW Communications, Inc., Framingham, MA 01701—Reprinted from *Computerworld*].

A tall order, no? It is often difficult to pinpoint those skills and attributes necessary to succeed.

Skills to Be Developed or Refined

Most systems analysts would agree that the following skills and attributes are essential:

- *Working knowledge of data processing techniques, technology, and computer programming.*
- *General business knowledge* *At least* a general knowledge of or experience with typical business functions of the organization. (Some typical business functions are listed in the margin.)
- *Problem-solving skills* The general ability to analyze and solve problems (Often, this requires considerable insight and creativity.)
- *Interpersonal communications skills* The ability to communicate effectively, both orally and in writing, with both technical and nontechnical people.
- *Interpersonal relations skills* The ability to work with many people of differing personalities, backgrounds, motivations, and attitudes.

Typical Business Functions

Accounting
Marketing
Finance
Personnel
Production
Inventory
Quantitative Methods

Most analysts would agree that the following are also highly desirable:

- Formal DP systems analysis and design skills
- Good old-fashioned experience

Let's look at these skills and attributes in more detail.

Working Knowledge of Data Processing Techniques, Technology, and Computer Programming The systems analyst should maintain current technical skills and knowledge. Technical skills include computer programming and software development tools and techniques. Technical knowledge includes computer equipment and software packages. The best way to keep up on what's happening is to develop an organized habit of skimming and reading various trade periodicals on data processing. Examples of helpful trade publications are listed in the margin. Most of these magazines should be available in your college or business library. If not, ask your librarian why they aren't.

Additionally, you should consider joining a professional association for data processors. Students and professionals alike are encouraged to join organizations such as the Data Processing Management Association (DPMA) and the Society for Information Management (SIM).

Trade Publications

Computerworld
Datamation
Computer Decisions
Infosystems
Byte
EDP Analyzer
Data Management

General Business Knowledge In most instances, the systems analyst need not be an expert in a specific business application or function area (such as accounting or production). However, this individual should be able to communicate with the business expert to gain knowledge of problems and needs. The type and level of business knowledge a systems analyst must obtain varies from one organization to another. Typically, the systems analyst will gain the necessary business knowledge while on the job. In the absence of specific business knowledge requirements, we suggest you include one course in each of the subjects listed in the margin. Specializations such as accounting or production can be very valuable in some instances. These subjects and others are taught in many colleges.

Business Subjects

- Financial Accounting
- Managerial or Cost Accounting
- Quantitative Methods (e.g. statistics)
- Marketing
- Production and Inventory Operations
- Personnel Management
- Business Finance
- Organizational Behavior

Problem-Solving Skills The systems analyst must have the ability to take a large business problem, break that problem down into its component parts, analyze the various aspects of that problem, and then assemble a system to solve the problem. This is not an easy task to learn. The analyst must also learn to analyze problems in terms of causes and effects rather than in terms of simple remedies. Recently, methodologies, such as structured analysis, have emerged for assisting the analyst in the problem-solving process.

Analysts must be able to creatively define alternative solutions to problems and needs. Creativity and insight are more likely to be gifts than skills, although they can certainly be developed to some degree. The following story is an example of creativity and insight in action.

> It was the custom of a primitive tribe in Africa to have their witch doctor determine the manner in which their captives were to die. Victims were told to make an affirmative statement. If the witch doctor believed the statement to be true, the victim would be shot with a poisoned dart. If the statement was considered false, the victim would die by fire. One day a missionary was captured by the tribe and condemned to death. The witch doctor told the missionary to make an affirmative statement. Death appeared inevitable to everyone except the missionary. The cunning missionary made a brief statement that so bewildered the witch doctor that the execution could not be carried out! What were the words the missionary spoke? [Adapted from Hart, 1939]

The missionary's statement was, "I will die by fire." Would you have been as creative in your solution? Insight helps the analyst understand the problem and create solutions.

Interpersonal Communications Skills An analyst must be able to communicate effectively, both orally and in writing. The analyst should actively seek help or training in business writing, technical writing, interviewing, presentations, and listening. A good command of the English language is essential. These skills are learnable, but most of us must force ourselves to seek help and work hard to improve them. Communications skills are probably the single most important ingredient to success. This is because of the number and complexity of the interpersonal relationships previously discussed. Some of the modules in Part IV of this book survey the importance of communications skills for the systems analyst.

Interpersonal Relations Skills It has been suggested that analysts "need to exercise the boldness of Lady Godiva, the introspection of Sherlock Holmes, the methodology of Andrew Carnegie, and the down-home common sense of Will Rogers" (Lord and Steiner,

1978, p. 349). In other words, systems work is people-oriented work and systems analysts must be extroverted or people-oriented people. Interpersonal skills help us work effectively with people. Although these skills can be developed, some people simply do not possess an extroverted personality. The interpersonal nature of systems work is demonstrated in the eight-part case study, "Analysts in Action," that appears at intervals throughout this book.

Formal DP Systems Analysis and Design Skills Most analysts could use formal training in systems analysis and design skills. Figure 1.4 illustrates a simple way of looking at systems analysis and design skills and their relationships to one another. The three sets of knowledge and skills depicted include:

- Concepts and principles
- Tools and techniques
- Methodologies

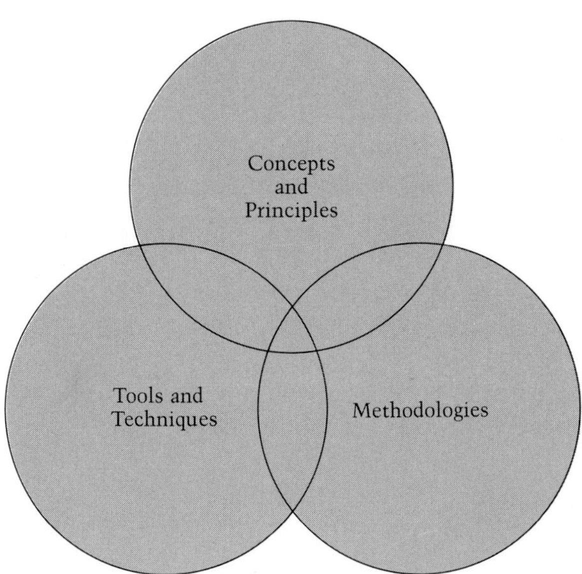

Figure 1.4

Formal systems analysis and design skills. This diagram depicts three sets of formal systems analysis and design skills. Note that each set overlaps the other skill sets to illustrate the dependence of one skill set on the others.

When all else fails, the systems analyst who remembers the basic concepts and principles of systems work will still succeed. No tool, technique, process, or methodology is perfect in all situations! Concepts and principles will help you adapt to new and different situations and methods as they become available. We have purposefully emphasized applied concepts and principles in this book. This is not a mechanical, "monkey see, monkey do" book! The concepts and principles in Part I will help you understand the product we are trying to build, the information system, and the process by which we build that system, the system development life cycle. We believe that if you study Part I carefully, you will be better able to communicate with potential employers, business users, and computer programmers alike!

Not too long ago, it was thought that the systems analyst's only tools were paper, pencil, and flowchart template. Over the years, several tools and techniques have been developed to help the analyst. The purpose of tools and techniques is to document information systems as they are developed. You can see from Figure 1.4 that tools and techniques are built on concepts and principles. As we present tools and techniques, we hope to show you this relationship. This book emphasizes two classes of tools. Classical tools have been used by systems analysts for some time now. They tend to be system design oriented because they are best suited to documenting the computer aspects of a system. Structured tools have recently evolved to overcome the weaknesses of many classical tools when applied to systems analysis. These tools are more suited to documenting the business problem and need. Contrary to some beliefs, classical tools have not become obsolete because of the newer structured tools. Indeed, you will learn that each class of tools has its advantages and disadvantages. And you will also learn that these tools can coexist and work together to build better systems! You can also see from Figure 1.4 that tools and techniques are often presented in the framework of specific methodologies.

Methodologies are specific strategies for applying specific tools and techniques in a disciplined manner to successfully develop systems. Besides using specific tools and techniques, Figure 1.4 illustrates that good methodologies should be installed on sound concepts and principles. There are numerous methodologies, and each has its own supporters. We will briefly discuss methodologies later in this book; however, we support no specific methodology. We believe you should learn to walk before you run. Therefore, this book will emphasize concepts, principles, tools, and techniques independent of methodology. We encourage you to study methodologies after you have mastered the concepts and tools in this book. Then you will be able to avoid the pitfall of blind devotion to any one methodology.

Good Old-Fashioned Experience Plainly stated, there is no substitute for good old-fashioned experience in systems analysis and design. Experience in applying the previous skills to an actual systems project is necessary for you to become a "good" systems analyst. No textbook can provide that experience!

SUMMARY

The data processing systems analyst is a professional who studies business problems and needs to determine how people, methods, tasks, and computers can best accomplish improvements for the business. When computers are used, the systems analyst is responsible for the efficient capture of data, the flow of that data to the computer, the processing and storage of that data by the computer, and the flow of accurate and timely information back to business users.

A systems analyst performs many duties including systems analysis, systems design, and systems implementation. Because of the emphasis on systems, the systems analyst must frequently apply the wisdom and insight attributed to the experienced business executive. The systems analyst is usually part of the data processing function in the business. Within the DP function, systems analysts are usually classified according to experience as lead analysts, senior analysts, analysts, and junior analysts. Systems analysts are organized into temporary teams, along with programmers, and are assigned to projects.

To properly prepare for a career as a successful systems analyst, you should develop or refine all of the following skills: your working knowledge of DP techniques and programming, your knowledge or experience with typical business functions, your ability to analyze and solve problems, your ability to communicate with others, your ability to work well with many types of people, and formal systems analysis and design skills. This book focuses primarily on formal systems analysis and design skills including concepts and principles, tools and techniques, and, to a small degree, methodologies. Finally, you need to seek out opportunities to gain experience with systems analysis and design methods.

PROBLEMS AND EXERCISES

1. What is the role of the systems analyst when developing a computer application? To whom is the systems analyst responsible?
2. Make an appointment to visit with a systems analyst or programmer/analyst in a local business. Try to obtain a job description from the analyst. Compare that job description with the job description provided in this chapter.
3. Using the definitions of *systems analysis, systems design,* and *systems implementation* provided in this chapter, write a letter to your instructor that proposes the development of an automated grade record keeping system. Tell your instructor what has to be done. Assume that your instructor knows nothing about computers or systems analysts. In other words, be careful with your use of new terms.
4. Mr. Gregg has been asked to reclassify his systems analysts. Most of his analysts do systems analysis, systems design, and computer programming. A few systems analysts work solely with the users to define problems, requirements, and possible solutions. Still other analysts perform systems analysis and design. How should Mr. Gregg reclassify his personnel?
5. Long ago, Allied Steel Products, Inc., adopted the policy of not promoting data processing personnel to the position of systems analyst. Instead, they staff the systems analyst positions with personnel who have a business degree or background and little or no technical, data processing background. Meanwhile, programmers in the DP Department perform all technical design tasks in addition to their programming responsibilities. Comment on this policy. What are the advantages and disadvantages of such a policy?
6. Smith & Smith, Inc., has followed a policy of promoting successful programmers to the position of systems analyst. Over the years, they've noticed a curious trend. The best of the programmers either left shortly before they were due for promotion or shortly after they were promoted. Futhermore, they've

noted that several not-so-good programmers left the company to accept positions as systems analysts (and these people seemed to be performing well as analysts). What is wrong with Smith & Smith's strategy? How can they reduce the number of good employees they're losing?

7. Coin Vending and Supply, Inc., has noted a proliferation of new microcomputers in their company. Users have been buying these microcomputers on their own initiative. In a sense, the business users of these microcomputers, who have little or no DP background, are developing their own application systems. Because of this, the DP manager has been asked to justify the continued growth of his programmer and systems analysis staff. There is even some feeling that the number of programmers and analysts should be reduced. How can the DP manager justify his staff? Will the roles of his programmers and analysts change? If so, how? Can the users completely replace the programmers and analysts?

8. The following letter to the editor appeared in a data processing magazine:

   > I have been reading your job advertisements with great interest. But I'm confused. Many ads offer jobs to qualified 'programmer/analysts.' I am a programmer. I carefully analyze the structure and logic of every program I write. Am I a 'programmer/analyst?'

   Respond to this letter.

9. The students in an introductory programming course would like to know how systems analysis and design differs from computer programming. Specifically, they want to know how to choose between the two careers. Help them out by explaining the differences between the two and pointing out factors that might influence their decision.

10. Several data processing magazines and journals, available at your local library, publish annual surveys of data processing jobs, salaries, experience levels, and so forth. Investigate the opportunities for a career as a systems analyst.

11. Your library probably subscribes to at least one big-city newspaper. Additionally, your library, academic department, or instructor may subscribe to a data processing newspaper such as *Computerworld* or *MIS Week*. Study the job advertisements for systems analysts and programmer/analysts. What skills are

being sought? What experience is being required? How are these skills and experiences important to the role of the analyst as described in this chapter?

12. Make an appointment to visit a local data processing installation. Where does the systems analyst fit into the organization? How many levels of systems analyst positions exist? Compare and contrast those levels with the levels of responsibility presented in this chapter.
13. You need to hire two systems analysts. Explain to a Personnel Department recruiter the characteristics and background you seek in an experienced systems analyst.
14. Prepare a curriculum plan for your education as a systems analyst. If you are already working, prepare a statement that expresses your personal need for continuing education to become a systems analyst.

ANNOTATED REFERENCES AND SUGGESTED READINGS

DeMarco, Tom. *Structured Analysis and System Specification.* Englewood Cliffs, N.J.: Prentice-Hall, 1978.

Hart, Harold. *Invitation to Fun.* New York: Frederick A. Stokes, 1939.

Lord, Kenniston W., Jr., and James B. Steiner. *CDP Review Manual: A Data Processing Handbook.* 2d ed. New York: Van Nostrand Reinhold, 1978. A review manual for the Certificate in Data Processing examinations. Chapter 8, "Systems Analysis and Design," traces the history, functions, and responsibilities of the systems analyst.

Martin, James. *Application Development Without Programmers.* Englewood Cliffs, N.J.: Prentice-Hall, 1982.

Wood, Michael. "Systems Analyst Title Most Abused in Industry: Redefinition Imperative." *Computerworld,* April 30, 1979, pp. 24, 26. This article sums up our feelings about systems analysts and what it takes to be successful as analysts. It has become our battle cry for the need to train analysts to develop their interpersonal relations and communications skills.

Analysts in Action

An Introduction to American Automotive Parts, Inc.

This is the continuing story of Cheryl Mason and Douglas Matthews, systems analysts for American Automotive Parts (AAP), Inc.

Episode 1

Systems analysis and design is more than concepts, tools, techniques, and methods. It is people working with people. Although experience is the best teacher, you can learn a great deal by observing other systems analysts in action. Ed Earl Jones, Director of Computer Information Systems (CIS) for American Automotive Parts, Inc. (AAP), has kindly consented to let you watch two of his analysts on a typical project.

Cheryl Mason, a senior systems analyst and project manager, has volunteered for this demonstration. She has successfully implemented several information systems for AAP and should be able to provide you with a valuable learning experience. Doug Matthews, Cheryl's partner, is a new programmer/analyst at AAP. In fact, today is his first day! Doug has to go through orientation today, and Ed Earl has invited you to observe the orientation. It'll be a good way for you and Doug to get acquainted with AAP.

Welcome to the Cincinnati Distribution Center

The Cincinnati Distribution Center (DC) is one of thirty-five AAP warehouses in the country. The Cincinnati DC is unique in that all computer information systems for AAP DCs and headquarters are developed and tested at the Cincinnati DC. We begin the preview by joining Doug in Ed Earl's office.

"Hi, Doug!" Ed Earl extended his hand. "It's great to have you aboard. My name's Ed Earl Jones, and I'm the director of Computer Information Systems. I didn't get a chance to meet you when you interviewed last month. Why don't you tell a little about yourself?"

Doug was having those first day jitters, despite Ed Earl's easy-going personality. "Well, I just graduated from college. I received a Bachelor's Degree in Information Systems from State University. I spent the last two summers as an intern programmer for the Executron Corporation in Dayton, Ohio. I was also president of my local student chapter of the Data Processing Management Association, and I hope to get involved in Cincinnati's professional chapter. My career goals are oriented toward applying the systems analysis and design skills I learned in college. That's the main reason I accepted your job offer. It looked like I'd get a chance to do some analysis and design here — not just programming."

"That's why we hired you Doug," replied Ed Earl. "In fact, your buddy will be Cheryl Mason, a senior systems analyst who is very familiar with ▸

the tools and techniques you learned in college."

"What's a buddy?" asked Doug.

Ed Earl answered, "A buddy is an experienced partner who is assigned to show you the ropes and help you learn about AAP and our way of doing things. You'll meet Cheryl soon. Are you all squared away with Personnel?"

"Yes," said Doug. "I think I've filled out all the forms."

Ed Earl stood up and motioned Doug to the door. "Okay, let's take a tour of the Distribution Center."

As Doug and Ed Earl walked down the corridor, Ed Earl continued his orientation. "This corridor leads to the warehouse. These offices are part of the Administrative Services Division. We do more data processing for that division than any other.

"I don't know how much you know or remember about AAP, so I'll give you a quick overview. AAP is a nationwide distributor of automotive parts, supplies, and accessories. We buy our products from the companies that manufacture those products. Then we sell those products to automotive supply stores. Most of those stores are AAP franchise stores. These franchises pay a fee to use the AAP name and logo. We also sell to some smaller non-AAP automotive supply store chains and independents."

"How many customers are there?" Doug asked.

"About 1,475 franchised stores," replied Ed Earl. "Of that total, this DC supplies about 125 franchise stores. And we also supply 25 or so non-AAP stores. This DC, like all DCs, is an independent operation. Although we report to AAP headquarters in Little Rock, Arkansas, we are fully responsible for our own sales, operations, finances, and management. The office on your left belongs to the DC Manager, Roger Miller. We kid him about having the same name as the country singer. Let's stop in and introduce you."

Roger Miller was standing in the receptionist area. Ed Earl called out. "Roger? This is Doug Matthews, the new programmer/analyst I told you about. Doug, this is Roger Miller."

"I'm glad to meet you, Doug. Ed Earl really twisted my arm to approve your position. You must have made some kind of impression on the interviewer."

Everybody moved into Roger's office and took a seat. Roger handed Doug a piece of paper (see Figure 1) and continued. "This is our organization chart, Doug. As you can see, this DC is divided into four main divisions, including the Computer Information Systems Division. The offices you walked through on your way to this office belong to the Administrative Services Division. They handle all business functions such as purchasing, inventory control, personnel, and accounting.

"Ed Earl will soon take you through the warehouse where parts are stocked and orders are filled. The shipping and receiving dock is part of the warehouse. On the other side of the warehouse you'll find the Customer Services Division offices. That's where all orders are processed. Finally, you should notice that the Computer Information Systems Division operates at the same organizational level as the other three divisions. This is because the Cincinnati DP staff develops the computer systems for all AAP distribution centers.

"I hope you like working for us. You'll find that our merit pay raises truly reward those who achieve company goals. And you'll have a say in determining what your goals will be. We don't have a lot of training. You learn on the job. And we'll schedule performance appraisals every six months so you know exactly where you stand and we find out where you want your career to go. Again, I'm really glad you chose AAP, and I hope you stay with us a long time. Ed Earl? Why don't you complete your tour? I'm sure you ▶

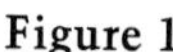

Figure 1

AAP organization chart. Because the Cincinnati DC develops applications for all other DCs and for AAP's corporate headquarters, the Data Processing Division (DPD) has been given a high position in the organization. Many other organizations would have placed DPD under what AAP calls the Administrative Services Division.

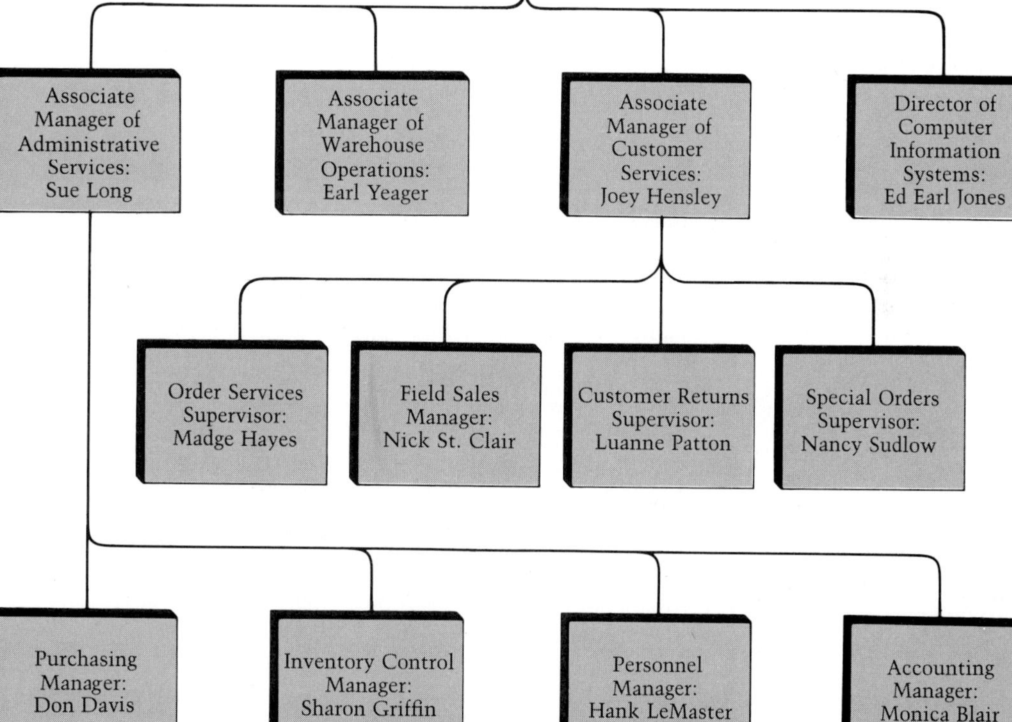

want to find some challenging work for this young man as soon as possible."

Doug responded, "It was nice to meet you, Mr. Miller." With that, he shook Roger's hand and left with Ed Earl.

As they walked through the double doors at the end of the corridor, Ed Earl said, "And this is the Warehouse Division. This is the heart of the DC—where the action is."

The warehouse is quite large. Indeed, it is so large that it has been divided into five product zones plus the shipping and receiving dock. Doug was somewhat surprised by the size of the operation. Trucks were being loaded and unloaded, and clerks were stocking shelves and filling orders.

As Doug and Ed Earl walked through the warehouse, Doug commented, "This must be a difficult operation to coordinate."

Ed Earl answered, "I wouldn't want to do it. We haven't done much in the way of data processing support for the warehouse. We're just starting to investigate that possibility. We do support purchasing and inventory control, but technically, those functions are part of the Administrative Services Division.

"This office area we are passing is the Customer Services Division. All those clerks are processing orders, back orders, follow-ups, and other customer transactions. That's where your first project is going to be. That's why I'm going to defer a tour of those facilities. Cheryl will be taking you there to meet your clients. So let's tour our own Computer Information Systems Division, and then I'll take you to meet Cheryl."

The Computer Information Systems Division at AAP

Doug and Ed Earl walked into the computer room where Ed Earl removed a sheet of paper from his pocket and handed it to Doug (see Figure 2). "This is an organization chart for Computer Information Systems, Doug. You might want to refer to it as we complete this part of the tour. We're in the Computer Operations Center right now.

"You're looking at our IBM 3033 mainframe computer. We have an audiovisual, self-study course that you'll take to learn more about the IBM computer and its MVS operating system. For now, it should suffice to say that this machine supports all of our computer processing needs. It has several disk drives capable of storing 100 million bytes of data. We also have a full complement of tape devices and printers. If you have any questions, just ask."

Doug replied, "I've never used this particular computer before. Is that going to be a problem?"

"No," answered Ed Earl. "You have a good, solid education in computers. Besides, that's one reason we assign a buddy to each new hire. You should be able to learn any new system fairly fast. Most people do. I don't know what your expectations were when you graduated, but I think you'll find that your education is only starting now that you're out of school. You'll catch on quickly, though. Trust me."

Doug and Ed Earl moved into an adjacent office area . Ed Earl said, "And this is where you'll be working. It's called the Applications Center. Different groups of systems analysts and programmers are located in different parts of the office. Each group supports a certain group of business users. You're assigned to the Customer Services Support Group."

Doug glanced at the center's organization chart, "I see a couple of groups on the organization chart that I'm not familiar with—Technical Support and the Information Center. What are they?"

"Good question," replied Ed Earl. "The Technical Support Group doesn't really serve users. It serves us. When you have a technical question or problem concerning the IBM computer system, that group will help you out. They're also ▶

Figure 2

The Data Processing Division's organization chart.

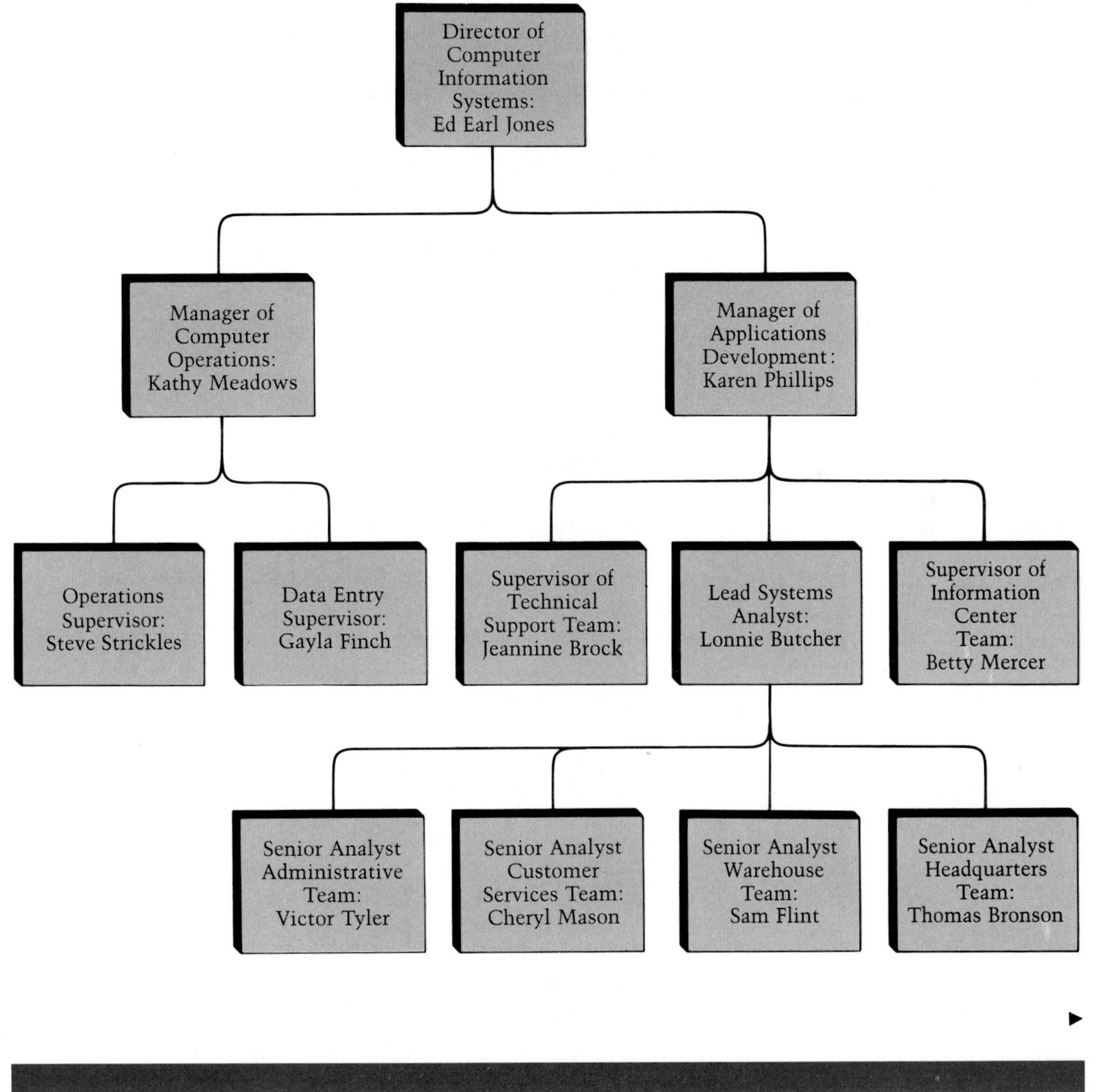

the people who will be teaching you about that IBM computer system. The Information Center Group is a new function. They're helping all AAP users learn how to apply microcomputers to do some of their own work. They teach the users how to do word processing, spreadsheets, and things like that. In other words, they teach the users how they can help themselves. That frees us up to do the really difficult projects. It's a novel concept for our operation!"

Doug and Ed Earl walked into an office. Ed Earl continued, "And this is your office—I wonder where. . . . Here she is!"

A young woman entered the office. Ed Earl continued, "Cheryl, I want you to meet Doug Matthews, your new partner."

"Doug and I met during his interview, Ed Earl." Cheryl extended her hand. "Welcome, Doug. I'm glad you accepted our offer. I really wanted to work with you—so much so that I asked to be your buddy. Has Ed Earl explained the buddy system?"

Doug nodded yes.

Ed Earl smiled. "Terrific! I didn't know you had already met. I don't know what you've told Doug about yourself, Cheryl, but I'd like to do a little biographical sketch.

"Cheryl has been with us for five years. Prior to joining AAP, she was a programmer with a small manufacturing company in Indiana. Cheryl was recently promoted to senior systems analyst because she's proven herself to be one of our most competent, progressive, and personable professionals. Cheryl has a Bachelors Degree in Business. She's had little formal computing education, but she's done well because she always seeks out opportunities to learn more through reading, seminars, and company training courses. Cheryl's credentials also include the Certificate in Data Processing, called the CDP. The CDP is awarded to data processing professionals who meet a five-year experience requirement and who pass each of five examinations that cover computer equipment, software and programming, data processing management, quantitative methods and accounting, and systems analysis and design. The CDP designation is roughly equivalent to the Certified Public Accountant, or CPA, designation for the accounting profession. So you see, Doug, you'll be learning from our best person!"

Doug nodded. "And I appreciate that fact!"

Ed Earl started to leave the office. "Once again, Doug, welcome! I'll leave you with Cheryl now. She'll help you get organized and start teaching you all the things you'll need to start learning. We'll sit down in a week or so to set some goals for your first six months. Bye!"

How to Use the Case Study

You've just been introduced to a case study that will be continued throughout this book. It's important that you understand the purpose of the case study:

> The purpose of the continuing case study is to show you that tools and techniques alone do not make a systems analyst. Systems analysis and design involves a commitment to work for and with a number of people.

When we started writing this book, we wanted to make sure that the chapters would teach you the important concepts, tools, and techniques. But we were also afraid you might begin to believe that, if you knew those tools and techniques, you'd have all the knowledge necessary to be a systems analyst. While Chapter 1 emphasized the importance of communications and interpersonal skills, this continuing case study has been designed to show you the people side of the job.

The case study is divided into episodes that represent ►

various stages of a typical project. Although each episode will introduce new tools and techniques, the episodes are not intended to teach the tools and techniques. Instead, they introduce a situation in which you will need to use a new tool or technique. The episodes show that need in terms of what Cheryl and Doug must do to develop a new computer information system for AAP. In almost all cases, you will see Cheryl and Doug working closely with their business users.

The chapters that follow an episode will teach you how to use the tools and techniques that were introduced in that episode. And those chapters will apply the tools and techniques to the AAP case study (as well as to other smaller examples).

A brief transition called "Where Do We Go from Here?" concludes each episode and introduces the chapters that follow it. We hope you'll find these demonstrations interesting and informative. We think they'll help you place the subject of systems analysis and design into its most practical setting—the world of business and work! ■

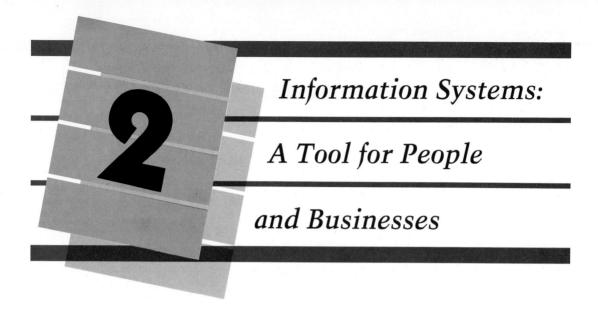

2 Information Systems: A Tool for People and Businesses

Minicase: Woodworld Designs

Woodworld, a large business specializing in customized cabinetry, was founded in Bob Earman's garage in Weiner, Arkansas, in 1972. By 1977, business had improved substantially and Bob Earman purchased a large warehouse to relocate his business. Employees were continually added to maintain an operating level sufficient to meet increasing customer demand. In 1982, Woodworld acquired an IBM PC/XT microcomputer and successfully automated many of its financial applications.

In 1984, Woodworld began experiencing its largest increase in business. The manual methods by which customer orders were processed were no longer effective, and customer orders were frequently backlogged, lost, or incorrectly processed. In the spring of 1984, Customer Services Manager, Mari Shadle, who was aware of the need to improve the order-processing operation, submitted a memo to Todd Browney, asking him to automate the current order-processing operations. Todd was a jack-of-all-computer-trades for Woodworld. He managed data processing and served as company systems analyst, computer programmer, computer operator, and computer technical support specialist.

After receiving the memo, Todd spent five months developing a new automated order-processing operation. He purchased IBM's latest microcomputer, the PC/AT, on which to implement the new system. After implementing the system, Todd scheduled a meeting to discuss it with Mari. At that meeting, the following conversation took place:

Todd Good morning, Mari. How are you doing?

Mari Just fine, thank you. I hear you've completed automation of our order-processing operations.

Todd That's right. Now I just want to discuss what I've come up with, and if it meets with your approval, we can begin conversion from the current order-processing system to the new system.

Mari That sounds just great! The sooner we can get the new operations installed, the better.

Todd proceeded to explain the new automated order-processing system to Mari. Impressed with the documentation that had been developed, Mari told Todd that this was the first time she had ever been able to actually read and understand documentation prepared by a computer expert. Overall, Mari was satisfied with the system Todd had developed. She was especially impressed with how easy the new system (and particularly the microcomputer) was to learn and use — not at all what she had feared! Todd had obviously spent a lot of time making the new system friendly to her staff, most of whom had never used a computer. Mari felt her order-processing staff would surely be excited when the new operations were installed. Let's listen in on the end of the meeting:

Mari I must say, I'm very impressed with what you've come up with. This should certainly solve a lot of our order-processing problems. There's one more small thing I'd like you to do for me. Could you make the computer generate me a couple of special reports?

Todd No problem. What type of reports would you like to have?

Mari Here are a couple of samples of reports I sometimes prepare to help myself make some important decisions. This is the most essential one. Mr. Earman [the company president] has informed me that our company is going to start becoming more aggressive in the retail market. By the end of 1987, we hope to capture 25 percent of the retail market. This report summarizes the company's monthly sales according to our different sectors of that retail market. It will help me track our progress toward our sales goals, both product by product and store by store. This other report gives me some idea of the volume of business we've handled during a given month. It summarizes the sales orders according to their type. I use this report to keep track of the volume and type of orders our department is handling.

Todd Okay, I see no problem with writing a couple new programs. It doesn't effect the programs that have already been written. But one last question. What do you mean by type of order?

Mari You know, we classify orders according to type of product and whether the product is a regular stock item, customized product, or modified regular stock item.

Todd Gee, I didn't realize you could distinguish between different types of orders. Should I have handled these different order types differently?

Mari I don't really know. I can't tell you exactly how they are processed, but my staff can. I tell you what, why don't you make the additions to the system operations and then go talk to my assistant, Ed Thorpe. He'll be very interested in knowing what we're up to. He might also be able to tell you about differences in the order types.

Todd That's a good idea. I talked to the order clerks and the supervisor, but I didn't talk to Mr. Thorpe. I think I'd better talk with him right now.

Todd went straight to Ed Thorpe's office, where he talked with Ed about the new plans for the order-processing system. Todd learned that the system he had created accommodated the bulk of all orders — those for regular stock items. But the processing of the other order types was slightly different. Otherwise Ed, who had been struggling to improve the productivity of his staff to efficiently handle the increasing number of custom product orders, was very enthusiastic. He saw the potential for decreasing order-processing time, reducing customer backlogs, and improving order-processing accuracy. The following is a portion of the conversation that took place during their meeting:

Ed This system sounds terrific. I particularly like the fact that the computer will be doing a lot of the work. I'm short on staff. Besides, they do make a lot of common mistakes like arithmetic and copying errors.

Todd You can be assured I included a lot of error-checking routines in the programs. The programs will catch any bad data they might key in.

Ed That's great. We've had a lot of inconsistencies in our credit-checking on customer orders. Sometimes we find we've approved credit sales that exceed the customer's credit limit.

Todd They won't be able to do that anymore.

Ed Actually, sometimes they should do it and other times they shouldn't. It all depends upon the customer's credit history.

Todd Looks like I've made some incorrect assumptions. I had no idea the credit limit should be extended in certain instances. You'd better explain to me how credit checks should be done. I have to make some modifications to one of my programs.

Ed Sure, I'll send you a write-up that describes how my staff checks customer credit orders. Hey, I noticed you have a note on your documentation that states you're going to have the computer generate a few reports for Mari. Do you suppose I could send you a description of a few reports I would like to have? I have some ideas for reports that would be very beneficial. They'd help me a lot more than those two reports that my staff requested for me.

Todd But they told me those are the reports they're supposed to send you!

Ed They are. But you should see what I have to do to get the information I need from them. It takes me several hours every week.

Todd I guess I'll just have to make the modifications and additions. I'm going to get back to work now. I'll be expecting your notes concerning the credit checking guidelines and about those reports you'd like.

Todd spent several weeks making the corrections and additions. Not only did he have to change computer programs; he also had to change the procedure manuals for the order-entry staff! Todd had meetings with Mari and Ed to obtain their final approval before proceeding to install the new system. Both of them eagerly encouraged Todd to begin installing it. One month later the automated order-processing system was up and running.

Unfortunately, the new system was something less than an unqualified success. Many problems did not show improvement. Some of the order-entry clerks—those dealing with the non-stock-item orders—found the new system cumbersome and unacceptable. They insisted that several atypical processing steps had been omitted. Ed's boss had called to complain that the reports approved by Ed were unacceptable to upper management. The Accounts Receivable manager had called to complain that credit checking policies were not entirely consistent with corporate policy. Todd didn't understand. He wondered why Ed and Mari had been so positive about the system and now other company personnel were so negative.

Discussion

1. Why wasn't Todd able to implement acceptable automated order-processing operations?
2. Whose fault is it that the automated order-processing operations proved less than completely acceptable?
3. What should Todd have done before he developed the initial automated order-processing system?
4. Why didn't Ed recognize that the proposed automated order-processing system would not work?

WHAT WILL YOU LEARN IN THIS CHAPTER?

Systems analysts build information systems for businesses. In this chapter, we learn about the benefactors of the information system — the business and its knowledge workers. You will know that you understand the business and knowledge-worker dimensions of information systems when you can:

1. Define *information system.*
2. Identify knowledge workers in an organization system or subsystem and characterize them as clerical and service staff, supervisory staff, middle-management and professional staff, or executive-management.
3. Describe how an information system serves knowledge workers.
4. Using the suprasystem/system/subsystem concept, explain the relationship between the business system, information system, computer system, and knowledge workers.
5. Describe the mission of a business by defining the purpose, goals, objectives, and policies for a simple business subsystem.

There is a tale that suggests that the first systems analyst appeared on the scene some six thousand years ago, during the construction of the Egyptian pyramids. This self-made systems analyst, concerned about the inefficient methods used to construct the great monuments, offered the following suggestion to Khufu, builder of the Great Pyramid at Cheops:

> "O Noble Khufu, it's time we got organized. We've been pushing this rock through the desert in the wrong direction for seven years. What we need is this Pyramid Erection and Routing Technique." Rumor also has that he was flogged on the spot and never heard from again — at least not until the mid-20th century [Lord and Steiner, 1978, p. 349].

That first systems analyst was looking for a better way to do business — building a product (the pyramids). The systems analyst of the industrial revolution also looked for a better way to do business — through better manufacturing methods. These analysts were called industrial engineers. Today's computer-systems analyst

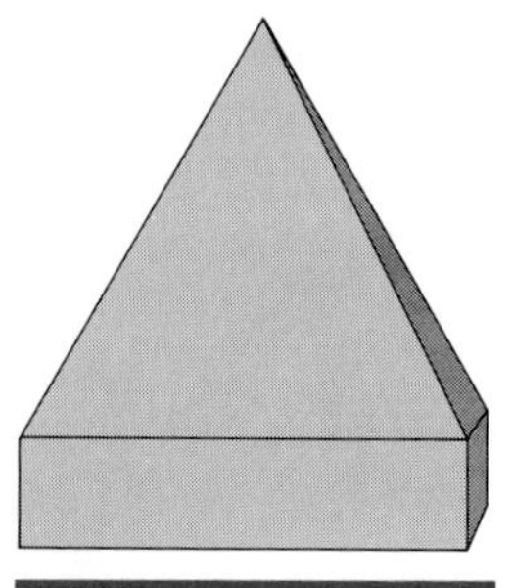

Information System Pyramid

is also looking for a better way to do business—building a new product (information systems) to improve business productivity and decision making.

As a tribute to that first systems analyst, we use a pyramid to illustrate information system concepts. Each face of the pyramid represents a different dimension or point of view and raises issues that you, as an analyst, must consider when analyzing or designing a system. The pyramid is designed to serve as a framework for understanding the complexities of modern information systems. Each face of the pyramid can be related to its other faces to demonstrate important trends and philosophies. The pyramid model is a simple and effective tool to use to understand the modern information system.

The pyramid model appears throughout the book to help remind us about important issues to be considered when we're doing systems analysis and design. As we go through each step of a process to develop information systems, we'll look at each face of the pyramid to consider what we should be doing in that step. When we learn a new tool or technique, we'll refer to the pyramid to consider how that tool or technique helps us build more effective information systems.

This chapter presents the knowledge-worker and business-mission faces of the pyramid model. Chapter 3 presents the information-support and input-process-output faces of the pyramid.

WHAT IS AN INFORMATION SYSTEM?

If you want to be a systems analyst or work with systems analysts, you begin to think like a business professional. Most businesses must make a profit to survive (nonprofit organizations must at least break even). The sum of a business's profitability is easily calculated:

EQUITY = ASSETS − LIABILITIES

What are the assets and liabilities of the modern business?

When you think of assets, you usually think of money, land, employees, buildings, and equipment. But today, businesses are recognizing another important asset: information. Companies that have the best information seem to make better business decisions and realize greater earnings. Information does more than report financial condition. It identifies trends, potential problems, and issues and helps managers identify and analyze alternative business decisions.

Typical liabilities include long- and short-term debts owed to creditors. But in a less tangible sense, many organizations consider lack of management information to be a crippling liability. Why? Well, if the competition has better information, the competition seems also to have the upper hand in market share and earnings!

In order to get better management information, systems analysts are charged to develop information systems. Information systems generate information. Let's define an information system before we examine its benefactors—knowledge workers and the business itself.

Some people will tell you that an information system can't be defined but you'll know one when you see it. Not being able to precisely define the product you are trying to build can make communicating with business users difficult. Indeed, if you can't define an information system, how can you justify its cost to management—or for that matter, your salary as an analyst? Fortunately, classical systems concepts exist to help us define an information system. We can begin with the definition of *system:*

> A **system** is a set or arrangement of things or components so related or connected as to form a whole.

There are two types of systems, natural and fabricated. The solar system and the human body are natural systems. They exist in nature. Fabricated systems, on the other hand, must be built by people. A manufacturing operation, an accounting system, and an information system are all examples of fabricated systems. Presumably, you wouldn't build a system unless it served a purpose. The purpose of our information system is to collect, process, and exchange information among business workers. More specifically, an information system should support the day-to-day operations, management, and decision-making information needs of business workers. This leads us to a definition of *information system:*

> An **information system** is an arrangement of components that interact to support the operations, management, and decision-making information needs of an organization.

Notice that the computer has yet to play a role in our definition. Information systems exist in all organizations. Whenever knowledge workers get together in an organization, they work out some sort of system to collect, process, and exchange information. These systems are usually implemented without the aid of the computer. Although manual systems usually get the job done, they are often inefficient and error prone. Therefore, manual systems are frequently computerized. Why does computerization help? Because the computer amplifies the potential of the information system by increasing efficiency, reducing errors, and increasing effectiveness. The computer complements rather than replaces the business worker (most of the time). With this in mind, we suggest the following definition:

> An information system is a person/machine arrangement of components that interact to support the operational, managerial, and decision-making information needs of an organization.

Information systems that use the computer are sometimes called **computer information systems.** In this text, we use the term *information system* to describe both computerized and noncomputerized systems.

Given our definition of an information system, let's study the people who use and benefit from that system.

KNOWLEDGE WORKERS, THE USERS OF INFORMATION SYSTEMS

The term **knowledge worker** has been coined to describe those people whose jobs involve the creation, processing, and distribution of information. Their livelihoods depend on information and the decisions made from information. Who are the knowledge workers? How many are there? Where do they come from and where are they going? And most important, why are knowledge workers important to the systems analyst? In this section, we examine the knowledge worker in today's business.

The Information Society and the Knowledge Worker

In his bestselling book, *Megatrends: Ten Directions Transforming Our Lives,* John Naisbitt (1982) analyzes today's society to paint a convincing picture of our future. The most explosive of the ten megatrends is our dramatic shift from an industrial society to an information society. Just as the early agricultural society gave way to a more advanced industrial society, so the industrial society has been replaced by an information society. We are now part of an economy built on the production, distribution, and usage of information. This is not to say we are not still manufacturing goods and growing crops. But today, the majority of workers are actually creating, using, or distributing information rather than manufacturing products or providing services. Indeed, many companies exist only to manufacture or transport information (such as overnight mail, computer service bureaus, and consulting firms) and information technology (such as computers and software). Today, the information services sector paces the economy.

Naisbitt points out that the change to an information society did not occur overnight. It was so subtle that most of us didn't even notice. It began in 1956, when white-collar workers first outnumbered their blue-collar counterparts. White-collar workers include managers, engineers, technicians, clerks, secretaries, civil servants, professionals, and money managers. They earn their living by creating, processing, using, and exchanging information instead of producing tangible goods. Hence, they have been described as *knowledge workers.* We also refer to them by their data processing nicknames, *users* or *clients.*

Knowledge workers, or users, are the new majority. Experts suggest that at least 60 percent of today's workers are knowledge workers. And as Figure 2.1 shows, this trend is expected to continue. Is this significant? You bet! If ever there were a watchword for today's economy, that watchword would be *productivity.* Although much attention is currently directed to automating our factories with robots and computers, we should also be asking ourselves how we can improve white-collar productivity.

The productivity of knowledge workers depends on information. Timely and correct information must be created, processed, and exchanged. Better information may lead to better decisions. An information technology revolution has propelled the information society, and the computer is the heart of this revolution. True, the computer was invented as a calculating machine, but it has evolved into an information machine. And we, as systems analysts, are responsible for harnessing the computer's power to produce better information that then increases knowledge-worker productivity.

The existence of the knowledge worker is vital to the systems analyst. If and when systems analysts stop improving the produc-

Figure 2.1

Knowledge workers: The new majority. (Reprinted with permission from *Changing Times* Magazine, © 1983 Kiplinger Washington Editors, Inc., August 1983.)

The Changing World of Work

This look at how the makeup of the U.S. work force changed between 1950 and 1980 and how it is expected to change by 1990 shows clearly that the shift from a blue-collar to a white-collar service economy has already largely taken place. In the years immediately ahead, only the farm sector is expected to experience further significant change.

Occupations	% of work force 1950	1980	1990	Projected % growth in number of jobs 1980–1990
Service Workers	10.2	15.2	15.8	30.1
white-collar	35.9	50.4	50.7	25.9
sales workers	6.8	6.7	6.9	28.5
clerical	12.0	18.5	18.7	26.8
professional, technical	8.4	16.0	16.2	26.4
managers, administrators	8.6	9.2	8.9	21.3
blue-collar	40.1	31.8	31.7	24.9
craft workers	13.9	12.1	12.3	27.4
operatives	19.8	13.9	13.8	23.9
laborers	6.4	5.7	5.6	21.9
Farm Workers	11.6	2.6	1.9	−9.8

Sources: *Historical Statistics of the United States; Occupational Outlook Quarterly* [From "Get the Jump on Tomorrow's Jobs," *Changing Times*, August 1983, p. 28]

tivity of knowledge workers, analysts will become obsolete. That is another reason we should study and attempt to understand our business users. They need us. But we need them also!

Who Are the Knowledge Workers in a Business?

The principle component in the information system is the user or knowledge worker. Different knowledge workers have different information needs. Because systems analysts work with knowledge workers to define their problems and needs, it is useful to know their characteristics and responsibilities. We can classify knowledge workers into four groups: clerical and service staff, supervisory staff, middle management and professional staff, and executive management. Most organizations have a formal structure that

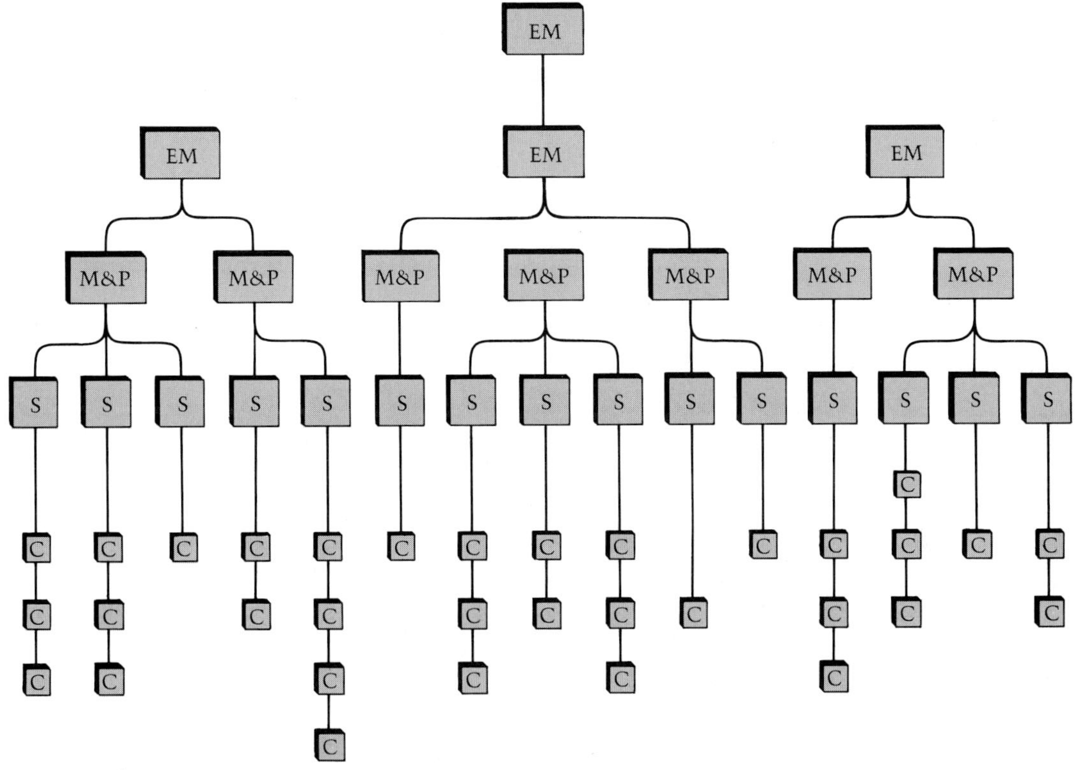

Figure 2.2

Knowledge workers in a typical organization chart. Four types of knowledge workers can be identified in most organizations: *executive managers* (EM) plan and control the long-term, strategic operations; *middle management and professional staff* (M&P) plan and control the short-term, tactical operations; *supervisors* (S) manage the day-to-day activities; and *clerical and service staff* (C) perform those day-to-day activities.

can be documented with an organization chart. An organization chart identifies responsibilities and authority for knowledge workers. Most current organizations are hierarchically structured as depicted in Figure 2.2.

Clerical and Service Staff

Secretaries
Office Workers
Clerks
Tellers
Salespersons
Bookkeepers

Clerical and Service Staff Clerical and service workers perform the day-to-day information activities in the organization; these include screening and filling orders, typing correspondence, and responding to customer inquiries. Examples of clerical and service staff are listed in the margin. Data are captured or created by these workers, many of whom perform manual labors in addition to their information roles. For example, the warehouse clerk who fills an order is both packing the products and recording valuable data about the transaction. The order-entry clerks in the Woodworld Designs minicase would be classified in this group of knowledge workers.

In addition to clerical and service knowledge workers, there are three generally recognized levels of managerial knowledge workers. Management performs the planning, organizing, controlling, and decision-making activities in a business. The three levels of management differ in the time frame of their activities, ranging from day-to-day operations to extremely long-range planning.

Supervisory Staff

- Foremen
- Supervisors
- Group Leaders
- Union Stewards

Supervisory Staff Supervisors represent the lowest level of management. They plan and control the day-to-day operations in the business. Examples of supervisory staff are cited in the margin. Most supervisory managers are concerned with no more than the current day's or the next week's operations.

Supervisors are users of day-to-day detailed information about those activities performed by their subordinates. For example, an order-entry supervisor might need an order register that indicates the status of all orders recently processed. A production foreman might need the detailed production schedule for any given day. Supervisors also frequently prepare reports that summarize the activities performed by their subordinates. For instance, a sales manager may prepare a report that summarizes the sales generated by each sales representative. When studying the needs of supervisors, the systems analyst should seek to understand the day-to-day activities supervised and how they can be measured and improved. Can you identify anyone in the Woodworld minicase who can be classified as supervisory staff? If you guessed Ed Thorpe, you are correct.

Middle Manangement and Professional Staff

- Operations Managers
- Industrial Engineers
- Accountants
- Marketing Specialists
- Engineers
- Business Lawyers
- Personnel Managers
- Sales Managers

Middle Management and Professional Staff Middle Management and professional staff consists of workers who are concerned with relatively short-term planning (sometimes called tactical planning), organizing, controlling, and decision making. They are not interested in the detailed, day-to-day operations that involve the supervisor. Instead, they are concerned with a longer time frame, perhaps a month or a quarter. Some of their functions include gathering operating information for higher levels of management, developing tactical strategies and plans that implement executive management's wishes, and designing products and services. Examples of middle management and professional staff are listed in the margin.

Middle-level managers buffer executives from having to deal with the day-to-day operations of the business.

In the Woodworld minicase, Mari Shadle is an example of middle management. That explains why Mari was unable to tell Todd how special and regular customer orders were processed. She was more concerned with how order-processing operations functioned as a whole than with the detailed step-by-step activities that occurred.

Executive Management Executive management is responsible for the long-term planning (sometimes called strategic planning) and control for the business. Executive managers frequently look a year or more into the past and future. They establish long-range plans and policies for the business and then evaluate how well the business carries them out. They allocate the scarce resources of the business, including land, materials, machinery, labor, and capital (money). Because they are concerned primarily with the overall condition of the business, executive managers usually want highly summarized information to support important decisions. Examples of executive managers are listed in the margin. In the Woodworld minicase, Bob Earman was representative of executive management. As president of Woodworld Designs, Bob was making long-range plans and important financial decisions.

Executive Management

- Board of Directors
- Presidents
- Chief Executive Officers (CEOs)
- Vice-Presidents
- Partners
- Any Executive Manager
- Comptrollers

Notice that the shape of the organization chart in Figure 2.1 is roughly triangular. If we overlay a triangle on the typical organization chart, we can illustrate the first dimension of our pyramid (see Figure 2.3). We'll call this the *knowledge-worker* (or *user*) *dimension of the information system.*

We should point out a very important trend in the knowledge-worker hierarchy. The organization chart triangle is becoming flatter due to reduction in the number of middle management workers needed. This has caused a dramatic middle manager unemployment crisis that will escalate through much of the next decade. Business is moving toward fewer levels of management with more direct communication between executive managers and the supervisory staff. Much of this trend is the direct result of increased computer use by executive management, which allows them to directly bypass middle management. Many members of middle management are perceived as information gatherers whose jobs can be more efficiently performed by computers (*Note:* computers *can* replace unproductive jobs). Only the real problem solvers and decision-making middle managers have secure jobs.

Figure 2.3

The knowledge-worker dimension of the information system. When developing any information system, the systems analyst should identify the knowledge workers and their responsibilities. This is the first dimension of our information system pyramid model. The other faces of the pyramid are discussed later in this chapter and in the next.

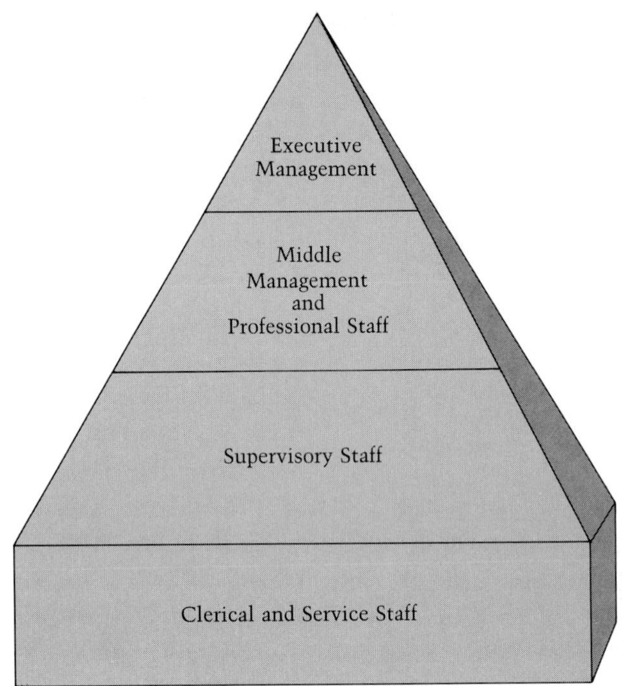

Knowledge Worker Dimension

The Knowledge Worker's Importance to the Systems Analyst

Systems analysts must be responsive to the needs of their knowledge-worker colleagues. The overriding philosophy of systems analysis and design must be that *the system is for the knowledge worker*. This is one lesson Todd Browney should have learned in the minicase. Todd made the mistake of not identifying the knowledge workers and their needs before proceeding with development of the new order-processing information system. As a result, he had to make major additions and modifications to the automated system to fulfill the requirements of Mari Shadle and Ed Thorpe. Even then, the system was inadequate. Why? Because, not realizing that Mari and Ed did not understand the detailed tasks performed by the order-entry clerks, Todd had failed to involve all the order-entry clerks when he was investigating needs.

The ultimate value of any information system is not determined by the analyst or by any computing professional. These people only build information systems. Knowledge workers are served by the information system, and only they, as users, can determine the system's worth!

The Next Generation *An Electronic Desk for the Knowledge Worker*

Knowledge workers have traditionally been at the mercy of data processing when obtaining a majority of their information needs. And for the most part, knowledge workers were content to let data processing professionals develop all computer applications. But three factors are changing this situation. First, there is a critical shortage of data processing professionals; the supply of expertise is not adequate to meet the growing demand for computer applications. Second, microcomputers have brought the technology of computing down to a physical size and cost that make computers in the office an attractive option. Third, managers are becoming more and more computer literate — and they are no longer afraid to use the computer! Also consider, if you will, that today's children are being raised on computers; their computer expectations will be more sophisticated than ours.

Common Knowledge-Worker Functions

It has long been recognized that knowledge workers, especially managers, engage in some common functions and activities that are independent of their business specialties; included among these are accounting, marketing, personnel, and production. What are these common knowledge-worker functions? The following list is typical:

- Preparation of letters, memos, and reports
- Preparation of financial data, such as budgets and cost/benefit analyses (this does not include accounting reports)
- Organization of data into small, local-office files, such as file folders, logs, and reports
- Management of projects (scheduling, progress reporting, and the like)
- Use of graphic and visual aids to present facts, conclusions, and proposals

The computing industry has responded to this by developing microcomputer software to help managers write (word processors), budget and analyze (spreadsheets), organize data (file managers), draw pictures (graphics), and manage project schedules. Each capability is provided by a separate software package. Using the packages in conjunction with one another has been very difficult . . . until recently. Now we are beginning to see the emergence of integrated management software for microcomputers. When all these management tools are combined into a single package, managers are provided with the equivalent of an electronic desk. Early examples of these products include Lotus Development Corporation's *SYMPHONY* and Ashton-Tate's *FRAMEWORK*. The question to be ▶

In the Woodworld minicase, one gets the impression that Mari Shadle and Ed Thorpe thought the new automated order-processing system would be the greatest thing since sliced bread. That's easy to understand because both of them saw the need for an improved order-processing system and because Todd had met with each of them and agreed to make their requested modifications to the new

The Next Generation (continued)

addressed in this "Next Generation" segment is "What impact will the electronic desk have on the systems analyst?" But first, let's briefly examine the state of the art in electronic desk capability (realizing, of course, that the technology is improving even as this book goes to press).

Electronic Desk Capability What can a knowledge worker do with an electronic desk? An electronic desk allows a manager to create, modify, and analyze information using a combination of text, tables, files, and graphs. Ashton-Tate's *FRAMEWORK* even allows you to organize your thoughts into an outline format from which each element in the outline will eventually be turned into text, tables, files, or graphs. Electronic desks may also offer a full complement of arithmetic or statistical functions especially suited for business managers. The individual components of the electronic desk include:

- **Word Processing** Software that helps the user create, edit, and reformat letters, memos, and reports. It gives the user complete control over documents, making it possible to change margins; move words, paragraphs, and sections; and insert and delete text — all effortlessly, at least when compared with paper-and-pencil work.
- **Spreadsheets** Software that creates rows and columns of cells that can contain numbers and text. The power of spreadsheets is derived from a cell's ability to hold an arithmetic formula where the operators are the numbers stored in other cells. Thus, the user can set up ledgers, forecasts, estimates, budgets, and projections. As numbers are entered into cells or changed within cells, the formulas are automatically recalculated in the arithmetic cells. This allows the user to play "what if" games for decision making without having to perform arithmetic with paper, pencils, and calculators.
- **File Managers** Also called database managers, file managers allow users to store facts in a flexible format and then retrieve those facts in a variety of formats suitable to business analysis and decision making.
- **Graphics** Software that converts facts from spreadsheets and files into pie charts, bar charts, line charts, and other graphical formats is called graphics. Knowledge workers find pictures useful for displaying trends and conclusions not immediately apparent in tables composed of numbers.
- **Project Managers** Software that helps managers keep track of the numer- ▶

system. On the other hand, the order-entry clerks were frustrated with the new system and thought it less than satisfactory. Why? Because, by their standards, the new system was unworkable.

As a footnote, you may be surprised to discover that the systems analyst is also a knowledge worker. Do you have any idea where the analyst is in our hierarchy? If you guessed professional staff, you are

The Next Generation (continued)

ous tasks involved in various projects. Calendars and schedules can be maintained and "what if" questions can be asked about possible project delays.

These menu-driven software products claim to be user friendly. Certainly, they will become friendlier and easier to use over time. The integrated software packages allow the user to choose the tool(s) needed to solve a particular problem. And the use of the tools can be integrated. Let's say a manager is preparing a budget request for higher-level management. That manager can call up historical cost data from the database function. This data can be placed into a spreadsheet set up to report the budget. Using the spreadsheet, the manager makes a variety of assumptions about sales and costs and can immediately project their impact on the budget. Several alternative budgets might be calculated and tested. To help sell the budget to higher management, the data might be translated into a pie chart to show what proportions of the budget are allocated to different expenses. Finally, the word processor is used to write up the proposed budget, cutting and pasting the spreadsheet(s) and graph(s) into the document. This ability to combine the common functions is where the name *integrated* software came from. Integrated software can be expected to include more and more functions in the future.

A Look Toward the Future
How will the electronic desk impact the systems analyst developing future applications? For one thing, analysts who become involved with developing microcomputer applications will have to consider the use of this integrated software to support those applications. Let's speculate a little. How long will it be before management insists on tapping the enormous power of large computer files and databases through their electronic desks? They are already asking for this ability. You see, it doesn't make sense for everybody to store common data on every microcomputer. It is more sensible to maintain common data centrally on the larger, mainframe computers. Management will eventually want applications that allow them to transfer that data to their microcomputers and then place that data into their spreadsheets, local databases, word processing documents, and graphs. Systems analysts will help develop these corporate databases and help users tap them. At the time of this writing, the technology is immature. But the problems of linking microcomputers and mainframe computers are being addressed by numerous companies. The ultimate in integrated computer information systems may be just around the corner. ■

correct! Systems analysts are professional staff workers. Along with other knowledge workers, analysts are responsible for increasing their own productivity. Keep this in mind as you study systems analysis and design methods. Remember, the business world will eventually eliminate unproductive jobs (for example, today's middle managers)—the systems analyst is not immune!

INFORMATION SYSTEMS SHOULD SUPPORT THE BUSINESS MISSION

So far, we've learned that knowledge workers use an information system. These knowledge workers are part of another system, the business itself. Like other fabricated systems, the business system serves a purpose. We'll call that purpose the *business mission.* The purpose of an information system should be compatible with the business mission. What is the relationship between the information system, the business system, and knowledge workers? What is a business mission? Why is the business mission important to the analyst? These questions are answered in this section.

Some Fundamental Systems Concepts

Many people have confused the terms *business system* and *information system.* They are not one and the same! To appreciate the difference, we need only examine a few simple system concepts.

Earlier in this chapter, we stated that a system is a set of components so related or connected as to form a whole. One of the difficulties involved in understanding any kind of system is overcoming its size and complexity. System concepts help us deal with size and complexity by showing us the general characteristics that *all* systems have in common. Let's examine some fundamental system concepts and apply them to the business as a system.

All systems, save perhaps the universe, have a **boundary** that separates the system from its **environment.** For all but the simplest systems, that boundary is somewhat artificial—you cannot see or touch it. The boundary of an information system is defined by the scope of the business activities to be supported by that information system. For example, a small information system may support only a few of the business activities in a single department, say, Accounting. A somewhat larger information system could be built to support all of the activities of the Accounting Department. And an even larger information system could be built to support several business departments, including Accounting.

This brings us to an important system concept—the concept of subsystems and suprasystems. Any system may contain numerous **subsystems,** each of which is a complete system within the larger system. For instance, in Figure 2.4, we see depicted a manufacturing system that contains four subsystems: production scheduling, pro-

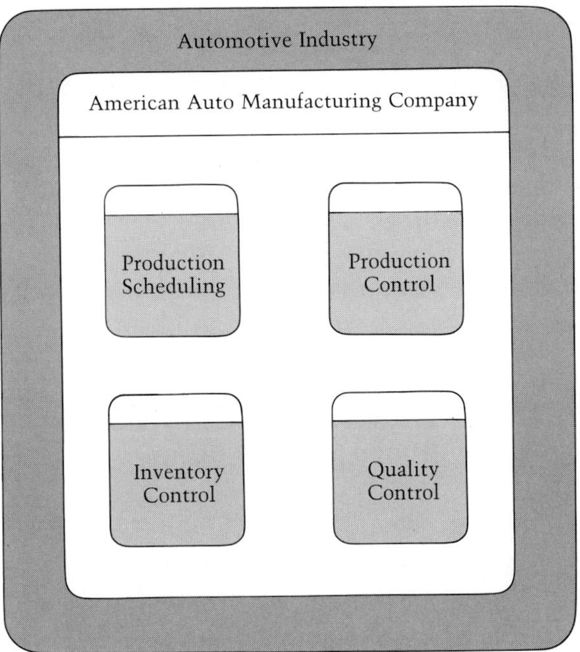

Figure 2.4

The suprasystem, system, and subsystem. Production scheduling, production control, inventory control, and quality control are subsystems of the American Auto Manufacturing Company (AAMC) system. AAMC, in turn, is a subsystem of the automobile industry. Along similar lines, the automotive industry is a suprasystem of AAMC. And AAMC is a suprasystem of each of the four lowest-level systems.

duction control, inventory control, and quality control. These subsystems, in turn, may consist of other subsystems. The concept also works in reverse. Any given system may be part of a larger system called a **suprasystem.** For instance, the manufacturing system in Figure 2.4 is part of a suprasystem called the automotive industry.

Why is this concept important? Remember, one of the questions we want to address is the relationship between the information system and the business system. As it turns out, the information system is a subsystem of the business system. In fact, a business system normally contains several information systems, each supporting some subset of the business's activities (see Figure 2.5 for an example). Along the same lines, the business system is a suprasystem of each information system. Any given information system

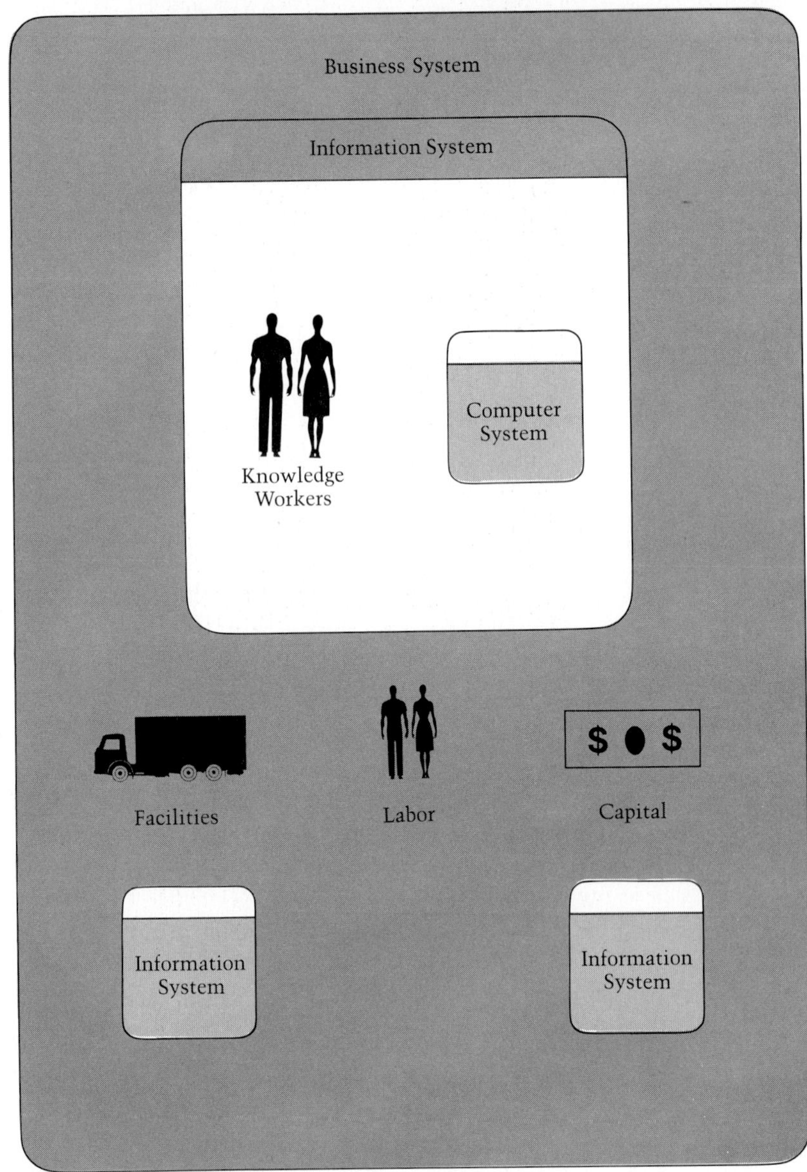

Figure 2.5

The relationship between business system, information system, computer system, and knowledge workers. The information system is a subsystem of the business system. Most businesses have several information systems. The knowledge worker is a component in both systems. The computer system is an optional subsystem of the information system.

may, of course, have subsystems, which in turn, may have more subsystems.

What is the relationship between the business system, the information system and knowledge workers? Recall that systems consist of components. Knowledge workers constitute one of the key components of the information system. Because the information system is a subsystem of the business system, the knowledge worker is also a component of the business system. This is illustrated in Figure 2.5. Are there other components in these two systems? Yes. We learn about them in Chapter 3.

Where does the computer system (computers, programs, data processing personnel, to name a few of its components) fit into this model? Referring again to Figure 2.5, you will see the computer system depicted as a subsystem of the information system. Recall that we said a computer system is not a mandatory part of an information system. It only amplifies (when properly used) the power and capabilities of the information system. When a computer system is used in an information system, the term *computer information system* is often used to describe the system.

Information System: A Refined Definition

Now that we've considered system concepts, let's make another refinement to our definition of an information system:

> An **information system** is a subsystem of the business. Specifically, it is a person/machine arrangement of components that interact to support the operational, managerial, and decision-making information needs of knowledge workers.

Notice that we've specifically recognized knowledge workers as the business people most interested in the information system. We've also specifically identified the information system as a subsystem of the business system. Because the information system must support its business suprasystem, we now examine the business mission as an important issue for the systems analyst.

What Is a Business Mission?

A business *system* is directed toward what we call its business mission. A **business mission** can be stated in terms of the business purpose, goals, objectives, and policies. To fully understand the needs of the knowledge workers in a business system, the systems analyst must understand the business mission.

The **business purpose** of a company is a general statement of the reason for its existence. Purpose usually addresses who the company's customers are and what products or services the company provides its customers. The systems analyst should always be aware of strategic plans relative to the business's primary purpose. Will the purpose change? For example: Is the company planning to change or add to its customer base? Is the company planning to add or delete products or services? Will such changes dramatically impact the information needs of knowledge workers? Does the company plan to add new knowledge workers with new and different information needs? A good analyst keeps abreast of the strategic direction of the business (as it becomes known).

You probably have some idea of what goals and objectives are, but they are terms that are commonly confused. **Goals** are very general statements of the degree to which the business purpose is to be realized. For example, does the business want to maximize profit, maximize market share, or maximize return on investments? These are all broadly stated goals. **Objectives** are specific targets that are directed toward goals. In order to maximize profits, we will likely establish many objectives, such as "Decrease production costs by 10 percent by August 30." It is interesting to note that one knowledge worker's objective may be another's goal. The previous cost reduction objective may not be specific enough for a lower-level knowledge worker who considers it a goal. One of this worker's objectives may be to reduce scrap and waste of materials at the turrent-lathes by 15 percent by August 30. Objectives should specify the activity and the performance criteria. Most objectives are defined at the work-unit level. That is, each work unit, such as Accounting or Personnel, will have separately defined objectives.

Goals and objectives are important because they typically motivate knowledge workers. Some firms practice a management technique called **management by objectives (MBO)**. Using this technique, knowledge workers help define their own objectives, carefully ensuring that the objectives achieve business goals. Bonuses and pay raises are awarded or withheld to motivate knowledge workers to achieve their objectives. Thus, goals and objectives motivate knowledge workers and frequently define their information needs.

Most organizations have adopted policies that must be followed in fulfilling objectives. A **policy** is a set of rules that governs the

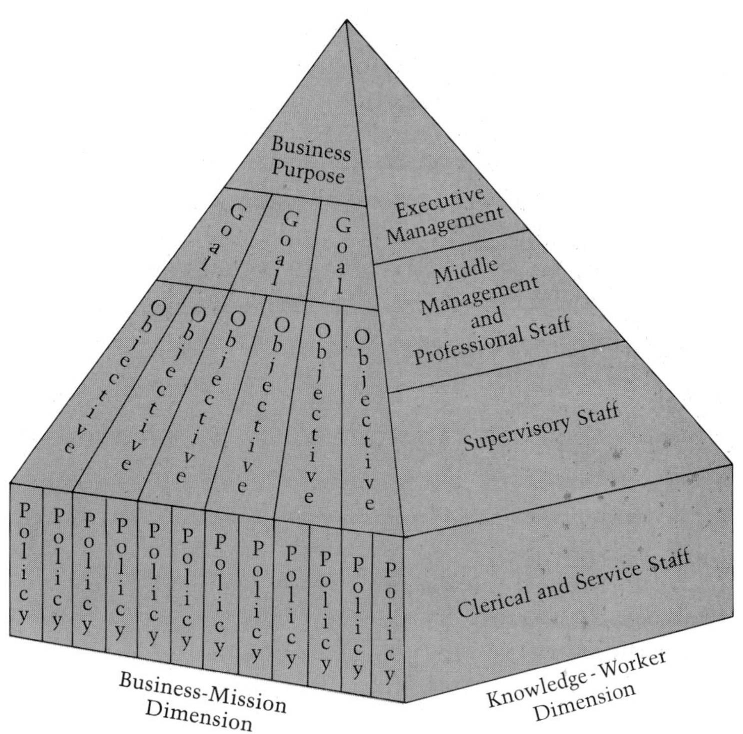

Figure 2.6

Business-mission dimension of the information system. When building an information system, the systems analyst should clearly understand or define the purpose, goals, objectives, and policies of the business. If you also look at the knowledge-worker face of the pyramid, you will see that goals come from executive and upper-middle management, objectives and policies are defined by lower-middle management and supervisors, and policies are carried out by clerical and service staff.

activities involved in achieving objectives. For instance, most companies have a credit policy for determining whether to accept or reject an order. The Woodworld company in our minicase did. And Todd, like any other systems analyst, should recognize that policies may place restrictions on how a system can function. To ensure that they don't deter achievement of the goals and objectives, policies must be set *after* goals and objectives have been determined.

We can now rotate our information system pyramid to show the business-mission dimension. The hierarchy in Figure 2.6 shows the correlation between the components of the business mission and the various levels of knowledge workers within the business. The business purpose is established by the highest levels of executive management. Goals and high-level objectives are developed by middle- to executive-level managers. Detailed objectives are established by middle managers. Policies are set by middle- to supervisory-level managers. Clerical and service workers must perform operational activities in accordance to company policies. It is vitally important that the analyst develop an understanding of the organization's purpose, goals, objectives, and policies.

The Business Mission's Importance to the Systems Analyst

The importance of thoroughly understanding the purpose, goals, objectives, and policies of an organization should be clear. The analyst should work closely enough with the different levels of knowledge workers to understand the full business implications of any information system project. The value of any information system is ultimately a function of compatibility with the business mission. Most organizations evaluate the activities and performance of their knowledge workers with respect to the purpose, goals, objectives, and policies of the business. Doesn't it make sense to evaluate information systems according to the same criteria? Information systems must support the business mission!

SUMMARY

An information system is a business subsystem. Specifically, it is a person and machine arrangement of components that interact to support the operational, managerial, and decision-making information needs of knowledge workers.

The overriding theme of this chapter is that the information system is for the knowledge worker. Knowledge workers are those individuals whose jobs involve the creation, processing, and distribution of information. Because these people represent the majority of today's work force, much attention is being placed on improving their productivity by building more effective and efficient information systems. When building an information system, the systems analyst should address the problems and needs of all involved knowledge workers, including clerical and service staff, supervisory staff, middle management and professional staff, and executive management.

The systems analyst must understand the relationship between the business system and the information system. The business represents a much larger system (suprasystem) within which the information system functions. Along the same lines, the information system is a subsystem of the business. Because of the close relationship between business and information systems, the information system must support the business mission. The business mission can be stated in terms of the purpose, goals, objectives, and policies of the business. The effectiveness and value of an information system is dependent on its fulfillment of this mission.

Knowledge workers are an integral component of the information system. The computer system is an optional but popular subsystem of many information systems. Information systems that contain computer components are often called computer information systems. Additional components of the information system are introduced in Chapter 3.

PROBLEMS AND EXERCISES

1. Define *information system.* Information systems are all around you. Give an example of a completely manual information system. Describe how a computer might improve that information system.
2. Identify a computer-based information system with which you are familiar. Any computerized application will suffice. If the computer were not used, how would the information system have to be implemented? What sacrifices would have to be made?
3. For each of the following job titles, identify the worker as clerical or service staff, supervisory staff, middle management, professional staff, or executive management. Defend your answer.
   (a) Production control manager
   (b) Computer programmer
   (c) Receptionist/secretary
   (d) Financial analyst
   (e) Department store manager
   (f) Systems analyst
   (g) Full-time terminal operator
   (h) Shop floor foreman

(i) Salesperson
(j) Employees who fill orders in the warehouse
(k) Major stockholder (owns more than half the stock)
(l) Chairman of the board of directors
(m) Product design specialist
(n) Industrial engineer

4. Give three examples of knowledge workers from each of the following classifications: clerical and service staff, supervisory staff, middle management and professional staff, and executive management. Explain the job responsibilities of each example you provided and state why your example represents that particular classification of knowledge worker.

5. The president of Grant Insurance Company is puzzled. He was under the impression that computerization of his clerical and service functions would effectively reduce the size of that staff. Since installing computer support eight years ago, he has seen his clerical and service staff increase 10 percent, while business has remained steady. His friends in the local Chamber of Commerce have experienced the same phenomenon. Why does this happen?

6. The president of Grant Insurance Company (introduced in problem 5) has noticed another curious trend. Although the use of computers did not decrease his need for clerical and service staff, it has reduced his dependence on middle level management and professional staff. This seems exactly the opposite of his expectations; however, it is typical. Why does this happen?

7. Obtain an organization chart from a local company (or at your library). Classify each person and/or job position appearing on the chart according to the type of knowledge worker represented (such as clerical and service staff).

8. Consider a business by which you were, or are, employed in any capacity. Identify the knowledge workers at each level in the knowledge-worker hierarchy. (*Alternative:* Substitute your school for the business. Students are part of the clerical and service staff classification. Do you see why?)

9. Identify an information system with which you are somewhat familiar. Remember, information systems are everywhere, so you shouldn't have to look far. What is the suprasystem of your information system? What are some of the possible subsystems of your information system?

10. Obtain an organization chart from a local company (or from your library). What are some of the subsystems you see on the organization chart? Do those subsystems have subsystems? An organization chart is, by definition, a chart of systems and subsystems.

11. A systems analyst for Grady Business Supply has uncovered a sensitive problem while working on a purchasing and inventory control project. The purchasing manager's job performance is based on minimizing purchase cost per unit on all products (all products are purchased direct from various manufacturers). She does this by taking advantage of large-quantity discounts offered by suppliers (in other words, the suppliers offer lower per-unit prices for large order quantities). Meanwhile, the inventory manager's job performance is based on minimizing inventory carrying costs while avoiding stockouts (running out of stock). He wants to keep the quantities of each product to a minimum. These managers have conflicting goals and objectives that prevent the analyst from suggesting a system that at least one of the managers is certain not to accept. What should the analyst do?

12. Select a typical business, and identify its purpose. What are some goals this business might establish? Identify some objectives that may direct the business toward reaching those goals. What are some of the policies that might exist within the business?

13. Make an appointment to discuss your curriculum with your advisor or an instructor. Consider your curriculum to be a system. (It is!) What is the purpose of your major? What are the goals? Choose a specific course in your major. What are the objectives of that course? Are those objectives consistent with some of the goals of your curriculum? Finally, identify a few policies that have been established in the course. Are those policies consistent with the course's goals and objectives?

ANNOTATED REFERENCES AND SUGGESTED READINGS

Changing Times staff. "Get the Jump on Tomorrow's Jobs." *Changing Times* 37 (August, 1983), pp. 26–31.

Davis, Gordon B. "Knowing the Knowledge Workers: A Look at the People Who Work with Knowledge and the Technology That Will Make Them Better." *ICP Software Review,* (Spring, 1982), pp. 70–75. This article provided our first exposure to the concept of knowledge workers as the new majority.

Davis, Gordon B., and Margrethe H. Olson. *Management Information Systems: Conceptual Foundations, Structure, and Development.* 2d ed. New York: McGraw-Hill, 1985. This is our all-time favorite book on information systems concepts and principles.

Lord, Kenniston W., Jr., and James B. Steiner. *CDP Review Manual: A Data Processing Handbook.* 2d ed. New York: Van Nostrand Reinhold, 1978.

Naisbitt, John. *Megatrends: Ten Directions Transforming Our Lives.* New York: Warner Books, 1982. A bestselling book that discusses, in considerable depth, the impact technology has had and will have on our society and business.

Sprague, Ralph H., Jr. "A Framework for the Development of Decision Support Systems." *MIS Quarterly* 4 (December, 1980), 1–26. This paper presents the forerunner of our information systems pyramid model.

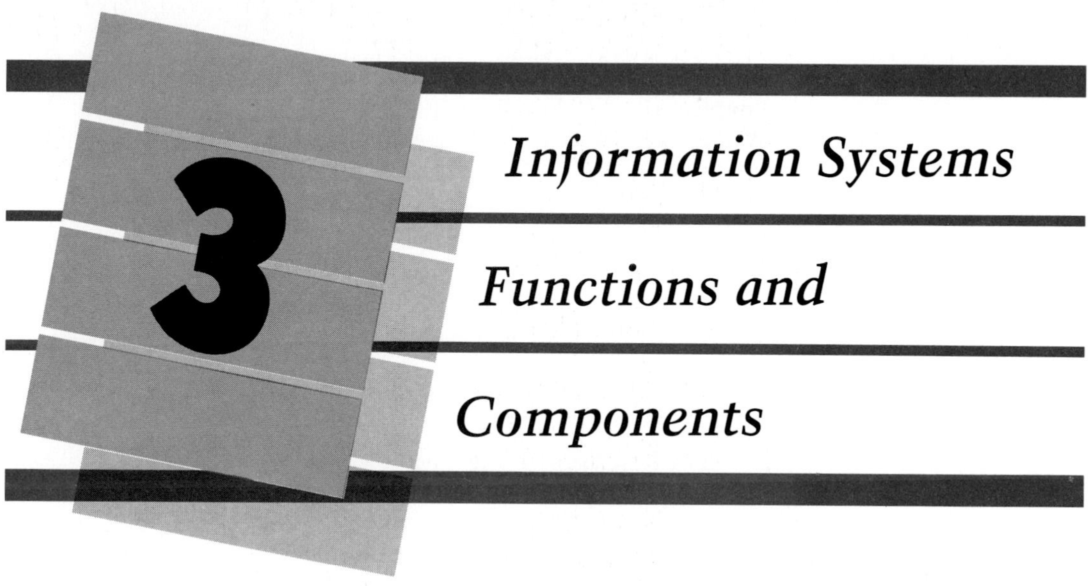

3 Information Systems Functions and Components

Minicase: Outland Engine and Hightech Electronics, Inc.

Larry Dunam, the Information Systems manager for Outland Engine, was attending his first meeting of the local chapter of the Data Processing Management Association (DPMA). During the meeting, Larry met John Becker, the MIS manager of Hightech Electronics. John was the chapter's membership chair, and he was encouraging Larry to join the chapter. We'll listen in on the conversation between the two men:

Larry I had no idea DPMA had so much to offer me. I'd like to join, but I'm concerned that problems that pop up at work will restrict the time I can devote to DPMA activities. It seems I'm always working on some major system.

John Everyone in this room is a computer professional and can certainly appreciate your concerns. But that's just one more good reason to join DPMA. You'll meet other data processing professionals who may have faced the same problems or situations. You might learn from their experiences.

Larry I'd like to meet some of those people. We're trying to computerize our manual inventory control system right now.

John Maybe I can help you. I've had some experience with inventory control systems. We have about twenty minutes before our guest speaker makes her presentation.

Larry Terrific! The project involves automating a manual purchasing system to replenish inventory. I didn't know much about inventory systems until I talked with the inventory staff. If I describe the manual system, maybe you could give me some feedback on what we're trying to do.

John I'll help any way I can.

Larry Currently, a purchasing clerk does a daily physical count of inventory and prepares a list of items that are low in stock.

John That's very time consuming. I assume you're thinking about automating the inventory file and having a computer program generate the report?

Larry Yes. Right now, it takes the clerk approximately three hours to do this inventory check. Anyway, the manager uses that list of items low in stock to initiate purchasing decisions. For each item listed on the report, he scans through a notebook containing copies of purchase order forms that were prepared and sent out in the previous week. If the item doesn't appear on any of the outstanding purchase orders, that item must be ordered. I'm convinced we should store this notebook in a computer file and have a program search the file for the outstanding purchase orders. The manager shouldn't have to spend time leafing through that notebook.

John I agree! And don't forget the potential that file has for generating other useful reports for your managers and staff. We've really implemented a super inventory reporting system. For instance, you mentioned a report that identifies items low in stock. We also created a report that identified items that were both low in stock and currently on order. Our warehouse people found the second report reassuring because it gave them an idea when new stock might be received.

Larry I didn't think of that. Do you generate many other reports?

John Sure! I'll bet we generate fifteen different reports off a file similar to your notebook. Different reports are intended for different clerks and managers. Some reports are very detailed, and others summarize those details. Still others report situations that different people in the company want to be aware of. When we develop a new system, we try to study the responsibilities and activities of all levels of management. Then we brainstorm different types of reports that management might need. It really gets them thinking about computer support, and they start recommending very useful reports on their own initiative! I'll introduce you to Holly Carter, one of my analysts, when she shows up. She can describe some of those reports.

Larry I'm beginning to appreciate the benefits of this organization. Getting back to my manual system — After the manager identifies items that need to be ordered, he then checks through another notebook containing information about suppliers and their products to determine the ideal supplier from which to order the item. Now this is the tough part. I'm not sure I can automate this step. I know this notebook could also be stored in a computer file but the data is volatile. Each day, I'd have to reproduce the equivalent of the notebook so that managers can make their decisions.

John Why?

Larry Well, first of all, a variety of information is needed to determine which supplier to order the part from. For example, the manager needs to know which suppliers carry the item, the supplier's price for that item, the supplier's ability to meet our requested delivery date, and any discounts the suppliers might offer. But I just can't justify printing that report every day.

John We were faced with the same problem, Larry. We, too, decided a report with that information was a waste of paper. Our people wanted to be able to get at the information for only the items they needed to order. So we gave them an online system. The workers use the system's inquiry function to retrieve needed information on demand. The program can provide the user with a menu of inquiries the user can perform, such as inquiries to obtain supplier, product, or purchase order information. If you have an on-line operating system, I'd put this portion of your system on-line.

Larry It would be a more difficult system to develop, but we could do it. In fact, I suppose I could also have the program provide the manager with the option of entering the final decision on supplier. But I still have a tricky problem to solve and I'll bet this one isn't similar to your system.

John Really?

Larry Yes. You see, we don't want to generate a purchase order right when the supplier decision is made for the item. Let me explain the steps we currently go through. After the manager makes a decision for an item, he transfers information about that item and supplier to something called an order pad. The order pad is given to a purchasing clerk who generates the final purchase order. The purchasing clerk uses the order pad to generate a list that consolidates those items that are to be ordered from the same supplier. This way, we don't send multiple purchase orders to the same supplier. Once this list has been prepared, the clerk completes the purchase orders. Additional information to be written on the purchase orders, such as the supplier address or unit of measure for an item, would have to be obtained from the supplier notebook. If I put the supplier selection decision on-line, how do I continue consolidating items into single purchase orders for individual suppliers?

John You're right, that is different from our system. Why not store the supplier selection decisions in a pending purchase orders file? New items could be added to a pending purchase order as decisions are made. Then . . .

Larry I get it! Then, at the end of the day, the computer could print the final purchase orders. It looks like the new system will work. Of course, with all these new files, I do have to make sure that there are mechanisms for capturing all the data used to create, modify, and delete records for files. The accuracy of reports and inquiries will be dependent on that data.

John Larry, I think you're going to have one fine inventory replenishing system. I also hope I've talked you into DPMA membership.

Larry I feel pretty optimistic now. I tell you what, why don't you give me a handful of those DPMA membership application forms? I'm going to encourage my entire MIS staff to join DPMA.

Larry successfully implemented the automated inventory purchasing system. The new system proved to be more efficient and effective than the old system. Each person involved with the inventory purchasing system was pleased with the support the new system provided.

Discussion

1. Did you notice that Larry and John were primarily focusing on the procedures for preparing purchase orders? Why were they primarily discussing how purchase orders were generated? How will an understanding of those procedures help Larry generate new and useful reports for management?
2. What are some examples of reports that Larry's new system might provide purchasing clerks and managers? Where would the data for those reports come from?
3. Why was it important to Larry to define the mechanisms for capturing all the data used to update the automated files?
4. Who were the knowledge workers mentioned in the inventory purchasing system? Did the new system serve each of the knowledge workers? How?

WHAT WILL YOU LEARN IN THIS CHAPTER?

In this chapter,we learn more about the information system itself — specifically, about information system functions and about the input, process, and output components of an information system. You will know that you understand the functional capabilities and input-process-output dimensions of an information system when you can:

1. Explain the relationships between data, information, input, processing, and output, and give examples of each item.
2. Recognize, describe, and give examples of the following three types of information support an information system can provide to knowledge workers: transaction processing, management reporting, and decision support.
3. Recognize, describe, and give examples of the input, process, and output components of an information system, including data, information, knowledge workers, methods and procedures, data storage, hardware, software, and internal controls.
4. Describe the importance of keeping up with information system trends and explain several current trends in modern information systems.

In Chapter 2, you learned that an information system was a tool created by businesses to generate operational, managerial, and decision-making information for knowledge workers. Ideally, that information also supports the business mission. But so far, we've said very little about the specific capabilities an information system can provide. In this chapter, we look at the types of information functions a modern information system can offer its knowledge workers.

Also recall from Chapter 2 that we defined an information system as *an arrangement of components.* So far, however, we have not identified those components. Because the systems analyst plays a major role in selecting and designing the components in an information system, we take time in this chapter to carefully examine the input, process, and output components of an information system.

We continue to unveil our information system pyramid model in this chapter, rotating the pyramid to reveal the last two of its faces—the information system functions and the input-process-output (IPO) components. Remember, we plan to use the pyramid to remind ourselves of important issues and concerns as we study systems analysis and design tools and techniques.

INFORMATION SYSTEM FUNCTIONS

The purpose of an information system is to fulfill the information needs of knowledge workers. But what is information? Is it the same as data? What information support functions should be considered by the systems analyst? These questions are addressed in this section.

Data and Information

Many people use the terms *data* and *information* interchangeably. Even software products frequently ignore the fundamental difference between data and information when naming their products. For example, IBM's *data*base management system is called *Information* Management System (IMS). But data and information are not the same thing. Throughout this book, we use a classical definition for each term:

> **Data** is raw facts in isolation. It describes the business system. These isolated facts convey meaning but generally are not useful by themselves.
>
> **Information** is data that has been manipulated so it is useful to someone. In other words, information must have value, or it is still data. Information must tell people something they don't already know or confirm something that they suspect.

It should be noted that one person's information may be another person's data. For example, consider a report that lists all customer accounts. If customers call to find out their current balance due, a clerk can answer their questions by looking at the report. To the clerk, this report is information. But, suppose a manager wants to know the total dollar amount of delinquent accounts. The manager would have to identify delinquent accounts on the report and sum their balances. Thus, the report (as it is) represents data to that manager.

What about the items-low-in-stock report that was mentioned in the Outland Engine/Hightech Electronics minicase? Did the report represent data or information to the manager? When the report was produced manually, it probably represented data. Sure the report told the manager what items were low in stock, but it did not tell the manager which items needed to be ordered. The manager had to check the purchase order notebook to determine whether or not the item was already on order. If the report had included only those items both low in stock and not currently on order, then that report would have been information (to the manager).

Data describes the fundamental components and events of the business system: assets, liabilities, accounts, products, materials, customers, suppliers, transactions (such as orders and invoices), and so forth. Each of these business components and transactions can be described by data attributes. For instance, a customer can be described by the following data attributes: CUSTOMER NUMBER, CUSTOMER NAME, CREDIT RATING, and/or BALANCE DUE.

An information system creates, collects, and stores data and processes that data into useful information. This is the single most important concept of systems analysis and design:

INFORMATION = f(DATA, PROCESSING)

Information is a function of data and processing. This formula is as important to the systems analyst as $E = mc^2$ is to the physicist, and you will find most systems methods easier to apply if you commit it to memory.

The concepts of data and information will be useful as we study different information system functions and capabilities. These support capabilities include transaction processing, management reporting, and decision support.

Transaction Processing

Transactions are business events such as orders, invoices, requisitions, and the like. Some organizations consider their **transaction-processing** systems as being separate from their information systems. But we've just learned differently! To produce information, we must first capture data. Business transactions represent 90 percent or more of all data that describes a business. If we capture that data, we can support most information needs imaginable. That explains why, in the Outland Engine/Hightech Electronics minicase, Larry was so intent on being sure that he identified the mechanisms for capturing the data used to update the files. Were he to fail to do so, the data used to prepare the various system outputs would be either inaccurate or nonexistent. Transaction processing is the means by which most business data is captured and maintained.

There are two types of transaction processing. The most familiar of these is the processing of *input transactions.* Examples of input transactions are listed in the margin. Each of these transactions inputs new data into the information system. For example, the order data input may consist of an ORDER NUMBER, CUSTOMER NUMBER, ORDER DATE, PRODUCT NUMBER (or NUMBERS), and QUANTITY (or QUANTITIES). In this chapter's minicase, the input transaction that was being processed was the manager's decision to place an order for an item.

Another type of transaction is the *output transaction.* Output transactions trigger responses from or confirm actions to those who eventually receive those transactions. Examples of output transactions are listed in the margin. In each case, the output transaction confirms an action or triggers a response (such as confirming that you're booked on a flight or acknowledging receipt of your payment of a bill). In this chapter's minicase, the purchase order forms that were being generated and sent to suppliers represent an output transaction.

An example of transaction processing is illustrated in Figure 3.1, which portrays an inventory purchasing system similar to the one envisioned in the Outland Engine/Hightech Electronics minicase. Do not concern yourself that the system is incomplete. We have tried to keep it simple enough to demonstrate only the concepts you've just learned.

Transaction processing includes more than the processing of input and output transactions. Because of the importance of complete and accurate data capture of transactions, there is a historical reporting requirement for most transaction-processing systems. These reports provide information on all transactions processed and serve as an audit trail that confirms transaction processing and ensures that the data can be recaptured in case it gets lost somewhere in the system. For example, in addition to generating purchase orders, Figure 3.1 shows the output of a purchase order register, which is a historical report.

Computer-based information systems generally support transaction processing for clerical and service knowledge workers. To some extent, the clerical tasks performed by these workers can be replaced by automation, which is faster and more accurate. These workers can, in turn, assume more stimulating and productive assignments. It should be noted that the reduction of clerical tasks is frequently offset by an increase in data-entry tasks and clerks to perform these new tasks. One trend in automated transaction pro-

Input Transactions

- Customer Orders
- Accounting Vouchers
- Course Registrations
- Time Cards
- Airline Reservations
- Payments
- Charge Card Slips
- Bank Deposit Slips

Output Transactions

- Customer Invoice (Bill)
- Course Schedule
- Paycheck
- Airline Reservation Confirmation
- Airline Tickets
- Payment Receipt
- Sales Receipt

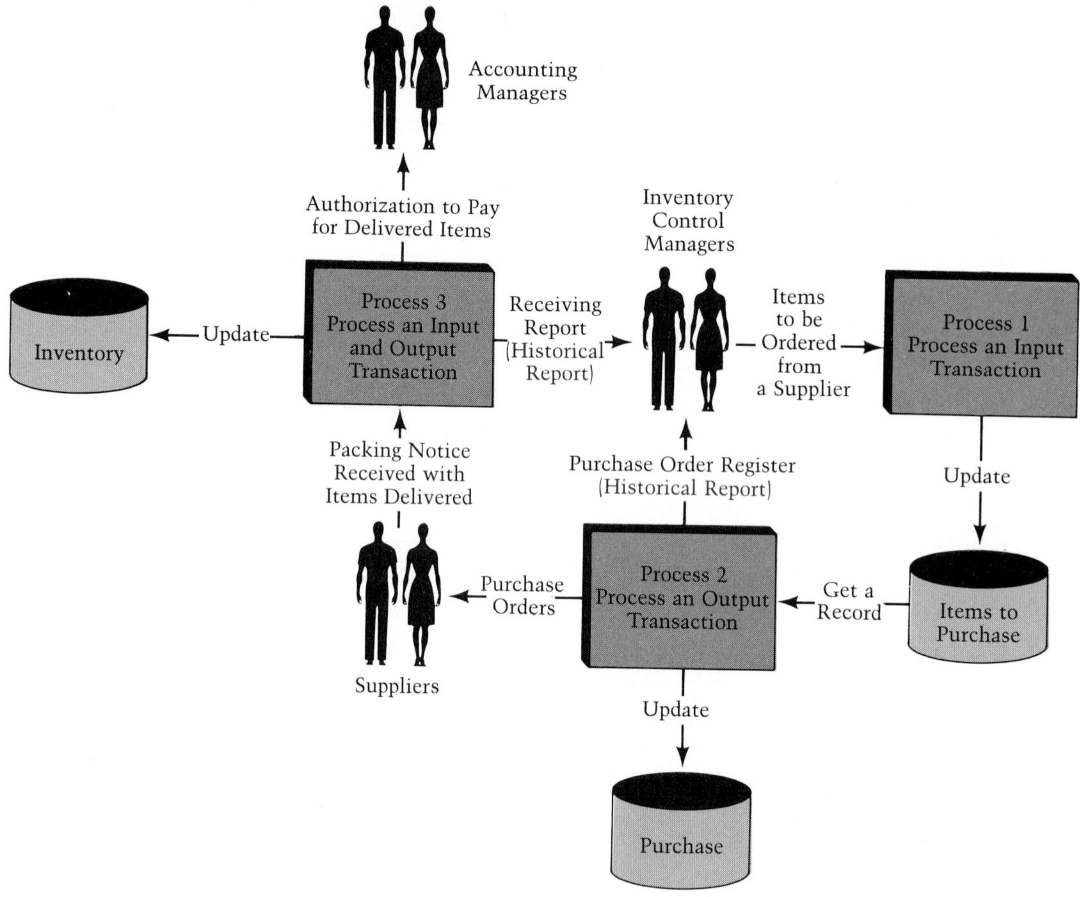

Figure 3.1

Transaction processing. Two types of transaction processing are illustrated. In process 1, we see an input transaction being captured and processed. In process 2, we see an output transaction being generated. Note the historical report. In process 3, we see an input transaction being processed *and* an output transaction being generated. Another historical report was also generated.

cessing is on-line support. On-line systems displace fewer workers because clerks must operate the computer terminals that are on-line with the computer. The advantage of on-line transaction processing is that data can be captured and processed immediately. It also permits discretionary decisions to be handled by people rather than machines. For example, credit decisions are often better handled by people. The computer provides the information, and a clerk or manager makes the decision.

Because of the large volume of data that must be captured and stored by most firms, transaction processing is the most visible type of information system support. Computer-based transaction-processing systems represent the first generation of information system applications. This generation is frequently referred to as electronic data processing (EDP). Data is the important commodity in such applications. Because EDP systems have been around for some time (they were the first systems developed), they are generally the most mature computer applications. However, many EDP applications are still being converted to on-line processing or on-line input with deferred processing.

Management Reporting

Management reporting is the natural extension of transaction processing. Data that was captured and stored during transaction processing can be used to produce information for management. By applying the computer to this process, we can produce reports that do more than confirm transactions. No longer is the computer solely used for speed and accuracy. Because the information produced is intended for the three levels of management (discussed in Chapter 2), the term **management information system** (MIS) was coined to describe this type of application. The information is used to plan future business operations and to monitor and control business operations.

MIS was the second generation of information system applications. The term *MIS* was much more popular in the 1970s than it is today because it never really lived up to its advanced billing. The cornerstone of the MIS concept was the idea that a single, large-scale, integrated system could be developed to support all levels of management. Few, if any, companies were able to achieve this goal. The basic fault rested in the assumption that members of management could identify all of their information needs; this simply was not (and is not) true.

Fortunately, many information needs were definable, particularly at the middle-management levels. This is because many middle-management functions and decisions occur frequently enough that we were able to define rules and information requirements for those activities. These include such planning and control functions as production scheduling, inventory control, and quality control. Other information requirements are regulatory, such as Equal Employment Opportunity Commission and Internal Revenue Service reports. It is these remnants of the MIS concept that we will refer to as *management reports.*

Management reporting systems typically produce three types of information: detail reports, summary reports, and exception reports.

Detail reports present information with little or no filtering or restrictions. Examples include a detailed listing of all customer accounts or products in inventory. These reports may be similar to the historical reports described for transaction processing, except that they are frequently organized differently. They also serve a different purpose, assisting management planning and controlling by generating schedules and analysis. Detail reports of all types have lost favor because managers don't wish to scan large reports to extract specific facts of interest.

Summary reports categorize information for managers who do not want to wade through details. The data is categorized and summarized to indicate trends and potential problems. Summary reports can be tabular (tables of numbers); however, graphics is rapidly gaining acceptance because of its ability to show trends at a glance. Many computer-based systems can easily generate graphical information from raw data. An income statement is a summary report that summarizes the income and expenses for a business. Another example of a summary report is a sales analysis report that summarizes sales according to salesperson, region, and product. Larry in this chapter's minicase might be asked to have the new system produce a report that summarizes the outstanding orders for different suppliers. Summary reports are very popular with modern managers.

Exception reports are the most exciting information alternative. They filter data before it is presented to the manager as information. Only exceptions to some condition or standard are reported. A classic example of an exception report is the items-low-in-stock report that was to be generated in this chapter's minicase. The information system examines data on all materials and reports only those materials for which the quantity on hand is less than is desired. This allows the purchasing manager or clerk to concentrate on only those materials that require immediate attention. Another exception report may tell a sales manager which salespersons are 10 percent or more below their sales quotas. The concept of exception

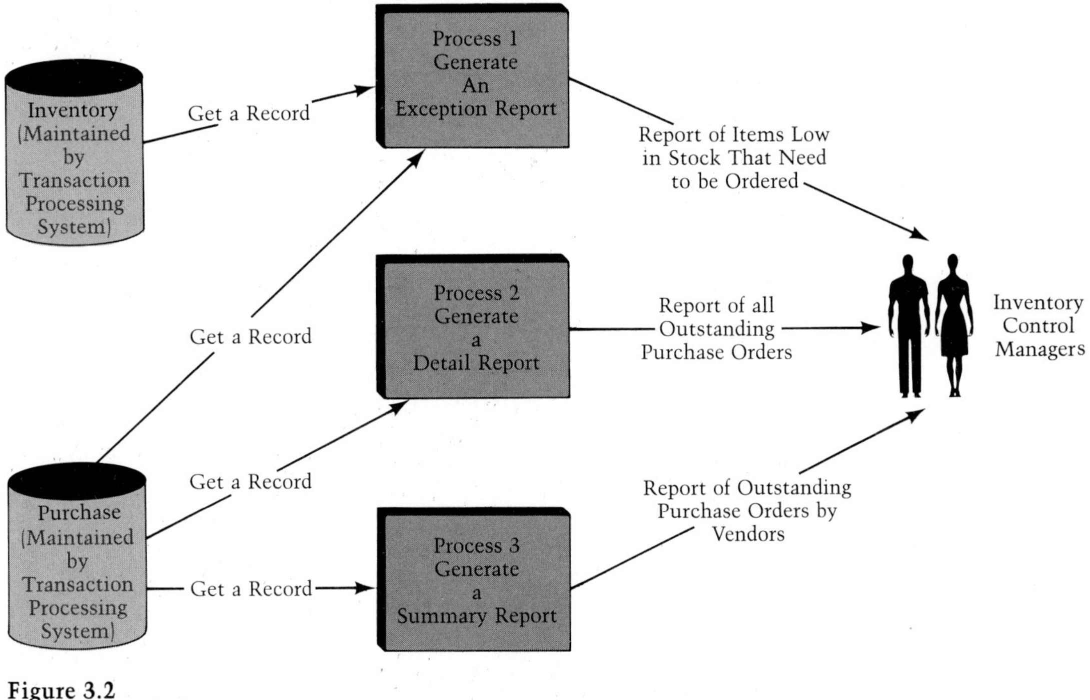

Figure 3.2

Management reporting. Management reporting systems typically produce three types of reports: detailed, summary, and exception. These reports are produced from the data that were originally captured and stored in files or databases by the transaction processing system. Notice that the exception report triggers a decision.

information has led to a new management philosophy, *management by exception.*

Figure 3.2 illustrates the management reporting capabilities of a typical information system. The management reporting subsystem receives its data from the files maintained by the transaction-processing subsystem. Management reporting capabilities will continue to be developed for modern information systems. There will always be new, useful reports that can be defined by managers.

Decision Support Systems

You have just learned that MIS never fully lived up to its expectations because managers cannot precisely define all their information needs. Sometimes managers don't know what information will help them until the need to make a decision arises. A **decision support system** (DSS) provides the knowledge worker with decision making information when a decision-making situation arises. DSS is the third generation of information system applications. It is not just a buzzword! We will not, however, bother to argue whether DSS is a new concept or an extension or realization of the MIS concept. This is not important. Instead, let's study decision making and determine how the information system can be made to support it.

There are two types of decisions, structured and unstructured. **Structured decisions** are those we can predict will happen. We can't always predict when they will happen, but we can predict that they will happen. Managers can usually define the information requirements to support a structured decision. For example, we can provide an on-line credit check to help a manager or clerk decide whether or not to let someone charge a sale at a local department store. We know charge sales will occur even though we can't predict when someone might say, "Charge it." We can also define what information is needed to check a person's credit.

Unstructured decisions cannot be predicted. We don't know when the decision-making need will occur, and we also don't know the nature of such a decision. Can you think of an unstructured decision? Stop! Think about it! If you could think of such a decision, it wouldn't be unstructured! Because the unstructured decision can't be predefined, you can't define what information will be necessary to assist the decision-making process. DSS is primarily intended to support the unstructured decision. Does this seem impossible?

One concept behind DSS is that the data for many unstructured decisions has already been captured and is being stored someplace. The data was captured by the transaction-processing and management-reporting systems. Additional data may be available in national and international databanks around the world. It should be noted that managers frequently have to input additional data that isn't stored in any files. The objective of DSS is to make it easy for managers to get at needed data and manipulate it when a decision must be made.

We have seen two types of decisions. How are decisions made? Ideally, a DSS should support the way decisions are made. A classic model of decision making used by managers is known as the Simon model. It suggests that most decision situations pass through three steps before the decision is made:

1. The **intelligence stage** identifies that there is a decision to be made. This usually involves searching for problems and opportunities.
2. The **design stage** identifies alternative courses of action and evaluates each alternative.
3. The **choice stage** selects the best decision alternative.

Consider the purchasing decision for our current minicase. During the intelligence stage, we must identify the need to purchase materials that are low in stock. The design stage identifies potential suppliers of the needed materials. Each supplier is analyzed with respect to price, discounts, delivery time, and so forth. In the choice stage, the best supplier is chosen.

How does a DSS support decision making? DSS provides the knowledge worker with tools for accessing databases and files with relative ease. We can use the Simon model to categorize these tools.

Intelligence support tools include query languages, report generators, statistical analysis packages, graphics tools, and the electronic desk (see "Next Generation" feature in Chapter 2). These tools allow the knowledge worker to search the files and database for potential problems and decision opportunities. Query languages allow the user to ask questions such as LIST ANY PRODUCTS THAT HAVE A QUALITY CONTROL REJECT RATE PLUS CUSTOMER DEFECT RETURN RATE THAT EXCEEDS 5 PERCENT. Clearly, the response to such a query identifies a decision opportunity. Report generators allow the user to use old data to quickly design and receive a new report. Such a report may confirm or deny a suspected problem or identify a different problem. Statistical analysis packages analyze data to isolate or confirm problems. Graphics generators can frequently summarize data into charts and graphs that trigger decisions. These tools currently exist and are becoming easier to use every day.

Design stage support tools include all of the same DSS tools just discussed as well as simulation and modeling tools. Query languages and report generators are useful for generating alternative choices and pertinent data concerning those choices. Statistical and graphics support can help analyze those alternatives. *Simulators* and *modeling* tools allow knowledge workers to play "what if" games. A project management model can answer the "what if" question, "If phase 14 is delayed by a week, how much will the delayed task delay the total project?" The most popular financial modeling tools are available to managers on microcomputers. The

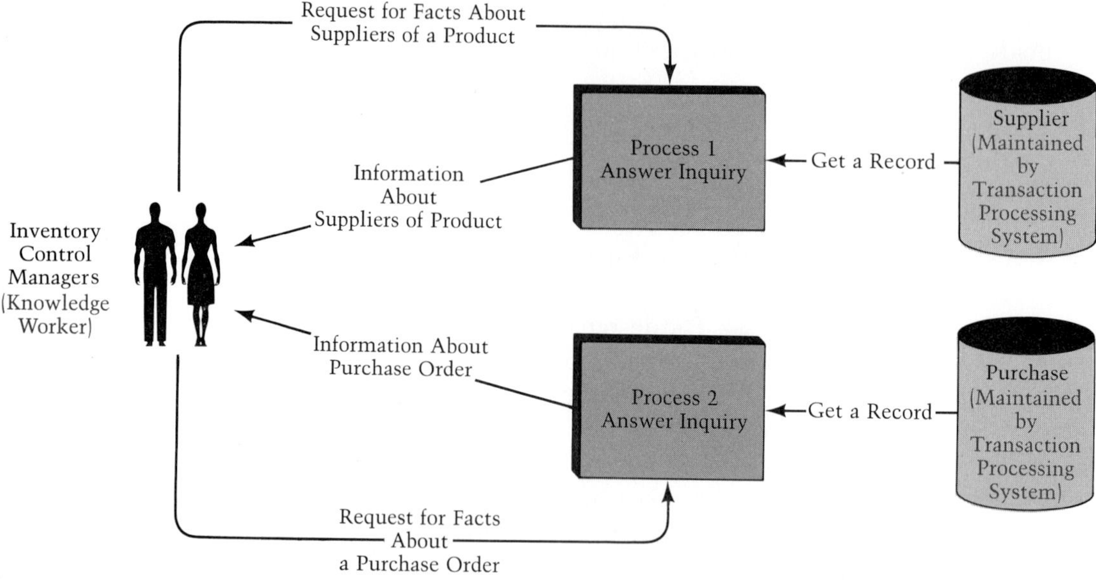

Figure 3.3

Decision support system (DSS). Decision support allows the knowledge worker to obtain information needed to solve a problem. Data needed to support the decision is obtained from the files or databases created and maintained by the transaction-processing and management reporting systems.

tool *VISICALC,* the first popular spreadsheet, has triggered a whole generation of tools that allow the manager to play "what if" games. More sophisticated simulators allow knowledge workers to predict the outcome of major decisions with respect to productivity, costs, profits, and return on investment.

The *choice stage* is only beginning to be supported by DSS. Artificial intelligence is believed to be the key to choice-oriented DSS. **Artificial intelligence** is the ability of a machine to perform certain human functions, such as reasoning, learning, self-improvement, and decision making. The technology is very young (see the "Next Generation" feature). An example of decision support is illustrated in Figure 3.3. •

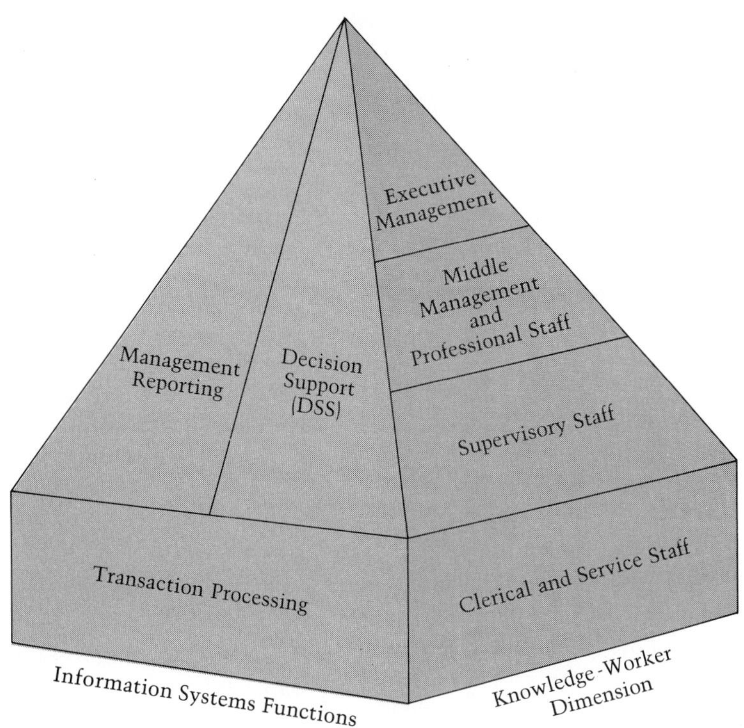

Figure 3.4

Information support provided by the information system. The systems analyst should design information systems that provide complete information support to knowledge workers including: transaction processing, management reporting, and decision support (DSS).

Integrating Transaction Processing, Management Reporting, and Decision Support for Information Systems

We can now rotate our information system pyramid to reveal its *information system functions* face (Figure 3.4). Notice that transaction processing is the foundation on which the information system is built. Looking over to the right-hand face, we also see that transaction processing primarily serves the clerical and service knowledge workers in the business.

Next, you should note that the management reporting and decision support systems (DSS) support all three management levels of knowledge workers—supervisors, middle managers and professional staff, and executive managers. Think about it, and it will

The Next Generation *Two Trends in Information Systems*

Typically, computer information systems are described as providing three levels of support to knowledge workers: *transaction processing, management reporting,* and *decision support.* But that's today! What do future information systems have in store for us? In Figure A, we speculate on two trends for future information systems applications: (1) Integrated Office Systems and (2) Expert and Programmed Decision Systems. We have used our pyramid model to illustrate where these future applications might fit into information systems support functions.

Integrated Office Systems Office automation has been with us for some time now. The trend toward office automation is due, to a large extent, to the decreasing cost of microcomputers, printers, and office-oriented software. The original idea was to provide computer support for secretarial staff, and the most often mentioned capability was word processing. But the concept has extended beyond secretarial support. Today, we are seeing a proliferation of office-oriented software including the following:

- *Word Processing* Software that helps workers develop and edit memos, letters, and reports. Most people are familiar with this technology.
- *Electronic Calendars* Software that helps office personnel coordinate their schedules, appointments, and project due dates.
- *Electronic Mail* Software that allows all office workers to transmit and receive messages, requests, and documents between secretaries and their bosses as well as between offices.
- *Electronic Filing* Software that computerizes office filing systems.
- *Voice Store and Forward* Software that converts voice messages to a computer format, stores that message, retrieves the message (by the intended receiver), and translates the computer-coded message back into the sender's voice.

These tools can be valuable to any knowledge worker! How far will office automation go? Some people believe we will see a day when the typical office is run without paper! Only time will tell if this concept can be realized.

Integrated office systems refer to the integration of office automation and other information system support capabilities. Historically, office automation tools have been *standalone* tools — that is, they did not interface with traditional information systems. But the trend now is toward integrating the use of these tools with our transaction-processing, management reporting, and decision support systems. When you think about it, this trend is inevitable. Office activities are part of the business and support the same business mission that traditional information systems do. It doesn't really make sense to provide office workers with separate office and information systems.

What is the implication of the integrated office system for the future systems analyst? Systems analysts will have to better understand the traditional office environment and activities. As new information systems are developed, analysts will be forced to consider both how the data and information generated in those systems can be shared with office automation tools and when such sharing will be appro- ▶

The Next Generation (continued)

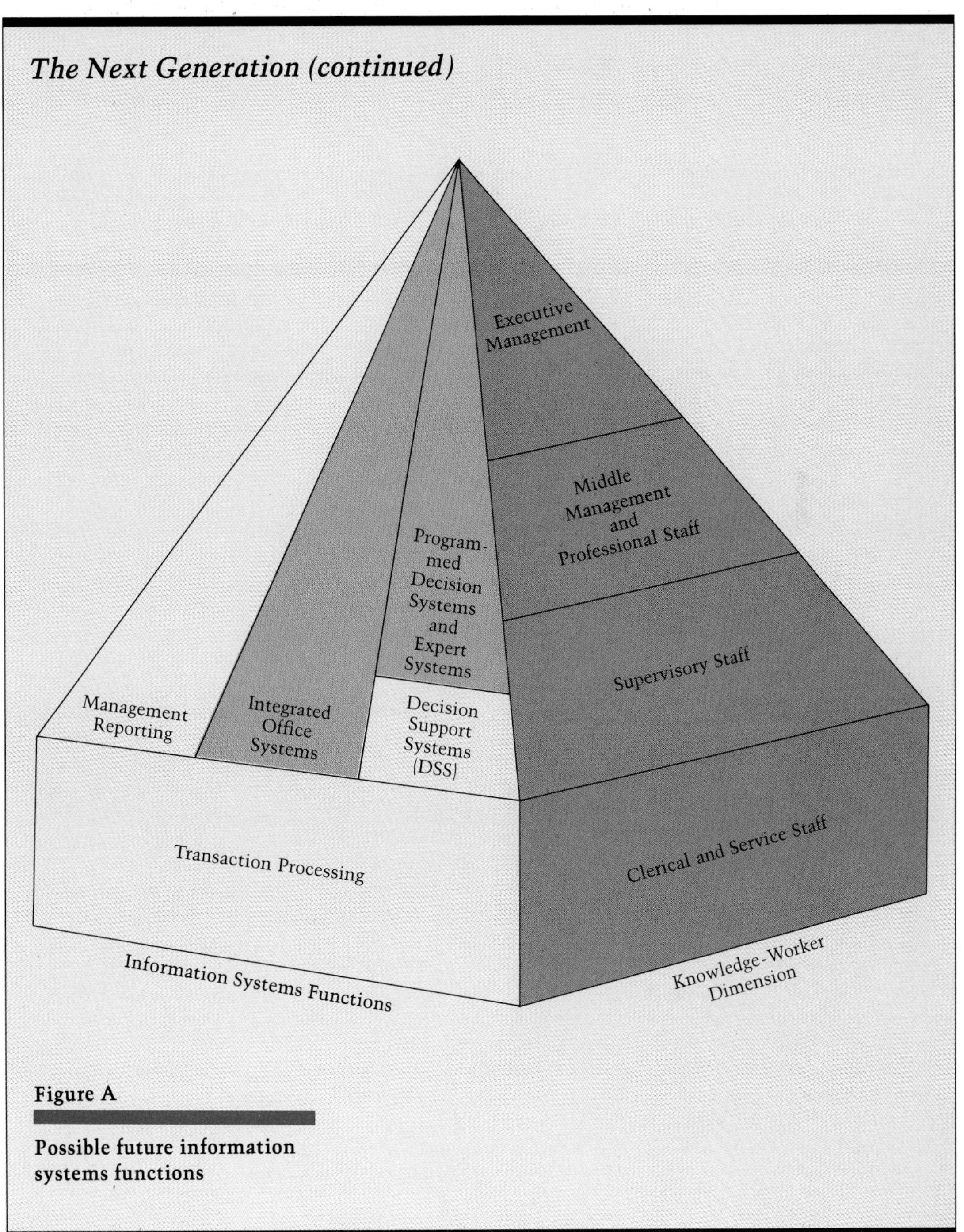

Figure A

Possible future information systems functions

The Next Generation (continued)

priate. Analysts may become more involved in the selection of office automation tools that are compatible with traditional information systems.

Expert Systems and Programmed Decision Systems
A second trend relating to information systems capabilities is the emergence of expert systems and programmed decision systems. As Figure A depicts, expert systems and programmed decision systems are extensions of the decision support system. They are primarily intended to support middle-management, professional-staff, and executive-management decision making. The key to these future systems is advancement of the technology of artificial intelligence (AI). AI systems are systems that can learn and reason in a manner similar to humans—a little scary, right? We won't debate the pros and cons of machine decision making; however, we would like to consider how this technology might affect the future of information systems and systems analysts.

Expert systems are computerized consultants. The combined expertise of a pool of experts in a particular subject (for instance, medicine, engineering, law, finance, or production methods) is collected and stored in a database. That database or access to that database is then sold as expert systems to interested businesses. There are, for example, expert systems available to help businesses mix and match computer systems that are appropriate for specific business problems. The computer staff inputs data that describes work load, size of the computer room, budget, and other factors. The system may prompt the user for important factors that the user might fail to consider (and that an expert would not forget). The system will then identify alternative computer system configurations.

What impact would the expert system have on the analyst? Well, for one thing, the analyst might be required to identify the potential for an expert system to support a specific DSS. The analyst would have to cost-justify the system and select the best system available. Finally, and because of the trend toward integration of capabilities within information systems, the analyst may have to develop appropriate interfaces between the expert system and DSS, management reporting, and transaction processing systems.

Programmed decision systems are systems that store not only data but also decision-making models. A decision-making model is a set of rules and guidelines for making a specific type of decision (called a *structured decision* in this chapter). A programmed decision system will regularly and automatically scan files and databases to look for conditions that require decisions *(intelligence)*. When such a situation is identified, it will call up the appropriate decision-making model(s) to identify alternative solutions *(design)*. Then it will either make the decision or recommend the decision to the knowledge worker *(choice)*.

Systems analysts will be heavily involved in the design of programmed decision systems. Analysts will define opportunities for such systems, design the decision-making models, determine how those models are stored, and interface those models with the appropriate databases and files (which also have to be designed). ■

make sense to you. *All* managers can make use of appropriate management reports. These reports differ only in their level of detail. Along the same lines, *all* managers make decisions — some operational, some tactical, and some strategic. Management reporting applications can be designed for managers at all levels of the organization.

The systems analyst should become familiar with all of the potential support capabilities of the modern information system. The systems analyst is responsible for educating the knowledge worker about these support capabilities and for choosing the best support for fulfilling their needs. For example, a detail report should not be designed when an exception report would better support the knowledge worker's task. It is important to note that the three levels of functions described in this section are not separate systems. They can and should be integrated, especially because they all share the fundamental data that describes the business system. This theme will be reinforced throughout this book.

INPUT, PROCESS, AND OUTPUT COMPONENTS OF AN INFORMATION SYSTEM

Do you recall the definition of an information system?

> An information system is a subsystem of the business — specifically, a person/machine arrangement of components that interact to support the operational, managerial, and decision-making information needs of knowledge workers.

It's time now to address a very important question — When we talk about arrangement of components, what components do we mean? How are these components arranged? What trends should we be aware of? The answers to these questions complete our introduction to the information system.

Information System Components

Most systems can be described in terms of inputs, outputs, and processes. In fact, the purpose of systems is frequently stated as the processing of inputs into outputs. In the case of a manufacturing system, the inputs are raw materials, the outputs are the finished products, and the processes are the machines, tools, and people that transform raw materials into finished products. And all of these inputs, outputs, and processes make up the arrangement of components that we call the manufacturing system.

System components can always be classified according to this input-process-output model. What about the information system? Recall our fundamental formula,

INFORMATION = f(DATA, PROCESSING)!

Information is output. Data is input. Therefore, we could modify our formula to read:

OUTPUT = f(INPUT, PROCESSING)

This is an appropriate way to look at any system. Reordering these components to appear in the order in which they occur, we get: INPUT, PROCESS, OUTPUT! Rotating our pyramid, we introduce its last face, the input-process-output (IPO) components for an information system (see Figure 3.5). Data makes up the input component, and information the output component. Because the information system is a subsystem of the business system, the net data input to the information system comes from the business system itself. Along the same lines, the net output from the information system will return to the business system.

The process that transforms the data into information may itself consist of a number of components including:

- Knowledge workers (you already knew they were a component)
- Methods and procedures
- Computer equipment or hardware
- Computer programs or software
- Data storage

Data is often input before the final information is needed. For example, a credit card agency inputs your charge slips and payments on a daily basis. The output is your account statement for that month. Consequently, we often need a place to store data for later use. We call this component *data storage.*

Computer hardware, software, computerized data storage, and data processing methods are components only in *computer-based* information systems. We sometimes have a tendency to view the computer as an *end* rather than a *means to an end.* Good systems analysts take particular delight in the design or modification of

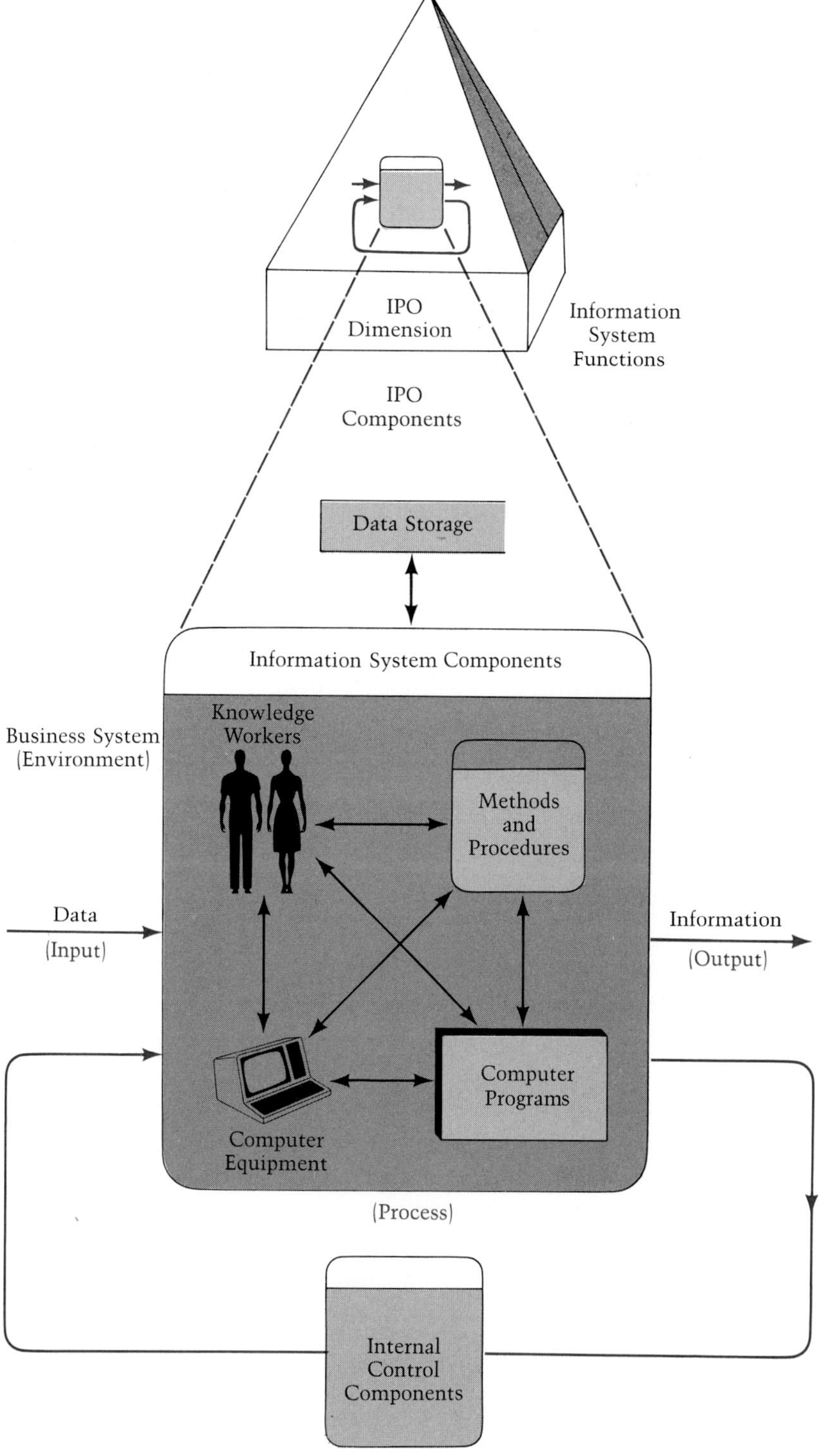

Figure 3.5

The input-process-output components of the information system. When studying or building an information system, the systems analyst should consider all of the illustrated input, process, and output components of the information system.

information systems that require little or no computer technology on the part of the user. A manual system should never be labeled as inadequate simply *because* it is manual.

Good information systems have another component we haven't yet mentioned—a set of internal controls. These controls are installed to ensure that the information system operates properly (see Figure 3.5 for their relationship to the information system). Let's examine each of the internal components of the information system.

Knowledge Workers The computer is important, but the people who use and work with the information system are the most vital and most overlooked aspect of the system! We are not referring only to data processing professionals. We are talking about the users of the information system. Information systems are for knowledge workers! How often have you referred to your latest project as "my system (or program)?" Is the system really yours? Hardly!

We must actively involve our users in the information system development process and educate them about the capabilities and limitations of modern technology. But most important, we must learn to ask questions and listen thoughtfully when working with users. They are the business experts. You've heard the motto, "the customer is always right." Well, the user is our customer.

This book is about *tools.* Many of the tools we study are people oriented, and many of them could be *more* people oriented. Some tools have a bad reputation because they've been used in an undisciplined or sloppy way. We'll emphasize the disciplined and proper use of these tools to maximize their communication value to users.

One of the most exciting trends on the people front of information systems involves knowledge workers' participation in information systems development. Part of this trend is caused by an ever worsening shortage of systems analysts and computer programmers. Users who are being forced to help themselves, are turning to decision support tools that are friendly and easy to learn and use. Whatever the causes, the knowledge workers are becoming more involved in systems development.

To support this new generation of computer-literate, computer-competent knowledge workers, a company may establish an information center. Through the information center, knowledge workers are taught how to use the computer to fulfill their own information requirements, specifically those for decision support. The information center is a place where knowledge workers go to get help from analysts and consultants. The knowledge workers are encouraged to build their own DSS applications.

Methods and Procedures Methods and procedures are also underemphasized in many information systems. Methods refer to how the information system works. More specifically, methods address how the input, processing, and output functions are fulfilled in an information system. Procedures describe how knowledge workers perform their jobs and make decisions. Procedures do not refer to computer programs. There is an important relationship between methods and procedures because the choice of methods can affect procedures carried out by people. Let's talk about methods first.

Methods typically refer to data processing techniques employed in computer information systems. Computer-based information systems generally process data into information by one of two methods, batch processing or interactive processing. Under **batch processing** methods, data must be accumulated into batches and processed periodically (usually on a specific schedule). For example, we could collect orders into batches and process them once or twice each day. On the other hand, using **interactive processing** methods, data is processed either as it occurs or as it becomes available. For instance, we could use computer terminals to enter and process each order as soon as it is received. Batch and interactive processing are not mutually exclusive. You could collect data interactively and process it as a batch. This is referred to as **deferred processing.** There are many implications of data processing methods, and we discuss them in Chapter 15.

It is important to realize that any data processing method will impact the business system and its knowledge workers. How will the data be collected and entered? How will the reports be distributed? What decisions and activities will the worker still be responsible for? What is the sequence of activities? What new forms are required to make the system work? These are all *procedural* questions that must be addressed by the systems analyst. Thus, business procedures are also very important, so much so that many businesses spend considerable time and effort standardizing their manual and computerized procedures.

In any system, there will always be tasks that are best performed by people. The procedures for these tasks should be spelled out explicitly to help the knowledge workers do their jobs. The key is *human engineering.* We are slowly learning that technological improvements must be counterbalanced with improved human elements. One of John Naisbitt's (1982) megatrends is our shift from *forced technology* (which we resist) to a *high tech/high touch* approach to balancing mechanization of our jobs with human engineering. Human engineering is the design of anything that is easy to use, appreciated, and nonthreatening. A key factor in resistance to new systems is poorly designed procedures. Does this sound familiar:

> Before the computer system, all we salesmen had to do to get our expenses was to complete a form, get it authorized and present it to the cashier at virtually any time. Now we have to complete the form with all sorts of codes, once a month. We have to put the form in by the last Friday of the month. Then, we eventually get a cheque [check]—up to three weeks later. Some service those computers give [London, 1976, p. 41].

Such a situation is not unusual. It indicates poorly designed procedures, misunderstandings, or both. Some of the tools you will learn about in this book are used to document methods and procedures.

Computer Equipment or Hardware Information systems may include a variety of hardware components including duplicating machines, calculators, and computer systems. In this discussion, we concern ourselves mainly with the computer system. You've already learned that the computer system is a subsystem of the computer-based information system. Computer system components include such peripheral devices as optical scanners (input), line printers (output), CRT terminals (input and output), magnetic disk drives (data storage), and central processing unit (processor). Data processing personnel are also a processing component since they perform a number of manual tasks for the equipment and software. We are assuming that you are familiar with these components, either from your first data processing course or through personal experience.

It's always frustrating to try to predict trends in the fast-changing world of computer technology. But most certainly, one trend that will continue is the proliferation of microcomputers. Knowledge workers will acquire and apply microcomputers in their offices. Today's microcomputers are powerful enough to handle complex business applications previously reserved for larger, centrally located computers. Furthermore, microcomputers bring a number of productivity tools to the average knowledge worker (for instance, word processing and spreadsheets). Another trend, supported by advanced telecommunications and networking technology, will be the continued emphasis on distributed data processing, in which processing power, in the form of mini- and microcomputers, will be located closer to the knowledge workers. These distributed systems will maintain local data. Shared data, of interest to many areas, will be maintained on larger computers that can be accessed through the minis and micros.

Computer Programs or Software Computer programs have been the responsibility of the computer programmer. There are many application programs that support specific business functions. There are also system programs that run the computer itself and allocate resources to the computer users. Programmers are responsible for the programs, and systems analysts are responsible for program specifications. You should, however, be aware of two significant software trends: the use of software packages and applications development without programmers.

Software packages are computer programs that are purchased rather than built. The concept is "why reinvent the wheel?" If a software package meets all or most of your needs, then programmers can be reassigned to projects for which software packages do not exist. Because programmers are a scarce commodity, this concept makes sense. Most packages require some modification before they operate properly. Many such packages are flexible and adaptable so they can be more easily customized. The systems analyst's job frequently requires the selection of a software package(s) for an information system.

Applications development without programmers? That's right! We've already discussed this idea somewhat. Many decision support needs are so spontaneous that data processing professionals cannot hope to respond quickly enough. Often, data processing cannot justify the analysis and programming cost of a one-time information requirement. But today we are seeing fourth-generation programming languages (see margin for examples) that fulfill these needs. These languages assume or construct an appropriate database. They provide easy-to-learn, friendly, concise syntax for answering queries and writing new reports. They do not replace third-generation languages (such as COBOL, BASIC, PL/I, and RPG). Third-generation languages are still more efficient (in terms of execution speed) than their fourth-generation counterparts.

Fourth-Generation Programming Languages

FOCUS
RAMIS
DBASE III
NOMAD
ON-LINE ENGLISH

Data Storage Data storage is another fundamental component of the information system. The internal data of the information system is stored in files and databases. These data stores can be either manual (for example, a file cabinet) or automated (a computer disk). We focus our attention on computerized data stores because significant trends are developing in this area.

The terms *file* and *database* are frequently and incorrectly used as synonyms. Because these terms are not interchangeable, it is important for you to learn the distinction between them at this time. Traditional information systems have been built around separate files of data. Each file is designed and structured for the application programs that will use it (see Figure 3.6). The file is specifically designed for that application. If a newly conceived program requires the file's data to be structured differently, then appropriate programs extract, sort, merge, and create a temporary file for that purpose. The existing file cannot be changed without forcing costly changes on the programs that use that file. In other words, the data in traditional files is dependent on the programs that use the data (and vice versa).

Each **file** is a collection of record occurrences of a single record type. For example, an ORDER file consists of all occurrences of the record type called ORDER. Each ORDER record is described by the same data elements or fields (for example, ORDER NUMBER, ORDER DATE, CUSTOMER NUMBER, SHIPPING ADDRESS, and for each part ordered, PART NUMBER and QUANTITY ORDERED). Because other applications frequently require some of the same data to appear in different formats, data elements are frequently duplicated in other files. For example, CUSTOMER NUMBER may be recorded in the ORDER file, the ACCOUNTS RECEIVABLE file, and several other files. These redundant data elements take up storage space and can present numerous update problems when data element values change.

A database is an extension beyond the file concept. The traditional notion of *files* as they were just defined disappears. A **database** is an integrated collection of data that serves a number of applications. Thus, database and files are very different. Data is stored with a minimum of redundancy in a common, integrated data store. Programs and applications share this integrated data store. Each program is given access to an appropriate subset of the total database. These subsets overlap (see Figure 3.7). Ideally, the data is structured independently of the programs that use them.

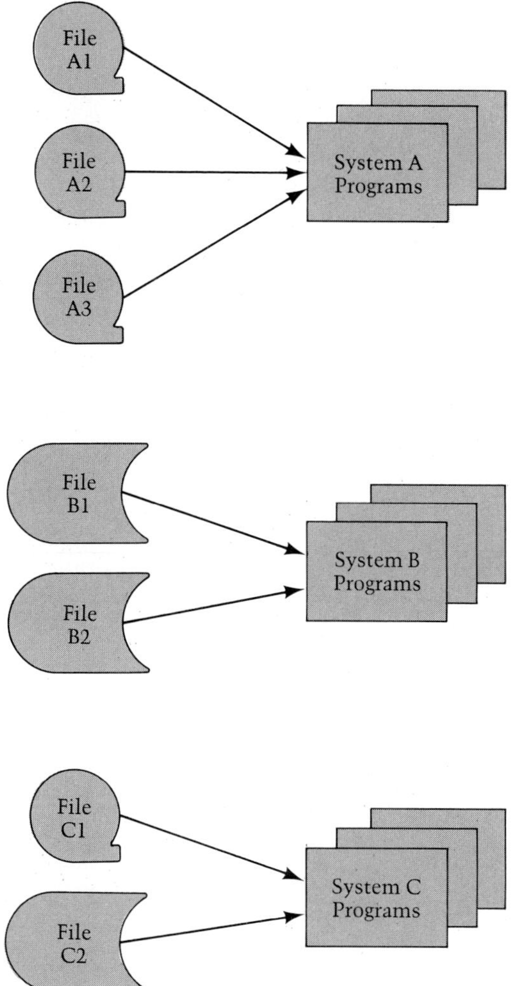

Figure 3.6

Traditional file processing. Files are developed for individual programs or applications. They are especially structured to support those applications. If a new program is added to the application, the file must often be converted to a new structure through additional sorts, merges, and extraction to create a file in the required format. Additionally, the files used by different applications usually contain considerable redundant data.

This allows data structure to be changed without having to change the existing programs that use the data.

How is database accomplished? Dissimilar types of records, such as ORDER, CUSTOMER, and PART, can be stored in a single database. Each type is described by its own unique data elements, with little or no redundancy. Related types are linked together so you can access specific occurrences of one type of record from a different type of record (see Figure 3.8). For example, given any specific occurrence of the PART record, we could directly access all occur-

Figure 3.7

Database processing. The notion of files disappears in the database environment. Instead, data is stored with a minimum of redundancy and shared by application programs. Each program has its own subset of the database with read-only or read-and-update access privileges.

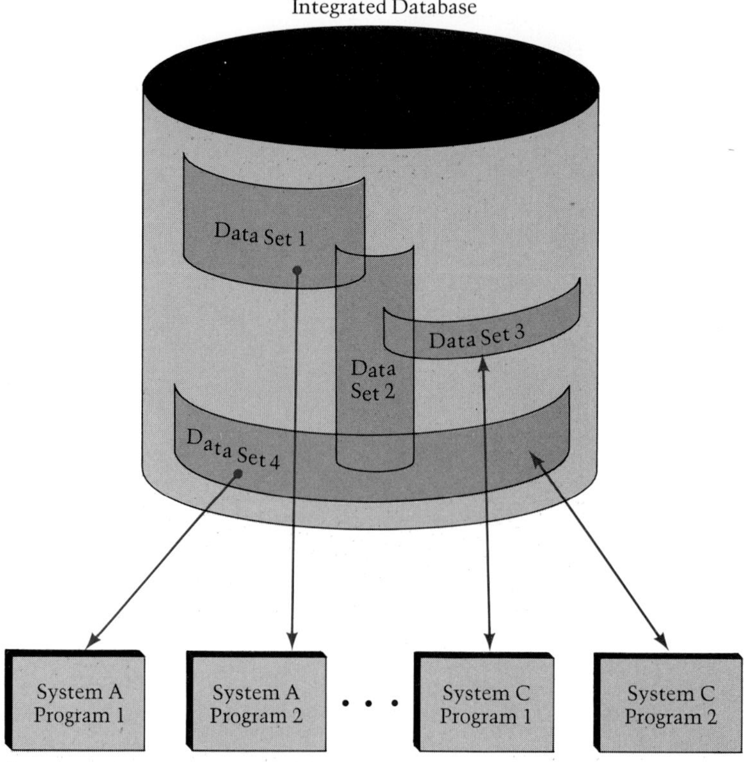

rences of the ORDER record where that part was on the order. Furthermore, given any specific occurrence of the ORDER record, we could access all occurrences of the PART record that are on that order. This is the power of a true database.

You may be thinking, "Why bother with files if a database is so powerful." The technology of database often requires significant resources and is frequently less efficient than files. Furthermore, great numbers of file-based information systems were developed before database technology was available, mature, or affordable. The use of conventional files is still common. The tools and techniques covered in this book are generally oriented to files. Database design is introduced as a separate, optional module in Part IV of this book. However, database is a subject that deserves greater attention than any introductory systems analysis and design textbook can provide. This is an exciting area in which future systems analysts must be competent!

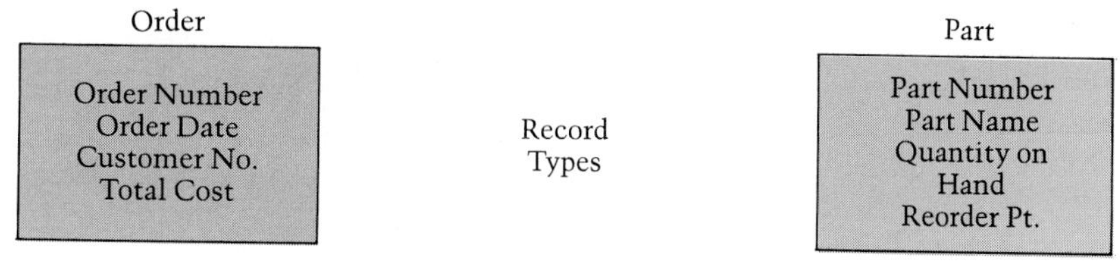

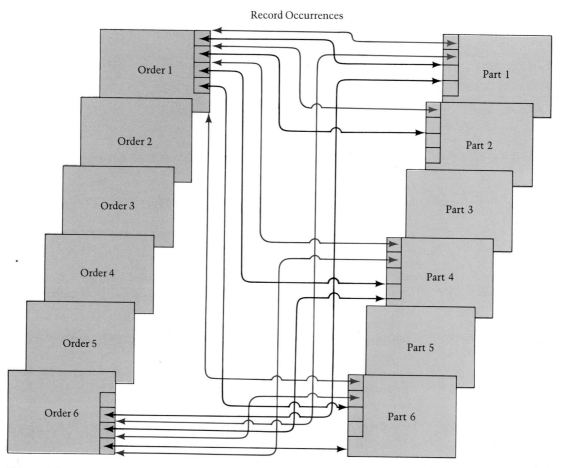

Record Occurrences

Order 1
Order 2
Order 3
Order 4
Order 5
Order 6

Part 1
Part 2
Part 3
Part 4
Part 5
Part 6

Figure 3.8

Database systems. In a database system, different record types, such as ORDER and PART, can be related using pointers. In addition to being able to retrieve any or all orders or all parts, a database system will allow you to retrieve all parts for an order or all orders for a part. Incidentally, you can have many more than two record types in a database. For example, you could add a CUSTOMER record type to this example and link all orders to the customers who placed them.

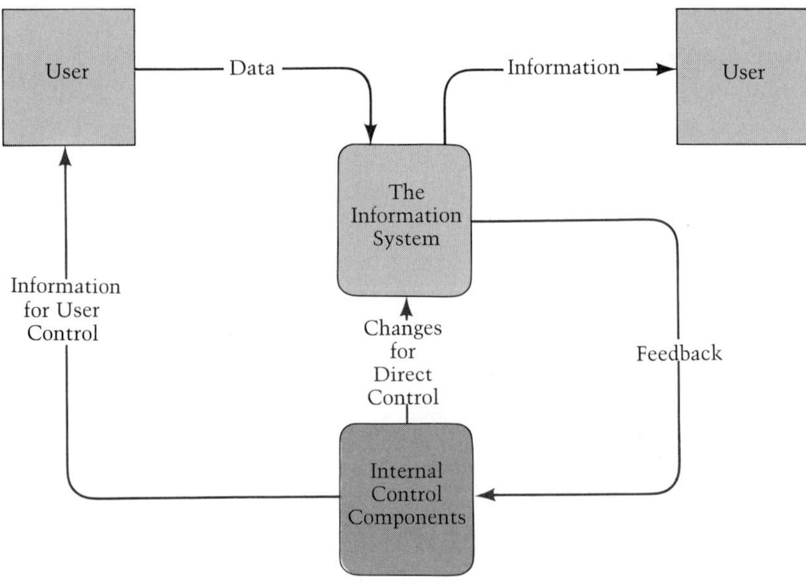

Figure 3.9

Internal controls for an information system. Good information systems contain a subsystem of components (knowledge workers, methods and procedures, data stores, hardware, and software) that make sure the system is properly operating. These components react to feedback from the information system and make or recommend changes for the information system.

Internal Controls Feedback and control is a system concept and feature that must be added to any system to ensure proper operation. In Figure 3.9, you can see a feedback and control model for our information system. As you can see, the **internal control** component is an information subsystem in and of itself. It consists of knowledge workers, methods and procedures, data storage, and possibly hardware and software. It reacts to information generated by the information system (which is data to the internal control subsystem). The internal control subsystem either directly implements change to the information system or notifies the user that the system is not functioning properly.

Input controls ensure that the input data is valid before they are processed, that file and database data are protected against unauthorized access and update, that recovery procedures are available for a system catastrophe, that output information is disseminated to proper knowledge workers, and that other relevant conditions are met. Again, controls ensure that the system works properly! We discuss controls throughout Part III of this book.

The Importance of Input-Process-Output Components to the Systems Analyst

The implications of the IPO components of information systems are profound. Although it is easy to become caught up with the computer components in a system, the knowledge workers, methods and procedures, manual data storage, and internal controls are equally important. And when computer hardware, software, files, and databases are used, they impact the other components. The analyst must ensure that the arrangement of components, both manual and computerized, work together to support the business mission.

SUMMARY

In addition to the knowledge-worker and business-mission dimensions of an information system, there exist information support and input-process-output dimensions. To understand these dimensions, it is important to differentiate between data and information. Data is raw facts in isolation. Information is data that has been manipulated so that they are useful to someone. An important concept of systems analysis and design is the formula

INFORMATION = f(DATA, PROCESSING).

An information system is capable of providing knowledge workers with three types of information. Transaction processing is the means by which most data is captured. There are two types of transactions, *input* and *output.* In addition to processing input and output transactions, transaction processing also fulfills a *historical reporting* role. Management reporting is another type of information support. Management reporting involves producing a variety of reports designed to fulfill the defined information needs of managers. Three types of reports can be produced: *detailed, summary,* and *exception* reports. Each report is produced from the data that was captured and stored during transaction processing. The third type of information support is the decision support system (DSS). A decision support system provides knowledge workers with the ability to obtain needed information when a decision-making situation arises.

In addition to providing different types of support in information systems, an analyst must design and select the working components of the information system. The components that make an information system work can be classified according to an input-process-output (IPO) model. The input component of an information system is data. The output component of an information system is information. The process components that transform the data into information consist of knowledge workers, methods and procedures, data storage, computer equipment, and computer programs. Information systems also include the component internal controls. Internal controls ensure that the information system is operating properly. A systems analyst must consider each of these components when developing an information system.

PROBLEMS AND EXERCISES

1. Identify each of the following as data or information. Explain why you made the classification you did.
   (a) A report that identifies, for the purchasing manager, parts that are low in stock.
   (b) A customer's record in the Customer Master File.
   (c) A report your boss must modify to be able to present statistics to his boss.
   (d) Your monthly credit card invoice.
   (e) A report that identifies, for the inventory manager, parts that are low in stock.
2. Give two examples of a report or document that might be considered information to one person but data to another. What would have to be done to transform the report into information for the second person?
3. Identify the type of information support provided for each of the following applications.
   (a) A customer presents a deposit slip and cash to a bank teller.
   (b) A teller gets a report from the cash register that summarizes the total cash and checks that should be in the cash drawer.

(c) Before cashing a customer's check, the teller checks the customer's account balance.
(d) The bank manager gets an end-of-day report that shows all tellers whose cash drawers don't balance with the cash register summary report.
(e) The system prints a report of all deposits and withdrawals for a given day.

4. Give an example of a transaction (input or output). What data describes that transaction? Now, describe a management report that might include that data. Finally, describe a decision that might require access to that data.

5. What is the relationship between data, information, input, processing, and output? Give an example of this relationship.

6. Last year, Hologram, Inc.'s Comptroller purchased an IBM PC and the spreadsheet, LOTUS 1-2-3. He learned how to use the product to support his own budgeting and cost control decision-making needs. He likes LOTUS, but he's getting tired of re-entering the same data into different spreadsheets. He wants to know why he can't store the data in a database on his microcomputer. Better still, he knows that much of the data currently resides on the Burroughs mainframe computer in data processing. Why not tap that database to minimize the amount of data he has to input personally? In terms of the information systems functions model, what is the comptroller requesting? Ignoring technical implications, are his expectations reasonable?

7. Identify the transaction-processing, management-reporting, and decision support functions that were discussed in the Outland Engine/Hightech Electronics minicase at the beginning of this chapter.

8. Make an appointment to visit a systems analyst at a local data processing installation. Discuss one of the information systems projects the analyst has worked on. What were some of the transaction-processing, management-reporting, and decision support provisions in the system?

9. Give an example (or better still, collect an example) of each of the following: a detail report, a summary report, and an exception report. *Hint:* Examples of reports are everywhere. They are in your programming and data processing textbooks, the places you work (DP or otherwise), your mail, on your teacher's or secretary's desk, and in all sorts of other places.

10. Liz, an account collections manager for the bank card office of a large bank has a problem. Each week, she receives a listing of accounts that are past due. This report has grown from a listing of 250 accounts (two years ago) to 1,250 accounts (today). Liz has to go through the report to identify those accounts that are seriously delinquent. A seriously delinquent account is identified by several different rules, each requiring Liz to examine one or more data fields for that customer. What used to be a half-day job has become a three-days-per-week job. Even after identifying seriously delinquent accounts, Liz cannot make a final credit decision (such as a stern phone call, cutting off credit, or turning the account over to a collections agency) without accessing a three-year history on the account. Additionally, Liz needs to report what percentage of all accounts are past due, delinquent, seriously delinquent, and uncollectable. The current report doesn't give her that information. What kind of report does Liz have—detail, summary, or exception? What kind of reports does Liz need? What kind of decision support aids would be useful?
11. Identify all of the information components discussed in the Outland Engine/Hightech Electronics minicase at the beginning of this chapter.
12. Define a decision that you (or your boss or a friend) have recently made (or are making). The decision can be either personal or business. Describe the decision-making process for that decision. What information or facts might help you make a better decision?
13. The knowledge worker is the most important and overlooked component of an information system. Explain why.
14. Visit a systems analyst at a local data processing installation. Discuss one of the information systems projects the analyst has worked on. Who were some of the knowledge workers supported by the information system? What were some of the automated and manual processing methods and procedures of the system? What types of data storage were being supplied? What computer equipment or hardware was being used? What were some of the application programs? What type of internal controls were installed in the system?
15. Why is it important to keep up with information trends? Explain how you plan to keep abreast of information trends.

16. Knowledgable University plans to support course registration and scheduling on a computer. The following user community has been designated:
    (a) Curriculum deputy—one per department, responsible for estimating demand by that department's own students for each course offered by the university. This person may revise demand estimates from time to time.
    (b) Schedule deputy—one per department, responsible for deciding which courses from that department will be offered, at what times, and by what teachers and what enrollment limits will be. These parameters may change during the registration period. This is the only person who can increase or decrease enrollment limits for a course (including adding or deleting a course to or from the schedule).
    (c) Schedule director—in charge of allocating classroom and lecture hall space and time to departments. Also prints the schedule of classes to show students what will be offered and when.
    (d) Students—submit course requests and revisions and receive schedules and fee statements.
    (e) Counselors—advise students and approve all course requests and revisions. Also help students resolve time conflicts (where student has registered for two courses which meet at exactly the same time).

    This is the cast of characters (which may be revised or supplemented by your instructor to more closely match your school). For each knowledge worker, brainstorm input and/or output transactions, management reports (especially summary and exception reports), and decision support inquiries.

ANNOTATED REFERENCES AND SUGGESTED READINGS

London, Keith. *The People Side of Systems.* New York: McGraw-Hill, 1976. Includes numerous examples of what can happen when information systems are not designed for ease of use by people.

Martin, James. *Application Development Without Programmers.* Englewood Cliffs, N.J.: Prentice-Hall, 1982. A classic! This book is recommended to those who want to take a closer look at several trends described in our Chapter 3. These include information center, fourth-generation programming languages, decision support tools, and application development without programmers.

Naisbitt, John. *Megatrends: Ten Directions Transforming Our Lives.* New York: Warner Books, 1982.

Sprague, Ralph H. "A Framework for the Development of Decision Support Systems." *MIS Quarterly* (December, 1980), 1–26. This paper presented the forerunner of our pyramid model. We are especially indebted to this paper for our *information system functions* face of that model.

Wetherbe, James. *Systems Analysis and Design: Traditional, Structured, and Advanced Concepts and Techniques.* 2d ed. St. Paul, Minn.: West Publishing, 1984. This book has an excellent systems concepts chapter that inspired us to look at what we called the IPO components of an information system. Although our IPO components model differs somewhat, the same fundamental system concept is being applied.

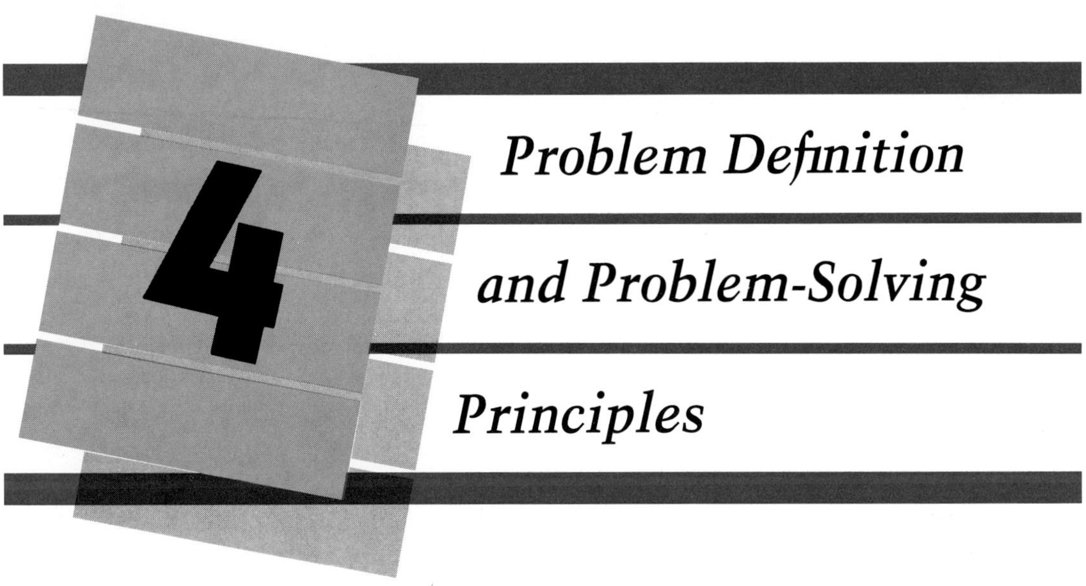

4 Problem Definition and Problem-Solving Principles

Minicase:
Rowinski Heating and Cooling

As Julie and Tony walked into an empty room, Tony spoke nervously. "This is not going to be a good meeting, Julie. We have a lot of explaining to do."

"Tell me about it. How often does Mr. Rowinski himself take such an interest in data processing projects?" replied Julie.

Tony knew the question was rhetorical, but he answered it anyway. "He does when the results are this bad."

Tony was the assistant inventory control manager at Rowinski Heating and Cooling, a distributor and servicer of furnaces, air conditioners, heat pumps, and spare parts. Julie was a systems analyst for the Data Processing Department. Julie had been project manager for the recently implemented inventory control system. The new system was a dismal failure, so much so that Robert Rowinski III, president and owner of the company, had called this meeting.

Preston Roberson, the inventory control manager, entered the room. His face was grim. He hadn't supported the project since it started. Tony looked very nervous. And for good reason—he had suggested the new system and been given responsibility for seeing that it succeeded. Both men took their seats. Mr. Rowinski entered the conference room shortly thereafter. He shut the door and spoke calmly.

"Let's get started. This inventory control system has turned out worse than any nightmare. It has cost the company more than $225,000, not to mention the lost sales revenues and increased inventory carrying costs. I can't afford this when I'm fighting my competitors tooth and nail for every sales dollar. I want some answers. What happened?"

Preston spoke first, "I was never in favor of this project in the first place. Why did we need this computer system?"

Tony replied defensively, "Look, we were experiencing *stock-outs.* We couldn't afford to run out of stock when trying to fill orders. Our customers were starting to complain. Some were threatening to take their business elsewhere. I was told to solve the problem. And I considered data processing to be a viable solution."

Rowinski asked, "Preston, why were you against the computer system?"

"Don't get me wrong. I'm not anticomputer," replied Preston. "It's just that Tony or Julie decided to computerize—just like that! I don't remember anyone analyzing other alternatives. To my mind, you should always analyze options. And let's suppose that the computer is our best option. Why did we have to build our system from scratch? I understand that there are some pretty successful inventory systems available for purchase. Did anyone look at that alternative? Did anyone consider microcomputers? I was against the project, not against the computer."

Rowinski responded, "Bob has a point, Tony! Still, the system you did propose was defended as feasible. And still it failed! I'd like to know what went wrong. That's why I wanted Julie here. You were assigned to this project from the outset, right?"

Julie answered, "That's right, sir."

Rowinski continued, "This is the feasibility report you submitted early in the project. It proposed a computerized inventory control system. This report suggests a system that would require Tony to hire five new clerks. Each clerk would have a CRT terminal connected to Data Processing's IBM System 34 [a small, business computer system]. The System 34's internal memory and disk storage would have to be expanded and the CRT terminals would have to be acquired. An on-line operating system would have to be acquired to support the system."

"Excuse me, sir," interrupted Julie. "Strictly speaking, we didn't need the on-line operating system."

"The report says you needed it," replied Rowinski.

"Bill made that recommendation," answered Julie. Bill Rowinski, Bob's younger brother, was data processing manager.

Rowinski continued, "In any case, the bottom line in this report is that the benefits outweigh the costs over the lifetime. You projected a 2.4 year payback period. I'd like to know what went into this report."

Julie answered, "I met with Tony four times—about six hours total, I'd say. Tony explained the problems. We documented the requirements, made suggestions, and projected the costs and benefits in the report."

Tony continued the story, "The new system would allow CRT clerks to enter inventory changes such as new stock [add to inventory], filled orders [subtract from inventory], and damages [subtract from inventory]. Once each day, the system would check inventory counts and generate purchase orders for those items low in stock—end result? No stockouts!"

Rowinski responded, "But that didn't happen, Tony. Why not?" When Tony didn't respond, Rowinski directed his next question to Julie. "What happened after this feasibility report?"

Julie answered, "We spent the next ten months developing the system."

"How much did you have to do with that, Tony?" asked Rowinski.

"Not a lot, sir. Julie occasionally popped into my office to ask a business question, something she didn't understand. She might show me a sample report or file—That's about it. Obviously, she was making progress, and I had no reason to believe that the project was off schedule. I didn't push Julie."

"Were you on schedule, Julie?" asked Rowinski.

"I don't believe so, Mr. Rowinski. My team and I were having some problems with certain business aspects of the system that Tony was unfamiliar with. Tony would have to go to the clerks and the purchasing officers for answers. We had to wait."

Rowinski replied, "I don't get it! Why didn't you go straight to the clerks and officers?"

Preston responded, "I can answer that. I designated Tony as Julie's contact. I didn't want her team wasting my people's time—They have jobs to do, you know."

"Something about that bothers me, Preston. Not only did your policy delay the project, it may have caused some of the resulting system failures. When this project got seriously behind, Tony, why didn't you consider canceling the project—or at least reassessing the feasibility?"

"We did," answered Tony. "Preston started complaining about progress about ten months into the project. With two months remaining, he hadn't seen any documentation. We called a meeting with Julie and her team. At that meeting, we learned that the new operating system wasn't working properly. One of Julie's programmer's had had to take a month off to fix some problems in an accounting system, and the new CRT terminals hadn't been ordered yet. And to top it off, Julie and her staff seemed to have little understanding of the business problem."

Julie interrupted, "As I already pointed out, I wasn't permitted contact with the users during the first ten months. I wanted to get my people programming so we'd have something to show for my efforts."

Tony continued, "As I was saying, we considered canceling the project. But I pointed out that $150,000 had already been spent. It would be stupid to cancel the project and see all that money wasted. With Julie's help, I did reassess feasibility, and we determined that the project could be completed successfully—with four additional months and another $50,000."

"But nobody asked me if I wanted to spend the extra money," argued Rowinski. "I would have insisted that the cost/benefit numbers be refigured. Go on."

Julie continued, "We worked extra hard, often ten- to fourteen-hour days. We brought in extra help. We even got a few chances to speak directly to users. The project was finished on time, according to the revised schedule, and only slightly over the revised budget—end of story."

"Wrong, Julie. Let me read you some excerpts from Preston's monthly report. Inventory records have mysteriously disappeared, deleted without explanation. Reports generated by the system have been characterized as late, inaccurate, and inadequate. Stockouts have *increased* by 13 percent! My sales manager claims that customers are not just complaining, they're doing increased business with my competitors. Somebody forgot to tell the Sales Department to send all the filled order notices to Tony's clerks. Somebody forgot to tell the inventory stock boys to record actual counts on shipping notices before having the notices sent to Tony's clerks. Do you have any idea what happens in an inventory system that doesn't capture all inventory transactions? Incorrect counts and stockouts! You tell me, what would you do if you were in my shoes?"

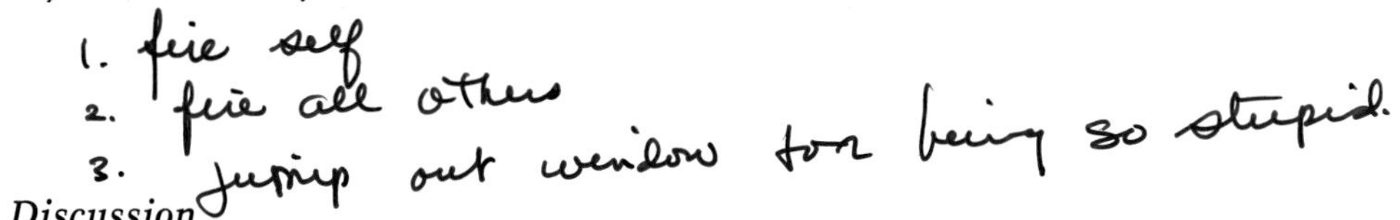
1. fire self
2. fire all others
3. jump out window for being so stupid.

Discussion

1. Did Julie have a reasonable chance to succeed? What did she do wrong? What did Tony do wrong? Did the project seem well organized? Why or why not?
2. How do you feel about those early meetings that led to the feasibility report? Did Julie and Tony meet often enough? Did they focus on the important issues?
3. What about the solution? Was the on-line system chosen for appropriate reasons? Were alternatives investigated? Did the team commit to a solution too early?
4. What do you think about the feasibility report? Can you accurately assess a problem and solution before a project begins? Can such a feasibility report encourage unjustified optimism and overcommitment?
5. Why did the system fail to satisfy business requirements? Did programming begin too soon? Why were Julie and her staff uncomfortable with the business problem?
6. Was the system properly documented? How do you know? Why do you suppose documentation was scarce?
7. Should the project have been canceled? What about the $150,000 investment that had already been made?
8. What would you have done differently? What would you do if you were in Julie's shoes? Tony's? Mr. Rowinski's?

WHAT WILL YOU LEARN IN THIS CHAPTER?

This chapter introduces some fundamental principles for problem identification and problem solving. You will know that you understand the implications of problem solving and information system development when you can:

1. Describe where information systems development projects come from.
2. Describe a typical information systems problem in terms of its performance, information, economic, control, efficiency, and service implications.
3. Explain, by example, three serious problems that often prevent successful information systems development.
4. Use seven fundamental principles of problem solving and describe their relevance to system development.

Systems development is not a hit-or-miss process! The stakes are high. The moral of the Rowinski minicase is that information systems don't just happen. As with any other product (such as bridges and automobiles), they must be carefully developed. Had the inventory control project been better controlled, the result might have been different. The systems development process is not magical. It is a businesslike process with businesslike origins. And successful system development is governed by some fundamental, underlying principles. Systems development is problem solving! Where do system projects come from? Why does systems development often fail? What basic principles can improve the possibility of success? These questions are answered in this chapter.

PROBLEM DEFINITION: WHERE DO SYSTEMS PROJECTS COME FROM?

Projects to improve information systems can be suggested by either knowledge workers or systems analysts. Most projects are identified by knowledge workers because they are closer to the business activities that need improvement. When requesting such improvements, many organizations require the knowledge worker to submit a standard form, such as the Request for Systems Services illustrated in Figure 4.1. Systems analysts, on the other hand, are frequently expected to survey the business system for possible improvements. The analyst will normally initiate a project by means of a brief memorandum that suggests the possibility for changing the system.

The impetus for most projects is a problem, opportunity, or directive. Problems may be either current or anticipated. **Problems** are undesirable conditions or situations that prevent or can be expected to prevent the business from fully achieving its business purpose, goals, objectives, and policies. For example, an increase in time required to fill an order can trigger a project to reduce that delay. An **opportunity** is a chance to improve the business system even though the existing system is performing acceptably. For instance, management is always receptive to cost-cutting ideas, even when high costs are not currently considered a problem. A **directive** is a new requirement that is imposed by management, government, or some other external influence. For example, the Equal Employment Opportunity Commission, a government agency, may mandate that a new set of reports be produced each quarter. Or management may dictate support for a new product line or corporate policy.

Let's clarify a subtle difference between two of our terms. Students often get hung up on the difference between problems and opportunities. There really isn't a whole lot of difference. The same situation could be either a problem or opportunity. For instance, consider the following request:

> Reduce the costs of processing an order.

Does this represent a problem or an opportunity? It depends. If management has determined that the costs of processing an order are too high, it's a problem. On the other hand, if management hasn't suggested that order-processing costs are too high, we have an opportunity for improvement. In other words, don't agonize over the difference between problems and opportunities. The examples we give for each of the following discussions could be either problems or opportunities.

There are far too many potential problems, opportunities, and directives to list them in this book. However, James Wetherbe (1984, p. 114) has developed a useful framework for classifying

```
REQUEST FOR SYSTEM SERVICES                                    FORM 100

SUBMITTED BY ___Barbara Rushin___________ DATE ___7-25-86___

DEPARTMENT ___Transportation Fleet Services_______________________

TYPE OF REQUEST  [x  ] New System
                 [   ] System Redesign
                 [   ] System Modification

PROBLEM STATEMENT (attach additional documents if necessary)

We would like a cost accounting system that makes every
vehicle in the fleet a cost center. Currently, we have no
way of attributing all direct and indirect departmental costs
to any vehicle. Hence, we are unable to determine when a
vehicle's costs are exceeding their benefits for that vehicle.
__________________________________________________________

REQUEST FOR SERVICE TO  Develop a system that allows all direct
and indirect costs incurred by this department to be assigned to
specific vehicles. System should generate monthly vehicle
costing reports and summaries.
****************************************************************

ACTION (to be completed by Steering Committee)

   [xx] Request Approved    Assigned to ___Wayne Tatlock______

                            Start Date ___as soon as possible___

   [  ] Request Delayed (backlogged) Until ____________________

   [  ] Request Rejected for Reason: ____________________
        _______________________________________________
        _______________________________________________
```

Figure 4.1

A typical request to develop or modify an information system. This is a typical information systems project request. Many data processing shops receive far more requests than they can possibly handle. Therefore each request is evaluated for priority.

problems, opportunities, and directives. He calls it the PIECES framework because the first letter of each of the six categories of problems, opportunities, and directives spell the word *pieces.*

P erformance
I nformation
E conomy
C ontrol
E fficiency
S ervices

The PIECES framework is significant because it teaches you an important lesson. Always examine problems, opportunities, and directives in terms of their bottom-line impact on the business. Given any problem, opportunity, or directive, you can evaluate it in terms of these six bottom-line categories.

The Need to Improve Performance

In Chapter 2, you learned that information systems are supposed to support the business purpose, goals, objectives, and policies of the business. And in Chapter 3, you learned that information systems perform tasks that process data and produce information. Performance problems occur when business tasks are performed too slowly to achieve business goals and objectives. Performance opportunities occur when someone recognizes a way to speed up a business task that is otherwise achieving business goals and objectives. A performance directive may occur if management decides that all transactions are to be done *on-line* to the computer to improve performance.

Performance is measured by throughput and response time. **Throughput** is the amount of work performed over some period of time. Most throughput projects are concerned with transaction-processing throughput. Consider the following scenario:

> A local credit union has been studying data about consumer loan applications. Over the past year, loan applications have increased 124 percent. The manager realizes that, if this growth rate continues, the current loan officers will not be able to keep up with the demand. The throughput of the current system must be increased.

Response time is the average delay between a transaction and a response to that transaction. The following example illustrates the point:

> A construction company has been contracted to perform repairs and improvements for a large corporate site consisting of many buildings. The corporate site submits work orders to the construction company. The work orders go through a processing cycle that may include data processing, purchasing, accounting, personnel, and operations. Currently, an average delay of sixty-two days occurs between the submission of the order and the arrival of the work crew to fulfill the order. Management wants to reduce this response time as much as possible.

Although throughput and response time are considered separately in the preceding discussions, they should also be considered jointly. For instance, one way to improve throughput in our credit union example would be to improve the loan officers' average response time for each loan application by giving those officers timely credit information.

The Need to Improve Information Available to Management

We've already learned that information is a crucial commodity for the knowledge worker. The information system's ability to produce useful information can be evaluated for problems and opportunities. Improving information is not a matter of generating large volumes of information. In fact, a major problem in many businesses is information overload. This is a situation in which too much information is given to the knowledge workers and the recipients are overwhelmed by the large volume. A characteristic of information overload can be seen in many businesses — piles of computer outputs!

Situations that call for information improvements include:

- *Lack of any information concerning the decision or current situations.* For example, the Accounting Department suspects that air travel reimbursements do not reflect minimum costs and bargains that could be obtained. However, they have no information to support their suspicions; therefore, they cannot justify possible changes to their procedures.

- *Lack of relevant information concerning the decisions or current situations.* For example, a personnel manager must allocate scarce overtime dollars to the supervisors of three manufacturing departments. The report that predicts the amount of work to be done does not break the information down to the department level.
- *Information that is not in a form useful to management.* For example, an inventory control clerk for a large printing business must reorder paper and supplies each Monday. The clerk is given an inventory report. However, the report includes all 3,000 inventory items. The clerk has to compare quantity in stock and projected usage for each item on the report—just to identify items that must be reordered. An exception report that has already made the comparison between supply and demand and reports only those items which need to be reordered would be more convenient.
- *Lack of timely information.* Consider this example: A hotel chain allows customers to make reservations for any hotel in the chain from any other hotel in the chain. However, when a reservation is made or canceled, it takes three days to get that information to the hotel that is affected. Meanwhile, that hotel may overbook or underbook rooms because the information is not timely.

Information can also be the focus of a directive. The classic example of this is a new reporting requirement imposed by a local, state, or federal government agency.

Economics: The Need to Track and/or Reduce Costs

Economics is perhaps the most common motivation for projects. The bottom line for most managers is *dollars and cents.* Economic problems and opportunities pertain to costs. There are two types of economic improvement projects, cost monitoring and cost reduction.

Cost monitoring seeks to identify and track the costs of business tasks, products, and services. The information generated by the system (notice the overlap between this category and the information category) summarizes budgeted and actual costs, possibly reporting cases in which cost overruns are occurring. Consider the following example:

> The Marketing Department needs to establish the new prices for products in their catalog. In order to establish a price that will recover manufacturing costs and overhead and provide an acceptable profit margin, they need a cost breakdown by product, including materials, direct labor, and overhead (for instance, utilities, plant maintenance). Although they have access to budgeted cost standards, they need historical data on actual costs because those costs may be exceeding the budgets.

Cost reduction projects seek to lower the costs of one or more business activities. For example:

> A purchasing manager has been ordered to reduce the costs of raw materials. There are two ways to reduce costs. First, by carefully comparing the alternative pricing structures offered by different suppliers. Second, by taking advantage of bulk quantity discounts. However, we must strike a balance between reducing purchasing costs and increasing inventory costs (yes, it costs money to store and handle inventory!). An information system can greatly assist the decision-making process.

The Need to Improve Control

Business tasks must be monitored and corrected when substandard performance is detected. Controls are installed to improve system performance, prevent or detect system abuses or crime, and guarantee the security of data, information, and equipment. Two types of control situations trigger projects — *too few* controls and *too many* controls.

A system that has too few controls may result in discrepancies between the information system and the business system. The following example is typical:

> A distribution warehouse for farm machinery parts is experiencing a stock problem. The computer information system is releasing orders after checking the inventory file to ensure that the products ordered are in stock. However, when the warehouse clerk tries to fill the order, the parts are not always in stock. An analysis reveals that, when the stock clerks place new inventory on the shelves, they do not count that inventory. They simply accept the supplier's word that the quantity

shipped is accurate. This system has too few controls to ensure the accuracy of inventory counts.

But we can go overboard! A system with too many checks and balances slows the throughput of the system. The red tape associated with decision making in some firms causes long delays and other problems.

Society's greatest concern about the Information Revolution is the privacy and security of data and information. Data and information have become important resources. Access to data and information may be controlled to some extent by government legislation and corporate policy. Because policies and laws are in a constant state of change, many systems projects are triggered by such changes.

The Need to Improve Efficiency

Efficiency can be confused with economy. Where economy is concerned with the amount of resources used, efficiency is concerned with how those resources are used with minimum waste. **Efficiency** is defined as output divided by input; therefore efficiency problems and opportunities seek to increase output, decrease input, or both. The commodities to be increased or decreased can be people, money, materials, or any other resource. The idea is to get more from less or at least to get more out of what you have. Consider this example:

> A manufacturing facility consists of 125 workstations of various types. Different products go through different types of workstations during production. Management is concerned with the need to expand production, but there is no money to expand facilities (did you recognize the throughput nature of this problem?). Management has observed two major limitations in current operations. First, separate orders for the same product are not consolidated. This causes workstations to be set up and broken down for the same product several times each day. Second, management has noticed that some workstations seem to be idle during some parts of the day and overworked during other parts of the day. Obviously, the production scheduling and control system is not making efficient use of production workstations.

The Need to Improve Service

Service improvements are a diverse category. Projects triggered by service improvements seek to provide better service to the business, to its customers, or to both. Improved services are intended to improve the satisfaction of customers, employees, or management. Like our other categories, service improvements may be intended to solve specific service problems, exploit opportunities to improve service, or fulfill a management directive. Service improvements are intended to improve one or more of the following:

- *Accuracy.* Accuracy is concerned with correctness of processing and results. For instance, a company may want to reduce the number of billing errors on customer invoices. We've all heard stories about customers who get a $100 thousand phone bill by mistake. Another example is order processing. Instead of sending a customer ten thousand pencils, the system sends ten thousand boxes of pencils, each box containing one hundred pencils. Or instead of sending part A-4666-L-G (man's tweed sportcoat, size 46 long, color gray), a customer receives D-4666-L-G (woman's dress, size 6, long sleeve, color gray).
- *Reliability.* No, reliability is not the same as accuracy. Whereas accuracy is concerned with *correctness,* reliability is concerned with *consistency* of processing and results. For example, an order-processing system may be denying credit to some customers but allowing credit to other similar customers (assuming equivalent credit ratings and payment histories).
- *Ease of Use.* Today, much concern is expressed about the *user friendliness* (or, as is more often the case, lack of user friendliness) of computer-based systems. A system, whether manual or computerized, should be as easy to use as possible. Many projects are initiated to improve the ease of use of computer systems. Similarly, many projects are initiated to overcome manual systems that have become too complex and awkward.
- *Flexibility.* Flexibility is concerned with a system's ability to handle exceptions to normal processing conditions. For instance, management may encounter a situation in which installment payments are promptly posted to customer accounts. However, prepayments or overpayments against accounts are sent through a lengthy process that delays customer orders even though those customers are not delinquent in their payments.

The system isn't flexible enough to respond to special payment alternatives.

- *Coordination.* A business system consists of many functions that must coordinate their activities to achieve goals and objectives. The desired result is *synergy,* meaning that the whole organization receives a benefit greater than the sum of the parts. A classic example of coordination occurs between the production and inventory functions of a business. When production is scheduled, it is important that raw materials be delivered to the workstations at the scheduled time. However, the workstations may not have enough floor space to hold an entire day's requisition for raw materials. Clearly, an information system is needed to coordinate the flow of raw materials to workstations.

It should be obvious from this discussion that the categories of the PIECES framework are related. Any given project can be characterized by one or more categories. Furthermore, the cause of any specific problem may be another problem itself. PIECES is a practical framework, not just an academic exercise! There are two ways to use PIECES. First, you can analyze a specific problem, opportunity, or directive against each of the six categories to get a better feel for its total impact on the business. Some categories may not apply, but by analyzing each category, you *know* which ones don't apply! Second, you can take a business system or information system and apply the PIECES framework to analyze that system. This approach may uncover problems and opportunities that the knowledge workers haven't realized existed.

PROBLEM-SOLVING PRINCIPLES FOR INFORMATION SYSTEMS DEVELOPMENT

Given that we have a problem, opportunity, or directive, we want to develop a new information system that improves the business. To do this, we use a process called a *systems development life cycle* (SDLC) that will take us from an existing information system to an improved information system (see Figure 4.2). The improved system will have solved problems, exploited opportunities, and fulfilled directives. Why is an SDLC needed? What makes information systems difficult to develop? We answer these questions in this section.

Figure 4.2

A system development process. Our goal is to present a generalized system development process whereby we can transform an existing information system into an improved information system.

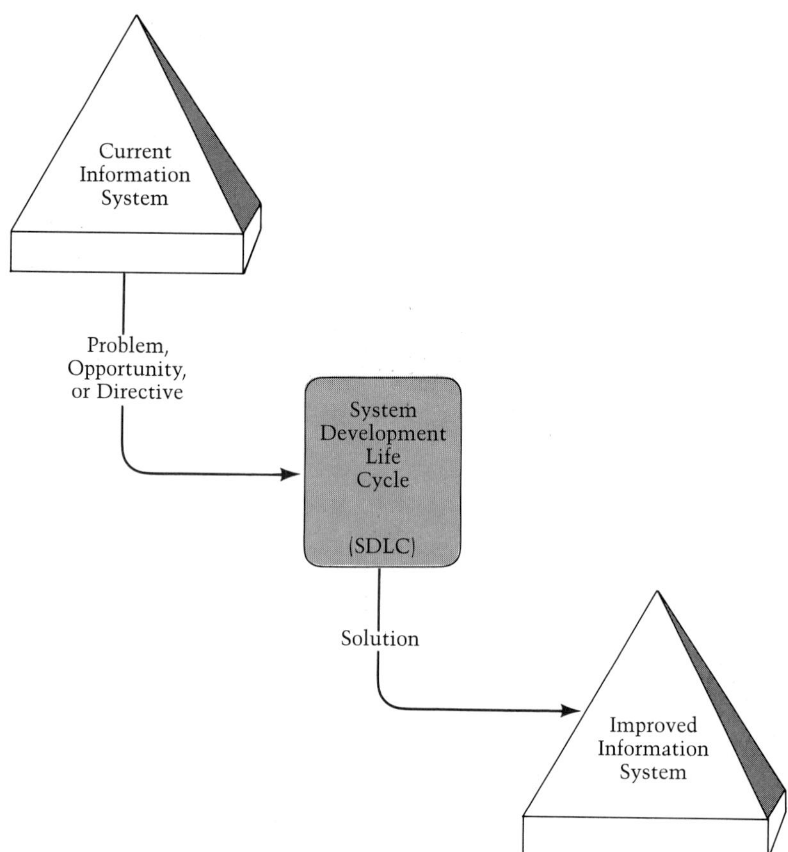

Roadblocks to Information Systems Development

Essentially, there are three possible barriers that can prevent us from successfully developing a new information system:

- The wide spectrum of business applications to which computing can be applied
- The dissimilarity between the business domain and the computing domain
- The lack of a common language for describing both the business domain and the computing domain

Let's make sure we understand these problems before we define our SDLC process.

1. The Scope and Complexity of the Business Problem The number of business applications to which computing can be applied has steadily increased. Much of this increase can be traced to the decreasing cost of the technology itself. Low-priced microcomputers enable the smallest of businesses to apply computers to business problems. Why is this a problem? Simple! No two business applications are the same. The typical systems analyst is faced with a new situation for each project. For example, the inventory control problems of the large corporation are very different from the inventory control problems of Ma and Pa's General Store. Furthermore, the analyst is practically expected to become an instant expert on the business application. Should we apply a different SDLC approach to problems of different sizes? We're going to have to address this question.

2. The Dissimilar Nature of Computing and Business Stated simply, we are trying to apply a very rigid, unforgiving technology to a very flexible and often unpredictable business situation. A classic system concept illustrates this problem.

Systems can be classified according to how *closed* or *open* they are. A **closed system** has a precise number of well-defined inputs and outputs. Its actions can be predicted with accuracy. For the most part, a *computer system* is a closed system. It acts predictably. It may not always do what we want it to do, but it usually does what we tell it to do! Furthermore, it is not programmed to respond to unplanned inputs. An **open system** doesn't have well-defined interactions with its environment. It is subject to random and unpredictable disturbances. Such is the case with the business system. In business, there arise situations that cannot be predicted; these include the actions of customers, vendors, and the government.

Our problem is clear. Systems analysts must develop a relatively open information system that adapts to the open nature of the business system. But that information system is to be supported by a relatively closed computer system that can react only to those situations for which it is programmed. This is almost a contradiction of goals — But nobody said this was easy!

3. Lack of a Common Language for Business and Computer Specialists The people who best know the business system and those who best understand the computer system talk entirely different languages. The cartoon in Figure 4.3 (page 118) is all too true. Those of

The Next Generation *The Changing Nature of Systems Projects . . . A Return to MIS?*

Most current information-systems-development projects are triggered by problems, opportunities, and directives. The scope of a project is limited to a rather small portion of the business's activities. Is this likely to change?

During the middle to late 1970s, the data processing industry became excited about the idea of building a single, integrated management information system (MIS) for any and all organizations. The concept was built on the growing enthusiasm for database technology. Unfortunately, the concept never really got off the ground. There are many frustrations and disenchanting stories to be told about those attempts. The systems were difficult to conceive, let alone build. Analysts would have to define the integrated database requirements for the entire business, a process that would consume many years in most businesses. Then they would have to reprogram numerous applications using the latest database technology. That technology, good as it was, was still immature. Database systems were grossly inefficient when compared to their file processing counterparts, especially when applied to transaction processing requirements. Furthermore, even if we could get the database up and running, data processing concluded that management's information needs were so numerous, volatile, and diverse that it would take an enormous staff of analysts and programmers to fulfill those needs. Thus, the concept of an integrated MIS gracefully exited from our dreams.

Or did it? Today, we are seeing evidence of a possible resurgence of the original MIS concept. However, the thinking of data processing management has matured. Few managers envision a single information system for the organization. But some managers see a federation of relatively few information systems as being an attainable goal. What has happened to change the prognosis? Well, the technology of database is getting better and more efficient all the time. But, the truth be known, we finally realized that the technology wasn't sufficient to get the job done.

For one thing, we had to improve the methodologies for applying database technology to business problems. Today, we are seeing the emergence of systems analysis methodologies built ▶

you familiar with basic computer technology are aware of the large number of acronyms and buzzwords that are used. Knowledge workers also have their own buzzwords, acronyms, standards, and procedures.

Systems analysts are responsible for bridging this communication gap. They must document the business problem and needs in the language of the knowledge worker and translate those needs into the language of computer programmers. This book is about tools and techniques for bridging this communications gap.

The Next Generation (continued)

around database concepts (for instance, *Information Modeling* and *Information Engineering*). Second, we have had to face facts: There will be a worsening of the shortage of programmers and analysts for many, many years! Solution? Get the end users more actively involved in fulfilling some of their own needs—especially those simpler needs, such as management reporting and decision support. But this requires that the technology become easier to learn and use. And this, too, is happening. Nonprocedural languages such as FOCUS, RAMIS, NOMAD, ON-LINE ENGLISH, and SQL have emerged to draw many end-users into doing some of their own programming.

Consequently, the projects to which systems analysts are assigned may change because of this new environment. Systems analysts and programmers would be assigned to fulfill transaction processing and data management functions. Their projects would not necessarily respond to small problems, opportunities, and directives. Instead, projects would respond to larger-scale opportunities to integrate and maintain a relatively small number of corporate databases (whether systems analysts would be called *systems analysts* in this environment remains to be seen). End-users would respond to their own management reporting and decision-support requirements. If the data is in the database, accessible, and flexibly structured, then the user need not perform systems analysis and design. Instead, the user only has to write programs (the simpler, the better!) in the new nonprocedural languages.

Will this really happen or will this be another dream-turned-nightmare? We don't know. Nobody does! But consider the following facts. First, microcomputers in business are proliferating, with no end in sight. This brings the computer age into the grasp of more and more knowledge workers. Second, each new generation of knowledge workers is more comfortable with computer technology. Today's children will consider the use of computers to be as natural as eating and sleeping. Third, database technology and nonprocedural languages are getting better and better. It all adds up to a *Brave New World.* ■

Problem-Solving Principles

We have learned that systems development is really problem solving. And that we must overcome the three critical system development problems described in the preceding section of this chapter. Experience has resulted in development of a number of problem-solving principles that should be incorporated into any system development life cycle. Let's return to the Rowinski minicase. What went wrong? For one thing, Tony and Julie violated most of the

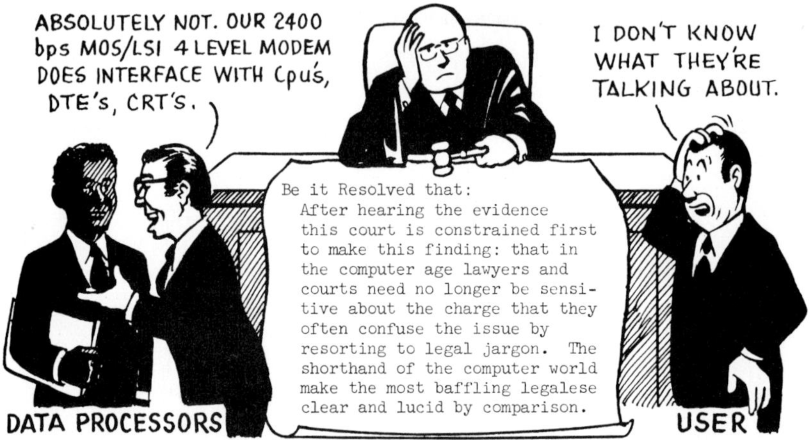
ABSOLUTELY NOT. OUR 2400 bps MOS/LSI 4 LEVEL MODEM DOES INTERFACE WITH Cpu's, DTE's, CRT's.
I DON'T KNOW WHAT THEY'RE TALKING ABOUT.
Be it Resolved that:
After hearing the evidence this court is constrained first to make this finding: that in the computer age lawyers and courts need no longer be sensitive about the charge that they often confuse the issue by resorting to legal jargon. The shorthand of the computer world make the most baffling legalese clear and lucid by comparison.
DATA PROCESSORS
USER

Figure 4.3

The data processing/user communication gap. (From Leslie Matthies, *The Management System: Systems Are for People.* Copyright © 1976 by John Wiley & Sons, Inc. Reprinted with Permission.)

fundamental principles of problem solving. Let's explore those principles (adapted from Benjamin, 1971) and use them to evaluate the systems development process that was used at Rowinski.

Principle 1: The System Is for the Knowledge Worker The information system belongs to the knowledge workers who will benefit (hopefully!) from it. Although the "my system" attitude motivates programmers and analysts to work hard to create technologically impressive solutions, those solutions often backfire—They don't address the business problems or they introduce new business or technical problems. Remember, long after the analysts and programmers have developed the system, the users must live with it! For this reason, user involvement is an absolute necessity for successful systems development. We must make time for users, insist on user participation, and seek agreement from users on all decisions that may affect them.

The Data Processing Department at Rowinski failed to recognize this principle. Two critical errors were made. First, a single user contact (Tony) was established. This minimized the time lost by users to assist Tony, but it created numerous problems. Inventory control personnel didn't get to see the system until it was too late to make inexpensive changes. They also missed the chance to suggest opportunities and problems unknown to Tony. Serious business errors went undetected. We can all learn from the

Rowinski minicase mistakes. When developing information systems, the systems analyst should involve *all* affected personnel.

The systems analyst would be wise to remember that "when a system succeeds, the credit must be apportioned among many participants, but failure (at least the most dramatic kind) belongs completely to the analyst" (DeMarco, 1978, p. 9). Words of wisdom for your career? Think about it.

Principle 2: People Education Is Essential People continue to be a significant problem in systems development and problem solving. All people — knowledge workers, systems analysts, programmers, manual laborers — must be educated about the problem and possible solutions. We are not talking about formal, classroom education. We are suggesting that system development requires on-the-job education. Knowledge workers need to learn what an information system is and what it can do for them. Did *you* study Chapters 2 and 3 carefully enough to be able to teach knowledge workers what an information system is and what it can do for them?

Systems analysts also need to educate themselves about the business applications for which they will build information systems. Additionally, they need to educate programmers about systems tools and techniques that will be used to specify the programs they will be asked to write. And systems analysts will have to teach users and managers how to use any new information system that is implemented. Analysts, however, aren't the only knowledge workers responsible for education. The users, themselves, must assume responsibility for educating the analyst about the business applications, requirements, policies, and so forth.

The Rowinski staff apparently failed to recognize the importance of education. The DP staff was too concerned with computer technology. Their SDLC appears to have been "code, implement, and repair," with little attention paid to understanding the inventory control business problem itself. Tony did not take the time to understand the implications of information systems and computing. And Julie should have assumed responsibility for educating Tony and his staff.

People education is also crucial to winning user acceptance of information systems. Because people tend to resist change, the computer is often viewed as a threat. Through user education, information systems and computers can be properly viewed by knowledge workers as a tool that will make their jobs less mundane and more enjoyable.

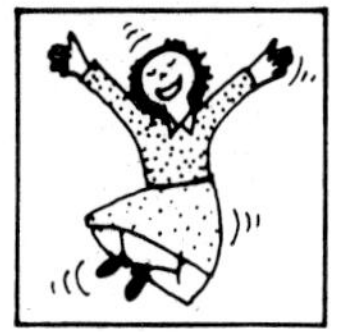
Wild Enthusiasm

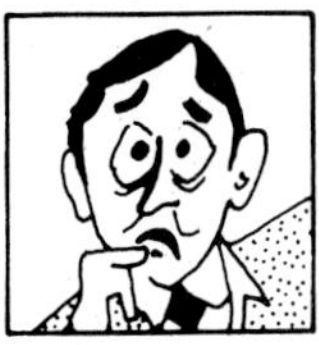
Disillusionment

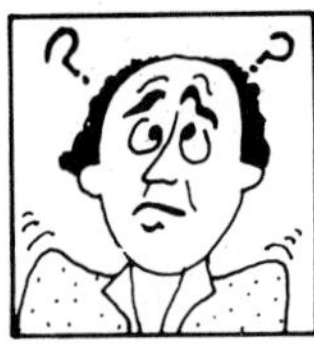
Total Confusion

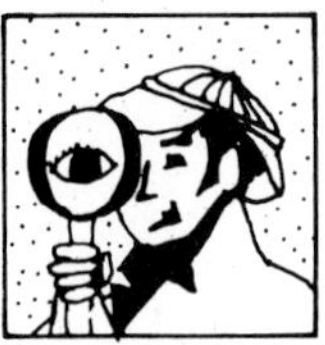
Search for the Guilty

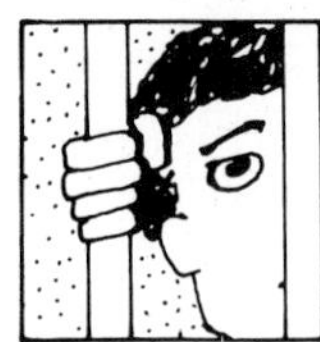
Punishment of the Innocent

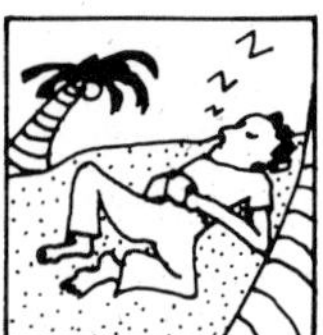
Promotion of Nonparticipants

The Rowinski system development process? (From William M. Taggert, Jr., *Information Systems: An Introduction to Computers in Organizations.* Copyright © 1980 by Allyn and Bacon, Inc. Reprinted with permission.)

Principle 3: Establish Phases and Tasks Large problem-solving projects can best be accomplished if they are divided into smaller, manageable tasks. Some people call this the Swiss cheese approach. You take a slice of cheese and repeatedly punch holes in it. Eventually, the cheese is gone. Most SDLCs consist of phases. Because each phase usually represents considerable work and time, phases are usually broken down into tasks that can be more easily managed and accomplished. In other words, each task is one more hole in the cheese. Phases and tasks are normally arranged into a sequence.

At Rowinski we see little evidence of a phased SDLC save perhaps the default phases illustrated in the margin cartoon. This haphazard approach is all too common — and the results are also common. Rowinski's DP staff was too anxious to start programming, which explains why the project got out of control. There were no milestones against which to measure progress (hence there were no progress reports). If nothing else, a phased approach to system development offers us the opportunity to measure our progress and ensure that important issues are not overlooked!

In Chapter 5, we identify phases for a representative SDLC. And in Chapters 6, 10, and 17, we examine typical tasks that should be included in each of the phases. Thus, this book will provide you with practical skills for using tools and techniques as well as the process by which you can apply those tools and techniques to a real project.

Principle 4: Problem Solving Is Not a Sequential Process This sounds like a contradiction of the last principle but it isn't! Generally speaking, the phases and tasks of a systems project should be completed in sequence. In reality, the phases and tasks overlap. System development life cycles often leave you with the impression that you must finish each phase or task before proceeding to the next. Textbooks are often to blame for this misconception. A book is a sequential device by nature. But just because we present output design before file design doesn't mean you must do output design before you begin file design! It may make sense to overlap those tasks. Remember, time is money in the business world. It pays to think and work ahead whenever it's practical. Just remember, if you do work ahead, that work is tentative. Until a previous phase or task is complete, there is no way of knowing whether that work may have to be changed.

In addition to opportunities for working ahead in the life cycle, we must also realize that we will make mistakes. At any point in time, we may have to return to a prior phase or task to correct mistakes or oversights. This necessity can be abused however. We must avoid infinite returns to any phase or task. A phase or task must end sometime, or the system will never be implemented. Perfection is rarely achieved, and if we try to achieve it, we will probably be frustrated. Sometimes it is best to put a change on hold until after the system has been implemented, unless that change is necessary to correct a critical error or oversight. This is often a judgment decision.

Did Rowinski violate this principle? It isn't really clear that the DP staff had an SDLC to begin with! Therefore, we don't really know if they approached their tasks sequentially. However, judging from the number of errors in the final system, we can guess that the Rowinski staff adopted the sequential attitude, "We can always fix it later." This approach is usually expensive because programs are more difficult to modify than design specifications.

Principle 5: Problem Solutions Are Capital Investments Most problem solutions (information systems in our case) are capital investments, no different from a fleet of delivery trucks or new manufacturing machinery. Even if management fails to recognize the system as an investment, you should not! When considering a capital investment, two issues must be addressed. First, alternatives should always be investigated. Second, the best alternative should be cost-effective.

Any time we spend money for one item, we lose the opportunity to spend that money on something else. Economists call this *opportunity cost.* For any problem, there are likely to be several possible solutions. The systems analyst should not accept the first solution that comes to mind. And after identifying alternative solutions, the systems analyst should evaluate each possible solution for feasibility. Obviously, users should be involved in this analysis.

Cost-effectiveness can be defined as striking a balance between the cost of developing and operating a system and the benefits derived from that system. Does management perceive that the lifetime benefits will exceed the lifetime costs? That is the important question.

Looking back at the inventory control project at Rowinski, it is not clear that alternatives were evaluated. In fact, it seems that the technology was selected early and that the decision was not motivated by the business application. Instead, the technology was selected by the DP manager, who had been wanting it. With respect to cost-effectiveness, the inventory-control-system costs were grossly underestimated, which leads us to:

Principle 6: Don't Be Afraid to Cancel A big advantage of the phased approach to problem solving is that it provides several "go" or "no go" decision opportunities. There is a temptation to *not* cancel a project because of the investment already made. Rowinski made this mistake and threw more money into a system that still failed! In the long run, canceled projects are usually less costly than implemented disasters.

We advocate a *creeping commitment* approach (Gildersleeve, 1976) to systems development. At any "go" or "no go" checkpoint, all costs are considered *sunk*—that is to say, the costs are irrecoverable and therefore irrelevant to the decision. The project is to be reevaluated at this point to determine if it *remains* feasible. The concept of sunk costs is familiar to most business managers, but it is often ignored by systems analysts. Rowinski paid dearly for ignoring this principle! Preston should have followed his first hunch to cancel the project.

Principle 7: Documentation Should Guide Problem Solving Failure to develop *working* documentation is one of the most frequent and critical errors made by systems analysts. Most students and practitioners talk about the importance of documentation. But talk is cheap! Most of you (alas, we are guilty too!) suffer from a disease called *postdocumentation syndrome*. We document after we finish the program or system. Come on! Be honest! When do you really place *comments* in your program? After you've finished, of course!

PRINCIPLES TO GUIDE SYSTEMS DEVELOPMENT

1. The system is for the knowledge workers. Get them involved.
2. People education is important. But don't forget the natural language barrier between data processing people and business people.
3. Establish phases and tasks.
4. Systems development tasks are not necessarily sequential. There is often a need to backtrack. And there are opportunities to overlap phases and tasks.
5. Information systems are capital investments. They should be economically justified as such.
6. Don't be afraid to cancel. Include checkpoints in your systems development process and reevaluate feasibility at those checkpoints.
7. Documentation should guide systems development, *not* follow it.

Figure 4.4

Problem-solving principles for systems development. These seven principles can be used to evaluate any systems development process or strategy, including the one we present in Chapter 5.

Unfortunately, we often carry this bad habit over to systems development, where we fail miserably.

Documentation should be a working by-product of the entire systems development effort. Documentation reveals the strengths and weaknesses of the system to others—*before* the system has been built. It can stimulate user involvement and reassure management that progress is being made. Be wary of any systems development life cycle or methodology that has a documentation phase. This is a planned postdocumentation approach and can cause numerous communication problems.

Rowinski's staff failed to document their efforts. They probably didn't even document their programs. Tony's problems can be traced to a lack of documentation that resulted from a lack of user participation. This book's primary emphasis is on documentation tools and techniques. We must learn to use the tools and techniques presented in this book to effectively communicate with users during the systems development life cycle.

There you have it! Seven principles that should guide any problem-solving or systems development project. These principles, summarized in Figure 4.4, can be used to evaluate any life cycle or methodology, including ours! After you study the systems development life cycle presented in Chapter 5, we'll evaluate that life cycle using the principles we've just presented.

SUMMARY

Information-system-development projects are usually triggered by problems, opportunities, and directives. Problems exist when the current system is not fulfilling the business's purpose, goals, objectives, or policies. Opportunities are chances to improve a system despite the absence of problems. Directives are decisions imposed on a system by management or government. All problems, opportunities, and directives can be evaluated in terms of their bottom-line impact according to the following categories: performance, information, economy, control, efficiency, and service. These analysis criteria can be easily remembered because they can be arranged so their first letters spell the word *PIECES.*

The development of information systems must overcome three major problems. First, we must recognize that the breadth of business applications to which computers can be applied is large and growing larger. If possible, we would like to deal with all applications in a similar fashion. Second, we must realize that the computer system is rigid and unforgiving. Because business systems are flexible and unpredictable, we need a disciplined approach to modeling business problems to be implemented on the computer system. Finally, we must be cognizant of the difference in languages spoken by the computing and business professionals. Our development process must allow for communication with both technical and nontechnical audiences.

To deal with these problems, we can apply seven basic principles of problem solving. First, we should actively involve the users in systems development. Second, we need to educate users, management, and ourselves throughout systems development. Third, we should use a phased approach to systems development. Fourth, we should recognize that phases can overlap and that we will also need to backtrack from time to time. Fifth, we need to install checkpoints in our systems development cycle. These checkpoints should allow us the option of canceling the project if it has become infeasible. And seventh, we should document a system while we develop that system. These fundamental principles should be incorporated into any system development process in order to increase our chances of success.

PROBLEMS AND EXERCISES

1. Differentiate between problems, opportunities, and directives. Give examples of each.
2. Characterize each of the following situations as problems, opportunities, or directives. Remember, problems and opportunities are sometimes hard to distinguish. In those cases, describe how the situation might be either a problem or opportunity.
   (a) Management has decided to offer credit to regular customers. Previously, all sales required prepayment.
   (b) A bank's manager wonders if bank machine transactions executed at other banks can be posted to customer accounts in fewer than the current average of two days. If so, the bank could save several thousand dollars worth of interest payments each day.
   (c) A baseball manager's competitive edge might be improved by access to information about a hitter's history against specific pitchers.
   (d) When a manufacturing work station breaks down, management finds it difficult to modify the production schedule to reassign work from the broken work station to work stations that might have capacity. Thus, products don't get produced.
   (e) Management has decided that all computer files should be integrated into databases to improve access to and flexibility of data.
   (f) Total cash from customer payments does not equal the sum of payments posted against customer accounts.
3. Make an appointment to visit a systems analyst at a local data processing installation. Discuss the analyst's current project. What triggered the project — a problem, opportunity, or directive?
4. Using the PIECES framework, evaluate your local course registration system. Do you see problems or opportunities? (*Alternative:* Substitute any system with which you are familiar.)
5. Apply the PIECES framework to each of the situations in exercise 2. Remember, the categories of PIECES overlap; therefore,

any given problem, opportunity, or constraint may have implications in more than one category.

6. Evaluate the following situations according to the PIECES framework. Do not be concerned that you are unfamiliar with the application. That isn't unusual for any systems analyst. Use the PIECES framework to brainstorm potential problems you would ask the client about.

   (a) The manager of the machining and tooling shop needs help with work order processing and management. Work orders are currently processed by hand. Initial office processing involves establishing a job number, making a job estimate, and scheduling the job. This is a time-consuming process, and delays are common. Store orders have to be issued for materials needed to respond to the work order (and if materials aren't available, the order has to be rescheduled). At this point, we lose all track of the costs for these materials. Time cards are completed in the shop when workers fulfill the work order. These time cards are used to charge back time to the customer. Time cards are processed by hand, and the final calculations are entered on the work order. The work orders are checked for accuracy and sent to DP where accounting records are updated and the customer is billed. Our basic problem is that the customer frequently calls to inquire on costs already incurred on a work order but we can't respond because DP sends a report of all work orders only once a month. Also, management has no idea of how good initial estimates are or how much work is being done in any given work center (or by any employee) in the shop.

   (b) The investments officer for ABC Co. has a problem. Currently, their bank contacts ABC's accounting department each day to relay information regarding deposits, check clearing, current and legal bank account balances, and float on recently issued checks. Accounting notifies the investments officer, who does a cash flow projection. Using pencil and multicolumn ledger sheets, this projection takes a couple of hours to complete. These projections are used to estimate capital available for investment (in stocks, bonds, futures, and real estate, among others). Investments are made on a daily basis. The trouble is that we are too dependent on the bank clerk phoning in the information. If the cash projections go too slowly, valuable time is lost (the stock market opens early in the morning, but ABC is rarely ready to make investments at that time). Considerable capital can be made or lost in less than one hour.

(c) The personnel department's retirement benefits counselor is having some problems. Her job is to counsel employees on their benefit package and options. The retirement package allows employees to supplement employer contributions and to exercise limited control over how all contributions are invested (for example, in stocks or bonds). She manually responds to employee requests for monthly retirement income projections based on several variables (such as contributions, income projections, and planned retirement age). Her problems are as follows. First, it often takes one full day to get salary data from the Data Processing Department. Second, employee data are stored in many files that are not always properly updated. When conflicting data become apparent, she can't continue her projections until that conflict has been resolved. Third, the computations are complex. It often takes one full day or more to create investment and/or retirement scenarios for a single employee. Fourth, there are some concerns that projections are being provided to unauthorized individuals (such as former spouses or nonimmediate relatives). Finally, the complexity of the variations in the calculations (there are a lot of "If this, do that" calculations) results in frequent errors, many which probably go undetected.

(d) National Fund Raising, Inc., an independent fund raiser for various nonprofit clients, has uncovered a problem. Their data is out of control. They keep considerable redundant data on past donors and prospective donors. This results in multiple contacts for the same donor—and people don't like to be asked to give a single annual fund multiple times! Contacts with donors and follow-up are not well coordinated. While some prospective donors are contacted too often, others are overlooked entirely. It is currently impossible to generate lists of prospective donors based on specific criteria despite the fact that data on hundreds of criteria have been collected and stored. Donor histories are nonexistent, which makes it impossible to establish contribution patterns that would help various fund-raising campaigns.

7. Make an appointment to visit a systems analyst in a local data processing installation. Discuss the analyst's current project. Evaluate the initial problem, opportunity, or directive in terms of the PIECES framework.

8. Apply the PIECES framework to each of the following situations. Remember, the categories of PIECES overlap; therefore, any given situation may have implications in more than one category.
   (a) During the processing of room assignment applications, many of the same data are typed onto different forms at different times.
   (b) A sales manager knows total sales for each region but can't tell how well each product line is doing in each region.
   (c) A new record-keeping system allows students to see their test and project scores for any course; however, the system also allows a student to see all of the scores for any student in the same course.
   (d) The cost of manufacturing a specific product has dramatically reduced that product's profit margin.
   (e) Warranty claims have increased because defective parts are being used in products.
   (f) Manufacturing produces too much of some products and not enough of other products.
   (g) The chief accountant's office must consolidate the accounting statements for several years, calculating a percentage change (plus or minus) for each item on the statements.
   (h) The cost-accounting office needs to determine what percentage of a product's increasing costs are attributed to higher pay scales (out of management's control) and what percentage to lower labor productivity (controllable by management).
   (j) The marketing department needs to improve the sales staff's ability to make changes to orders that haven't already been shipped.

9. Explain three serious problems that can prevent successful information systems development. Give examples of each problem.

10. What are the seven fundamental principles of systems development? Explain what you would do to incorporate those principles into a systems development process.

11. Go to the library and check out a book on introductory data processing concepts or systems analysis and design. Most of these books will present a *system development life cycle, project life cycle,* or similar system development process that consists of steps or phases. Analyze that process in terms of the seven fundamental principles of systems development. (*Alternative:* Analyze the real-life process used by a local data processing installation.)

Note: We present a system development life cycle in Chapter 5. Don't analyze that one. We do that analysis at the end of that chapter.

ANNOTATED REFERENCES AND SUGGESTED READINGS

Benjamin, R. I. *Control of the Information System Development Cycle.* New York: Wiley-Interscience, 1971. Benjamin's sixteen axioms for managing the system development process inspired our adapted principles to guide successful systems development.

DeMarco, Tom. *Structured Analysis and System Specification.* Englewood Cliffs, N.J.: Prentice-Hall, 1979. Chapter 1 describes many problems that plague projects.

Gildersleeve, Thomas. *Successful Data Processing Systems Analysis.* Englewood Cliffs, N.J.: Prentice-Hall, 1976.

London, Keith. *The People Side of Systems.* New York: McGraw-Hill, 1976.

Matthies, Leslie H. *The Management System: Systems Are for People.* New York: Wiley, 1976.

Taggart, William. *Information Systems, An Introduction to Computers in Organizations.* Newton, Mass.: Allyn & Bacon, 1980.

Wetherbe, James. *Systems Analysis and Design: Traditional, Structured, and Advanced Concepts and Techniques.* 2d ed. St. Paul, Minn.: West Publishing, 1984. We are indebted to Dr. Wetherbe for the PIECES framework.

Analysts in Action

A New Information Systems Project Is Started

Cheryl and Doug get an assignment, "How can we improve our order processing through improved information system support?"

Episode 2

Cheryl entered her office that Monday morning hoping something interesting would happen that day. Things had been pretty slow since the new Purchasing system had been placed into operation. Conversion to the new system had been unusually smooth. Very few errors had been made, and the users were happy. Cheryl was confident that the project would be a success. She had actively involved the Purchasing personnel in the project, and she had insisted that her team develop complete and meaningful specifications for the programmers and users. But she eagerly wished for a new project. She wouldn't have to wait long.

Debbie Lopez knocked on her office door at 8:45 that same morning. Deb was assistant manager for the DC and had triggered several previous information systems projects.

"Morning, Cheryl. How was your weekend?"

"Just fine, Deb. By the way, the tomatoes you gave me were delicious. We really enjoyed them. I sure hope that piece of paper you're holding is a project request. I'm ready to let go of this Purchasing project and get on with something new."

"I always aim to please!" responded Deb. "This is indeed a project request. And I wouldn't trust it to anyone but you. That Purchasing system is a godsend. Bill is so pleased with it that you'll probably get a free lunch out of him. Meanwhile, this one is just as important, probably more so. Joey handed this proposal to me last week. I think we ought to get some preliminary analysis quickly." She handed the project request form to Cheryl (see Figure 1).

"What do we have here?" Cheryl took a look at the project request form.

"Well, in a nutshell, we want to see what you can do to improve our order-entry and approval system. We need to be able to process orders faster. You know, get them out into the warehouse quicker. We need to know what products are out of stock much sooner and try to get large orders for stockout products shipped direct from supplier to customer—avoiding the DC altogether."

"This may be a stupid question," Cheryl countered, "but why don't you just hire more clerks."

"I'd love to, but I can't! Roger won't approve the additional payroll. Besides, we're convinced that the problem is information- and decision-oriented."

"Could you clarify that?"

"Well, the delays occur because we can't validate customer data, credit status, part numbers, part availability, etc., quick enough. Even if Roger gave me more people, where would we put them? And sooner or later, sales would increase to a point where the added staff would be inadequate again. You know how it is: Increase sales! More! More! ▶

Figure 1

Customer services project request.

```
REQUEST FOR SYSTEM SERVICES                                 FORM 100

SUBMITTED BY ___Debbie Lopez_____________  DATE ___July 25, 1986___

DEPARTMENT ___Customer Services Division  (Mgr: Joey Hensley)______

TYPE OF REQUEST  [ xx] New System
                 [   ] System Redesign
                 [   ] System Modification

PROBLEM STATEMENT (attach additional documents if necessary)
  Order transactions are expected to increase 25% over the next
  three years. Current order-processing and follow-up procedures
  cannot support this demand. The problem is inefficient
  transaction data capture, inadequate decision support, and lack
  of management information to support operations.
_________________________________________________________________

REQUEST FOR SERVICE TO  Implement an improved customer services
  system with immediate emphasis on order entry and order follow-
  up and with growth potential in the areas of special orders and
  reclass returns.
*****************************************************************

ACTION (to be completed by Steering Committee)
   [ ]  Request Approved    Assigned to ________________________
                            Start Date _________________________
   [ ]  Request Delayed (backlogged) Until _____________________
   [ ]  Request Rejected for Reason: ___________________________
        ________________________________________________________
        ________________________________________________________
```

▶

More!" Deb's tone was serious.

Cheryl was already gleaming with enthusiasm. "Let me get to Joey on this, Deb. I think we have a priority project here, but I'll know better when I've done the preliminary study and analysis."

"This one is sure to get through the Steering Committee," Deb responded. Cheryl knew that the results of a preliminary investigation were always reviewed by the DP Steering Committee to determine whether the proposed project was worthwhile and of a high priority. Deb continued, "I hear you have a new partner."

"Yes," answered Cheryl. "His name is Doug Matthews. He must have heard something about this project when he met Ed Earl [Director of Computer Information Systems]. He said something about a new project in Customer Services. You'll meet him soon, I'm sure."

"Well, I just wanted to deliver the request personally. See you later, Cheryl."

Cheryl studied the Request for System Services form carefully. Then she phoned Joseph (Joey) Hensley, the manager of Customer Services, who was responsible for the order processing and follow-up activities for the DC.

"Joey? Hi. Listen, Joey, I got your project proposal today. Can we meet over lunch to discuss this order-entry problem of yours? Say, about 11:30?"

"Great!" said Joey. "Have I got an earful for you! See you at 11:30. Bye!"

Cheryl invited Doug to join the luncheon meeting. She knew Doug was anxious to start a real project. And she wanted to give Doug a tour of the Customer Services Division's offices. The meeting started on schedule.

"Joey, I'd like you to meet Doug Matthews, my new partner. Doug, this is Joey Hensley, manager of Customer Services."

"I'm glad to meet you, Joey," said Doug. "How are you, today?"

"Just fine, Doug. So, Cheryl, you two received my project request? I've been talking to Bill about that Purchasing system you built. If you do half as well for me, I'll be grateful." Joey was openly enthusiastic.

They ate lunch and then directed the conversation to the proposed project. Cheryl opened the questioning, "Tell me something about how you do order entry and approval today. I'm just trying to get a general feel for your situation. We'll study the system in considerable detail later."

"Well," responded Joey, "I'll try to give you an overview. We process three kinds of orders: stock orders, emergency customer orders, and employee orders. Most orders are classified as stock orders; that is, customers are simply trying to replenish their own stock. Emergency orders are for small quantities of specific parts—probably needed by a service station for a specific vehicle being repaired. Employee orders are simply a service we provide to our own employees here at the DC."

"I didn't know I could order parts!" exclaimed Doug.

"Yes, and at wholesale prices!" replied Joey. "Anyway, orders are received via mail, phone, and sales reps. The orders are manually screened for accuracy and completeness. Some orders have to be transcribed to . . ."

"Transcribed?" asked Doug.

"Yes, copied to our standard order forms. Most orders are then sent to Computer Information Systems (we call it CIS) to be processed. CIS performs credit checks but cannot reject orders officially. Most orders pass the credit check and are split into multiple orders corresponding to the warehouse zones in which the products are located."

Cheryl reentered the conversation. "What kind of problems initiated your project request, Joey?"

"First off, I purposefully simplified my description of order entry and approval. You need to spend time in Customer Services to really appreci- ▶

ate the magnitude of my operation. But, to answer your question, I do have a few problems to share. First, I've got a big problem coming! Last week, I had a meeting with Roger [DC manager], Deb, and Joshua Vadir [company president, from the Little Rock headquarters]. I was told to expect an aggressive new marketing program over the next three years—TV, radio, newspapers, and magazines. Little Rock expects sales to increase at least 25 percent during that time. I can't handle that load with my existing staff. I have no place to put new staff, and I'm not sure that Roger thinks that's the answer anyway. Meanwhile, my response time to orders is getting worse each month. Orders are getting more complicated. New policies encourage customers to overstock high-volume products by guaranteeing full credit if they return the unsold portion of those products. My area has to handle those returns in addition to their normal orders. We also have to execute special orders for parts not normally inventoried in the warehouse, and those orders are becoming more frequent."

"I'm beginning to see your problem, and you're right, we're going to have to spend some time in Customer Services to fully understand. I'm a bit lost already. Can you explain to us what you think you need?" asked Cheryl.

"Yes," replied Joey. "I would like more significant support of order processing. I want to be able to do better follow-up on outstanding orders. I want some way to prioritize back-orders. I'd also like to get some decent information that shows me where I can improve my operation. I don't really know *what* information that'll be. I'm kind of hoping that you can help me figure that out. At least help me harness my data so I can get at it when I want to." Joey's tone indicated some frustration with his current operation.

"This sounds interesting," said Doug.

"Yes," agreed Cheryl. "Doug and I will need to gather some more facts. We should talk with you again very soon. We better get going, Doug. We have a review conference on the Purchasing system in fifteen minutes. Thanks for joining us, Joey. We'll get back to you soon!"

Doug and Cheryl completed their preliminary study with two more in-depth interviews with Joey. They presented their findings in a memorandum to the Steering Committee (Figure 2). The Steering Committee approved the project.

Where Do We Go from Here?
Cheryl and Doug now have a project. Where should they start? If you were assigned to write a proposal that outlines a step-by-step process to develop the new system, what would your steps be? Take a moment to jot down your ideas.

In Chapter 5 you will study a general process for developing an information system—Cheryl and Doug are being asked to develop an Order Information System. The process you'll be studying is called a systems development life cycle. The steps are called *phases.* Each phase may consist of several tasks. Those tasks are studied in Chapters 6, 10, and 17. The systems development life cycle is the basis for all of the tools and techniques you will learn about in the remainder of this book. ■

Figure 2

Feasibility survey report. Most systems projects begin with some sort of preliminary analysis that results in a feasibility assessment similar to this report. ▶

MEMORANDUM

DATE: August 3, 1986

TO: CISG Steering Committee

FROM: Cheryl Lynn Mason, CDP, Senior Systems Analyst
Douglas Raymond Matthews, Programmer/Analyst

SUBJECT: Proposed Order-Entry Information System: Preliminary Investigation Findings

We have just completed a preliminary investigation for a proposed order-entry and follow-up information system to support the customer services section of the warehouse. If a successful system can be developed (we think that is highly likely), then the system should prove invaluable for all AAP distribution centers.

Problem Statement: About 80 percent of order transactions are currently supported (partially) by a batch data processing system developed in 1973. Many procedures are still performed manually by order-entry clerks in the customer services area. The following problems in the existing system were identified:

1. Several order-processing tasks (such as screening, customer data update, and prepayments) are still performed manually. Delays can occur when information required is not readily available.

2. All emergency orders are processed manually. Twenty-four-hour turnaround is desired; however, forty-eight-hour turnaround is more typical. Credit screening and inventory checks take considerable time and are subject to delay-causing errors.

3. Orders for parts not normally stocked in the warehouse are subject to a time-consuming process to effect direct delivery from our supplier to the customer.

4. Orders for parts that customers can intentionally overstock and then return for full credit require special processing, which is currently performed by clerks.

5. Back orders are not receiving priority over new orders for the same products.

6. Orders are not traced after they leave customer services for the warehouse and are lost with increased frequency. When lost, they must be processed from scratch.

7. All types of orders and transactions are likely to increase 30 percent or more over the next three years. It is highly unlikely that the current system can handle such a workload.

Scope of the Proposed Project: The user is requesting a system that will:

1. Expedite the processing of all orders through improved data collection methods and decision support.

2. Provide improved information support for customer services managers and supervisors.

3. Provide a mechanism for prioritizing orders and following up on outstanding orders.

Analysts in Action

The primary users of the system would include the customer services manager and staff including: (1) order-entry supervisor and clerks, (2) order follow-up supervisor and clerks, (3) sales requisitions clerks, and (4) overstock clerks.

The proposed system could benefit or affect: (1) the Purchasing Department, (2) the warehouse, and (3) the shipping/receiving dock.

Constraints: The new system is needed within one year. At that time, the current system will be unable to maintain current order turnaround time to meet increased demand.

Preliminary Alternative Solutions: The final solution would be a function of a more detailed study of the current system's limitations and the user's requirements; however, the following potential solutions are presented:

1. Improved batch data processing support. The current system could be expanded to process all orders and provide improved management-reporting capabilities.

2. Implementation of an on-line order entry system to support the data collection and decision requirements of order processing. Management reports could be implemented on a scheduled or demand basis in such a system.

3. Supplement the current system by adding microcomputer support for some of the local data and information needs of the customer services section.

4. Expansion of current customer services facilities and staffing to support improved manual procedures.

Other solutions may become apparent during the project. All alternatives will eventually be analyzed for feasibility (at an appropriate time).

Recommendations: As a result of this preliminary study, we highly recommend a detailed study of the current system be approved. The volume of order processing and its associated costs make this application a high-priority project. A detailed study will more clearly identify problems and opportunities and set the stage for defining detailed user needs. Findings of the detailed study will be submitted to the Steering Committee, who can evaluate the project's desirability with greater certainty.

Resource Requirements: Doug and I can complete a detailed study of the current order entry system and present our findings and recommendations in two months. Joey Hensley should arrange for us to meet with and question key personnel in the system.

The detailed study will cost approximately $7,700.00, budgeted as follows:

2.5 person months for systems analysts	$4,750.00
1.0 person month user release time	1,775.00
0.5 person month secretarial support	500.00
overhead	475.00
	$7,700.00

The detailed study will include a budget for the requirements definition and feasibility analysis phases.

If you have any questions, feel free to contact me at 42560.

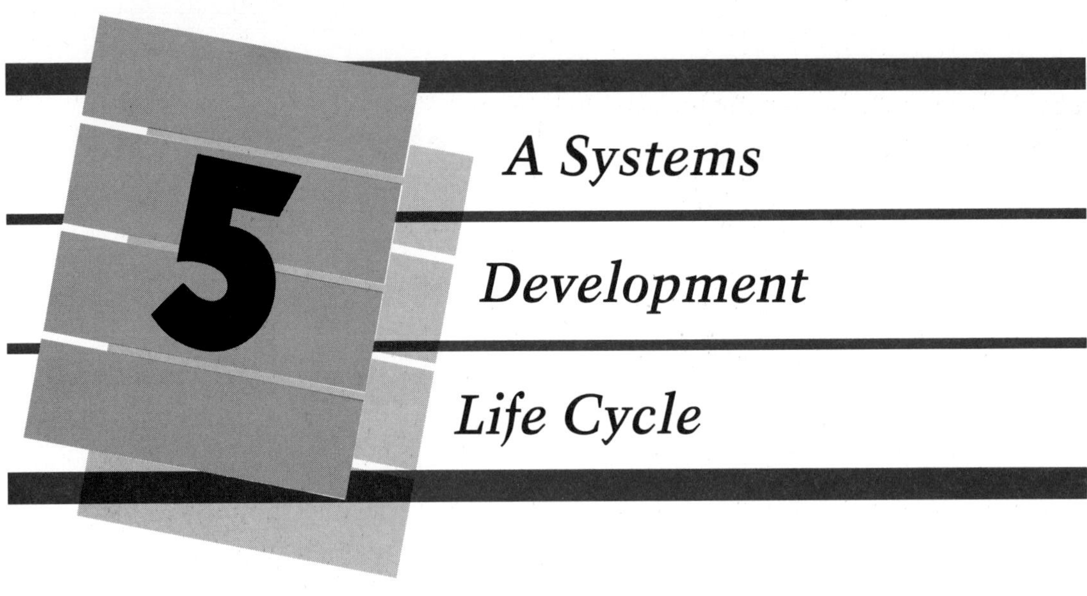

5 A Systems Development Life Cycle

Minicase: Americana Plastics, Inc.

Jeannine's intercom buzzed. "Your 3 o'clock appointment is here Ms. Matson. Shall I send him in?"

"Yes," answered Jeannine, an analyst with Americana Plastics, Inc.

Alan Springer, the Marketing manager, entered Jeannine's office. "Hi, Jeannine. I think I've got a big problem. I'm hoping you can hclp."

"I'll try my best," answered Jeannine.

Alan's face turned serious. "I'll make a long story short. Three months ago, our office bought a microcomputer. We aren't trying to go over your heads. We only want to do some things you haven't been able to do for us."

Alan continued, "Anyway, we decided to create a system to track and analyze sales of new products in test markets. I had each clerk and staff member list all the features they would like to see in such a system. Then I learned how to program in the database language that the computer store sold to us. I thought I did a pretty good job. But the system just hasn't lived up to the expectations of either my boss or my staff. I know you can't come over and bail me out. But I was wondering if you could tell me what I did wrong and how I might be able to fix it quickly."

Jeannine had stopped smiling. "Alan, I wish I had a dollar for every time I've heard a story like this. It's happened here at Americana, and my friends at other companies tell me similar stories. You've made a common mistake. Computers don't magically solve problems. You don't just flip the switch on and start reaping benefits. Not even with micros! The computer is a tool. Business applications have to be designed around the tool. But tell me, what's wrong with the system you built?"

"Where do I begin?" Alan responded. "The system just doesn't provide the information my boss and staff want. I used some of the sales reports generated by your computer system to update my database. My clerks don't particularly like the fact that they have to reenter that data, but I explained to them that it was a different computer and that we didn't have time to get an interface between the micro and your computer."

"I would have asked, Alan." replied Jeannine. "I'm not a data communications expert, but we do have people who are. Anyway, go on."

Alan continued, "It turns out that my people were using your data because that's all they had. Actually, those data are not considered adequate. When I found out a little more about what they really wanted, I discovered that my database isn't set up correctly. I can't figure out how to get the data out in a way that will support the necessary reports. And even if I could, they want to plug the data into tables and play 'what if' games to see the potential impact of different marketing strategies. They also want graphics, something my database system can't do. I could go on and on."

Jeannine spoke calmly, "Alan, I haven't got any easy answers for you. Your problems are the result of shortcuts taken through the system development process. When we develop a system for you, we do a detailed analysis of your current system and alternatives to improve that system. We carefully design the new system and get your approval. Then, and only then, do we start programming."

"Wait a minute!" Alan erupted. *"I only bought a microcomputer! It's not the same as that monster you guys use.* I figured that,because I was using a smaller computer, I didn't need to go through that ritual you guys go through when you build a system for us."

"That's the mistake, Alan. The size of the computer doesn't matter. These so-called micros are nearly as powerful as the mainframes in our not-too-distant past. And even if we ignore the technology, you were designing a system, not just a computer program. Computers and software are only a part of your total business solution. Analysis and design are important no matter what size computer you use. There is more to systems than computers and software."

Alan responded, "But I didn't have time for the ritual of systems development."

Jeannine responded, "You didn't have time to do it right? Then where are you going to find time to do it over?"

Discussion

1. Looking back to Chapter 4, what principles of systems development did Alan possibly violate?
2. Alan suffers from one of today's most common problems, the belief that systems development in the microcomputer era is, somehow, different from systems development in the big-computer era. Why do you suppose users fall into this trap?
3. What conclusions can you draw from Chapters 1 and 2 that might help Alan understand that microcomputer-based systems are not significantly different from their larger computer counterparts?
4. What would you recommend Alan do to improve his new system? Does your solution represent the same quick-fix that Alan took?

WHAT WILL YOU LEARN IN THIS CHAPTER?

This chapter introduces a basic system development life cycle (SDLC) and some implementation variations that you can introduce into that basic process. You will know that you understand the SDLC when you can:

1. Apply a problem-solving approach to identify the phases of a system development life cycle.
2. For each phase in our system development life cycle,
   (a) Describe the purpose of that phase.
   (b) Describe the inputs and outputs of that phase.
3. Describe three false phases found in many life cycles and suggest how those activities should be incorporated into the life cycle.
4. Compare and contrast alternative implementations of the system development life cycle.
5. Differentiate between systems analysis, systems design, and systems implementation.
6. Differentiate between the system development life cycle and a system development methodology, and describe three different types of methodologies.
7. Critique any given system development life cycle against the seven principles of system development (Chapter 4).

A **systems development life cycle** (hereafter called an SDLC) is a disciplined approach to developing information systems. Although such an approach will not guarantee success, it will improve the chances of success. Most experts agree that there is an SDLC. And most agree that a *phased* approach is appropriate. Beyond that, you'll find little agreement. There are as many SDLCs as there are authors and companies. They are more alike than different. The terminology differs, but the intent is the same. In this chapter we present an SDLC. Notice we did not say *the* SDLC. We don't claim that we're right and everybody else is wrong. But we'll start from scratch and try to avoid the terms that have frequently confused readers, namely *systems analysis, systems design,* and *systems implementation.* We'll discuss those terms after we've presented our SDLC.

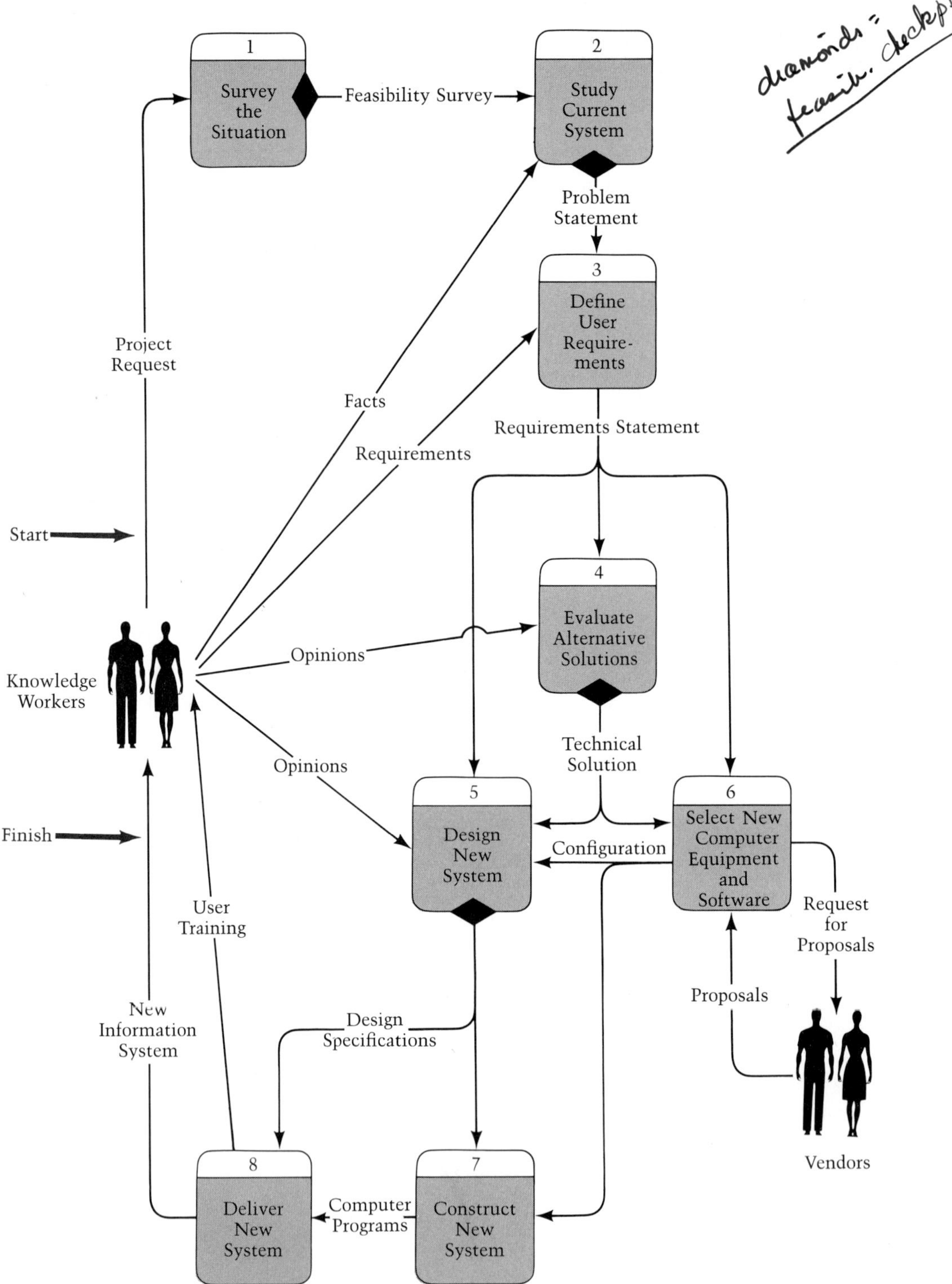
1
Survey the Situation
Feasibility Survey
2
Study Current System
Problem Statement
3
Define User Require-ments
Requirements Statement
4
Evaluate Alternative Solutions
Technical Solution
5
Design New System
6
Select New Computer Equipment and Software
Configuration
Request for Proposals
Proposals
Vendors
Design Specifications
7
Construct New System
Computer Programs
8
Deliver New System
Project Request
Facts
Requirements
Opinions
Opinions
Start
Knowledge Workers
Finish
User Training
New Information System

THE BASIC PHASES OF A SYSTEMS DEVELOPMENT LIFE CYCLE

An eight-phase SDLC is illustrated in Figure 5.1. The rounded rectangles represent project phases performed by the systems analysts and computer programmers. The arrows represent working inputs and outputs (documentation) for a phase. The person figures are people and organizations the analyst may have to interact with. Finally, the shaded diamonds indicate checkpoints at which management should reevaluate feasibility.

In Chapter 4, you learned that system development is triggered by *problems, opportunities,* and *directives* in the business system. We'll refer to these triggers as the **project request.** To understand the SDLC, we need a project request that you can relate to.

The Project Request

Don't you just hate it when you go to the grocery store to buy a few food items and the store is completely out of one or more of them? Well, the stores hate it too! Why? Because they know you're going to go to a competitor to get what they don't have. It may surprise you to learn that the grocery industry only realizes a few percentage points of net profit. This is largely because of their high inventory carrying costs. A store normally overstocks shelves to prevent stockouts. We have received the following request from the manager of a small grocery chain, J&W Food Mart:

> We are in trouble. Our competitors are using the latest in point-of-sale computer technology. Each item purchased by their customers is run across one of those bar-code readers in the checkout line. The item is automatically subtracted from inventory. Reorder reports are produced daily. This allows our competitors to carry lower amounts of inventory, which allows them to reduce their spoilage and lower their prices. We can't compete! We can only check inventory levels for most items

◄ **Figure 5.1**

An eight-phase systems development life cycle. Most firms have a systems development life cycle (SDLC). It is a phased approach to building information systems, computer-based or otherwise.

once a week, and we do it manually. We have to overstock our shelves or we'll run out of critical items. HELP! We need an improved inventory control system.

The great thing about this example is that you are part of this system because you are a prospective store customer. We'll walk through each phase of the SDLC for this problem, describing what you have to do in those phases. Throughout this discussion, we suggest you mark Figure 5.1 for quick and easy reference. And as we walk through the phases, we'll give you a sneak preview of the tools and techniques you'll learn to use in the rest of this book.

Please note: This is only a sneak preview. Don't try to completely understand the tools and techniques as you read this chapter. You'll learn those skills and more in Parts II, III, and IV of this book.

The SDLC: A Problem-Solving Approach

Given a project request, we can use a generalized problem-solving approach to complete the project. The problem-solving approach consists of eight steps or phases:

1. Survey the situation.
2. Study the current system.
3. Define user requirements.
4. Evaluate alternative solutions.
5. Select new computer equipment and software (if necessary).
6. Design the new system.
7. Construct the new system.
8. Deliver the new system.

Survey the Situation We begin our typical project by surveying the current situation. The **survey phase** is often called a preliminary investigation or feasibility study in other SDLCs. The term *feasibility study* may be misleading because it sounds so final — not consistent with our creeping-commitment approach to feasibility. In any case, the survey phase is a quick and dirty analysis of the problem, opportunity, or directive that triggered the project. The purpose of the survey phase is to determine whether or not significant resources should be committed to the other phases of the life cycle.

During the survey phase, you will define the scope and nature of the project, the knowledge workers in the system, and the preliminary feasibility of the project.

The output of the survey phase is a feasibility survey that presents the findings and recommendations of the analyst. It also includes a preliminary cost/benefit analysis that determines if the project is feasible. At this stage of the project, feasibility is rarely more than a statement that the problems, opportunities, or directives are worthy of being addressed. The findings must be reviewed by management to prioritize the project. Let's assume that our grocery system project has been surveyed and approved to continue to the next phase.

Study the Current System There's a saying that suggests, "Don't fix it until you understand it." You need to understand the existing inventory control information system before you design and build a new system. Therefore, the first major phase of our SDLC is to study the current system. Do the problems and opportunities really exist? If so, how serious are the problems and how important are the opportunities? Yes, you answered these questions during the survey phase, but with a minimum of analysis. During the study phase, you want to address the causes and effects of problems and opportunities.

To properly analyze problems, opportunities, and directives, you need to understand *how* the existing system operates. The study phase educates you about the business problem. How does the existing system operate? Where do limitations, problems, and opportunities exist? The study will frequently uncover problems and opportunities not originally reported by the users. Thus, you are trying to clarify the size and scope of the project.

To better understand the current system and its limitations, you may want to draw a data flow diagram (Figure 5.2). A **data flow diagram** traces the flow of documents and reports through a system and clearly identifies the work performed by people and computers along the way. You'll learn how to use this important tool in Chapter 7. Still, data flow diagrams are fairly easy to read, even without formal training. Do you see yourself in the diagram (as a customer)? After you have drawn the data flow diagram of the current system, you can analyze problems and opportunities. The findings of the study phase should be documented as some form of problem statement for the next phase of the life cycle.

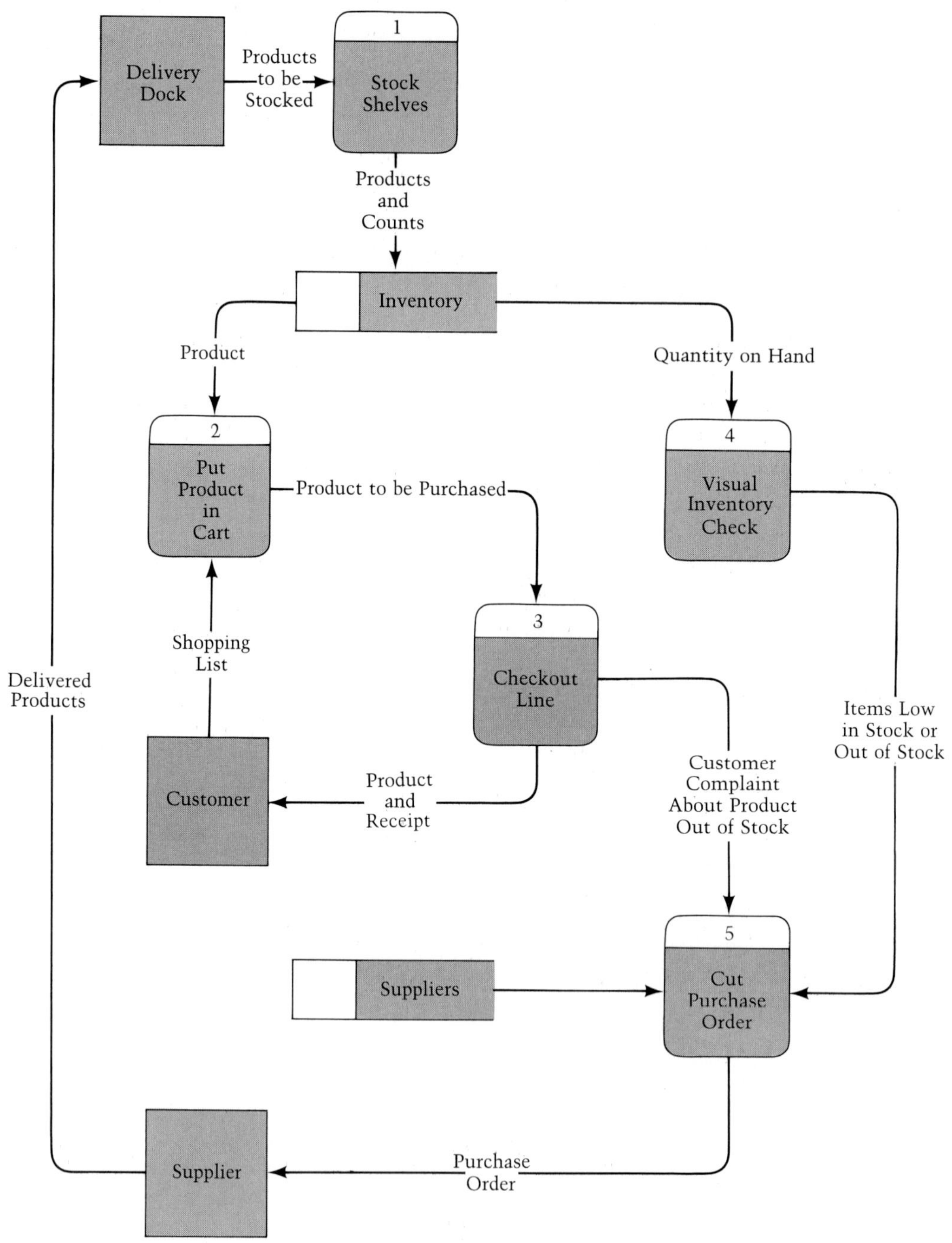
Delivery Dock
Products to be Stocked
1
Stock Shelves
Products and Counts
Inventory
Product
Quantity on Hand
2
Put Product in Cart
Product to be Purchased
4
Visual Inventory Check
3
Checkout Line
Shopping List
Delivered Products
Items Low in Stock or Out of Stock
Customer
Product and Receipt
Customer Complaint About Product Out of Stock
5
Suppliers
Cut Purchase Order
Supplier
Purchase Order

A useful analogy to an information systems development project is construction of a house. Consider the problem of building your dream home. The architect is the systems analyst of the housing industry. Does the architect do a study phase? You bet! The architect surveys the land and soil, studies other houses in the area, and learns about building codes that are pertinent to the property. Essentially, the architect, like the systems analyst, is studying the existing environment.

Define User Requirements Now you can design the new inventory control information system, right? No, not yet! What do you want the new system to do? What performance level do you expect? Careful! We didn't say *how*. We said *what*. The next phase of our SDLC is to define user requirements. You go to the users and find out what they need or want out of a new system. You will frequently find the user defining additional opportunities during this phase. Essentially, the purpose of the **definition phase** is to define the inputs, files, processing, and outputs for the new system, but to do so without expressing computer alternatives for implementing those requirements.

There is some controversy on the issue of requirements definition. A primary reason for the failure of many information systems is missed requirements. But can the systems analyst always define the user's requirements? Many analysts say "No, the user often doesn't know what information will be needed until a situation arises." Other analysts believe that most information needs can be determined by carefully studying the user's job. Actually, both views are correct. We believe that there are two categories of user requirements:

- *Information requirements.* By studying knowledge workers' jobs, we can identify information needs that either recur or are clearly required. We call these needs information requirements because we can define the specific output the user requires. For

◀ **Figure 5.2**

A sample data flow diagram for J&W Food Mart. A data flow diagram traces the flow of data and documents through a system. It depicts the work performed along the way. This diagram shows the flow of data through the existing grocery inventory system. A similar diagram could be drawn for an improved system.

example, users can identify specific reports or transactions that they need on a regular basis. Given the outputs, you can define the required inputs, files, and processes.

- *Data requirements.* For those information needs that cannot be predetermined, we return to a fundamental system concept: INFORMATION = f(DATA, PROCESSING). The information requirements may not be known; however, the raw data that describes the business function can be identified, collected, and stored in a database until some future time when the information requirement makes itself known. Although business policies and procedures constantly change, the types of data stored are more stable. The types of data we store today can be used to meet tomorrow's new information requirements.

Documentation tools play a significant role during the definition phase. Data flow diagrams can again be used to express the general requirements for the new system. But they illustrate requirements at a very high level. It is also useful to define details during the definition phase. For instance: What should the content of a certain report (information requirement) be? or What should the content of a specific file (data requirement) be? Detailed requirements can be documented in a data dictionary (Figure 5.3). The **data dictionary** records important details about content, size, number of occurrences, and other system parameters that may affect our choice of an ideal computer solution. You will learn how to construct a data dictionary in Chapter 8.

In addition to detailed data and information requirements, you will need to define policies and procedures for the new system. For example, our inventory control system may need to specify policies for reorder quantities, given the possible spoilage of products. Decision tables and Structured English (Figure 5.4) are two tools for describing policies and procedures. Given a set of possible conditions, the **decision table** tells us what actions should be taken under what conditions. **Structured English** is programming-like language oriented to those who have little or no programming background or interest. You'll learn how to prepare decision tables and write Structured English in Chapter 9.

The entire requirements specification is organized into a document called a **requirements statement.** This document should be reviewed with your knowledge workers.

Let's return to our house project. The architect will also define the homeowners' requirements before designing the house. How

```
ITEMS LOW IN STOCK  *    A report that identifies
                         products in inventory that are
                         low in stock or out of stock.
                    =        DATE OF REPORT
                    and      PAGE NUMBER
                    and      1 to 200 occurrences of:
                                  PRODUCT NUMBER
                             and  PRODUCT DESCRIPTION
                             and  TOTAL QUANTITY ON HAND
                             and  TOTAL QUANITY ON ORDER
                             and  REORDER POINT
                             and  REORDER QUANTITY
                             and  AVERAGE USAGE PER MONTH
                             and  USAGE LAST WEEK
                             and  USAGE LAST MONTH
                             and  UNIT OF MEASURE
                             and  LIFETIME TILL SPOILAGE
                             and  1 to 5 occurrences of:
                                  PEAK USAGE PERIOD
```

Figure 5.3

A sample data dictionary entry for J&W Food Mart. A data dictionary records details about data and information. It can be used to keep track of the overwhelming number of details an analyst must consider when developing a new system.

many people are in the family? What are their ages? How important is privacy? Where do the family members spend most of their time? The requirements can become more specific. How many full bathrooms are wanted? How many windows are desired, and where should they be located? This is only a sampling of questions the architect uses to learn the homeowner's requirements.

Evaluate Alternative Solutions Now can we design the new inventory control information system for our grocery chain? Let's think about it for a moment. Design is a detailed activity. We will spend considerable time designing detailed inputs, outputs, procedures, programs, files, and so forth. But there are numerous alternative ways to design the inventory control system. How much of the system should be automated? Should we design an on-line or batch system? Should we support the system on the chain headquarter's central computer or distribute the processing to a satellite computer in each grocery store? The next phase of our SDLC is to evaluate alternative solutions.

```
For each SALES ITEM, do the following:
     Given the PRODUCT NUMBER and SALES QUANTITY supplied by
     the cashier:

          Find the UNIT PRICE and PRODUCT CLASS in the
          INVENTORY file using the PRODUCT NUMBER.

          Calculate the EXTENDED PRICE using the following
          formula:
               EXTENDED PRICE = SALES QUANTITY X UNIT PRICE

          If the PRODUCT CLASS is "TAXABLE" then:
               Add the EXTENDED PRICE to the TOTAL TAXABLE
               SALES.

          Add the EXTENDED PRICE to the SALES SUBTOTAL.

          Record the PRODUCT DESCRIPTION, SALES QUANTITY,
          and UNIT PRICE on the SALES RECEIPT.

          Subtract the SALES QUANTITY from the QUANTITY ON
          HAND.

          Add SALES QUANTITY to the AVERAGE USAGE PER MONTH
          and USAGE THIS WEEK

     Calculate the SALES TAX
          SALES TAX = TOTAL T

     Record the SALES SUBTOT
     RECEIPT.

     Calculate the TOTAL SAL
     formula:
          TOTAL SALES AMOUNT

     Record the TOTAL SALES A

Give the PAYMENT supplied by
     Record the PAYMENT on th

     Subtract the PAYMENT fro
     the AMOUNT DUE.

     Record the AMOUNT DUE on
```

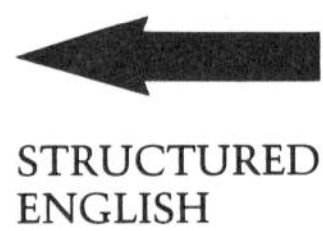

STRUCTURED ENGLISH

DECISION TABLE

PROCESS NAME CASH CHECK		RULES 1	2	3	4	5	6	7	8	9
CONDITIONS	TYPE OF CHECK	–	2	1	1	3	3	4	4	
	AMOUNT OF CHECK	G	–	L	L	L	L	L	L	
	IDENTIFICATION PROVIDED	–	–	Y	N	Y	N	Y	N	
ACTIONS	ACCEPT CHECK			X		X		X		
	REFUSE CHECK	X	X		X		X		X	

◀ **Figure 5.4**

Structured English and decision tables samples for J&W Food Mart. Structured English is a method for documenting business procedures, computerized or manual. Decision tables are used to document complex business policies and decisions.

The **evaluation phase** looks at *how* the new system is to be designed but only at a very high level — no details! We can document possible solutions with system flowcharts (Figure 5.5). **System flowcharts** show how the computer will be applied within a system, but they show a minimum of technical details. The sample system flowchart in Figure 5.5 shows one alternative solution for the grocery inventory system. You'll learn how to draw system flowcharts in Chapter 15.

After defining alternative solutions to the requirements, each alternative is evaluated according to three criteria:

- *Technical feasibility.* Is the solution technically practical? Will we need to acquire new or additional computer equipment or software? Does our staff have the technical expertise to design and build this solution?
- *Operational feasibility.* Will the solution fulfill the user's requirements? To what degree? How will the solution change the user's work environment? How do users feel about such a solution? Will the solution possibly create new problems?
- *Economic feasibility.* What will the solution cost to develop? What will the solution cost to operate? What are the tangible and intangible benefits of the solution? Is the solution cost-effective?

Infeasible alternatives should be eliminated from further consideration. More than likely, several alternatives will be feasible. However, you are looking for the *most* feasible solution, the one solution that offers the best combination of technical, operational, and economic feasibility. The evaluation phase is frequently documented as a proposal to management who will make the final decision.

Does our architect evaluate alternatives? Yes, indeed! The architect will examine the ranch, bilevel, and trilevel alternatives. Is the exterior to be finished in brick, stone, wood, or aluminum? Will there be gas or electric appliances? These decisions will affect the ultimate design of the house.

Figure 5.5

A sample systems flowchart for J&W Food Mart. A systems flowchart is used to document data processing methods and procedures for an information system. This system flowchart depicts a proposed computer solution for our grocery inventory system.

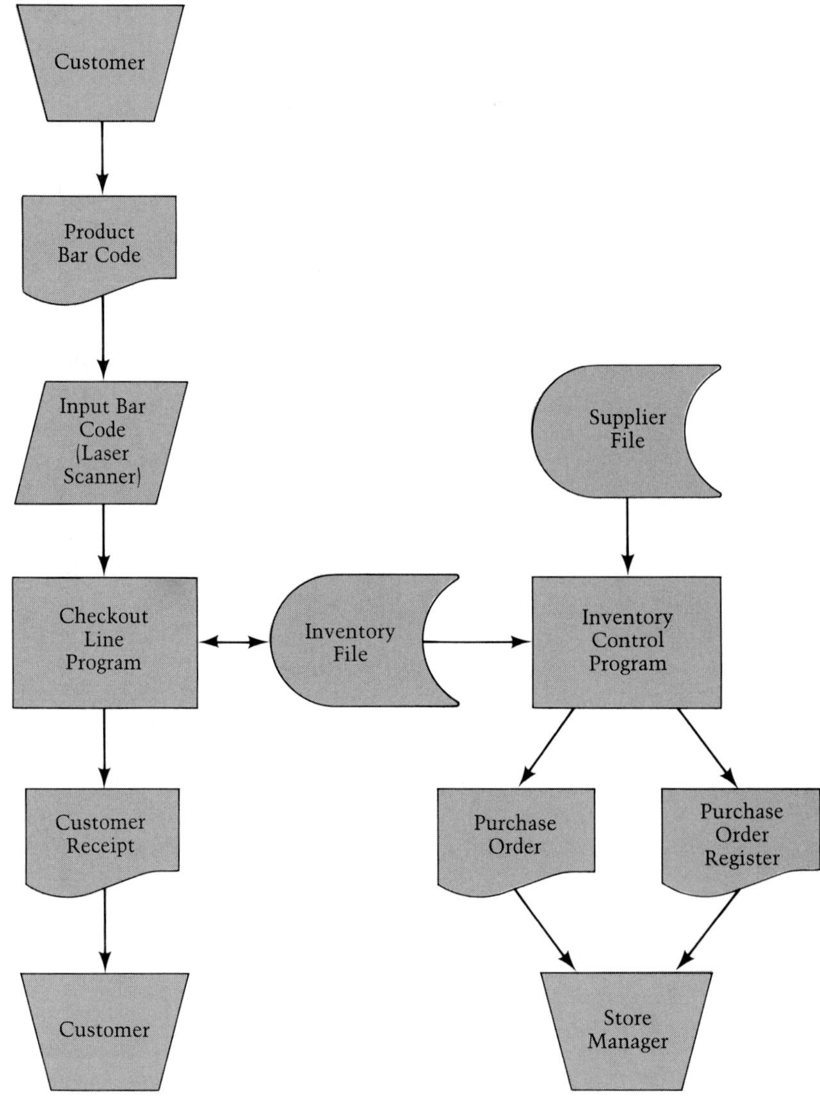

Select New Computer Equipment and Software (if necessary) Here is a phase that is missing from many SDLCs. College graduates are often shocked to discover the high percentage of computer software that is purchased rather than built. Furthermore, a new information system may present the need to acquire additional computer equipment (for instance, computer terminals). Our SDLC must provide for the selection of equipment and software.

It is a common mistake to abandon the SDLC when the system is to be purchased instead of built in-house. The study phase is still needed to analyze problems and opportunities. The definition phase is even more important—you usually get what you ask for when you purchase a system. The evaluation phase still determines the technical solution. The technical solution may indicate that no new technology is needed, but if the technical solution calls for new hardware or software, the selection phase becomes necessary.

During the **selection phase,** you need to determine which specifications are important for the equipment and software to be purchased. Needs are communicated in a request for proposals that is sent to vendors who may be able to fulfill those needs. After receiving proposals from the vendors, your job is to select the proposed hardware or software configuration (you are still looking at Figure 5.1, right?) that best meets your needs at a reasonable cost.

The selection phase has taken on special importance because of the increased use of microcomputers. The small business that buys a microcomputer cannot afford a full-time staff of systems analysts, computer programmers, and computer operators. Many microcomputer-based information systems depend on packaged software that can be bought off the shelf, loaded, and run—all without significant computer programming effort.

And what about our house construction analogy? Does it go through a selection phase? Yes, the architect and contractor must acquire building materials at the lowest possible cost without sacrificing quality. Thus, building materials must be carefully selected, usually through a bidding process similar to our request-for-proposals approach for selecting computer technology.

Design the New System Given a feasible technical solution from the evaluation phase, can you now design the new inventory control system? Yes! You understand *what* the requirements are (from the definition phase) and *how* you want to fulfill those requirements (from the evaluation phase). Now you can afford to spend time to design the new system, the next phase of our SDLC.

Computer outputs are normally designed first because output design can affect the design of computer inputs, files, and methods. You will normally document each output's format on a printer spacing chart (see Figure 5.6). A printer spacing chart communicates the content and format of a report or form to the computer programmer. You'll learn how to design computer outputs in Chapter 11.

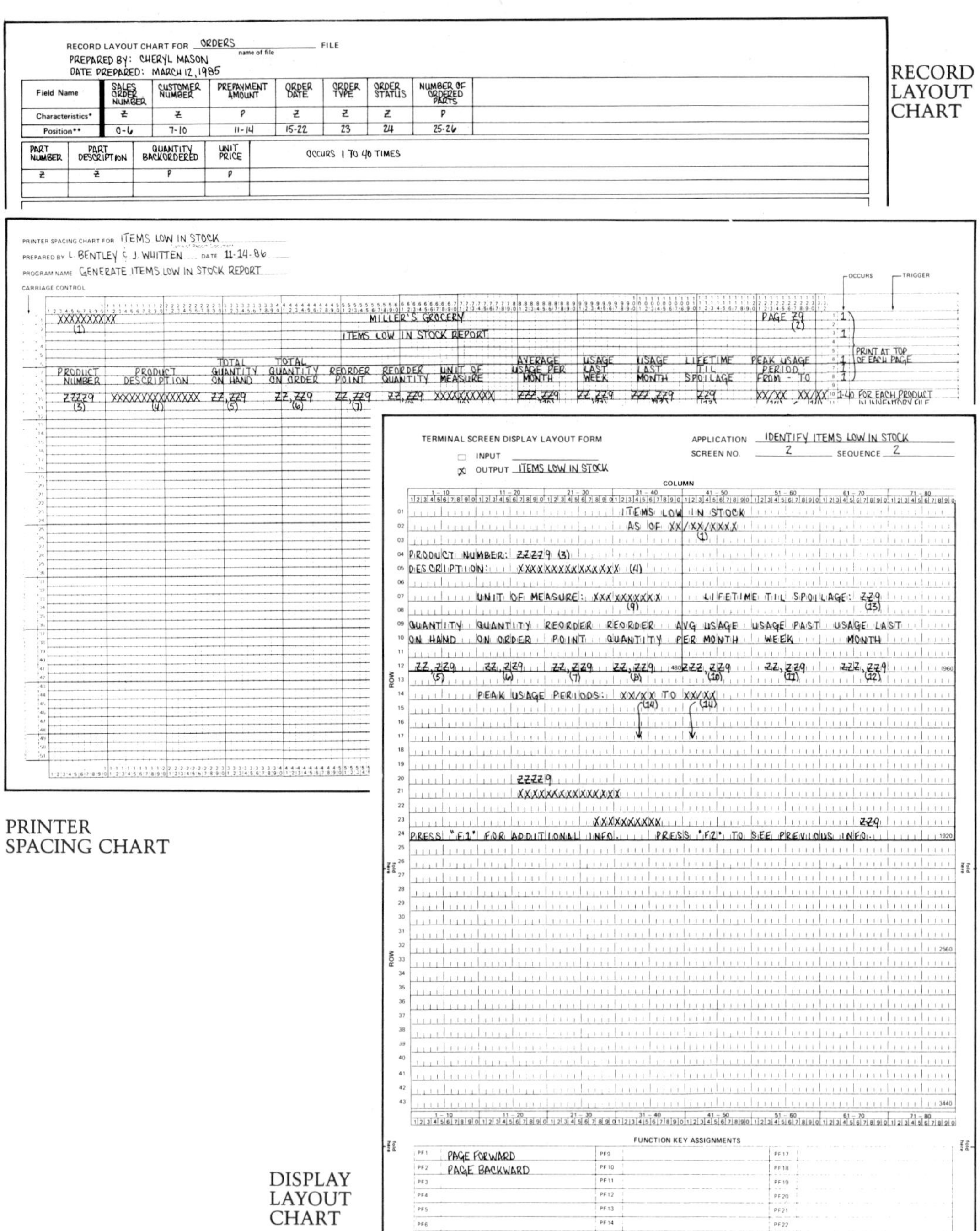

RECORD LAYOUT CHART FOR ORDERS FILE

PREPARED BY: CHERYL MASON

DATE PREPARED: MARCH 12, 1985

Field Name	SALES ORDER NUMBER	CUSTOMER NUMBER	PREPAYMENT AMOUNT	ORDER DATE	ORDER TYPE	ORDER STATUS	NUMBER OF ORDERED PARTS
Characteristics*	Z	Z	P	Z	Z	Z	P
Position**	0-6	7-10	11-14	15-22	23	24	25-26

PART NUMBER	PART DESCRIPTION	QUANTITY BACKORDERED	UNIT PRICE	OCCURS 1 TO 40 TIMES
Z	Z	P	P	

RECORD LAYOUT CHART

PRINTER SPACING CHART FOR ITEMS LOW IN STOCK

PREPARED BY L. BENTLEY & J. WHITTEN DATE 11-14-86

PROGRAM NAME GENERATE ITEMS LOW IN STOCK REPORT

CARRIAGE CONTROL — OCCURS — TRIGGER

```
XXXXXXXXXX                    MILLER'S GROCERY                    PAGE Z9      1
(1)                                                                    (2)
                         ITEMS LOW IN STOCK REPORT                                1
                                                                                  PRINT AT TOP
                      TOTAL     TOTAL                              AVERAGE    USAGE  USAGE  LIFETIME PEAK USAGE  1  OF EACH PAGE
PRODUCT  PRODUCT      QUANTITY  QUANTITY REORDER REORDER  UNIT OF  USAGE PER  LAST   LAST   TIL      PERIOD      1
NUMBER   DESCRIPTION  ON HAND   ON ORDER POINT   QUANTITY MEASURE  MONTH      WEEK   MONTH  SPOILAGE FROM - TO   1

ZZZZ9    XXXXXXXXXXXXXX ZZ,ZZ9  ZZ,ZZ9   ZZ,ZZ9  ZZ,ZZ9   XXXXXXXXXX ZZZ,ZZ9  ZZ,ZZ9 ZZZ,ZZ9 ZZ9      XX/XX XX/XX 1-40 FOR EACH PRODUCT
(3)      (4)          (5)       (6)      (7)                                                                      IN INVENTORY FILE
```

PRINTER SPACING CHART

TERMINAL SCREEN DISPLAY LAYOUT FORM

APPLICATION IDENTIFY ITEMS LOW IN STOCK

☐ INPUT

☒ OUTPUT ITEMS LOW IN STOCK

SCREEN NO. 2 SEQUENCE 2

```
01                                    ITEMS LOW IN STOCK
02                                    AS OF XX/XX/XXXX
03                                           (1)
04 PRODUCT NUMBER: ZZZZ9 (3)
05 DESCRIPTION:    XXXXXXXXXXXXXX (4)
06
07        UNIT OF MEASURE: XXXXXXXXXX          LIFETIME TIL SPOILAGE: ZZ9
08                            (9)                                     (13)
09 QUANTITY  QUANTITY  REORDER  REORDER   AVG USAGE  USAGE PAST  USAGE LAST
10 ON HAND   ON ORDER  POINT    QUANTITY  PER MONTH  WEEK        MONTH
11
12 ZZ,ZZ9    ZZ,ZZ9    ZZ,ZZ9   ZZ,ZZ9    ZZZ,ZZ9    ZZ,ZZ9      ZZZ,ZZ9
13  (5)       (6)       (7)      (8)       (10)       (11)        (12)
14        PEAK USAGE PERIODS: XX/XX TO XX/XX
15                              (14)      (14)
20                      ZZZZ9
21                      XXXXXXXXXXXXXX
23                                XXXXXXXXXX                        ZZ9
24 PRESS "F1" FOR ADDITIONAL INFO.    PRESS "F2" TO SEE PREVIOUS INFO.
```

FUNCTION KEY ASSIGNMENTS

PF1	PAGE FORWARD	PF9		PF17	
PF2	PAGE BACKWARD	PF10		PF18	
PF3		PF11		PF19	
PF4		PF12		PF20	
PF5		PF13		PF21	
PF6		PF14		PF22	
PF7		PF15		PF23	
PF8		PF16		PF24	

DISPLAY LAYOUT CHART

◀ Figure 5.6

A printer spacing chart, record layout chart, and display layout chart. Printer spacing charts are used to format computer-generated reports and documents. Record layout charts are used to lay out the contents of computer files and input records. Display layout charts are used to show what terminal screens will look like. All of these tools are used to communicate system specifications to the computer programmer.

You will also need to design the layout and structure of computer files and inputs. In Chapter 12, you'll learn about record layout charts (Figure 5.6) as a tool for documenting file designs. Input design may involve the design of forms on which data can be captured and the design of the input media (card, tape, disk, and the like). You'll learn all about input design in Chapter 13. If data are to be input via CRT terminals, you will need to design a friendly dialogue between the computer and the user. Display layout charts (Figure 5.6) are used to communicate the layout of terminal screens in a computer dialogue. You'll learn how to design friendly computer terminal dialogues in Chapter 14.

Finally, methods and procedures must be designed for the computerized aspects of the new system. Files must be backed up. Controls must be designed. Methods and procedures for computer processing are normally documented using system flowcharts (Chapter 15). To complete the design, computer program specifications that integrate all of the documentation just mentioned into a package of specifications for the programmer must be prepared. You'll learn this skill in Chapter 16. Program specifications should include the input, output, and file layouts as well as descriptions of each program's processing requirements.

The **design phase** should be somewhat familiar to those of you who are programmers. The specifications you work from are one of the products of the design phase. You may have found yourself redoing those specifications when they were incomplete or unclear. The design phase of the SDLC is the most typical entry-level analyst assignment. This makes sense because most analysts come from the programmer ranks and have at least seen design specifications, which are the output of the design phase.

And our architect can similarly design or blueprint a house to fulfill the homeowner's requirements.

Construct the New System Now we come to the SDLC phase with which you are probably most familiar: Construct the new system. Actually, you are most familiar with the principal activity of this phase, computer programming. The **construction phase** is frequently the most time-consuming and tedious phase of the life cycle. However, the time required for construction is often longer than it should be because the preceding phases were completed hastily or not at all. Programmers work from specifications that have been developed and refined through the study, definition, evaluation, and design phases. If the specifications are unclear, incomplete, inaccurate, or otherwise faulty, the construction phase will be complicated and time consuming! The output of this phase is computer programs that execute properly for our new inventory control system.

Alternatively, the construction phase may involve installation of purchased software packages. These packages, which were chosen during the selection phase, often must be modified to properly execute on your computer system.

Note that, in the construction phase, the principal figure is the programmer, not the analyst. If the analyst and programmer are not one and the same, the analyst is still involved to the extent that specifications may need to be clarified—the perfect specification probably doesn't exist. And just as the programmer replaces the analyst as the principal figure during information system construction, the contractor replaces the architect as the principal figure during house construction. The house is constructed according to the architect's blueprints.

Deliver the New System You've designed and constructed your new inventory control system. What's left to do? Now we must deliver the new system to our users: the clerks, cashiers, and store managers. What's so significant about the **delivery phase?** Remember, the new system solution represents a departure from the way things are currently done. You need to provide for a smooth transition or conversion from the old system to the new system and help the users cope with normal start-up problems. You may have to convert old file systems to new file systems. You will have to prepare user documentation and train the users.

That's just about it for the basic SDLC. The similarity between our SDLC and the design and construction of a house is striking, don't you agree? But the parallels are not mere coincidence. You see, we cannot take full credit for our SDLC. Then again, neither can the housing industry. Both the inventory control system project and the house project were problems. We wanted something we didn't have. Our SDLC and the house-building process are instances of a basic problem-solving process. Compare, for instance, the SDLC presented in Figure 5.1 with the building construction life cycle depicted in Figure 5.7. They are more alike than different.

You have just learned a basic system development life cycle. And as we saw in our Americana Plastics minicase, the need for an SDLC is independent of the size of computer to be used. In reality, the phases are not strictly sequential. There are opportunities for overlap, and we'll evaluate those opportunities in the next section of this chapter. And we acknowledge that we will have to backtrack through some phases when errors and oversights are identified. But the general flow through the SDLC is sequential.

Overlapping the Work Within the Phases

We have already learned that at any point in time, you may have to go backward in the SDLC to correct a mistake or oversight. This is unavoidable because we cannot be perfect. As a matter of fact, this is preferable because it improves the chances that we will discover errors *before* they become more expensive to correct. On the other hand, we've also stated that there are opportunities for working ahead in the life cycle and for overlapping two or more phases.

The opportunities for overlap within the phases are shown in Figure 5.8. This diagram, called a *Gantt chart,* clearly depicts opportunities for overlapping phases within our life cycle. A Gantt chart only shows *opportunities* for overlap. The ability to overlap phases will depend, to a great extent, on the size and complexity of the project and the number of analysts and programmers assigned to it. Let's take a look at some of these opportunities.

The Survey, Study, and Definition Phases We cannot recommend that the survey and study phases of the SDLC be overlapped. The entire purpose of the survey phase is to determine whether to commit resources to the study phase. Thus, we see that the survey and study phases are truly sequential.

Similarly, we cannot recommend that the study phase overlap the definition phase. It is extremely important that the final solution address the correct problems, opportunities, and directives. We cannot assume that the problems originally stated by the user are the critical problems. After studying the existing system, we

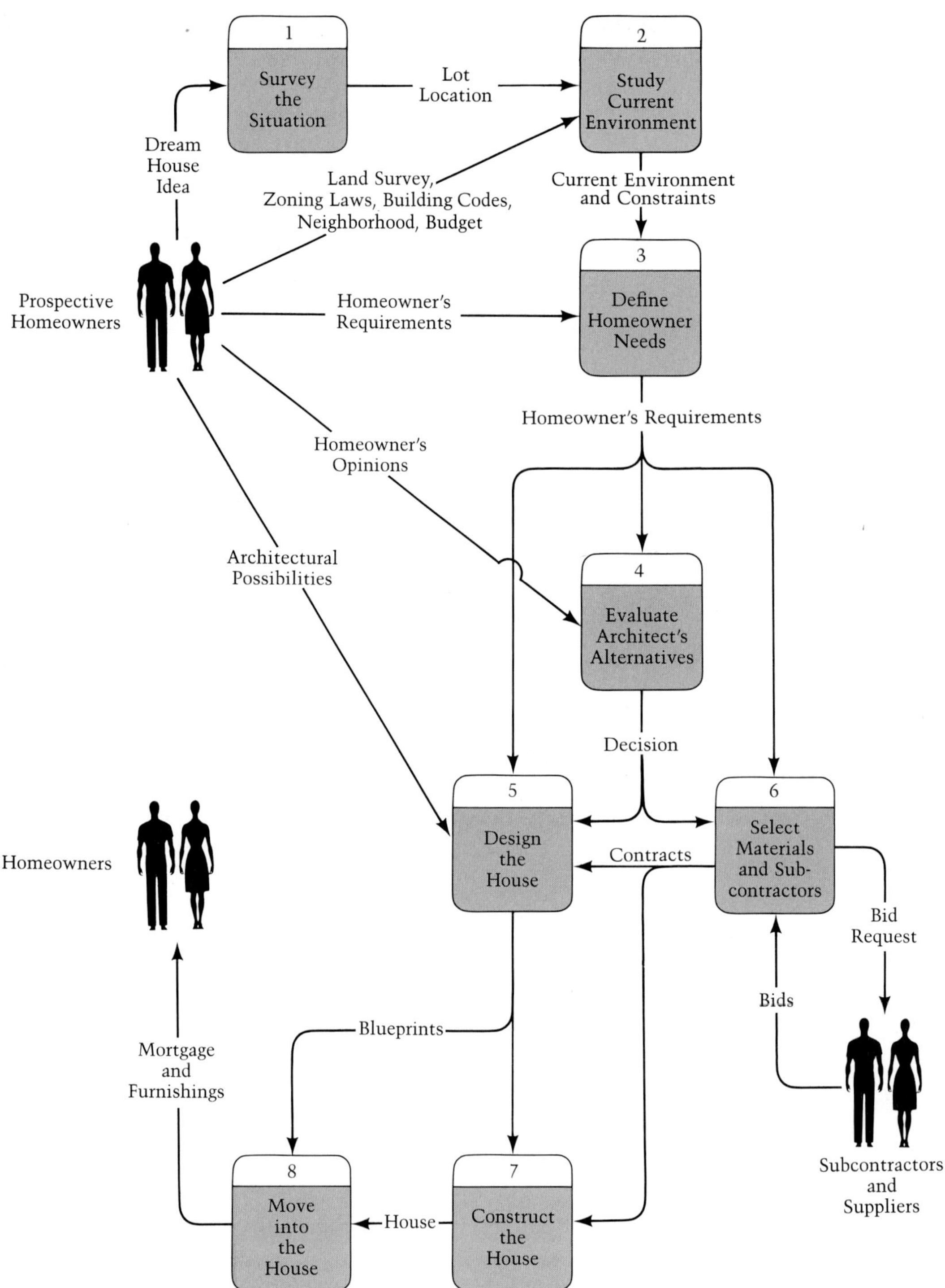
1
Survey the Situation
Lot Location
2
Study Current Environment
Dream House Idea
Land Survey, Zoning Laws, Building Codes, Neighborhood, Budget
Current Environment and Constraints
3
Define Homeowner Needs
Prospective Homeowners
Homeowner's Requirements
Homeowner's Requirements
Homeowner's Opinions
Architectural Possibilities
4
Evaluate Architect's Alternatives
Decision
5
Design the House
6
Select Materials and Sub-contractors
Contracts
Homeowners
Bid Request
Bids
Blueprints
Mortgage and Furnishings
Subcontractors and Suppliers
8
Move into the House
House
7
Construct the House

often find that the original problem is only a net effect or symptom of a more critical problem. The study phase defines the scope and magnitude of the project and should be completed before starting the definition phase.

The Definition, Design, and Evaluation Phases These three phases present numerous opportunities for overlap. As Figure 5.8 shows, the definition of user requirements must be somewhat complete before alternative computer and manual solutions can be evaluated. But notice that the evaluation of alternatives should be completed *before* any design work is done. Why? Design specifications are

◀ **Figure 5.7**

House-building example. Notice the similarities between our information systems development cycle and the activities required to build a house. The similarities are not coincidental. Both cycles represent problem-solving processes.

Figure 5.8 ▼

Opportunities to overlap SDLC phases. This chart depicts opportunities to overlap systems development phases. The horizontal axis is time. The phases are represented by bars. Where the bars overlap, the phases overlap. The actual overlap in any given project is dependent on the project's size and the resources committed to the project.

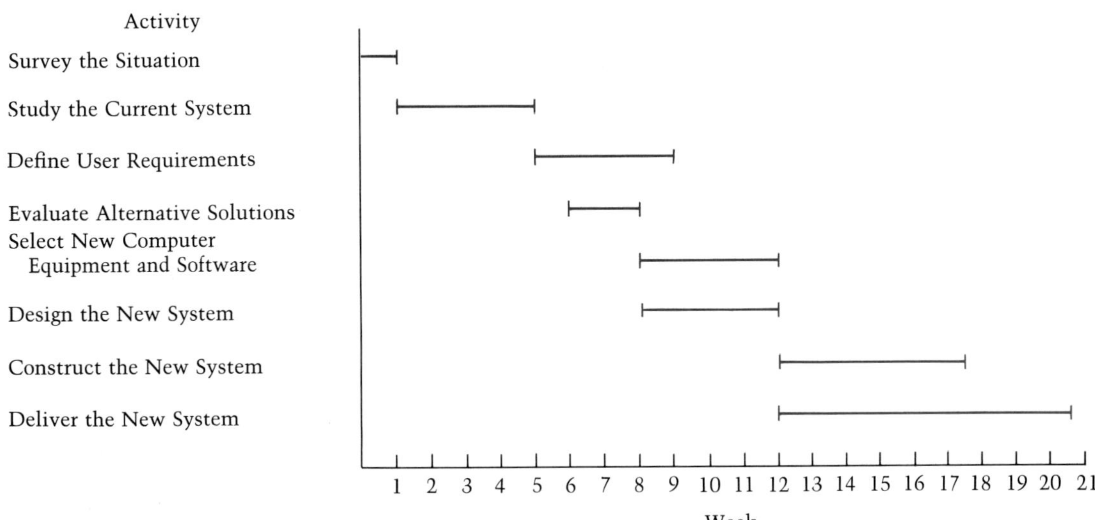

dependent on the decisions made during the evaluation phase. On the other hand, notice that once the evaluation phase has been completed, the definition and design phases can overlap. For example, it only makes sense that after we *define* a report we can *design* that report, even if the definition phase is not fully complete. It is important to realize, however, that the design of any component is subject to change until the requirements definition is complete and verified.

The Design and Selection Phases Computer equipment and software certainly can be selected, ordered, and installed while you are designing a new system. In fact, this is desirable because you would like to have the technology available by the time you complete the design. However, you need to recognize that the computer technology selected may impact the design of the system. For example, the selection of a terminal may affect the number of characters that can be displayed on the screen at any one time. This would certainly affect the design of terminal dialogue! Thus, the design and selection phases of our life cycle should nearly always overlap.

The Design and Construction Phases Generally speaking, however, the design specifications should be completed before the construction phase begins. We should avoid the temptation to program from incomplete specifications — such an approach causes numerous delays because programmers constantly find themselves accommodating change and correcting mistakes. The exception to this rule is properly conceived prototyping, which we discuss in the "Next Generation" feature for this chapter.

The Construction and Delivery Phases The construction and delivery phases always overlap. While the programmers are constructing the new system, the systems analysts can be preparing for final delivery. Specifically, the analysts can be writing user documentation and training manuals. Training courses can be taught. The implementation plan can be developed as can a final system test to ensure the system is ready to go. Obviously, the construction phase will end before the delivery phase ends because delivery isn't complete without properly executing programs.

IMPLEMENTING THE SYSTEMS DEVELOPMENT LIFE CYCLE

So now you'll be able to deal with any business's or book's SDLC, right? Well, not exactly. Earlier, we stated that there are as many SDLCs as there are authors and businesses. What we have given you is a powerful, basic SDLC. Each real-world SDLC will seem to be different, perhaps vastly different. How can you evaluate a real SDLC? First, you should look for false or *phantom* phases that show up in many life cycles. Second, any given SDLC is subject to modifications based on *systems development methodologies* that are in use at the time. The final evaluation, however, can be made by checking the SDLC against the seven system development principles you learned in Chapter 4. Let's examine all of these issues.

Phantom Phases: Activities That Overlap the Entire SDLC

If you have encountered any other SDLC, you may have noted that we did not include specific phases for:

- Fact finding
- Documentation and presentations
- Feasibility study

We left these activities out of the phased life cycle because they are phantom phases — they do not exist, at least, not as phases. These phantom phases are actually ongoing activities during the SDLC. Let's briefly examine each of these activities.

Fact Finding You may frequently encounter a phase called *fact finding* or *data collection* in an actual SDLC. The intent of such a phase is sincere: the analyst must collect facts about a system in order to document and analyze that system. Typically, if there is a fact-finding phase, it is inserted prior to what we call the *study phase* in our life cycle. This is inappropriate because fact finding actually occurs during several phases of the life cycle. Specifically, the analyst employs fact-finding techniques during the following phases:

- *Survey phase.* The analyst collects general facts about the problems, opportunities, directives, environment, knowledge workers, and so forth.
- *Study phase.* The analyst collects facts about how the current system functions.
- *Definition phase.* The analyst collects facts about the user's requirements and performance expectations.
- *Design phase.* The analyst collects facts about the user's preferences regarding format of reports, format of input documents, and dialogue between the computer and user.

Obviously, fact finding is an activity that overlaps many phases of our SDLC.

Documentation and Presentation Be wary of any life cycle with a documentation phase! It is a trap. A documentation phase supports the postdocumentation syndrome we talked about in Chapter 4. If you study Figure 5.1 carefully, you will see that documentation and presentations are clearly by-products of each and every phase. Each named arrow on the diagram represents documentation. Documentation *is* the life cycle, in a very real sense. Documentation provides continuity from one phase to the next. It is the standard against which we measure progress.

People don't like to document. The activity is time consuming. How much should you document? If you prepare too little documentation, you'll have to depend on verbal communication and memory and misunderstandings can occur. If you produce too much documentation, you'll slow down progress. Nobody wants to read a huge book full of specifications. You need to strike a balance (as with most things in life). Documentation and presentations are best served in small to medium-sized doses; a report here, a presentation there — not all at once.

Feasibility Study Earlier in this chapter, we stated that many organizations preface the SDLC with a feasibility study phase. We feel that this approach results in an overcommitment to the project. If we are so accurate in our feasibility estimates, why are so many information system projects late and over budget? Too many projects call for premature system development estimates. Systems analysts tend to be over optimistic during the early stages of a project. They underestimate the size and scope of a project because they haven't yet completed a detailed study. Many costs are out of their control. For this reason, we have suggested the creeping commitment approach that reevaluates feasibility at appropriate checkpoints during the SDLC (these checkpoints are indicated by diamonds in Figure 5.1).

We have seen that documentation, presentations, and feasibility analysis are ongoing activities of the SDLC, as illustrated in Figure 5.9 (p. 162). Are there any other ongoing activities? We can think of at least one, *project management.* Systems development projects frequently involve a large number of analysts and programmers who work together as a team. Project management is the ongoing process by which the team leader directs the team to develop an acceptable system within the allotted time and budget.

All of these ongoing activities of systems development are discussed in the *Modules* that make up Part IV of the book. These modules are:

Module A — Project Management

Module B — Fact Finding

Module C — Presentations (oral and written)

Module D — Cost/Benefit and Feasibility Analysis

As soon as you've completed this chapter, you will have sufficient background to study any of the modules, in any order. You may study entire modules or parts of modules.

Systems Development Methodologies — What Are They?

The systems development life cycle is a general process to follow when building information systems. The key word here is *general.* Systems development **methodologies** (SDMs) get more specific. An SDM is a specific, step-by-step strategy for completing one or more phases of the life cycle. Methodologies impose their own tools and standards on the SDLC. Some methodologies are available through textbooks. Others must be purchased from consulting firms. We have found that most methodologies can be classified according to which phases of the SDLC they emphasize. Let's take a brief look at systems development methodologies and how they should be used. Most methodologies tend to place emphasis on either *systems analysis, systems design,* or *systems implementation,* as they are defined in Figure 5.10 (p. 164).

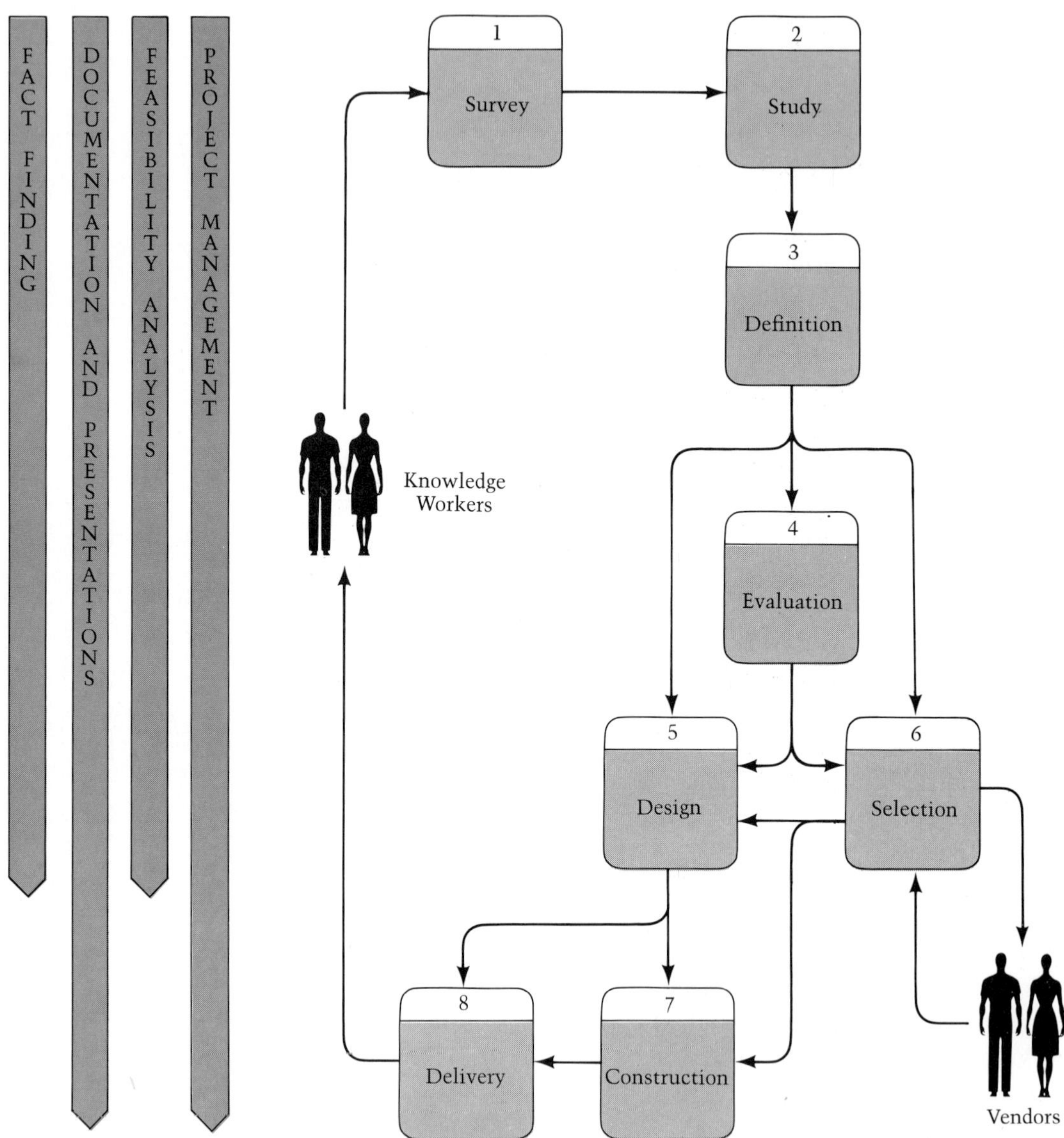

Figure 5.9

Activities that overlap several phases of the SDLC. Fact finding, documentation, presentations, feasibility analysis, and project management are activities that overlap several phases of the SDLC. The overlapping is depicted by bars that run in parallel with the SDLC phases on the right-hand side of the page.

Systems Analysis and Analysis-Oriented Methodologies Analysis-oriented methodologies have become very popular in recent years. Structured Analysis and Design, Information Modeling, and Information Engineering are popular methodologies that place greater emphasis on the systems analysis phases: study, definition, and evaluation. Advocates of analysis-oriented methodologies believe that user requirements can be specified in considerable detail. **Structured Analysis and Design** emphasizes the specification of what we called *information requirements.* **Information Modeling** and **Information Engineering** emphasize the specification of what we called *data requirements.* By spending more time in the analysis phases, advocates claim that design and implementation will go faster and result in better systems.

Systems Design and Design-Oriented Methodologies We included a design phase in our life cycle. Most early information systems and business data processing systems were developed with design-oriented methodologies. Design-oriented methods place systems emphasis on the design and construction phases. Minimal time is spent on the study, definition, and evaluation phases. Most early methodologies emphasized design because the analyst's tools were very computer-oriented. Because very few tools existed for the analysis phases, these phases were done quickly and documented narratively. The design-oriented approaches suffered from this lack of adequate analysis. As a result, considerable design and construction time is wasted to clarify problems and requirements that could not be or were not adequately specified during the analysis phases.

Systems Implementation and Implementation-Oriented Methodologies Implementation-oriented methodologies place greater emphasis on the systems implementation phases: construction and delivery. Considerable attention is now being paid to a new class of methodologies built on the concept of prototyping. **Prototyping** is an implementation-oriented approach because it aims, in a sense, to bypass design by quickly constructing a working prototype of the system. Details can be filled in after the prototype is approved by the users. For more about prototyping, see the "Next Generation" feature for this chapter.

The Problem with Methodologies Methodologies are the snake oil of the data processing business. We are constantly being introduced to the latest, greatest methodology for developing improved sys-

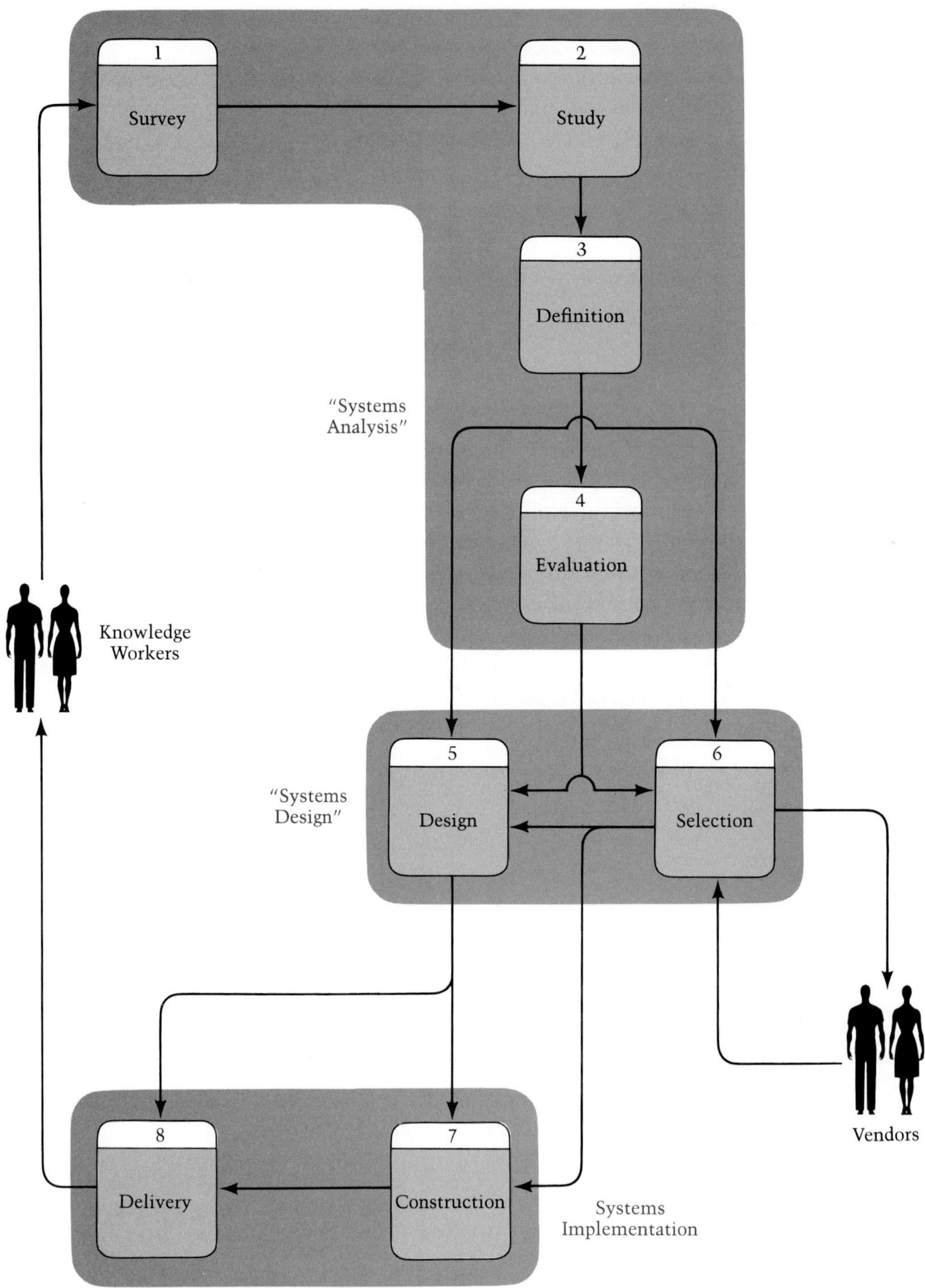
1
Survey
2
Study
3
Definition
"Systems
Analysis"
4
Evaluation
Knowledge
Workers
5
Design
6
Selection
"Systems
Design"
Vendors
8
Delivery
7
Construction
Systems
Implementation

◀ **Figure 5.10**

What are systems analysis, systems design, and systems implementation? The terms *systems analysis, systems design,* and *systems implementation* have numerous meanings. For purposes of this book, we use the definitions implied by this diagram. Systems analysis consists of the study, definition, and evaluation phases. Systems design refers to the design and selection phases. Finally, systems implementation includes the construction and delivery phases.

tems with lower costs and on time! Be careful. Most methodologies have something to offer, but you should not become a diehard devotee to any one of them. No single methodology can be all things to all people! Consequently, this book advocates no specific methodology. Instead, we present some of the successful tools utilized by the traditional design-oriented methodologies and by the currently popular analysis-oriented methodologies. Several of the "Next Generation" features highlight our expectations of implementation-oriented tools. Tools can complement each other. Regardless of which methodology you use, each tool fulfills a role in the systems development process.

After you have mastered the concepts, tools, and techniques presented in this book, you should study specific methodologies. We hope that you will then adapt these methodologies to the situations you encounter. You should look for opportunities to integrate old and new tools and techniques, just as we have. And you can integrate your methodologies right into the SDLC. Systems development is more satisfying and successful when you understand what you're doing and why.

How to Evaluate a Systems Development Life Cycle

One way to evaluate an SDLC, including ours, is to judge it against the seven systems development principles you learned in Chapter 4. In fact, we'll evaluate our SDLC against those principles right here. Refer back to Figure 5.1 during this evaluation.

The system is for the knowledge workers. The knowledge worker is part of the existing information system (recall the pyramid). Notice the interaction with the knowledge workers (for instance *facts, requirements, opinions*). Our SDLC does encourage user participation!

The Next Generation

Prototyping—The Fourth-Generation Methodology

Prototyping is one systems development methodology that is gaining rapid acceptance. Prototyping, an engineering-inspired approach to systems analysis, represents an interesting variation on our traditional systems development life cycle. Emphasis is placed on constructing a working model of the final system as quickly as possible. That model is called a *prototype.* The prototype system can be reviewed with users to determine if it is appropriate and adequate. If not, the prototype can be discarded (because it didn't take a lot of time to build) or modified. Gradually, the prototype is transformed into the final system.

Figure A illustrates the prototype methodology using our SDLC. Notice that the phases have been resequenced. The study phase is followed by the evaluation phase. The evaluation of alternatives is based on a very high-level set of objectives and requirements that were listed during the study phase. Notice that the construction phase incorporates what we have called the definition and design phases. In other words, the definition and design phases are accomplished by constructing the prototype—hence this approach has been called *design by prototyping.* Also notice that the prototype has replaced the more traditional paper documentation, namely the requirements statement and design specifications. The prototype is reviewed by the users, changes are noted, and a new prototype is developed. This might be called a *prototype loop.* Because documentation is still important, analysts should discipline themselves to develop comprehensive documentation during the delivery phase.

Why has prototyping only recently emerged as a viable methodology? For many years, most computer programming was done in languages like COBOL, FORTRAN, PL/I, and with the advent of microcomputers, BASIC. These languages are not suited to prototyping because prototypes developed with these languages take too long to develop. The structure and logic of the programs must be determined. Coding and debugging of the programs is usually time consuming. And as anyone who has done maintenance programming can testify, changes to the programs can be even more time consuming. The prototype approach accepts the necessity of change! It is assumed that the first prototype will require changes, and so will the second, and so on, until the system is accepted by the user. Thus, traditional languages served as a roadblock to prototyping.

Today, we are seeing new and exciting languages—often called **fourth-generation languages**—that are suitable for prototyping. Examples of these languages include FOCUS, RAMIS, DBASE III, and USER-11. End users are said to be able to write their own programs in these languages. That may be true for writing simple programs to generate new reports. However, the most significant trend is the use of these languages by systems analysts to rapidly develop prototypes of complete information systems. Analysts are trained to maintain a systems perspective and ensure that all aspects of the system (for instance, data maintenance and file backup) are properly developed. They can use prototyping to significantly decrease the time required to develop an information system.

When a prototype has been completed and approved, the analyst is faced with a decision. If the prototype, writ-

(continues on p. 168) ▸

The Next Generation (continued)

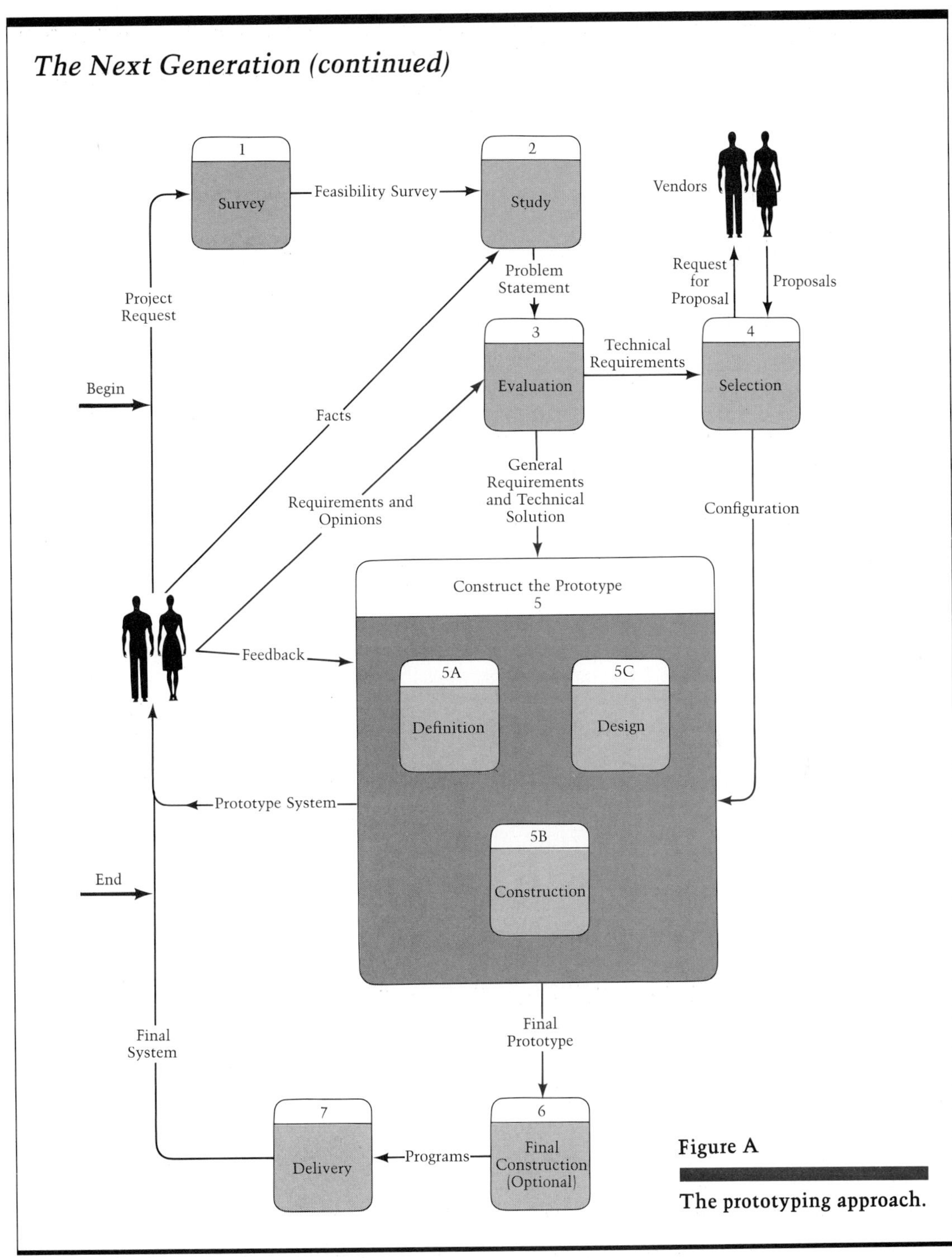

Figure A

The prototyping approach.

The Next Generation (continued)

ten in one of the prototype languages, is not efficient enough to be placed into operation, the analyst will have programmers rewrite the prototype in a more traditional and efficient language (such as COBOL). Otherwise, the prototype can actually become the programs employed by the end user.

One word of caution is in order: Prototyping should not be used as a shortcut for systems development. Unless the study phase is completed, the wrong problems can still be solved—just as can happen in a more traditional methodology. Also, unless alternatives are analyzed, the final solution may not be the best solution. And finally, remember that the prototype represents only two components of the information system: hardware and software. The analyst must still carefully consider the knowledge-worker, methods-and-procedures, and internal-controls components.

Prototyping is said to be the methodology of the future. In reality, you should probably aim to combine the best advantages of this approach with the best features of other methodologies. In any case, increased use of prototyping is inevitable. With the growing shortage of programmers and analysts, we must use any approach that can increase the productivity of those of us who have chosen to become computer professionals. Otherwise, management will be forced to look for a way to replace us! ■

People education is essential. Education is a two-way street. During the survey, study, and definition phases, the users are educating the analysts (concerning, for instance, *problems, facts,* and *requirements*). During the evaluation, design, and delivery phases, the analyst is educating the users (concerning, for example, *possibilities, implications,* and *training*). Thus, the education principle permeates our entire SDLC.

Establish phases and tasks. The phases of our life cycle have been discussed throughout this chapter. The tasks that comprise the various phases are discussed in Chapters 6, 10, and 17.

Phases and tasks are not necessarily sequential. Take another look at Figure 5.8. Clearly, our life cycle recognizes the opportunities to overlap phases.

Information systems are capital investments and *Don't be afraid to cancel.* These two principles are reflected in the many checkpoints installed in our SDLC (remember, the checkpoints are represented by diamonds on Figure 5.1). Each checkpoint gives us an opportunity to reevaluate feasibility and cancel the project.

Documentation should guide systems development. Every arrow on Figure 5.1 is irrefutable evidence of working documentation in our SDLC. The better part of the remainder of this book will develop your skills with the documentation tools!

Thus, our SDLC stacks up pretty well against the seven system development principles. Use these principles to evaluate and modify any SDLC you might encounter.

SUMMARY

A systems development life cycle (SDLC) is a disciplined approach to developing information systems. Given a problem, opportunity, or directive, a problem-solving approach can be used for an SDLC. Initially, the analyst should survey the situation.The purpose of the survey phase is to determine if system development resources should be committed to the project. Next, the analysts will study the current system. This is a detailed study of the current business environment to analyze the problems, opportunities, and directives. Once the current system is fully understood, the next phase is to define user requirements. User requirements are specified independently of the alternative ways that the computer might be used. Given the user requirements, the analysts can evaluate alternative solutions. Solutions are evaluated on the basis of *technical, operational,* and *economic* feasibility. If new computer hardware or software is required, the analysts may have to select new computer technology, interacting with computer vendors to select the best technology for the best price. At this stage of a typical project, the analysts can design the new system to fulfill user requirements and provide the most feasible solution. Then comes construction of the new system. This is the phase of the life cycle during which computer programs are written or modified. Finally, the analysts and programmers must deliver the new system, training users and providing for a smooth transition from the old system to the new system.

The implementation of an SDLC can introduce a number of variations on the basic life cycle. The analyst should be aware that certain false phases are part of many real-life SDLCs. For instance, fact finding, documentation and presentation, feasibility analysis, and project management phases are included in many SDLCs. In reality, these phantom phases are ongoing activities of the life cycle, not phases. SDLCs can also be modified to incorporate one or more systems development methodologies, which are step-by-step strategies for implementing the phases of the SDLC. Methodologies can be classified according to the phases they emphasize. Be careful not to become a diehard advocate of any methodology! No methodology can be all things to all people. The best way to evaluate any SDLC implementation is to judge it according to the seven principles of systems development that were introduced in Chapter 4.

PROBLEMS AND EXERCISES

1. Assume you are given a program assignment that requires you to make some modifications to a computer program. Explain the problem-solving approach you would go through. How is this approach similar to the phased approach of the systems development life cycle presented in this chapter? Are there any false phases incorporated in your problem-solving approach?
2. Which phases of the SDLC presented in this chapter do the following tasks characterize?
   (a) The physical layout of an employee master record is determined by the systems analyst.
   (b) The systems analyst observes the order-entry clerks to determine how customer orders are processed.
   (c) A systems analyst is demonstrating how the accounts payable manager can use the CRT to obtain information concerning a particular invoice.
   (d) The accounts receivable manager is describing a new summary report the systems analyst is being asked to have the new computerized billing system prepare.
   (e) The systems analyst is reviewing the company's organizational chart to identify the knowledge workers of an information system that is slated for improvement.
   (f) The systems analyst is brainstorming to identify ways to use the computer to generate purchase orders for the Inventory Control Department.

(g) A computer programmer is writing a data editing routine in COBOL.

(h) The systems analyst is comparing a variety of microcomputers and available software.

3. Visit a local data processing installation. Characterize the SDLC that the company follows when developing information systems. Compare that SDLC with the one introduced in this chapter. What phases in this chapter's SDLC represent analysis, design, and implementation phases of the local company's SDLC? Evaluate the company's SDLC with respect to the seven systems development principles presented in Chapter 4. Can you identify any false phases in the SDLC?

4. As an alternative to exercise three, substitute the SDLC used in another systems analysis and design textbook.

5. How would you defend the *creeping commitment* approach of an SDLC to top-level management who are primarily concerned with knowing the cost feasibility of a project up front?

6. Take one of the problem situations presented in Problem 6 for Chapter 4. You are an independent consultant. Write a letter of proposal that offers your services as a systems analyst and programmer to help solve the problem. Your client, who is skeptical of all computer-type people, is turned off by computer buzzwords. Be sure your proposal explains, step-by-step, how you will build a system that meets this client's needs.

7. You have a client who has a history of impatience, encouraging shortcuts through the systems development life cycle and then blaming the analyst for systems that fail to fulfill expectations. By now, you should understand the phased approach to systems development. For each phase, compile a list of consequences that you will present to the client when he suggests a shortcut through or around that phase.

8. The Stores and Supplies manager is tired of waiting on Data Processing to get around to building information systems for her needs. So she bought a personal computer along with a spreadsheet, a database, and word processing software. With these tools in hand, she plans to develop her own systems. Her strategy will be to learn how to program using the database and spreadsheet. The word processor is just for office writing needs. A data processing systems analyst has suggested she take a systems

analysis and design course before beginning to use the spreadsheet and database. The local computer store says she doesn't need any systems analysis and design training to be able to develop systems using the spreadsheet and database programs. Is the computer store correct? Why or why not? Can you convince her to take the systems analysis and design course? What would your arguments be?

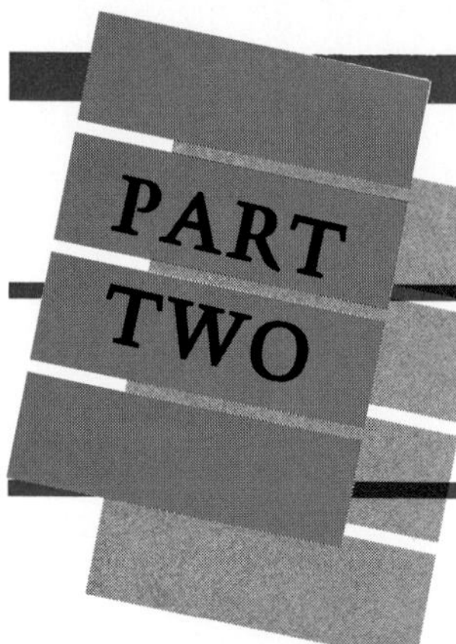

Systems Analysis Tools and Techniques

Systems analysis—a process performed by many but practiced by few. Does that sound like a contradiction? It really isn't. Systems analysis is considered an essential activity by most data processing professionals. However, few of those professionals practice systems analysis with rigor or according to well-defined standards. Why? Simply stated, because they don't know how. We tend to spend the least time on those activities with which we are the least familiar, no matter how important they are! How important is systems analysis?

Systems analysis is the most critical process of information systems development. It is during systems analysis that we learn about the existing business system, come to understand problems, define objectives and priorities for improvement, define business requirements, and evaluate alternative solutions. Clearly, the quality of the subsequent systems design and implementation is dependent on a good systems analysis. In fact, the best technical design and implementation is useless if it doesn't solve the correct problems, fulfill objectives, and meet requirements in a cost-effective fashion! So why is systems analysis the most short-changed of the systems development processes? Because most analysts are not well schooled in use of systems analysis tools and techniques, that's why!

The purpose of this unit is to introduce you to the systems analysis process and to some useful tools and techniques for performing that process. Four chapters make up this unit. The first chapter introduces the systems analysis process. That process consists of the four phases: survey, study, definition, and evaluation.

The next three chapters develop systems analysis skills in use of tools and techniques that are especially useful during systems analysis. These three chapters develop expertise with the following tools: hierarchy charts, data flow diagrams, data dictionaries, Structured English, and decision tables. Hierarchy charts are useful for breaking a system into subsystems and tasks for easier understanding. Data flow diagrams depict information system problems and solutions in terms of the flow of data through the system and the work performed on that data. Data dictionaries document the content and structure of data and information in a system. Finally, Structured English and decision tables are useful for documenting business policies and procedures. Although none of these tools are exclusive to the systems analysis process, they are most useful to it. We will also examine possible uses for systems design and implementation.

In addition to hierarchy charts, data flow diagrams, data dictionaries, Structured English, and decision tables, you may elect to skim or read (or you may be assigned one or more) of the modules in Part IV. These modules survey skills that are not restrictive to the systems analysis process but that are nevertheless extremely important to effective systems analysis.

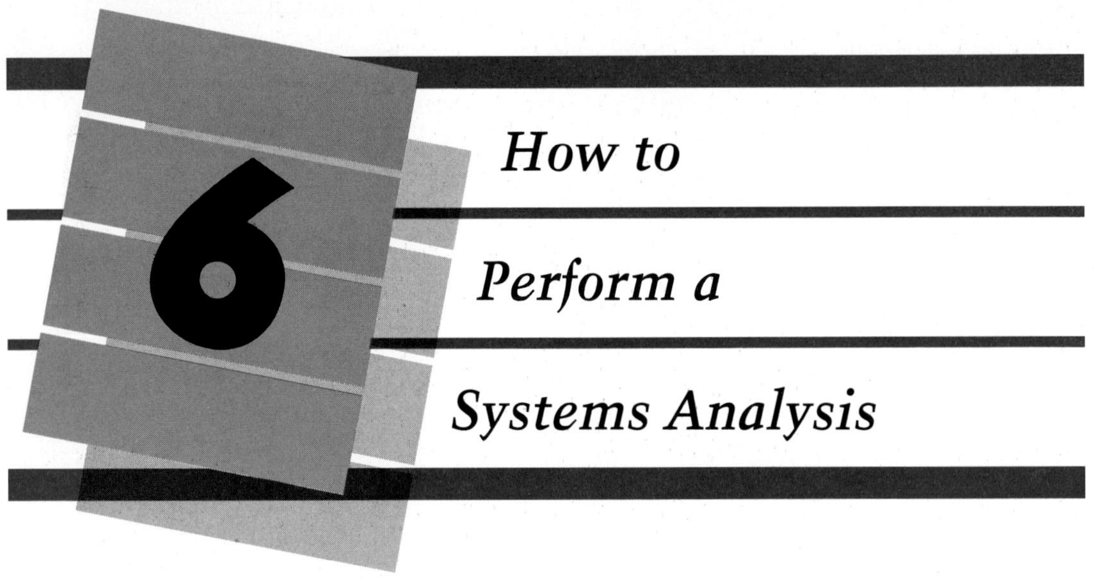

6 How to Perform a Systems Analysis

Minicase: Transport Pipe Company

Ken Hayes, the MIS manager at Transport Pipe Company, is conducting an annual performance review on Tim Stallard, one of his computer programmers. Tim received high praise for the work he'd done and was assured that a good pay raise would be coming. Near the end of their meeting Ken asked Tim what his career goals were. Let's listen in on the conversation that followed.

"I want to be promoted to systems analyst," Tim said as he slid forward to the edge of his chair. He had been looking forward to this opportunity to discuss his career. "I've been a programmer for five years now, and a darn good one I might add. I know I could do as good a job as your current analysts in preparing the systems design documentation."

Ken was quick to correct Tim. "A systems analyst does a lot more than simply document the design of an information system.

That design documentation you've been receiving is the end product of a very difficult and time-consuming process called *systems design*. But another process takes place before the systems analyst really begins systems design. That process is systems analysis. All of our systems analysts are required to spend a minimum of 50 percent of the allotted system project time doing systems analysis. What do you know about systems analysis?"

"That's where the systems analyst deals with the users to determine what their needs are. I'm sure that must be difficult because most users don't know anything about computers."

"On the contrary, we've found that more and more users are fairly knowledgeable about computing," Ken responded. "Besides, the users do have knowledge about something that is much more important than the computer—they know about their business operations. That knowledge is the focus during the analysis process. If our analyst doesn't obtain a clear understanding of the business as it pertains to the user, the chances of successfully identifying the user's problems and needs and implementing a new and improved information system are greatly reduced."

Ken realized that Tim's understanding of a systems analyst's job was restricted to his personal experience—to the interactions that take place between programmer and systems analyst. "You see we have our analysts go through a number of well-defined phases when they perform systems analysis for a systems project. Each phase serves a specific purpose. Let me pose a situation to you, and you tell me what your actions would be. A user confronts you with a problem in a particular area and asks you to solve the problem by automating a portion of his or her operations. What would you do?"

Tim thought for a moment and responded. "The first thing I would do is what we just talked about. I would meet with the user to obtain an understanding of the operations involved and how the computer could be used. Then I would prepare the systems design documentation for the programs so the new system could be programmed."

Ken replied, "You make it sound very simple. Let me ask you a few more questions. We receive a number of system project requests each day. We have limited resources and time. Would you implement each of the requests?"

"Obviously not." Tim realized he had jumped the gun. "I assume each would have to be evaluated and prioritized."

"Correct," Ken assured Tim. "We'd require you to perform the first of several feasibility assessments on the project. You'd be required to do a cost/benefit analysis, something that is repeated several times during analysis and design. Have you ever done a cost/benefit analysis?"

"No, but I'm sure I could learn," answered Tim.

Ken continued, "If the project proves feasible, what would you do?"

"Well," answered Tim, "I'd thoroughly study the business application, especially since I'm not a business expert. I'd try to determine what improvements are needed and how the users want to utilize the computer."

Ken interrupted, "What if the problems turn out to be more extensive or different than you or the users initially believed?"

"Does that happen very often?" asked Tim. Noting Ken's nod that it happens often enough, Tim went on, "Then I'd have to suggest a different or more extensive solution than the user initially suggested."

"But that could be more costly!" replied Ken.

"But the benefits may be greater also. I guess I'd have to reassess the cost/benefit situation at this point, huh?"

"You got it!" Ken exclaimed, pleased that Tim seemed to appreciate the activities the analyst must perform during systems analysis. "Some alternatives may not even involve a computer solution. Do you think you can exercise the creativity I expect of our analysts to envision solutions and assess their feasibility?"

"I understand what you've been saying," said Tim. "There's much I will have to learn, but yes, I think I can do it."

"I do too!" Ken stated encouragingly. "Tell you what I'm going to do. I just received this brochure offering a three-day cost/benefit analysis seminar. I'm going to send you to that seminar. I'd also like you to take our audiovisual course 'Structured Systems Analysis.' After those courses, I'll team you up with one of our senior analysts on a small project. I think we can both benefit from this career shift!"

Discussion

1. If Tim is an experienced programmer, why doesn't he know more about the job of the systems analysts he frequently deals with?

2. How would you have responded to the situation Ken posed to Tim?
3. Tim is determined to become a systems analyst. What should Tim do to help himself achieve this goal?

WHAT WILL YOU LEARN IN THIS CHAPTER?

In this chapter, you will learn more about four of the phases in the systems development life cycle: *survey, study, definition,* and *evaluation.* These four phases are collectively referred to as the systems analysis process. You will know that you understand the systems analysis process when you can:

1. Define *systems analysis* and relate the term to the survey, study, definition, and evaluation phases of the life cycle.
2. Describe the survey, study, definition, and evaluation phases of the life cycle in terms of
   (a) Purpose and objectives
   (b) Tasks or activities that must or may be performed
   (c) Skills you need to master to properly perform the phase
3. Describe the relationship between the systems analysis phases and cost/benefit analysis.
4. Explain how the time spent on systems analysis can be managed.

What is systems analysis? We already know what a system is. But what is analysis? If you consult your dictionary, you will find a definition similar to this:

> **a·nal·y·sis** 1: a separating or breaking up of any whole into its parts, esp. with an examination of these parts to find out their nature, proportion, function, interrelationship, etc. (*Webster's New World Dictionary of the American Language, Second College Edition,* Simon & Schuster, a Division of Gulf & Western Corporation, 1980)

For our purposes, *analysis* is the separation of an information system into its component parts for the purpose of identifying and evaluating problems, opportunities, constraints, and needs. But there is more to information systems analysis than just analysis.

During systems analysis, we must also identify a feasible solution to the problems and opportunities identified in the current system. In this chapter, we examine both aspects of the systems analysis process.

We examine four systems analysis phases: (1) surveying the feasibility of the project, (2) studying the current information system, (3) defining user requirements for an improved system, and (4) evaluating alternative information system solutions (see Figure 6.1). For each phase, we study the *purpose* and *objectives* of the phase, the *tasks* that should be performed, and important *skills* to be mastered. We also address the issue of cost/benefit and feasibility analysis, an important concern to management during the systems analysis phases. Finally, we discuss some project management implications of systems analysis — how to manage the time spent on analysis. Your study of skills in the subsequent chapters and modules will be easier if you understand the systems analysis process.

HOW TO SURVEY FEASIBILITY OF THE PROJECT AND STUDY THE CURRENT INFORMATION SYSTEM

An engineer would not design a bridge without thoroughly studying the environment that the new bridge will occupy. An architect would not design a building without studying the land and the laws that govern the use of that land. A good business manager will not impose numerous policy changes without understanding existing policies and their implications. Unfortunately, many data processing professionals try to build new information systems without thoroughly studying existing systems. As a result, many information systems fail to solve existing problems, meet the needs of its knowledge workers, or provide cost-effective solutions to problems.

Figure 6.1 ▶

The systems analysis process. Systems analysis is defined as the survey, study, definition, and evaluation phases of the system development life cycle.

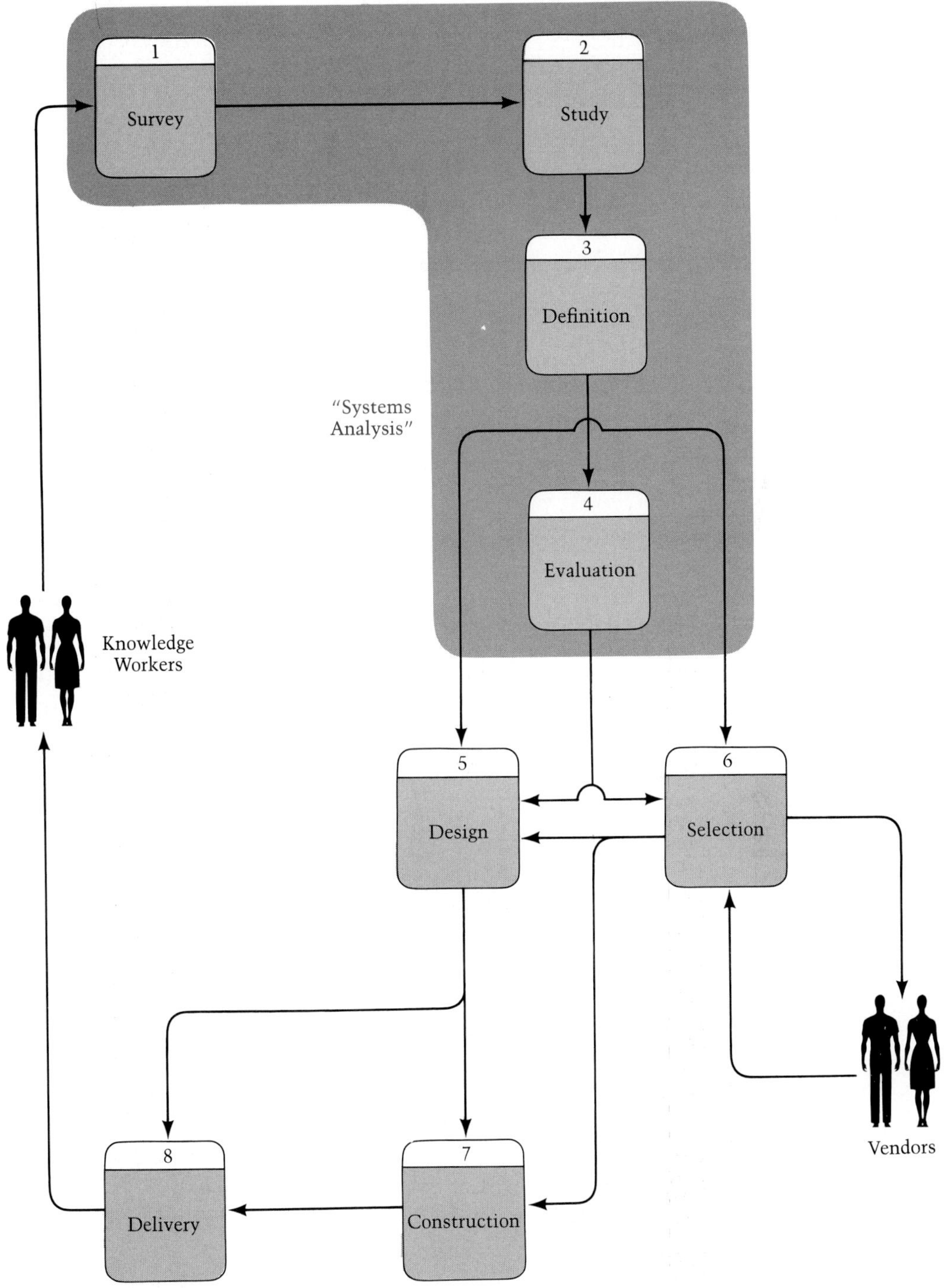
1
Survey
2
Study
3
Definition
"Systems
Analysis"
4
Evaluation
Knowledge
Workers
5
Design
6
Selection
Vendors
8
Delivery
7
Construction

Purpose and Objectives of the Survey and Study Phases

The survey and study phases serve the same basic purpose, that is, to understand the current system and its problems and to determine if solving the problems would be beneficial. The only difference between the two phases is the amount of time spent in each phase— the survey phase is a preliminary investigation of the system whereas the study phase is a much more detailed investigation. The survey phase establishes the initial feasibility of the project to determine if resources should be committed to the detailed study. Because of their similar purpose, these two phases are examined together in this section. Your information-system-pyramid model provides some specific objectives for understanding the current system. These objectives include:

- Identify all knowledge workers who use or are affected by the current system.
- Identify the purpose, goals, objectives, and policies of the current business and information systems, and analyze the extent to which this business mission is being achieved.
- Identify the information system functions provided by the current system, and analyze the extent to which these functions support the knowledge workers and the business mission.
- Separate the current information system into its components, and analyze how these components interact to provide the current information resources (notice that this goal is consistent with our classical definition of the term *analysis*).

Let's examine each of our four objectives in greater detail.

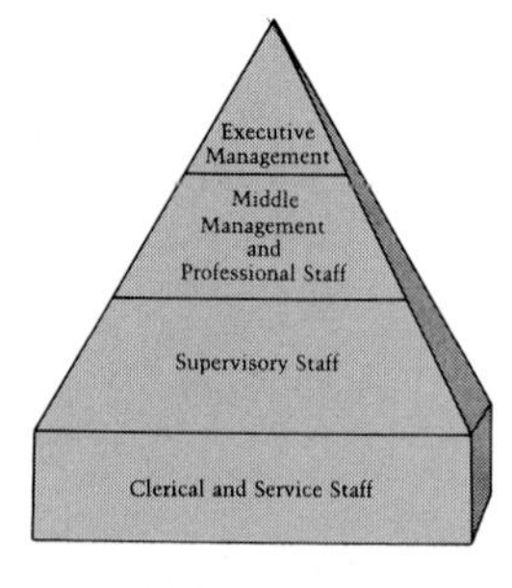

Knowledge Workers

Identify Knowledge Workers in the Current System During the survey and study phases, it is important to identify all the knowledge workers in the current information system. As a reminder, the knowledge worker dimension of your pyramid model is reproduced in the margin. The formal organization structure is frequently documented in the form of an organization chart. The analyst must be careful to update organization charts instead of accepting them as true indications of the reporting relationships in the business. It's important to note that most organization charts do not show the clerical and service staff workers.

Each worker's role and interest in the system should be understood. Finally, the analyst must identify two specific groups of knowledge workers: those who *use* the system and those who are or might be *affected by* the system. The latter group includes all those whose jobs are affected by the inputs and outputs of the system being studied. For instance, the accounting system in most businesses will be affected by virtually every other system. It is important to take these people into account because they may be affected by any changes you make to the current system. All of these people may offer valuable information.

Identify and Analyze the Business Mission of the Current System It is important for the analyst to identify and analyze the purpose, goals, objectives, and policies of business systems. Recall that these elements form the business dimension of your pyramid model (reproduced in the margin). Even more important, the analyst should determine how well the current information system supports that business mission. Are the objectives directed toward achieving the goals? If not, why not? Are the activities of the knowledge workers consistent with the mission? The objective of the study phase is to isolate points at which the information system is inconsistent with the business mission. For example, most production systems establish cost standards for labor, materials, and overhead. If these costs are being exceeded, the analyst should try to determine if the standards (goals) are reasonable or if production management's policies cause excessive costs through lack of control.

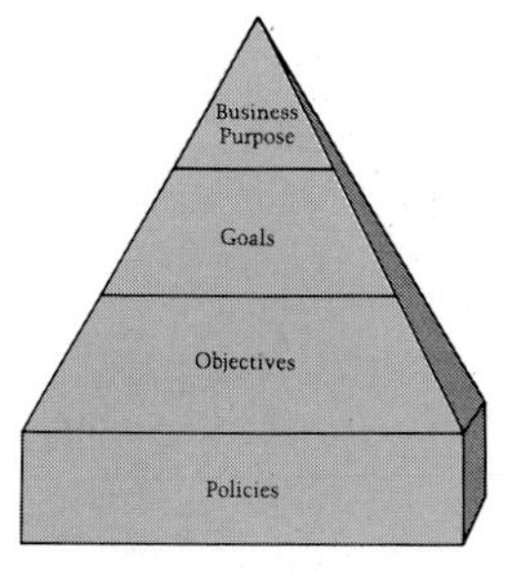

Business Mission

It is equally important to understand whether the business mission of the information system being studied is beneficial to the business as a whole. A system's mission might be *self-serving* and not in the best interest of the business as a whole. Consider, for instance, a purchasing system. To reduce inventory costs, a purchasing manager may be ordering excessive quantities of materials, thus obtaining lower unit prices via quantity discounts. This policy may adversely effect the inventory system, which will experience a higher inventory carrying cost because materials will remain unused for a longer period of time.

Identify and Analyze the Information System Functions Provided by the Current System During the survey and study phases, the analyst should identify and analyze the information systems functions (see margin) provided by the current system. The analyst must identify all of the transactions currently processed and any problems or opportunities that exist relative to these transactions. The analyst should not restrict the study to those transactions processed

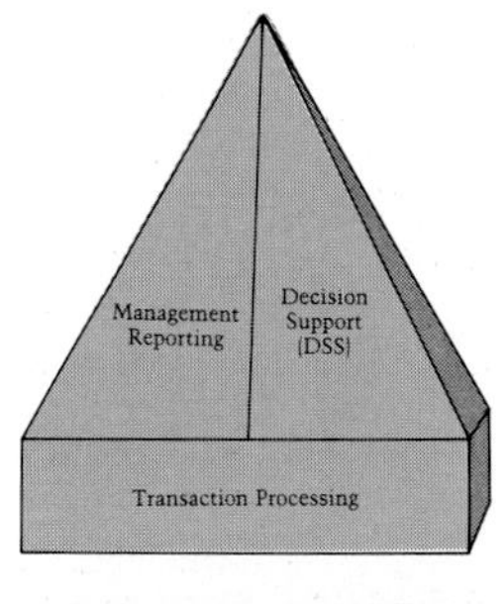

Information Systems Functions

on the computer. Manually processed transactions are equally important!

The analyst should also study all the information and reports currently being generated and used by and for knowledge workers in the current system. Emphasis should be placed on how the information is generated and used (or not used) as well as on specific problems with the information. For instance, information may be termed incomplete, inaccurate, untimely, or inadequate.

Finally, the analyst should study the decisions made by the knowledge workers when performing their jobs. How do these workers get the information needed to make those decisions? How do they use this information? Is the information sufficient for all decisions? Be on the lookout for data that are being collected and stored for no specific reason. These data may be necessary to support the ad hoc decision-making needs of the knowledge workers.

Identify and Analyze the Components of the Current Information System Recall that *analysis* is formally defined as the separation of a whole into its parts. The decomposition makes it easier to critique the whole. During the study phase, we'll perform analysis by identifying and evaluating the components highlighted below. What are

IPO Components

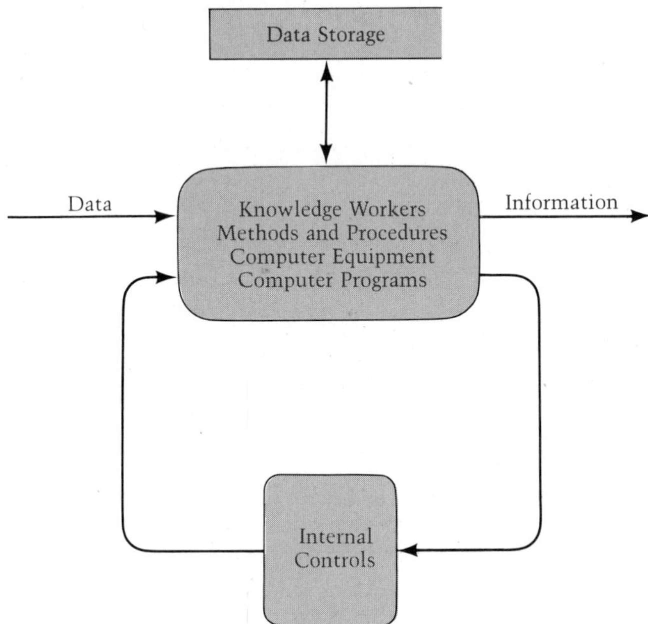

the responsibilities of each person in the system? How do all the knowledge workers interact? What methods (data processing and manual) are used to process data and information? What step-by-step procedures are used? What files and databases (manual and computerized) exist in the system? What hardware supports the existing system? Is the hardware adequately supporting the system? What software supports the current system? Are the users satisfied with these programs? If not, why not? It is most important to understand how all these components interact to make the current system work or not work.

How to Complete the Survey and Study Phases

So far, we've discussed *what* you need to do in the survey and study phases. In this section, we discuss *how* you perform the two phases. Let's identify and discuss the specific tasks, documentation, and skills for the survey and study phases.

Figure 6.2 depicts the survey and study phase tasks and their documentation. The rounded rectangles are tasks. Each task is numbered to guide you through the discussion that follows. The named arrows represent input and output documentation for the tasks. As we examine the tasks and documentation, we identify the skills you need to develop to be able to perform the tasks.

Task 1: Survey the Feasibility of the Project The survey phase was previewed in Chapter 5. Recall that the survey phase is sometimes called a *preliminary study* or *feasibility study.* In most organizations, the number of project requests submitted far exceed the number of projects that can be completed by data processing personnel. Therefore, we need to rank project requests so that time is spent on those projects most valuable to the business. In many organizations, a **steering committee** of business managers decides which projects will be developed and which will be backlogged for later dates. The purpose of the survey phase is to provide the steering committee with information with which to make those decisions. As you can see in Figure 6.2, the survey phase is triggered by the project request. The analyst is asked to present a feasibility survey to the steering committee. How is the survey phase accomplished?

The analyst normally conducts a first-contact interview or meeting with the key managers or users of the current system. At this meeting, the analyst attempts to "get a feel" for the current system

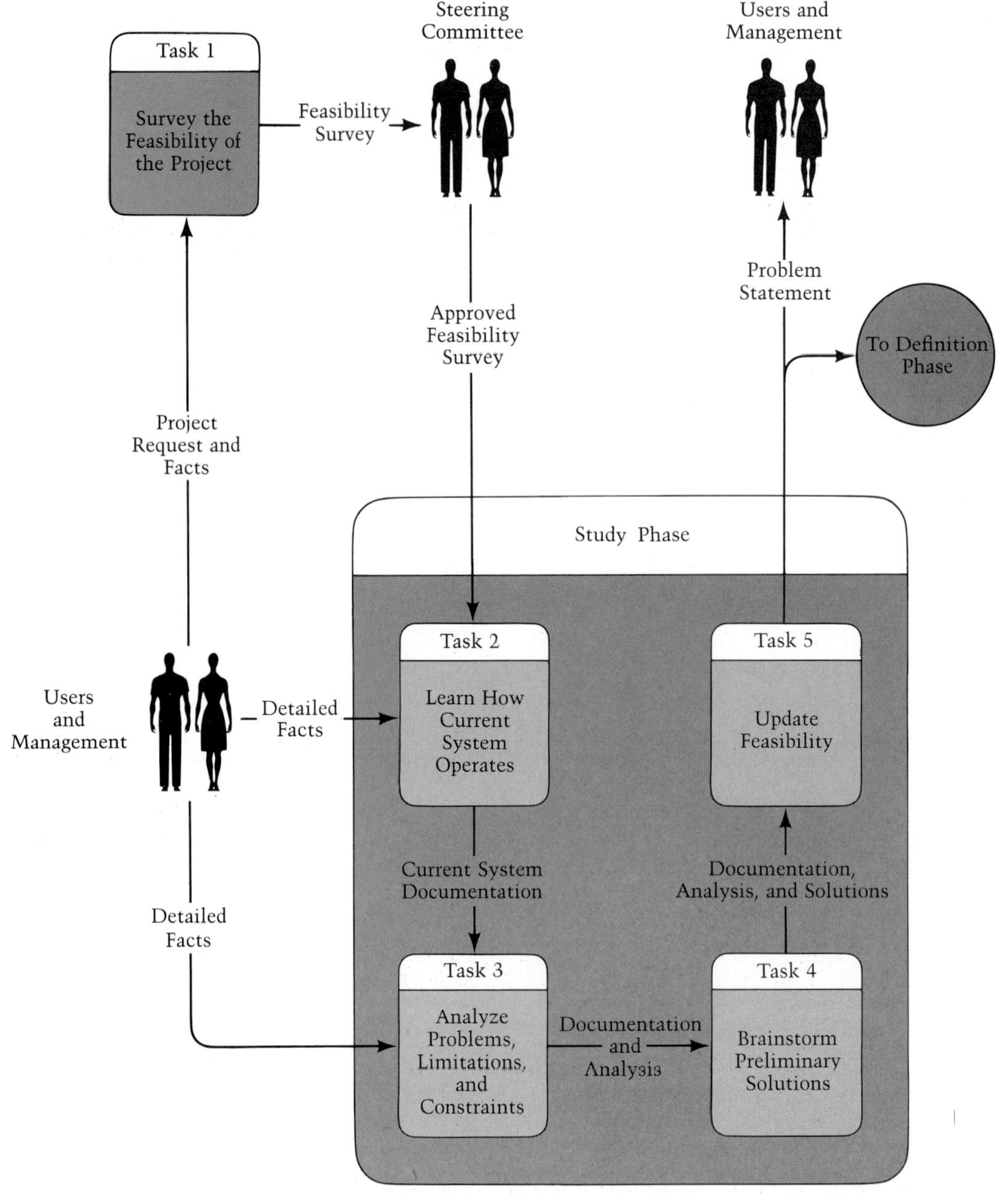

Figure 6.2

Feasibility survey and study phase tasks. The feasibility survey and study phases can be broken down into the tasks suggested on this diagram. The arrows depict documentation.

and the problems. Specifically, the analyst seeks answers to the following types of questions:

- What is the nature of the problems, opportunities, and requests? What led the user to make the request?
- What is the scope of the system? (This may change during the detailed study but you should try to define what you think the scope to be at this time.)
- What personnel are directly or indirectly involved with the system? Who will be the principal user contact(s)?
- What are the effects of the problem or the anticipated benefits of the opportunity? (To as great a degree as possible, quantify these effects and benefits; for example, express in dollars amounts.)
- Are there any constraints on the project, such as deadlines, policies, contracts that can't be broken, or computer systems that can't be changed?
- Does anyone have any potential ideas for solving the problems or exploiting the opportunities? (It is important to stress that any ideas will be treated as *preliminary* ideas!)

Given the answers to these questions, the analyst performs the first of many cost/benefit analyses on the project. The purpose of a cost/benefit analysis is to determine if the business benefits to be realized by continuing the project are greater than the costs that will be incurred if the project is continued.

At this early stage of the project, costs are difficult to pinpoint. Why? Because we haven't (and shouldn't have) addressed solutions. Still, we know how much the problems and limitations are costing the business. We can assume that, by solving the problems and eliminating the limitations, we will realize a benefit *at least* equal to those costs. And we can estimate whether those benefits, measured over some reasonable lifetime for the new system, will exceed the costs of developing the new system. If so, the project should be continued. Thus, the cost/benefit analysis for the survey phase is a measure of the urgency or worthiness of the project, both as a stand-alone project and relative to other proposed projects.

The feasibility survey phase serves several important purposes. It helps measure or establish the level of management commitment to the proposed project. Additionally, it establishes a preliminary statement of problems and objectives. The findings of the analyst should be presented to management or the steering committee in the form of a report (this is called a *feasibility survey* in Figure 6.2).

We have just identified three important skills necessary to complete this task: interviewing, report writing, and cost/benefit analysis. In the summary for this chapter, we show where in this book each of these skills is developed.

Fact-Finding Techniques

- Document Sampling
- Observation
- Questionnaires
- Interviewing

Task 2: Learn How the Current System Operates The next phase is a detailed study of the current system. The first task of the detailed study is to learn how the current system operates. We need to understand what the current system is doing and how the system is doing it before we try to analyze problems and opportunities or define solutions.

A significant amount of factual data about the current system, problems and opportunities, and needs is to be collected during this task. Because your users can't anticipate which facts you need and when you will need them, fact finding is a very important skill for this task! In particular, you should use the fact-finding techniques listed in the margin. To learn about the current system, keep in mind the objectives of the survey and study phases (discussed earlier in this chapter): identify the knowledge workers, identify and analyze the business mission, identify and analyze current information systems functions, and identify and analyze current system components.

Presentation Techniques

- Walkthroughs
- Verbal Presentations
- Written Reports

It is especially useful to document the current system in some fashion. Why document existing systems that will likely change? Information systems of any size are complex. Because there are many interacting components to be considered, you can quickly become overwhelmed by details and lose perspective. Therefore, one important skill you need to learn is how to draw useful pictures of the current information system. Existing system documentation will also help you verify your understanding of the current system. But you'll need to develop sound written and verbal communications skills for presenting your documentation and findings to your users. Appropriate presentation techniques are listed in the margin.

Task 3: Analyze Problems, Limitations, and Constraints in the Current System Referring again to Figure 6.2, you will see the next task: analyze problems, limitations, and constraints in the current system. During this task, you are responding to the facts you collected and the documentation you prepared during the last task. Problem analysis skills can be learned by applying cause and effect analysis to the problem categories of the PIECES framework you learned about in Chapter 4. The documentation from the previous task also assists with problem identification.

This task is often difficult for beginning analysts. Experience indicates that most new analysts try to solve problems without analyzing them. If we were to ask you to state a problem, your response would probably include the words *we need to* or *we want to*. Do you see what's wrong? You are stating the problem in terms of a solution. You must learn to state the problem, not the solution. Furthermore, you need to analyze the problem in terms of its causes and effects. This is a difficult skill to acquire, but you can begin by asking the right questions. What causes the problem? The answer often reveals a more fundamental or serious problem. What is the net effect of the problem? The answer tells us how serious the problem is and whether it is worth solving.

Task 4: Brainstorm Preliminary Solutions Even during this early phase of system development, it can be useful to generate some ideas about possible solutions to problems. There is no commitment at this time; there are just ideas. Therefore, we brainstorm preliminary solutions. By definition, *brainstorming* defines possible solutions without evaluating them. No solution is considered too outlandish or infeasible. Brainstorming helps you learn how much the users understand about the potential of the computer. And brainstorming can help you educate the user about that potential. Stress to the user that ideas generated during this task are not exhaustive and may change during later phases when more specific business requirements have been identified.

Task 5: Update Feasibility This is the second of our cost/benefit or feasibility analyses. Because the detailed study phase has taught us much more about the current system, we can now update feasibility estimates. Is the project still feasible?

We haven't committed to any solution, so we still don't know what the final system will cost. But we now have a thorough understanding of the problems, limitations, and opportunities for improvement. And we should have a better estimate of how much the problems and limitations in the current system are costing the business, including intangible costs. The sum of those costs, projected over the lifetime of the new system, equals the updated benefits to be derived from the new system.

Let's say, for example, that the new system will provide $100,000 per year of benefits. If the projected lifetime of the new system is five years, we can ask ourselves, "Will the solution likely cost us more than $500,000 [$100,000 × 5]?" Once again, we see that the ability to perform a cost/benefit analysis is an important skill for this task. As a result of a cost/benefit analysis, we can cancel the project, reduce the scope of the project to make it more feasible, or continue the project.

The end product of the study phase tasks is the **problem statement.** A suggested outline of a study phase report is presented in Figure 6.3. Once again, we see that presentation and communications skills are very important. The approved problem statement is passed on to the definition phase.

Study Phase Report

I. Introduction
   A. Purpose of the report
   B. Background of the project
   C. Scope of the project and the report
   D. Structure of the report

II. Tools and techniques used to complete the study

III. Findings
   A. Walkthrough and evaluation of the current system
   B. Summary of problems, limitations, and constraints

IV. Recommendations
   A. Preliminary solutions and ideas
   B. Updated feasibility assessment

V. Conclusion

VI. Appendices (may include detailed system documentation and sample forms)

Figure 6.3

The study phase report. This is an outline of a typical report written by an analyst at the end of the study phase.

HOW TO DEFINE USER REQUIREMENTS FOR AN IMPROVED SYSTEM

Historically, analysts have made a critical mistake after completing the study of the current information system! The temptation at that point is to begin looking at alternative solutions, particularly computer solutions. The most frequently cited error in new information systems is, "The system doesn't do what we wanted (or needed) it to do." Did you catch the key word? It's *what!* Analysts are frequently so preoccupied with the computer solution that they forget to define the business requirements for the solution. The *defining user requirements phase* is critical to the success of any new information system!

Purpose and Objectives of the Definition Phase

The purpose of the definition phase is to identify what the improved information system must be able to do without specifying how the system could or will do it. We can achieve the goal of the definition phase by accomplishing the following objectives:

- Identify all of the knowledge workers who will use or be affected by the new information system.
- Review and refine the business mission, establishing for the new system objectives that will help knowledge workers achieve the business mission.
- Define the information system functions that must be provided by the new system; these will include transaction processing, management reporting, and decision support.
- Define the noncomputer components of the new system, including data and information requirements, policies and procedures, and data to be stored.

Let's further examine each of these objectives. Once again, we will reproduce your pyramid model in the margin as a reminder of the concepts being applied.

Identify Knowledge Workers in the New Information System During the definition phase, the analyst should actively involve all of the knowledge workers (see margin) who were identified during the study phase. It is especially important to give knowledge workers at

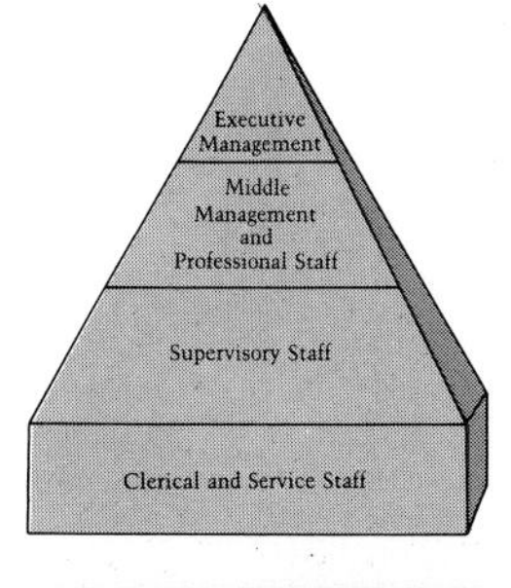

Knowledge Workers

every level of the organization the opportunity to define goals, objectives, and information system needs.

You will probably discover that, like you, knowledge workers will have difficulty specifying what they want or need without considering how to meet those needs. Don't discourage the discussion of computer alternatives, but filter those ideas into a mental suggestion box and focus on the underlying business requirements. Also, learn always to ask *why* something is needed or wanted. For instance, if a manager asks for a report that compares budgeted sales for each product against actual sales, ask why that information is needed and how the information will be used. If the reason is to identify those products not selling as well as projected, perhaps an exception report identifying only those products would be better.

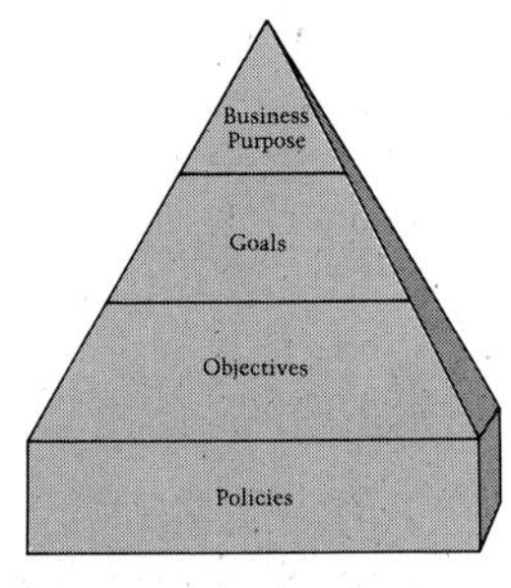

Business Mission

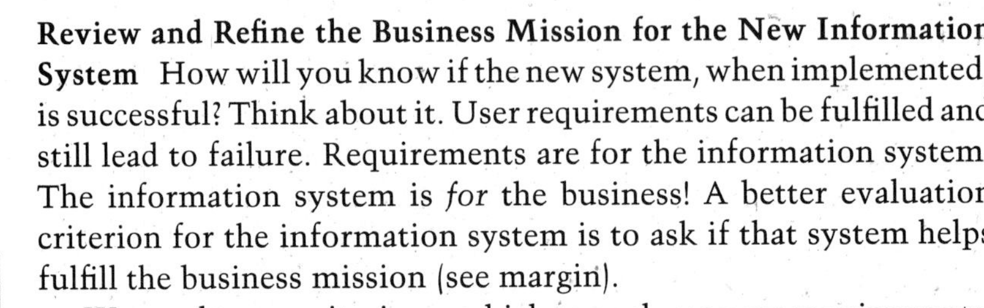

Review and Refine the Business Mission for the New Information System How will you know if the new system, when implemented, is successful? Think about it. User requirements can be fulfilled and still lead to failure. Requirements are for the information system. The information system is *for* the business! A better evaluation criterion for the information system is to ask if that system helps fulfill the business mission (see margin).

We need some criteria on which to evaluate user requirements. The data and information that the users request should be evaluated against those criteria. If a user says, "I need certain information on overdue accounts," you should ask why. The user may respond, "So I can identify and reduce credit losses!" The reduction of credit losses is a *business* objective, albeit general. By defining objectives, we can then measure the value of specific system requirements. Therefore, during the definition phase, the analyst should reevaluate and refine the business mission: purpose, goals, objectives, and policies. Then, we can define information system objectives that are consistent with the business objectives and policies.

Define the Information System Functions to Be Provided by the New Information System Can knowledge workers define their data and information requirements? For many of you, one of the most aggravating experiences you are likely to encounter will be the "I don't really know" response to your "What do you need?" question. Be honest! You've probably assumed that users *can* define their requirements (see margin). Right? Wrong. But don't panic! Users *can* define most *transactions* because they already exist. And many *reports* and *inquiries* can be defined because the users already use or know how they'll use the information. These are **information requirements** for the new system.

But there are reports and inquiries the users cannot define. Every manager encounters situations that could not be predicted and that call for decisions. Because the decisions that will be called for can't be predicted, the information needed to help the manager make those decisions can't be predicted. Fortunately, you probably can determine what types of data describe the business environment. Those data, in some format, will likely be the ingredient necessary to answer the manager's needs. These are the **data requirements** for the new system.

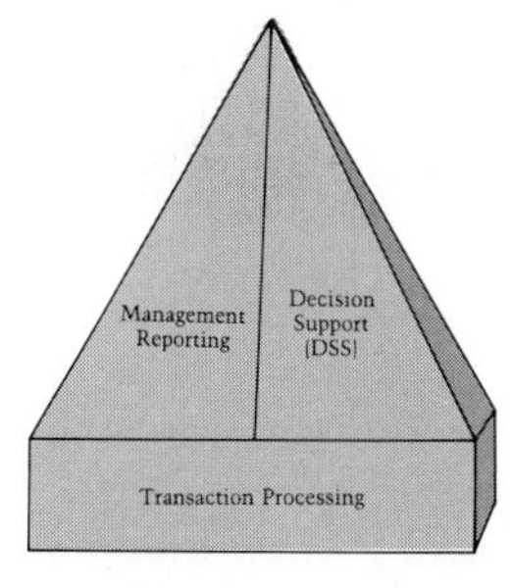

Information Systems Functions

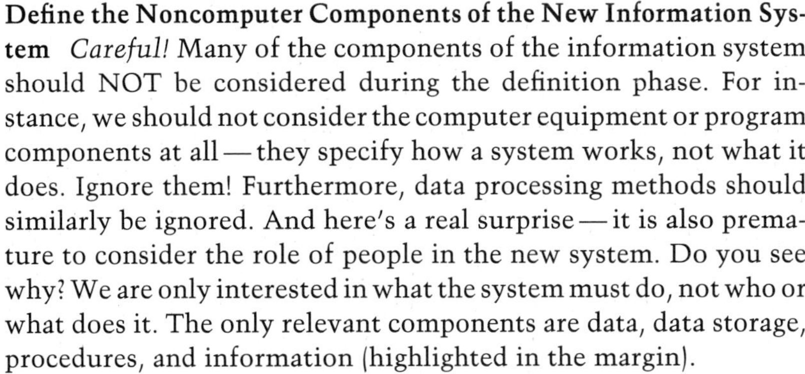

Define the Noncomputer Components of the New Information System *Careful!* Many of the components of the information system should NOT be considered during the definition phase. For instance, we should not consider the computer equipment or program components at all — they specify how a system works, not what it does. Ignore them! Furthermore, data processing methods should similarly be ignored. And here's a real surprise — it is also premature to consider the role of people in the new system. Do you see why? We are only interested in what the system must do, not who or what does it. The only relevant components are data, data storage, procedures, and information (highlighted in the margin).

What data (transactions) must be processed? What information (reports and inquiries) must be produced? What data must be stored? We do not consider how or where those data are to be stored! Finally, what procedures and policies transform the data into information? For instance, a credit policy may exist for approving orders. These are the only information system components that concern us during the definition phase.

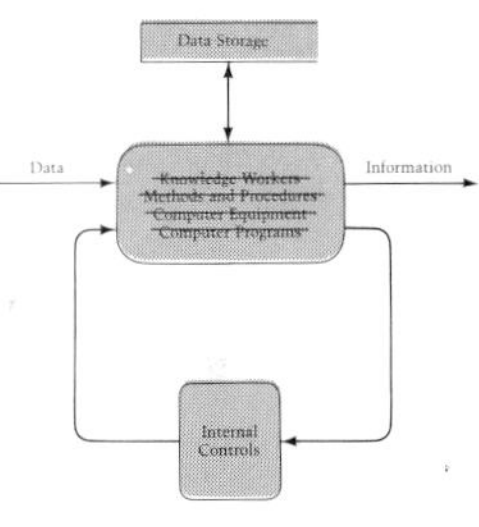

IPO Components

How to Complete the Definition Phase

In this section, we identify and discuss the specific tasks, documentation, and skills for the definition phase. Figure 6.4 illustrates the definition phase tasks and documentation. The tasks are numbered to guide you through the following discussion.

Task 1: Define System Objectives and Priorities Your attention should now shift from the current system to an improved system. Define system objectives and priorities first. The input to this task is the problem statement (included in the study phase report). The

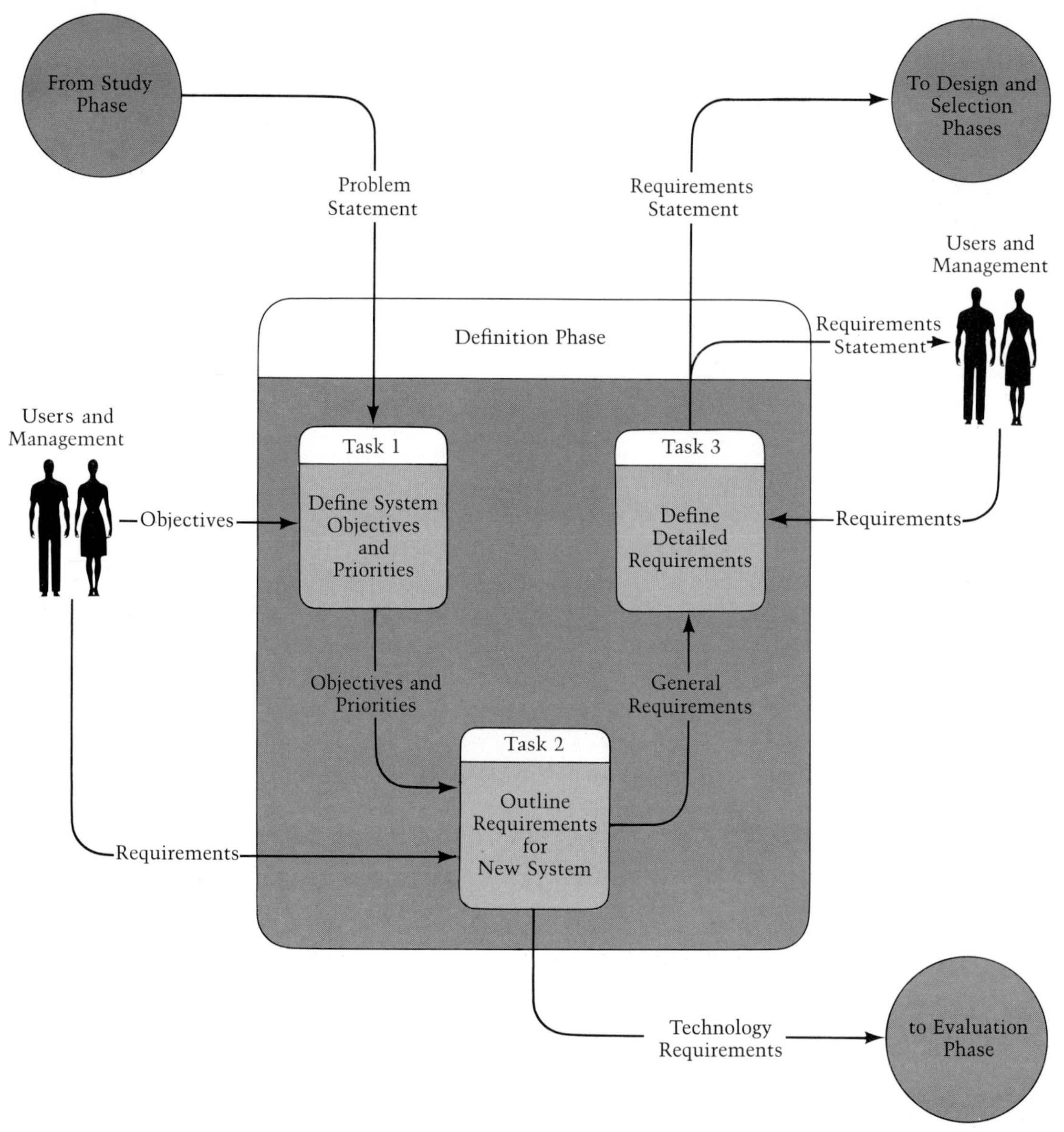

Figure 6.4

Definition phase tasks. The definition phase can be broken down into the tasks suggested on this page. The named arrows depict documentation.

problem statement identifies constraints that might limit the requirements and solutions. *Constraints* are situations that cannot be controlled or changed. Examples of constraints are listed in the margin. Given the constraints, identify specific objectives to support the business application and its knowledge workers.

Objectives should not be stated in terms of inputs, outputs, or processing. Instead, objectives should be precise, measurable statements of business performance. The objectives define the expected performance level of the new system. For example:

> Reduce the number of uncollectible customer accounts by 50 percent within the next year.
>
> Increase by 25 percent the number of loan applications that can be processed during an eight-hour shift.
>
> Decrease by 150 percent the time required to reschedule a production lot when a work station malfunctions.

Constraints

- Budget
- Deadlines
- Company Policies
- Government Regulations

Did you notice how the objectives state the desired performance? This gives us a ruler against which we can measure the data and information requirements that will be defined in the next task. Your objectives should address the problems and limitations identified during the study phase.

You also need to consider the possibility that not all objectives may be met by the new system. Why? The new system may be larger than expected, and you may have to reduce the scope to meet a deadline. Rank the objectives in order of importance. Then, if the scope must be reduced, the higher-priority objectives will tell you what's most important.

Task 2: Outline the Requirements for the New System How do you write an English composition or research paper? Hopefully, you outline the paper first. Why? So you can maintain a perspective on the *whole* paper. Otherwise, the paper may have no theme or direction. An information system presents the same dilemma. Therefore, the second task in the definition phase is to outline the requirements for the new system. Avoiding details, we define what inputs (data), outputs (information), and processes are needed in the new system. The outline can be narrative although a picture is more useful — especially if during the study phase, you drew a picture of the current system. The objectives and priorities identified in task 1 should be used to evaluate the general requirements.

What skills are necessary to perform this task? Because you need to solicit objectives and requirements from users, fact-finding techniques are once again essential. And we once again see some value in learning how to draw pictures of a system. Finally, because we need to review those pictures with the users, written and oral presentation techniques are also critical.

Task 3: Define Detailed Requirements for the New System Given the general requirements identified in task 2, we should define detailed requirements for the new system. We still want to place our emphasis on what the user wants rather than how to do it! For example, if the user identified a need for information on overdue customer accounts, we should now specify the details of this requirement. The following elements might be included in overdue account information:

CUSTOMER ACCOUNT NUMBER

CUSTOMER NAME

CUSTOMER ADDRESS

BALANCE DUE

DUE DATE

DATE OF LAST PAYMENT

PURCHASES SINCE LAST PAYMENT

Notice that we have not specified the media or format of the information. Similarly, we need to define the procedure for identifying the overdue accounts. For example:

> An account is considered overdue if there has been no payment in the past thirty days and there is a positive account balance due. Do not report accounts with a balance due that are being properly disputed by the customer.

Requirements are formatted as a **requirements statement** that is passed on to the design and selection phases of our systems development life cycle. At a minimum, a requirements statement should specify enough detail to proceed to the design and selection phases. Requirements statements are often believed to be large documents that are difficult to prepare and tedious to read. This is unfortunate. Complaints about the size and detail of many requirements statements can be traced to an overdependence on the English language for specifying requirements. Therefore, you need to learn how to use special tools for documenting and presenting requirements. Additionally, you need to learn how to present requirements in pieces, rather than in large, intimidating documents. Finally, it is important to document requirements in terms the user can understand.

HOW TO EVALUATE ALTERNATIVE INFORMATION SYSTEMS SOLUTIONS

Given the business requirements for an improved information system, we can finally address how the new system (including computer-based alternatives!) might operate. The final solution must also be feasible. Let's examine the evaluation phase as we did the survey, study, and definition phases.

Purpose and Objectives of the Evaluation Phase

The purpose of the evaluation phase is to identify the *best* solution (*possibly* computer-based) to our user requirements. We can define the following objectives for the evaluation phase:

- Define alternative solutions in terms of required information system components and interactions. (For the first time, these components include computer components, such as data processing methods, computer equipment, and programs.)
- Evaluate the impact of alternative solutions on the knowledge workers who will use or be affected by that system.
- Evaluate alternative solutions according to their ability to fulfill the business mission and information system objectives.
- Evaluate alternative solutions according to their ability to provide the required information system functions identified during the definition phase.

It is important to examine as many alternatives as time permits. The resulting feasibility analysis results in a major commitment (or noncommitment) to the expensive and tedious design and implementation phases. Let's examine each of these objectives further.

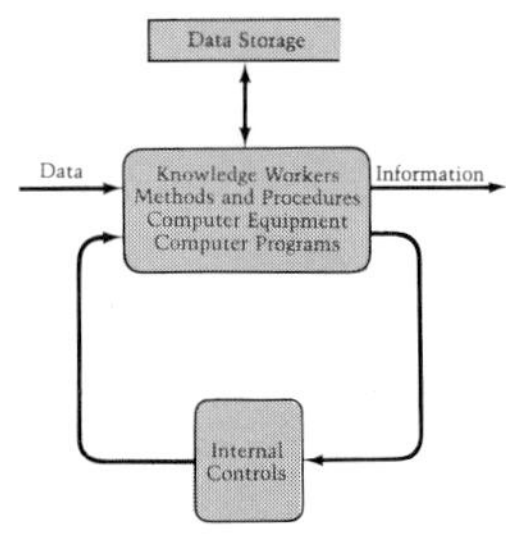

IPO Components

Define Alternative Solutions in Terms of Information System Components During the evaluation phase, we define those information system components (highlighted on your pyramid model in the margin) ignored during the definition phase. These include:

- The methods by which inputs and outputs will be implemented (for instance, an information requirement could be implemented as a printed report or a terminal screen display)
- The roles and functions of the knowledge workers in the system (How will job descriptions change?)
- Data processing methods and procedures (for instance, on-line versus batch processing)
- Computer equipment required to implement the alternative solutions
- Computer programs that must be programmed or purchased to implement the alternative solutions
- Files and databases that will need to be designed, built, and loaded for the alternative solutions
- Internal controls that need to be installed to ensure security and reliability of the solutions

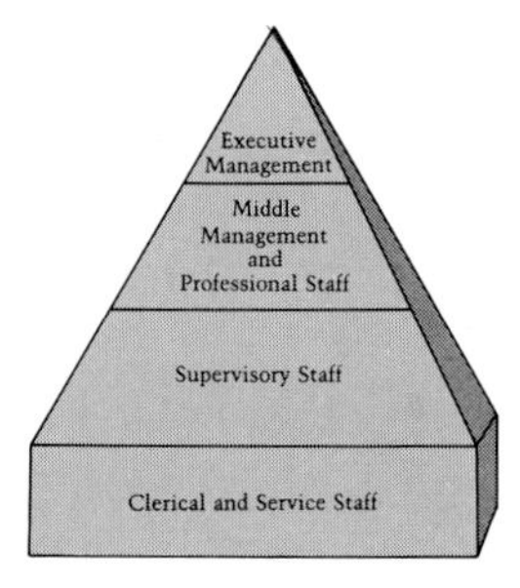

Knowledge Workers

Evaluate the Impact on the Knowledge Worker As was the case in the definition phase, all knowledge workers identified in the study phase should participate in the evaluation phase. In one sense, this can be more difficult. Why? Because this is the first phase in which we talk about how the computer might be used. And many knowledge workers are not familiar with the capabilities and limitations of the computer. Therefore, the analyst often must educate the knowledge worker during the evaluation phase. On the other hand, some users possess some knowledge of computers—perhaps too much knowledge. Such users often want to leap before they look. The importance of involving users in the feasibility analysis of alternatives cannot be overstressed! They must be willing to live with the solution. And they usually must justify the expenditure.

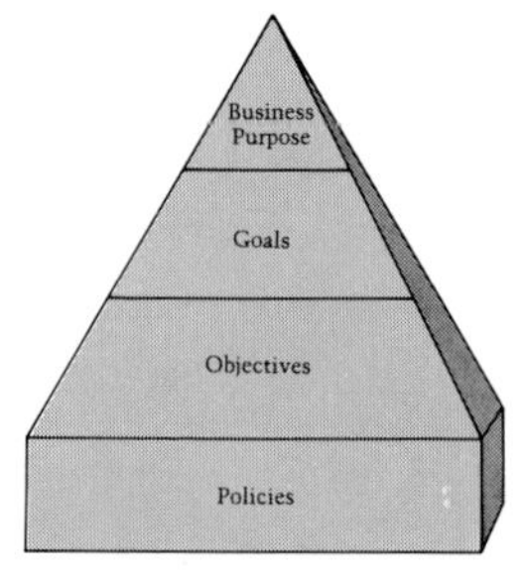

Business Mission

Evaluate the Impact on the Business Mission The analyst's principal concern with the business mission (see margin) during the evaluation phase is to ensure that the proposed information system fulfills goals, objectives, and policies of both the business and the project. This is made easier by ensuring that the requirements defined in the previous phase were also consistent with the business mission.

Evaluate How Well Alternative Solutions Provide Required Information System Functions The transaction processing, management reporting, and decision support requirements (see margin) were specified during the definition phase. In the evaluation phase, you are simply defining different ways to implement those requirements. For example, an information requirement might be fulfilled by a printed report or a terminal-displayed report. A specific transaction can be processed as a batch or directly processed on-line. Given such alternatives, you evaluate how well the solutions fulfill the functional requirements. This evaluation can be complicated by user preferences and conflicting interests.

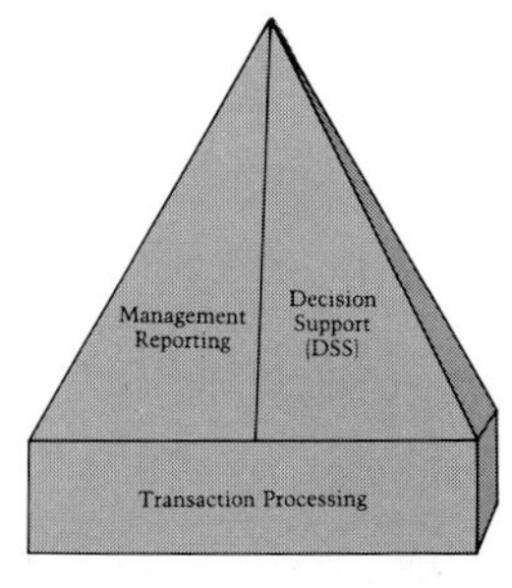

Information Systems Functions

How to Complete the Evaluation Phase

Let's identify and discuss the specific tasks, documentation, and skills necessary for the evaluation phase. Figure 6.5 depicts the tasks and documentation of the evaluation phase. The tasks have been numbered to guide you through the following discussion.

Task 1: Specify Alternative Solutions There's *always* more than one way to implement the requirements of an information system. Our first task is to specify alternative solutions. This normally involves defining alternative person-machine boundaries. A person-machine boundary separates those tasks that will be performed by people from those that will be performed by computer. At least four levels of decisions must be made:

1. Where should we draw the person-machine boundary? Different alternatives should define different degrees of automation. Which tasks will be manual? Which will be automated?
2. How should the person-machine interface of each individual alternative be handled? Will data be input as a batch or input on-line? Will the information be printed or displayed? There are numerous batch and on-line combinations possible in most information systems.
3. Will the solution be centralized or distributed? In other words, what portion of the alternative will be implemented on your mainframe or minicomputer? What portion will be done on mi-

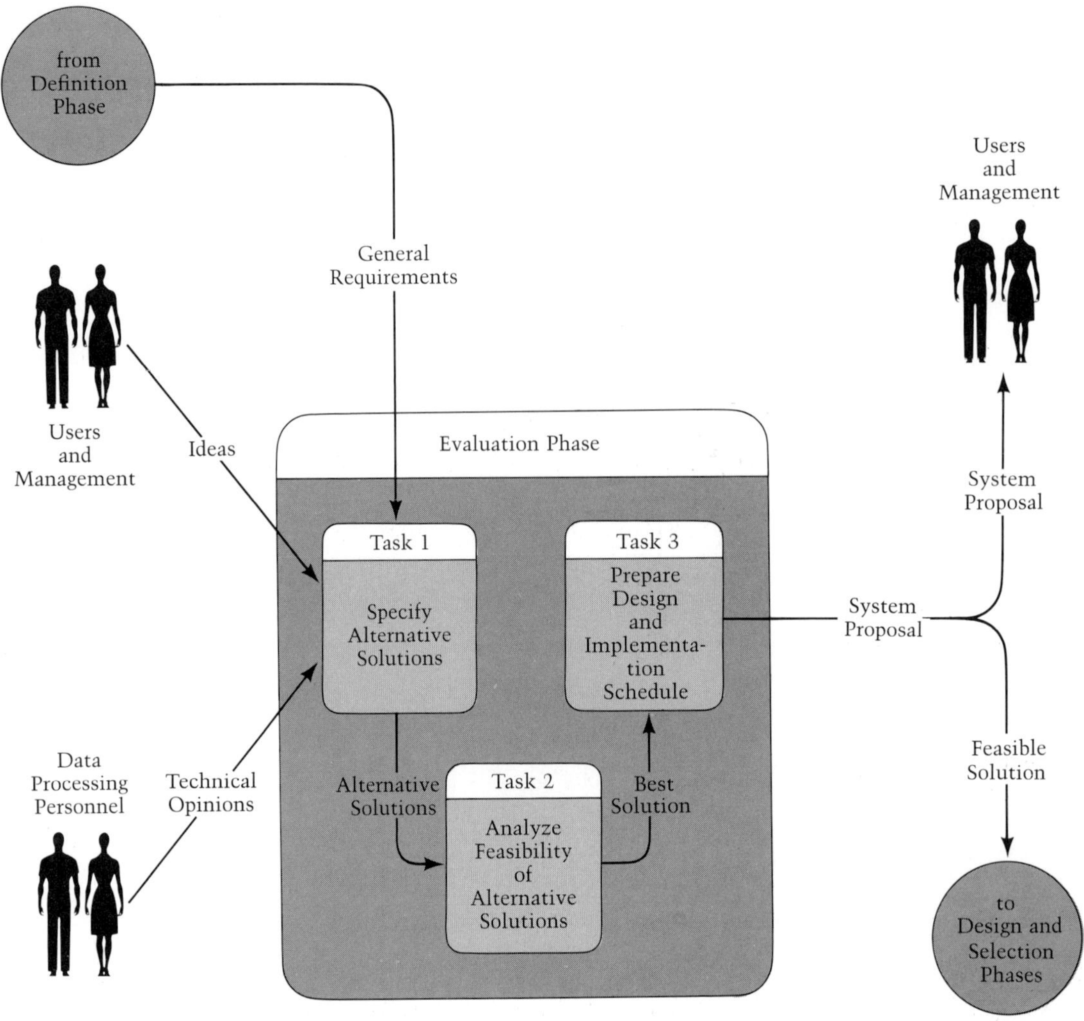

Figure 6.5

Evaluation phase tasks. The evaluation phase can be broken down into the tasks suggested on this page. The named arrows depict documentation.

crocomputers? Will data have to be passed between computers? If so, how will this be done?

4. What technology (hardware and software) must be purchased to support each of the alternatives? What technology (hardware and software) might be purchased to support the alternatives? Note that the make-versus-buy issue is first addressed at this time.

The media for all inputs and outputs should be specified. The hardware and software required should be specified. The manner in which data will be stored should be defined. And the methods and procedures for operating the system must be identified. Many of the skills developed for documenting the current system and defining the new system's requirements are also valuable for defining alternative solutions.

Task 2: Analyze Feasibility of Alternative Solutions The next task is to analyze the feasibility of each alternative solution. This is the third assessment of cost/benefit feasibility during systems analysis. Prior cost/benefit analyses were limited by our not having defined specific technical solutions. Consistent with our creeping commitment approach to feasibility, we can now perform a more thorough feasibility analysis.

But this feasibility analysis should not be limited to costs and benefits. How should you analyze the feasibility of a potential solution? Most analysts evaluate solutions against three sets of criteria:

1. *Operational feasibility* is defined as the suitability of the solution to the people who will have to use that solution.
2. *Technical feasibility* is defined as the availability of suitable technology to support the solution and adequate expertise to develop the solution. Also, it must be possible to implement the solution within a reasonable time frame.
3. *Economic feasibility* is the classical cost/benefit analysis. Because we are now looking at specific technical solutions, the costs to develop those solutions can be estimated with greater precision. Additionally, the costs to operate the new information system (supplies and expenses) can now be estimated. Finally, the benefits to the business can be estimated with greater precision. Whichever alternative solution offers the greatest lifetime benefits minus lifetime costs is the best *economic* solution.

The ability to perform a feasibility analysis, specifically a cost/benefit analysis, is a major skill you need to learn! Furthermore, the ability to present your feasibility analysis, both orally and in writing, is equally important.

Task 3: Prepare a Design and Implementation Schedule for the Recommended Solution Given a recommended solution, you should plan a schedule for the phases that are still to be completed in the project: design, selection, construction, and delivery. Experience will help you estimate the time required to complete the tasks in these phases.

Systems alternatives, their feasibility analysis, and the schedule are normally presented in the form of a **systems proposal** or **feasibility report.** This proposal or report is presented to the steering committee (or its equivalent) that determines whether or not to commit resources (people and money) to the design, selection, construction, and delivery phases of the project. A suggested format for the system proposal or feasibility report is presented in Figure 6.6.

HOW TO MANAGE THE TIME SPENT ON THE ANALYSIS PHASES

We conclude our discussion of the systems analysis process with a discussion of project management implications for the phases involved. The first issue addressed is the amount of time spent on systems analysis. Then we examine the sequencing and the degree to which the tasks of systems analysis can be overlapped.

How Much Time Should Be Spent on Systems Analysis?

Everybody has an opinion on this issue. Let's present the extremes and then focus on how you can decide. In Chapter 5, you learned that different methodologies emphasize different phases. Traditional or design-oriented approaches place less emphasis on systems analysis. Approximately 10 percent of the total system development effort would be devoted to the analysis.

Alternatively, more recent methodologies have suggested that, in order to reduce the number of design errors and expedite the design and implementation processes, greater emphasis should be placed on the analysis process. These methodologies (for instance, structured analysis) may increase the total analysis effort to as much as 30 percent or more of the total system development effort. It is believed that the subsequent design and implementation phases (which are more expensive) would require less time to complete!

The amount of time that should be allocated to the survey, study, definition, and evaluation phases will likely be a function of

System Proposal

I. Introduction
  A. Purpose of the report
  B. Background of the project leading to this report
  C. Scope of the project
  D. Structure of the report
II. Tools and techniques used
  A. Solution generation
  B. Feasibility analysis (cost/benefit)
III. Information systems requirements
IV. Alternative solutions and feasibility analysis
V. Recommendations
VI. Appendices

Figure 6.6

System proposal report. This is an outline for a systems proposal, the result of the evaluation phase. The system proposal presents the feasibility of alternative information system solutions and recommends a course of action that will guide system design and implementation activities.

the project's size, complexity, and importance to the organization and of the experience of the analyst. The larger the current system, the more important it is to study that system. The larger the target system, the more important it is to define requirements and alternatives. When allocating project time to systems analysis, consider the deadline and scope of the project. If the time allocated to the study, definition, and evaluation phases clearly appears inadequate, you and your users have a decision to make. The choices are simple:

- Reduce the scope of the project such that the systems analysis (and remainder of the project) can be completed on the original schedule.

or

- Extend the time required to complete the analysis and subsequently extend the deadlines for completing design and implementation.

The Next Generation — *The Systems Analysis Productivity Workstation*

Systems analysis has often been perceived as the *paperwork* part of systems development. The only tools required of the analyst are pencil, paper, and flowchart template. The work proceeds slowly, as the analyst manually draws and redraws numerous charts and diagrams that depict the current and proposed information systems. Furthermore, the analyst uses a myriad of interrelated forms to keep track of important system details. And a change in any one chart or form can impact several other forms and charts in the documentation package. It's easy to become overwhelmed by all of this, but help is on the way! New computer-based tools are emerging to improve the analyst's productivity and make the job of preparing and correcting documentation much less tedious.

The concept of computer-based tools to support the systems analyst is not new. The ISDOS Project at the University of Michigan developed such a tool—*Problem Statement Language/Problem Statement Analyzer (PSL/PSA)*—in the 1970s. With PSL/PSA, the analyst could draw diagrams and maintain a data dictionary for a systems development project. The software could provide numerous checks for completeness and consistency within the documentation. Furthermore, the impact of changes made to any part of the documentation could be minimized or, at the very least, itemized. The PSL/PSA software runs on larger, mainframe computers. Thus, any firm that uses PSL/PSA has to dedicate enough of its most precious resource—its main computer—to support the tool.

As you are no doubt aware, microcomputer technology has boomed in recent years. Today we are beginning to see an exciting new product emerge from that technology: the **systems analyst productivity workstation.** Essentially, the analyst's workstation is an extension of the original PSL/PSA concept—brought down to microcomputer size. At the time of this writing, two such workstations are available. They are Index Technology's *Excelerator* (designed to work on IBM Personal Computers) and Nastec's *MTC 2000* (built around a Convergent Technology microcomputer). Microcomputers are a natural for systems analysis productivity tools. The analyst can create and maintain documentation without affecting ▶

To What Degree Can the Phases and Tasks Be Overlapped?

The survey phase is completed before resources are committed to any of the subsequent phases of the life cycle. If the project is continued, the study, definition, and evaluation phases are essentially completed in sequence. Why? You cannot consider your requirements definition complete if you have not studied all of the current system's problems and opportunities. You cannot consider your evaluation of alternatives complete until you have defined all of the

The Next Generation (continued)

the business's main computers!

What can you do with a systems analysis workstation? One of the major advantages of these workstations is their graphics capabilities. The workstation does for the analyst what CAD (Computer-Aided Design) does for the engineer. Using the workstation, you can easily create and modify flowcharts, data flow diagrams, database charts, and other graphically oriented tools. If you make a mistake, you simply correct the existing chart and reprint it. Productivity workstations also include tools for cataloging data, procedures, and system details. These details can be printed in a variety of formats, depending on purpose and audience. Future workstations will also be able to (some already can) perform analysis similar to PSL/PSA.

Most workstations will also include standard productivity tools such as word processors (for writing reports to users and management) and spreadsheets (for budgeting and cost/benefit analysis). Some workstations may include comprehensive tools for project management, such as the ability to draw PERT and Gantt charts. And workstations will also include tools for enhancing productivity during systems design (see the "Next Generation" feature for Chapter 10). Most of the tools covered in this book can be implemented on both the Excelerator and MTC 2000 workstations.

What impact will these workstations have? Some early tests suggest a 50 percent or greater increase in analysts' productivity! The workstations also take much of the drudgery out of documenting systems. Given the shortage of programmers and analysts, any technology that maximizes their productivity and morale is a *can't miss* prospect. You can expect the number, sophistication, and use of these workstations to increase during the next few years. The graphics, data dictionary, project management, spreadsheet, and word processing capabilities will be (in some cases, already are) highly integrated. One of the manufacturers of this technology has appropriately labeled the systems analyst productivity workstation as "shoes for the cobbler's children," a reference to the fact that computer experts — in this case, analysts — are being the last to take full advantage of their own technology. ■

target system's requirements. Thus, there is a general sequence to the phases.

Still, the analysis phases offer some opportunities for overlap. Let's begin by suggesting that the study phase tasks be completed prior to beginning either the definition or evaluation phases. You should thoroughly understand the current system's operation and limitations before defining solutions! On the other hand, some of the tasks within the study phase can overlap. For example, you can analyze problems, limitations, and constraints as you are learning

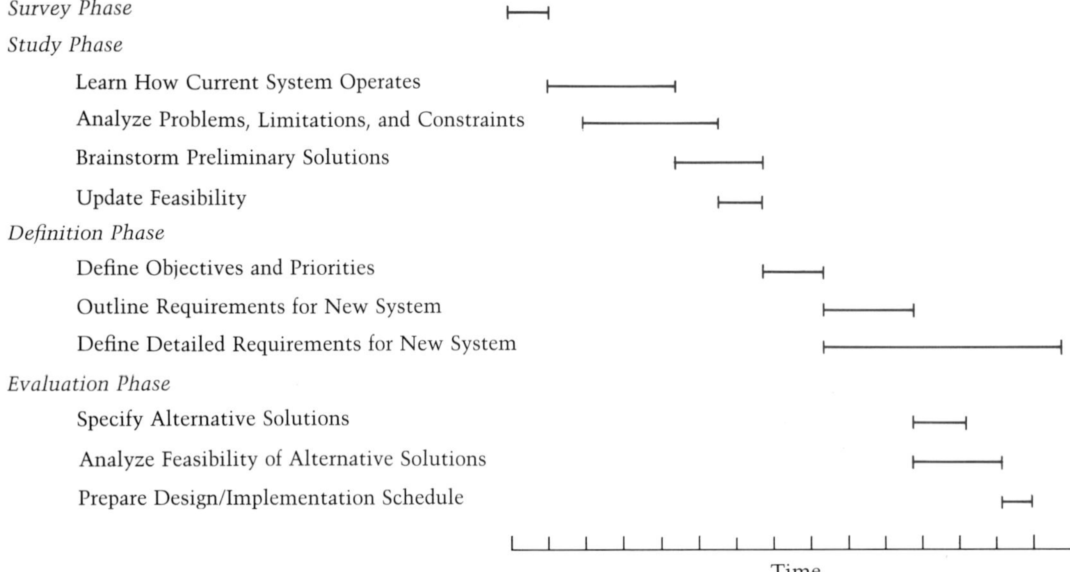

Figure 6.7

Opportunities to overlap analysis tasks. This chart shows opportunities to overlap the systems analysis tasks described in this chapter. The tasks are listed on the vertical axis. The horizontal axis represents time, which may be measured in days, weeks, or months, depending on project size and complexity.

about (and documenting) the current system. Also, it's hard not to brainstorm preliminary solutions during those tasks. The Gantt chart in Figure 6.7 illustrates the opportunity to overlap the study phase tasks.

The opportunities for overlapping tasks of the definition and evaluation phases are more extensive. These opportunities are also illustrated in Figure 6.7. Notice that the definition of objectives is completed before any other task is started. However, notice that the evaluation phase tasks can begin as soon as the general requirements for the new system are outlined. In fact, the chart clearly shows that the evaluation is usually completed before the detailed requirements are defined. Why? It is highly unlikely that the *detailed requirements,* as we have defined that term, will affect the alternative solutions. For instance, we usually don't need to know every element that must appear on a report before we determine the best way to implement the report.

SUMMARY

Systems analysis is the most critical process of information systems development. Systems analysis can be defined as the separation of an information system into its component parts for the purpose of identifying and evaluating problems, opportunities, constraints, and needs. Systems analysis consists of four phases that can be successfully completed by applying appropriate skills and carefully addressing each dimension of the information system.

The purpose of the survey—the project feasibility phase, also referred to as a *preliminary study* or *feasibility study*—is to determine the initial feasibility of a project request. The product of this phase is the feasibility survey that is presented to a steering committee for a decision on whether the project should be developed. If the project is approved, the next phase is the study of the current information system. The purpose of that phase is to learn how the current system operates. The analyst documents the current system in some fashion and presents the findings to users for verification. The analyst then studies the current system to identify problems, limitations, and constraints and brainstorms preliminary solutions. Finally, the analyst updates the feasibility estimates and presents the findings as a problem statement or formal study phase report.

The third phase of systems analysis is to define user requirements for a new information system. The purpose of this phase is to identify what the new, improved information system must be able to do. The problem statement from the study phase is used to define system objectives and priorities. General requirements for the new system are outlined in terms of inputs, processing, and outputs. These general requirements are verified with the users before adding specific details, such as content, timing, and volume. The product of this phase is the requirements statement.

The fourth phase of systems analysis is to evaluate alternative information systems solutions that fulfill the systems requirements. Several alternative solutions are identified and evaluated in terms of operational, technical, and economic feasibility. The analyst will recommend the best solution to the steering committee for approval. The recommendation may be presented in the form of a system proposal or feasibility report.

A cost/benefit analysis is an integral part of the survey, study, and evaluation phases. The cost/benefit analysis determines if the expected system development and lifetime costs for a new system

Tasks	Ch. 10 An overview of the systems design process	Ch. 17 An overview of the systems implementation process	Ch. 4 Problem-definition and problem-solving principles—Pieces framework	Ch. 7 Data flow diagrams—Picture of information system components and their interactions	Ch. 8 Data dictionary—Documenting data, information, and data storage requirements	Ch. 9 Structured English and decision tables—Documenting policies and procedures	Mod. A Project management guidelines—Tools and techniques	Mod. B Fact-finding techniques—Document sampling, observation, questionnaires, and interviews	Mod. C Oral presentations—Meetings, presentations, and walkthroughs	Mod. C Written reports—Business and technical reports	Mod. D Cost/benefit and feasibility analysis techniques
Learn how to survey and study the current system										•	
Survey the feasibility of the project			•					•	•		•
Learn how the current system operates				•				•	•		
Analyze problems, limitations, and constraints in the current system			•					•			
Brainstorm preliminary solutions			•					•	•		
Update feasibility									•		•
Learn how to define user requirements for an improved system										•	
Define system objectives and priorities								•			
Outline the requirements for the new system				•				•	•		
Define detailed requirements for the new system					•	•		•	•		
Learn how to evaluate alternative information system solutions										•	
Specify alternative solutions				•							
Analyze feasibility of alternative solutions									•		•
Prepare a design and implementation schedule for the recommended solution	•	•					•		•		

◀ Figure 6.8

Cross reference chart. This chart identifies the chapters and modules in this book that will help you develop the skills needed to perform the various systems analysis phases and tasks.

will be offset by the benefits of the new system. The repetition of a cost/benefit analysis allows management to gradually commit to the new system, thus reducing the possibility of implementing costly failures.

The systems analyst should consider project management implications for the systems analysis phases. More recent systems analysis methodologies suggest that greater emphasis be placed on the analysis process to reduce the number of design errors and expedite the design and implementation processes. The analyst should recognize that the survey phase must be completed before resources are committed to any of the subsequent phases of the life cycle. Although the study, definition, and evaluation phases should essentially be completed in sequence, there are opportunities for overlap.

In the following chapters, you will be introduced to tools and techniques for accomplishing the systems analysis tasks presented in this chapter. You may find the chart in Figure 6.8 a useful cross reference guide for locating chapters and modules that develop analysis skills against the analysis tasks that you learned in this chapter.

PROBLEMS AND EXERCISES

1. Explain why systems analysis is the most critical process in the systems development life cycle. List some potential consequences of a poor systems analysis.
2. Differentiate between the survey and study phases of the systems analysis process. Why not just begin with the study phase?
3. What skills are important in order for a systems analyst to be able to successfully perform systems analysis? How are these skills used in each phase of the systems analysis process?

4. How does the information systems pyramid model aid in systems analysis? Examine each face of the pyramid separately.
5. What is the end product of each systems analysis phase? Explain the purpose and content of each of these products.
6. Problem 6 in Chapter 4 provided several typical systems project scenerios. Assume that one of those companies is considering awarding your consulting firm a contract to develop a new and improved system. But at the beginning, they only want to commit to systems analysis. They are concerned about your ability to understand their problems and needs. And most of all, they want to see what kind of computer-based solutions you propose before they contract with you to do the design and implementation of a new system. Write a letter of proposal that will address their concerns.
7. You have been developing an improved sales tracking system for Bob Boring Auto Sales. You have already studied the existing sales tracking system to identify problems and opportunities. You have also defined new requirements for an improved system. Finally, you have defined two alternative solutions that will fulfill the requirements. The first alternative merely fulfills the minimum requirements, processing sales transactions as a batch and producing the required reports. The second alternative processes transactions on-line with the salesperson entering additional data about the negotiations that preceded the sale. The on-line option also provides immediate access to customer reports and inquiries about types of customers who buy cars, features that are selling well, negotiation strategies that do and don't seem to work, and so forth. After hearing the two strategies described, Mr. Boring immediately requested that the second option be designed and implemented. On what feasibility criterion was Mr. Boring's decision being made? Why is that decision based on incomplete analysis? What other criteria and questions should Mr. Boring address before making the final decision?
8. A systems project has been approved by a steering committee. The time allocated for completing the project is one year. How much time would you allocate to the analysis, design, and implementation processes? Explain your rationale for distributing the time.

9. If the time you allocated to the analysis process of the project in question 8 proves to be inadequate, what decision would you make? What are your alternative choices?
10. Explain how the time spent completing the systems analysis of a project can best be managed.

ANNOTATED REFERENCES AND SUGGESTED READINGS

EXCELERATOR. Index Technology Corporation, Five Cambridge Center, Cambridge, MA 02142. This is one of the systems analyst productivity workstations mentioned in the "Next Generation" feature for this chapter.

MTC 2000 Nastec Corporation, 24681 Northwestern Highway, Southfield, MI 48075. Nastec manufactures this systems analyst productivity workstation mentioned in the "Next Generation" feature for this chapter.

Analysts in Action

The Existing Customer Services System is Studied

When we left Cheryl and Doug, they had concluded a preliminary study into the order-entry problem at AAP. Now they must do a more thorough study of the current order-entry system.

Episode 3

This episode begins shortly after the steering committee has approved Cheryl and Doug's preliminary study report and authorized a more detailed study of the current system.

Fact-Finding Strategy

Cheryl and Doug are plotting strategy with Joey in Cheryl's office.

"Good morning Joey!" Cheryl was genuinely excited about starting the new project. "I asked you here so Doug and I could review our strategy for the first phase of our project. This will only take a couple of minutes."

"Terrific! How's this going to work?" Joey asked as he took a seat.

"This phase is accomplished in four steps," explained Cheryl. First, we review the document and work flow in your current order-entry system. To accomplish this, we will have to gather significant factual data from you and your people. After verifying the facts, we can begin the second step, which is an analysis of problems and constraints. The third step will be to define some preliminary solutions. But, please, we cannot overemphasize that these solutions are only *tentative* at this point in the project. Finally, we will reevaluate feasibility to determine if the project is still feasible. This entire phase will take no longer than three weeks."

Joey shifted in his chair. "This sounds great, but I should bring up a concern I have at this time. My people have jobs to do. Their jobs come first. We'll give you all the time we can afford, but when push comes to shove, we have to get those orders processed."

Doug joined the conversation, "I'm glad you brought that up! Cheryl and I wanted to address that issue with you at this meeting. We have a fact-finding strategy that will minimize the time your people will have to sacrifice. We won't just barge in and ask for interviews. First, we want to collect as many facts as possible without interviews. We'd like you to get us copies of all the forms and documents used in order entry. If you have existing procedure manuals or instruction guides, we'd like copies of them too. It would be helpful if the sample forms you give us are in various stages of processing. We can learn a lot about the current system by studying these forms."

"Not to mention the fact that my people don't have to give up any of their time! I'll personally put that package together and have it to you today."

Cheryl nodded, "That'll be great. After we've studied the ▶

forms, we'll ask you for permission to observe a couple of your clerks as they perform their jobs. It would be nice if you explained that we're not evaluating their performance. We just want to observe how they process the orders."

"I don't think that'll be a problem," said Joey. "I've already explained that the proposed system will not eliminate anybody's job. They seem excited about the prospect of using the computer."

Cheryl continued, "We should point out that questions will be minimized during the observations. After we've looked at the documents and spent some time observing the system, we'll collect additional facts by using questionnaires and holding interviews. The questionnaires will help us prepare for the interviews. And the nice thing about questionnaires is that they can be completed when your clerks aren't busy. We'll turn all the questionnaires over to you and ask that you distribute them among your clerks. We'd appreciate two- to three-day turnaround on the questionnaires. After collecting as many facts as possible by observing and by studying the questionnaires, we'll conduct interviews. We hope you can see how this strategy tries to minimize direct user-contact time while still achieving our goals."

"I like what I'm hearing!" exclaimed Joey. "I suspect you'll also need to verify your facts. Correct?"

"Indeed!" Cheryl answered. "We'll definitely verify our facts. We'll be drawing pictures of your system. We'll schedule review sessions with you and with one or more of your people. And we'll walk through the pictures and make any corrections you indicate. Any questions?"

"Sounds good!" Joey grinned. "Let's get started."

[*We pick up our story one and a half weeks later.*]

The fact-finding strategy has been working well. Indeed, with the notable exception of Cheryl and Doug's more frequent presence in the Order-Entry Department, there has been no noticeable difference in day-to-day operations.

By studying the sample forms, documents, and procedures Joey provided, Doug and Cheryl were able to find the general *shape,* as they like to call it, of the system. They were able to clearly document the normal procedure for tracking an order through the system, provided there were no abnormalities. Observation of two clerks over an eight-hour period cleared up some misconceptions and identified a number of the exceptions and abnormalities that can occur in the system. To collect additional facts, questionnaires were distributed. Some clerks failed to respond, but the responses that were returned were helpful. Questionnaires were intended only to eliminate some of the need for direct interviews. Additionally, the responses helped Cheryl and Doug profile the attitudes of the personnel involved.

A couple of interviews had been conducted. Throughout the entire review process, Doug and Cheryl had noted problems, complaints, bottlenecks, and constraints. But they had not discussed these issues, nor had they offered any opinions or solutions. The *big picture* had unfolded very nicely. With documentation in hand, Cheryl and Doug joined Joey, Madge, Karen, and Ted for a walkthrough of the current system. Let's sneak in on the meeting . . .

Review of the Current System
Cheryl called the meeting to order, "Well, it's 3:30, and it looks like we're all here. Doug tells me there is a special place in heaven for people who start and end meetings on time. So we'll end this meeting at precisely 4:30, no matter where we stand. Is that agreeable?"

Noting that everyone was nodding approval, Cheryl continued. "The purpose of this ▶

meeting is to review the current data and work flow of sales orders in the order-entry operation. Doug and I have drawn some pictures of the system as we understand it. Some of you have seen us sketching these pictures during our previous discussions. What we want to do today is walk through the pictures with you. We ask that you point out any errors, omissions, or contradictions that you see." (Note that Cheryl did not refer to the pictures by some fancy name (such as data flow diagrams) that could have intimidated the users.)

Cheryl placed a picture on the overhead projector (see Figure 1, which is annotated with circled numbers to help you follow this discussion). "This is a picture of the document and work flow for order entry. The picture isn't really a step 1, step 2, step 3 picture. All of the activities shown here are being done simultaneously. Let's walk through our picture. The entire process is handled by five or six clerks, one of whom is the bonded payments clerk who handles all money. Most orders are received in the mail, but some smaller orders are phoned in [see ① on Figure 1]. Only AAP franchises are permitted to phone in orders [see ②]. Other customers are ineligible. First, the order must be screened . . ."

"Excuse me, Cheryl," interrupted Madge. "Some mail orders don't come in on our standard AAP order forms. They may come in on stationery, telegrams, or non-AAP order forms. When they do, the first thing we have to do is to transcribe the order to AAP's order form, Form 50."

"Now that's a new one on me. Thanks Madge! That's exactly the kind of thing we're trying to find out during this walkthrough. But I'm not sure I understand the idea of non-AAP order forms." As she spoke, Cheryl was modifying the picture so the change could be made formally on the next set of pictures.

"That's because," Madge went on, "some of our customers are not AAP franchises. They use their own forms for submitting orders."

Cheryl continued, "I see. That makes sense. Okay, I've added a transcription process here. Let's continue. All orders must be screened [see ② on Figure 1]. And as Madge explained a moment ago, they must be on Form 50 before they can be screened. As we understand the screening process, a single clerk screens each order. Is that correct?"

Karen replied, "That's right."

"Good. That's why we showed the screening as a single process. The screening consists of a number of items. You verify the customer data [③]. You also verify that the parts ordered are valid [④]. For any part that isn't valid, you request clarification via a form letter. Then you log the order into the Sales Order Log on the clerk's desk [⑤] and place the order into the out box for data processing [⑥]. Have we forgotten anything?"

Ted noted, "Yes, sometimes an order will contain a part that we don't stock in the warehouse. We find this out when we check the ordered parts against the Parts Master Catalog [④]. When this happens, we fill out a purchase request, Form 66. At the end of the day, all purchase requests are forwarded to the Purchasing Department for processing."

Cheryl was embarrassed. "I should have known that. I just finished a Purchasing System project. Those requests are used to generate orders that'll be delivered directly to the customer, bypassing this Distribution Center, right?"

"That's right," answered Ted. Cheryl was already making the change to the diagram.

"Pardon me," Joey spoke up. "It's not clear on your diagram that orders that have problems are placed into an in/out box that we call Pending Orders. At the end of the day, we send those orders to the Order Follow-Up Group for subsequent processing." (to page 216) ▶

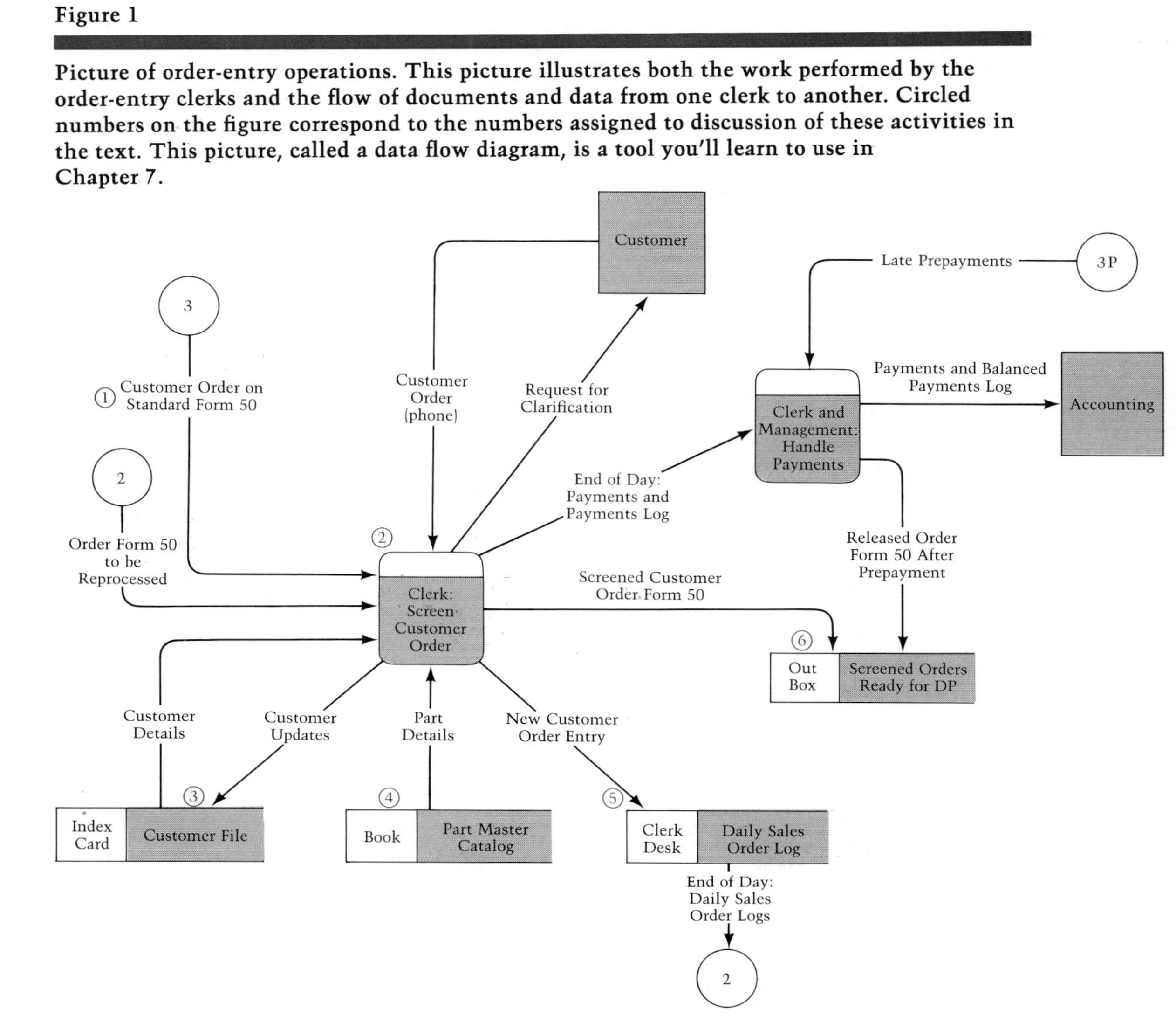

Figure 1

Picture of order-entry operations. This picture illustrates both the work performed by the order-entry clerks and the flow of documents and data from one clerk to another. Circled numbers on the figure correspond to the numbers assigned to discussion of these activities in the text. This picture, called a data flow diagram, is a tool you'll learn to use in Chapter 7.

Cheryl shook her head. "We goofed. We knew about that and just forgot to draw it. Doug, will you sketch that on the picture? Moving right along, we see that payments are stripped during the screening process and sent . . ."

[*You should get the idea by now. We can quietly sneak out of the meeting.*]

Analyzing Problems and Opportunities

Four more days have passed. Doug and Cheryl have completely drawn and verified the Customer Services System. Let's join Cheryl and Doug in their office and see what they're doing now.

"Well, Doug, that's just about it for documenting the current system. Do you think we should discuss some of the current system's problems and limitations before we write our report?"

"Yes! Let's take it one subsystem at a time, beginning with the order-entry function, and let's brainstorm some of the problems we've uncovered. I'll take notes for the report."

Cheryl was ready to start. "It seems to me the biggest problem that occurs with orders is the delay incurred during the screening process. Let's analyze the problem in terms of causes and effects. What causes the problem?"

"A major cause is the large number of manual files that have to be accessed. Those index card files for customers are frequently shuffled out of numerical order and are not always up to date. The Parts Master Catalog suffers from the same problem. I noticed that one clerk was using an old catalog because the most recent edition had been misplaced. Furthermore, the customer data and part data are *reverified* by data processing—it seems redundant."

"Well, Douglas, you've identified three causes! What about the effects of this problem?"

"I'm not through with this delay thing, Cheryl. I observed five phone orders, and the average credit check took five minutes. Sometimes the credit check took ten minutes. I wonder how many orders are phoned in during the time that phone is tied up?"

Cheryl was pleased with Doug's in-depth analysis. "Nice pickup. Anything else?"

Doug shook his head, and Cheryl took over. "Did you get a sense that any significant numbers of errors are being made while processing transactions?"

"No," answered Doug. "The clerks seem to do a fairly good job of transcribing orders. However, between 10:00 A.M. and 2:00 P.M., the clerks appear to be consistently busy. They don't stop for lunch. Also, Fridays and Mondays are busier than other days. Unfortunately, this is the period when it takes Accounts Receivable longest to perform a credit check."

Doug offered the next question. "What about management? How would you rate management's role in the order-entry system?"

"What management?" asked Cheryl. "Joey and Madge supervise and fill in, but they don't seem to manage in the classic sense of the word."

Doug replied, "I don't think we want to say that in our report—not if we want to get our next paycheck."

Cheryl laughed and replied, "I didn't mean it in a bad way anyhow. How can there be effective management without information? There is very little data collected to help managers do a more effective job for planning, control, and decision making. I don't think Joey knows the potential value of the information we can provide him."

Doug nodded. "Actually the system works fairly well, except for the increasing order processing time. Let's be sure to say that in the report."

"And," Cheryl added, "we should note the problem of lost orders. Remember? Karen said that orders occasionally get lost between Order Entry and the ▶

warehouse. Nobody follows up on those orders until the customer complains. It usually costs the company a sale, especially for smaller orders that the customer needed filled promptly."

[*We leave the room.*]

Cheryl and Doug will do a similar analysis on each subsystem and prepare a formal report in which they present their findings to management. The report will include an update of their tentative alternative solutions and a feasibility update. The feasibility update will focus on each alternative's ability to solve the problems identified during the study phase. Costs will not become a significant issue until the evaluation phase.

Where Do We Go from Here? This episode of the running case previewed some of the skills that are important during the analysis of the current system. Before Cheryl and Doug begin trying to figure out what's wrong with the system, they are trying to learn as much as possible about how the system works.

First, they collected facts about the system. Fact finding is an important skill for you to learn. Because fact finding is not done *only* during systems analysis, we have chosen not to include training on this skill in this systems analysis unit. Instead, you will find the necessary material in Part IV, Module B: "Skills Which Overlap Systems Analysis, Design, and Implementation." You have all the prerequisites needed to study that module at this time.

Second, in order to learn about the system, Cheryl and Doug drew a picture. In Chapter 7, you will learn that the picture they drew is called a *data flow diagram*—a very important tool for every systems analyst to master! But data flow diagrams are only tools. That's easy to forget when you are learning about data flow diagrams in Chapter 7, but try to keep in mind that systems analysis is a people-oriented activity.

And also note that Cheryl and Doug had to make a presentation of their findings (two presentations if you count the written report that they will soon submit). Presentations, like fact finding, require skills not restricted to systems analysis. Therefore, you will find the module on presentations in Part IV of the book. Again, you already have the necessary prerequisites for reading and understanding this material, which is presented in Module C: "Communications Skills for the Systems Analyst." ■

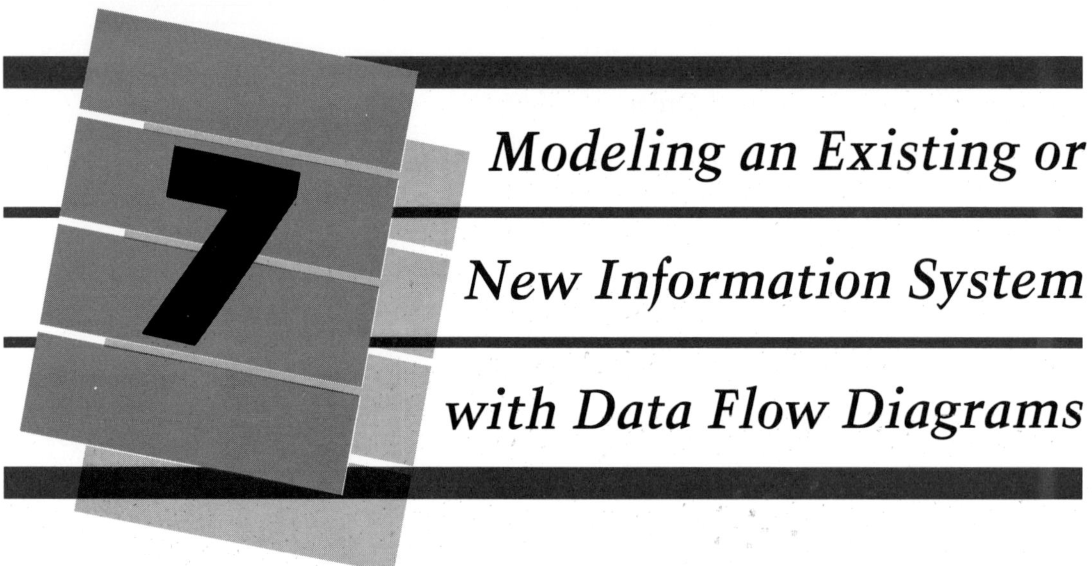

7 Modeling an Existing or New Information System with Data Flow Diagrams

Minicase: Platters by Mail Record Club

The Platters by Mail Record Club advertises records and albums in a variety of magazines. Most orders are submitted by magazine subscribers who complete and send coupons to the mail order company. All mail arrives at the receptionist's desk. The receptionist sorts and distributes the mail to the appropriate departments. Mail orders and letters requesting order cancellations are forwarded to an order-entry clerk in the Sales Department.

The order-entry clerk initially checks the availability and price of the ordered items, possibly mailing a back order notice to the customer. This clerk also takes orders from customers directly by phone and forwards all fillable order forms to the credit clerk.

When the order-entry clerk receives a letter requesting an order cancellation (or a cancellation by telephone), the status of the order is first determined. If the customer order has not been invoiced, the order-entry clerk informs the warehouse that the order should be canceled and then informs the customer that the cancellation has been completed.

When fillable orders are received by the credit clerk, the customer's credit status is checked. Orders are approved and an order-confirmation letter is sent to those customers with good credit standing. Customers with bad credit standing are sent a payment overdue notice requesting prepayment. The credit clerk forwards approved orders to the warehouse.

The warehouse fills the approved order and updates the inventory availability. A packing slip is sent with the packaged order to the customer, and a shipping notice is sent to the Accounts Receivable Department.

Accounts Receivable bills the customer for the products shipped. This department also maintains the invoice data files, updating them to reflect charges or payments received. Payments are received in the mail and delivered to Accounts Receivable by the receptionist. A payment receipt is sent to the customer.

The assistant sales manager is responsible for answering frequent customer inquiries concerning product prices, customer credit, and invoice data.

Challenge

One of the challenges for systems analysts is to communicate their understanding of an existing system or to propose and sell the users on a proposed system. To this end, analysts have learned that pictures communicate better than words. On a single eight-and-a-half- by eleven-inch sheet of paper, draw a picture to describe the business flow explained above. If you have difficulty, don't be too concerned. This chapter introduces you to a tool that will suit your purpose.

WHAT WILL YOU LEARN IN THIS CHAPTER?

In this chapter you will learn how to use a popular system modeling tool, the *data flow diagram,* to document the flow of data and information through a system. You will know you have mastered the use of data flow diagrams as a systems analysis tool when you can:

1. Factor a system into component subsystems, functions, and tasks and depict its structure using a hierarchy chart.

2. Document the interfaces between subsystems, functions, and tasks using a data flow diagram.
3. Describe how data flow diagrams document an information system and how they can be used during the systems analysis phases.
4. Develop a set of leveled data flow diagrams for an existing or proposed information system.
5. Differentiate between physical and logical data flow diagrams and explain when to use each.

Recall that the primary purpose of systems analysis is to study a problem situation, define solution requirements, and evaluate alternative solutions. But how do you know if you truly understand an existing information system? How do you know if the information system you are proposing will fulfill the knowledge worker's needs? Obviously, you need some way to communicate your understanding of the system to the knowledge workers. But *how?* An information system is very complex and contains many components that interact to capture data and produce information. We cannot reasonably expect an English narrative to communicate our understanding of a system. An English narrative might explain what you know, but it will not necessarily indicate what you *don't* know. If the reader or listener fails to realize what you've left out, the omission may go unnoticed until too late. We need a better tool!

How about a *picture* of the system? In this chapter, we study the data flow diagram (DFD), a tool for drawing a picture of an information system without concern for *excessive* details, whether they be data processing or manual. Data flow diagrams can be *the* most important tool available to the analyst during the analysis phases. Let's study this tool, its conventions, and its uses.

DATA FLOW DIAGRAM CONVENTIONS AND GUIDELINES

Even after the analyst has identified the user community, spoken to those people, gathered sample documents and reports, determined goals and objectives, and so forth, *the analyst often does not have a clear picture of the total system!* A **data flow diagram (DFD)** illustrates the flow of data through a system and the work performed by that system. In fact, we like to describe this tool to users as nothing more than a picture of their business operation. This tool's popularity is an outgrowth of a systems analysis methodology called *Structured Analysis and Design.* This book doesn't cover the methodology; however, the tool is useful to any system development strategy.

Data Flow Diagram Symbols

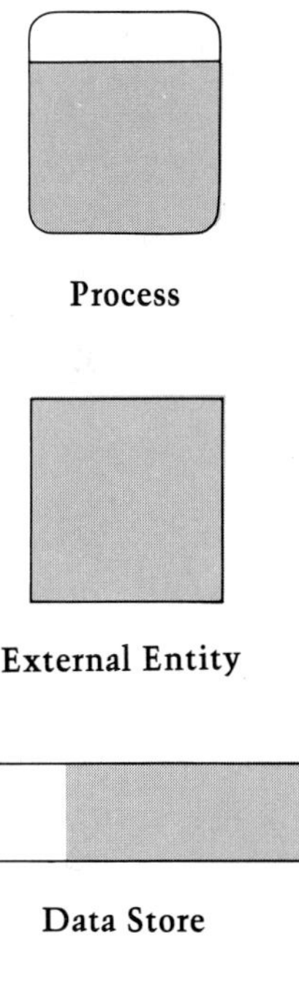

Data Flow

Figure 7.1 (see p. 222) demonstrates the basic symbols of a DFD. We have chosen to diagram a familiar system, personal finance. We all must pay our bills, balance our checkbook, budget our money, and so on. DFDs are pretty easy to read and understand.

In a DFD, the emphasis is placed on the process, which is represented by a rounded rectangle (symbols are also depicted in the margin). Processes transform input data flows into output data flows. The details of the transformation are not shown. Therefore, you can immediately conclude that DFDs do not show as much procedural detail as computer program flowcharts. The open-ended boxes depict data stores, which are collections of data used and maintained by the system. In Figure 7.1, bank statements are being saved for future reference (hence BANK STATEMENTS is in an open-ended box). We also depicted the checkbook as a data store because all transactions are recorded in that book, and those entries are used to balance the account at a later date. The squares on our picture represent external entities in the system's environment that input data to the system or receive information from the system. These entities define the boundary of the system. Finally, the named arrows depict the data flows. Data flows can depict reports, forms, entries, updates, and any other data or information flow.

Don't confuse DFDs with flowcharts! Most of you are reading this book after some exposure to computer programming. Part of programming centers around the use of flowcharts. *Data flow diagrams are very different from flowcharts!* Let's summarize the differences:

- Processes on a DFD can operate in parallel. Thus, several processes may be working simultaneously. For instance, you may be balancing your checkbook at the same time as your partner is paying the bills. This is a key advantage over flowcharts, which tend to show only sequential processes. In a realistic business system, activities and processing overlap one another.

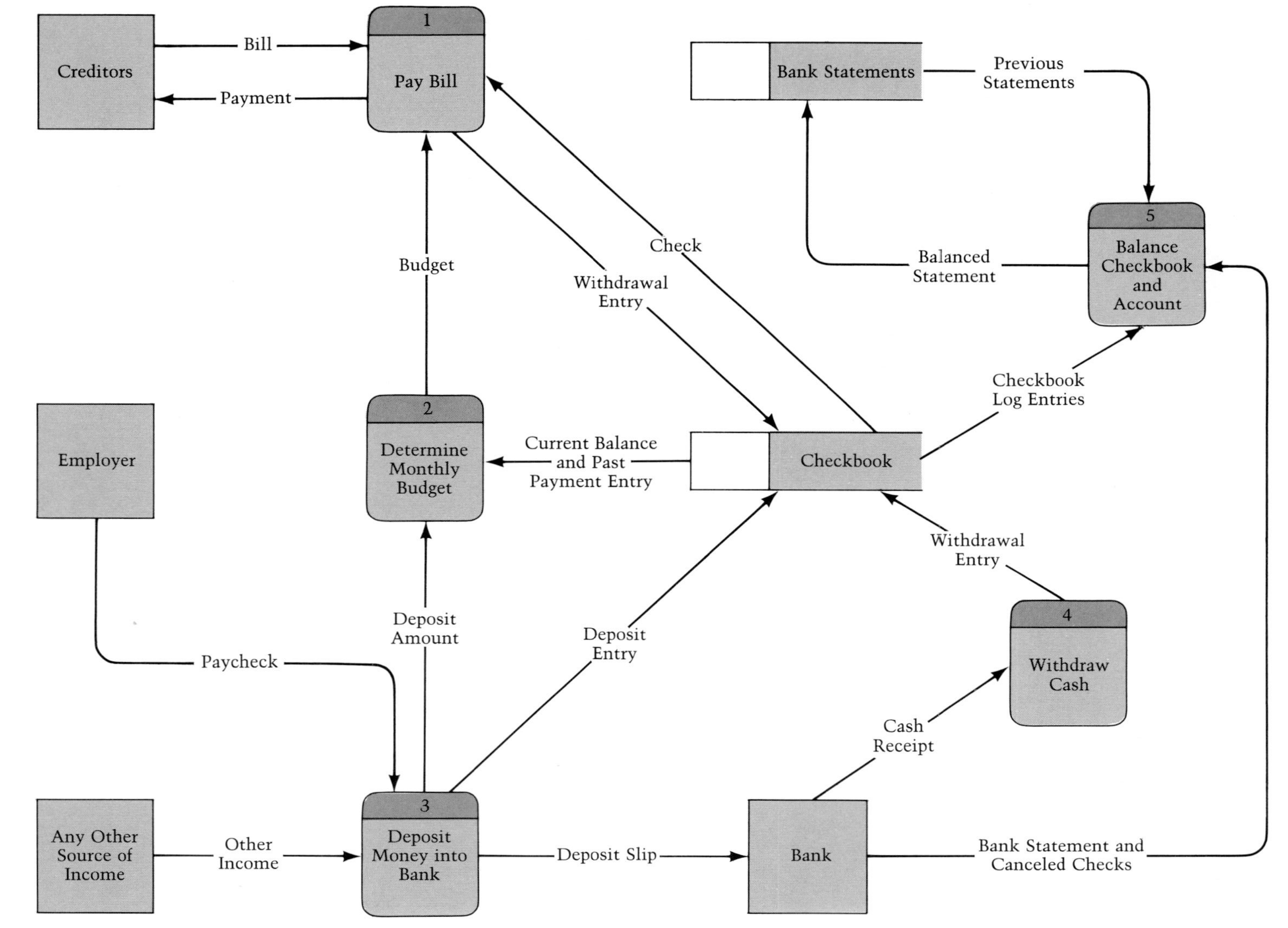
Creditors
Bill
Payment
1
Pay Bill
Bank Statements
Previous Statements
5
Balance Checkbook and Account
Balanced Statement
Budget
Check
Withdrawal Entry
Checkbook Log Entries
Employer
2
Determine Monthly Budget
Current Balance and Past Payment Entry
Checkbook
Withdrawal Entry
Deposit Amount
Deposit Entry
4
Withdraw Cash
Paycheck
Cash Receipt
Any Other Source of Income
Other Income
3
Deposit Money into Bank
Deposit Slip
Bank
Bank Statement and Canceled Checks

◄ Figure 7.1

Simple data flow diagram. This is a simple data flow diagram for a personal finance system. Notice that some of the processes can occur on several days of a month (such as processes 1, 3, and 4). Other processes usually occur only once each month (such as processes 2 and 5). Also, more than one process may execute simultaneously. For instance, you may pay a bill at the exact same time as your partner makes a deposit. Finally, there is no true starting point on a DFD. These features differentiate data flow diagrams from systems flowcharts.

- DFDs show the flow of data through a system. Flowcharts show the sequence of steps in an algorithm. DFDs, unlike flowcharts, do *not* explicitly show looping and decision (if-then-else) constructs.
- DFDs can show processes that have dramatically different timing. For example, you make many deposits and withdrawals to your bank account before you balance your account.

Noting these differences, let's study the DFD symbols and conventions in greater detail.

The External Entity or Boundary Every system has a boundary. The boundary separates a system from its environment. And most systems exchange inputs and outputs with their environment. External entities are people, organizations, and other systems in a system's environment. An external entity is almost always one of the following:

- An office, department, or division within your company but external to the system being studied or designed
- A person or persons within your company but outside the scope of your system (such as a specific manager or administrator)
- An organization or agency that is altogether outside your company (for instance, customers, suppliers, government agencies)
- Another information system (possibly computer-based) outside the scope of your system but with which your system must interact
- The original source of an input transaction
- The final recipient of a report

Services and processing performed for your system by data processing are always part of your system. *Data processing support is not an external entity.* Do you understand why? Think about it for a moment. Your knowledge workers are ultimately responsible for the work performed for it by data processing. If DP is processing your orders and the computer becomes unavailable, who would have to process the orders? That's right, the knowledge workers in your system. Therefore, DP support is *not* shown as boundary. Instead, it is shown as processes on your DFDs.

The Data Flow What is a data flow? Think of the **data flow** as a highway down which *packets* of data of *known composition* are allowed to travel. Data flows travel between processes, data stores, and external entities. Data flow packets may include the following:

- A business form or document
- A printed report (not necessarily computer generated)
- A computer terminal display of a report or form
- A computer input
- A spoken communication (of fixed, well-defined content)
- A form letter or memorandum
- Data retrieved from or stored in a file
- An entry being recorded in a logbook or on a data sheet
- A data transmission from one computer to another

Data flows can be inputs or outputs. In any case, the key to defining a data flow is *known composition.* Occurrences of the data flow must contain data. This principle is one of the most consistently violated rules of DFDs! Why? The temptation is to use a data flow to illustrate step 1, step 2, and so on. This is *flowchart* thinking! Such thinking results in unnamed data flows with no data composition. How can you avoid this mistake?

1. Label or name all data flows, that's how! If you can't name the data flow, it probably doesn't exist. For example, look at Figure 7.2. What should we name the data flow in question? How about GET NEXT REQUISITION? That won't work. Why? Because GET NEXT REQUISITION is not data—it is an instruction.
2. Try to describe the data elements that make up the data flow. If you can't name or describe those elements (for example, REQUI-

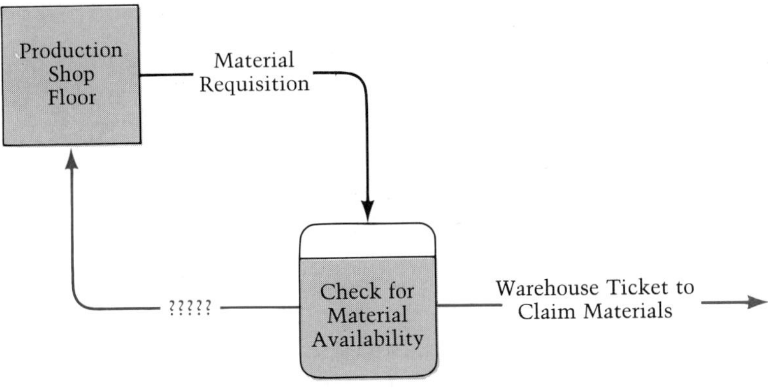

Figure 7.2

Data flows should have data content. All data flows should contain data. If they don't, they are probably not data flows and shouldn't be shown. The questioned data flow on this diagram is probably not data—It looks as though it might be an instruction such as "get next requisition." If this is the case, it should be deleted.

SITION NUMBER, DATE, MATERIAL REQUESTED, QUANTITY) then the data flow doesn't exist.

Data flow names should be descriptive and meaningful to your users (who will have to be able to read the DFDs). Sometimes it is appropriate or desirable to use buzzwords or form numbers familiar to your users. "We fill out a '23' in triplicate and send it to . . ." is a common user explanation of their data flow. The real name of the '23' may actually be COURSE REQUEST FORM. Which name should you use in your DFD? Well, that depends on whether you are using the DFD to describe *how* the system works (called physical DFDs) or *what* the system does (called logical DFDs). Later in this chapter we discuss when to draw which kind of DFD. The point we want to make here is that names on the DFD should be meaningful!

A more subtle problem is also common. Recall that we described a data flow as a *packet* of data. The packet concept is critical. For example, suppose the phone company sends you an itemized INVOICE of your charges for the month *along with* a PAYMENT CARD that must be returned with your PAYMENT. The INVOICE and PAYMENT CARD should be depicted on the DFD as a *single* data flow (see Figure 7.3). Why? Because they travel together as a packet! Data that travel together should be shown as one data flow, no matter how many documents are involved.

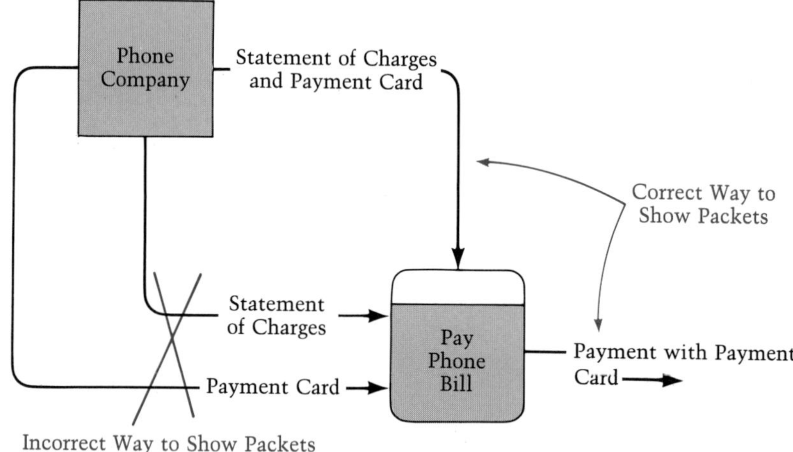

Figure 7.3

The data flow packet concept. If two or more documents travel together, they should be shown as parts of a single data flow.

General Process Names

ACCOUNTS RECEIVABLE SYSTEM
BILLING SUBSYSTEM
CREDIT FUNCTION
PROCESS PAYMENT
HANDLE DISPUTE

Detailed Process Names

CREDIT CUSTOMER ACCOUNT
RECORD AMOUNT IN DISPUTE
UPDATE CUSTOMER CREDIT RATING
IDENTIFY POOR CREDIT RISKS
SUMMARIZE RECEIPTS

Figure 7.4 illustrates two more data flow concepts: *diverging* and *converging* data flows. Diverging data flows, represented by ① on Figure 7.4, are very useful for illustrating a common business practice, multi-part business forms or multiple copies of a report being distributed to different destinations. In Figure 7.4, you see an ORDER form that is *burst,* with the copies sent to various destinations. Converging data flows (② on Figure 7.4) are less common. They represent portions of a single data flow that originate at different processes or external entities. For example, suppose that the packing copy of the ORDER must be consolidated with the BILL-OF-LADING for shipment.

Finally, *all data flows must begin and/or end at a process because data flows either initiate a process or result from a process!*

The Process Processes are work that is performed by people, machines, or computers on incoming data flows to produce outgoing data flows. Every process should be given a reference number (recorded at the top of the symbol) and a descriptive name. Naming should not be taken lightly. Names should clearly and completely describe the process. Process names are recorded below the reference number in the symbol. Sometimes you draw high-level DFDs to show the general flow or big picture of the system, omitting

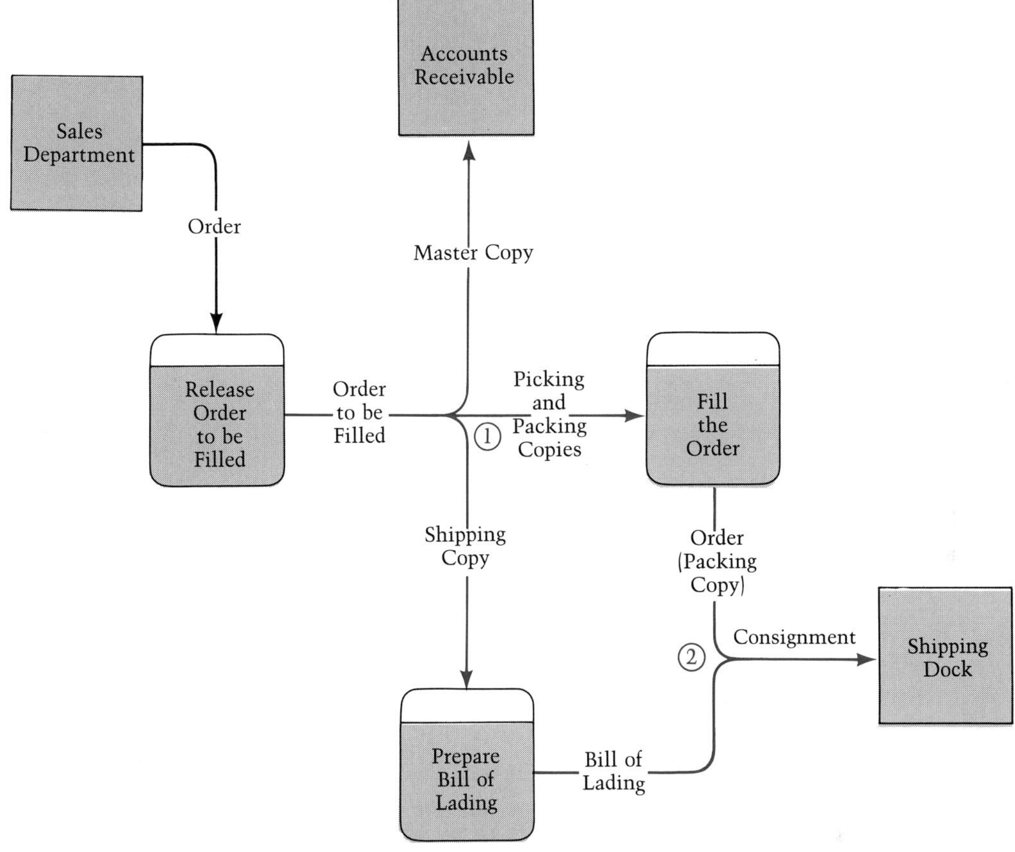

Figure 7.4

Diverging and converging data flows. Diverging data flows represent copies or subsets of the same data flow that go to different destinations. Converging data flows represent separate data flows that have separate origins and come together to travel as a single packet.

detailed and exceptional data flows. Process names on these general DFDs will have to be equally general. Examples of general process names are listed in the margin on the previous page. On the other hand, the processes on detailed DFDs should be given more specific names consisting of a strong action verb followed by an object clause that describes what the action is performed on or for. Examples of more specific names are listed in the margin. The process name should be recorded below the reference number. In some

Reference #

Name of Processor: Description of Process

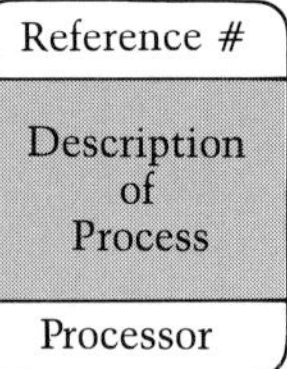

Reference #

Description of Process

Processor

Three Ways to Label Processes

cases (specifically, physical DFDs described later), it is useful to also record who or what performs the process or where the process is performed. Examples of the labeling conventions and their alternatives are illustrated in the margin.

When drawing DFDs, don't worry about the policies and procedures that underlie the processes. Some processes do nothing more than move or route data, leaving the data unchanged. For example, Figure 7.5 shows a secretary forwarding a variety of documents to their next processing location. Other processes actually work on incoming data flows, changing the composition or nature of those data flows. This change takes *one or more* of the following forms:

- Performing a computation using the incoming data flows and producing entirely new data flows (Figure 7.6a, p. 230)
- Splitting an incoming data flow into two or more outgoing data flows, each one a subset (possibly overlapping) of the incoming data flows (Figure 7.6b)
- Combining two or more incoming data flows into a lesser number of outgoing data flows (Figure 7.6c)
- Verifying one data flow against another (Figure 7.6d) (The output data flow has not been physically changed. Only the nature of the data flow is changed—we know something after the processing that we didn't know before the processing.)
- Reorganizing incoming data flows (Figure 7.6e) (In this case, the incoming data flows may be filtered, reformatted, or sorted. The data isn't changed, but it's structure is different.)

You may have noticed that a process can have many incoming and outgoing data flows. Some may occur every time the process is executed. Others may occur optionally, under certain conditions. The DFD does not show which data flows are mandatory and desirable or in what combinations they occur. These details are deferred until the procedures for the processes have been specified (Chapter 9).

We conclude our discussion of processes by pointing out two common errors, black holes and miracles. Look at the DFD in Figure 7.7, p. 231. What is wrong with process 1? The process has inputs but no outputs. We call this a *black hole* because data enters the process and disappears. If you encounter a black hole, you probably forgot the output. What is wrong with process 2? You probably

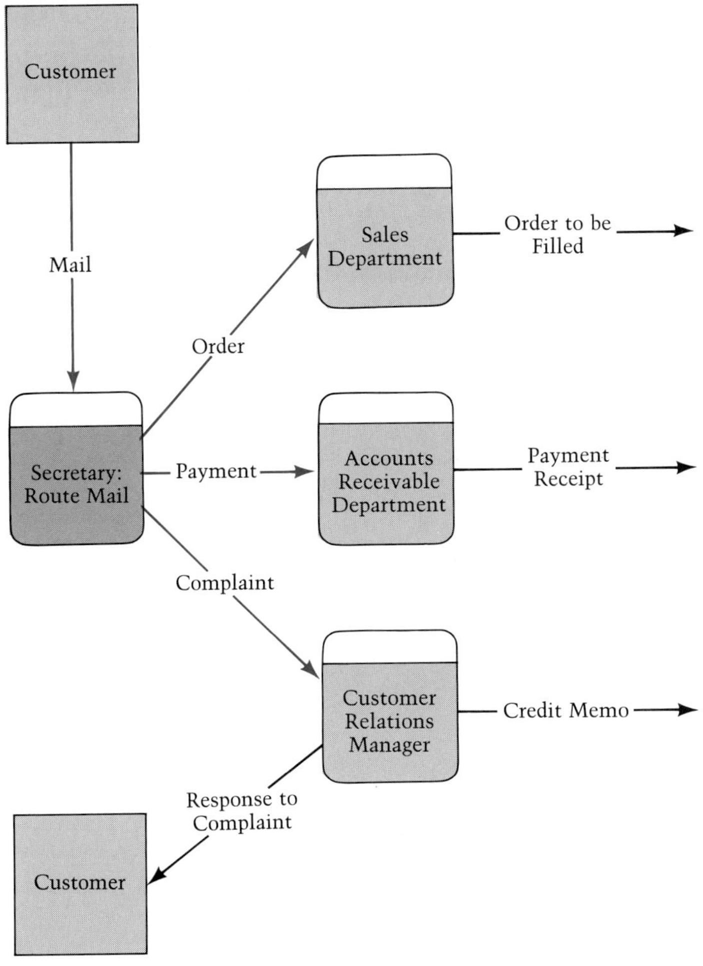

Figure 7.5

Routing or forwarding processes on the DFD. Some processes on a DFD do not change data. They simply route or forward data to another process that will change the data.

guessed it. The process has output but no input. Unless you are Merlin the Magician, this is a *miracle!* In this case, the input data flows were forgotten. Remember, information must be produced by using data. All processes must have at least one input and one output. Furthermore, the inputs must contain all the data necessary to produce the outputs.

Figure 7.6

DFD processes that change or transform data. Most DFD processes either physically change incoming data flows or change the nature of those incoming data flows—all before producing their output data flows.

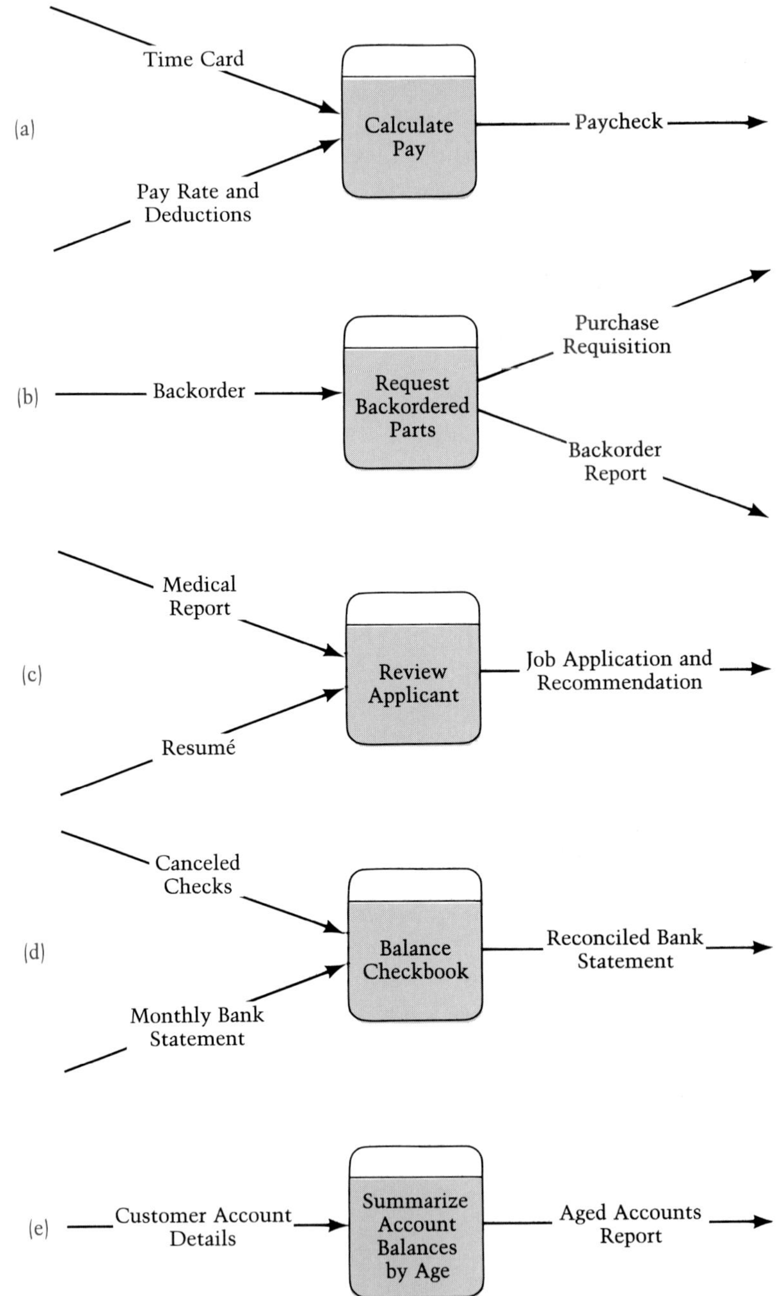

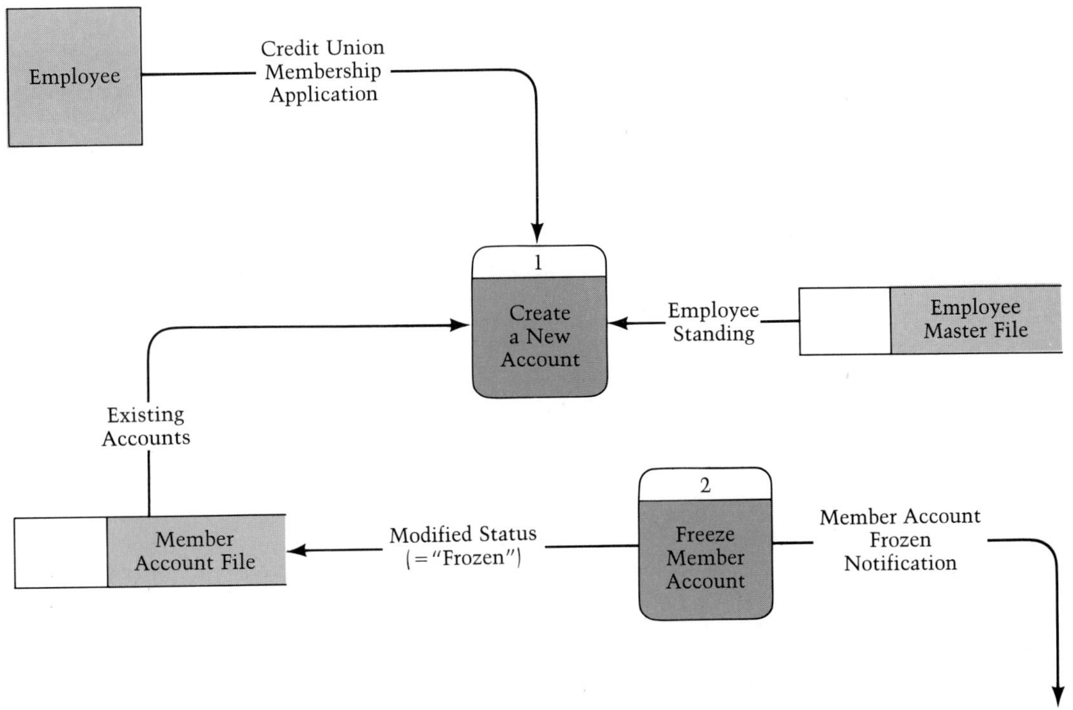

Figure 7.7

Common DFD errors. Process 1 has inputs but produces no outputs. This is called a *black-hole* error. Process 2 produces outputs but receives no inputs. This is called the *miracle* error. All processes must have at least one input and one output.

The Data Store **Data stores** are inventories of data that can take on many forms including:

- A computer file or database
- A file cabinet of records
- An index card file
- An in/out box on someone's desk
- A frequently referenced book or binder of reports or tables
- A log sheet or anything onto which entries are recorded (recall the checkbook in our personal finance DFD)

Medium	Name of File

Name of File
(Medium)

Two Ways to Label Data Stores

Let's first look at the notation we suggest for data stores. (These are illustrated in the margin.) Data store names should represent the data being stored. The term *data* should not be part of the name because it is implicit that the data store stores data (in fact, the terms *data* and *information* should be avoided for all DFD symbols). On some DFDs, the data store name is all we want to record in the box. On other DFDs, we might also be interested in the medium of the data store (such as disk, diskette, book, or box).

Data flows to and from data stores are significant and sometimes difficult to grasp. The trick is to forget thinking in computer terms. Our guidelines, illustrated in Figure 7.8, are as follows:

1. Only processes may interface with data stores. This makes sense because the use or update of a data store requires a person (for a manual data store) or a computer program (for a computerized data store).
2. The use of double-ended arrows for data flows is discouraged on detailed DFDs because the direction of arrows is significant. Data flow direction is interpreted as follows:
   (a) A data flow from a data store means that the process uses those data. Notice that we said *uses,* not *reads.* Of course we have to read a file to use it! The *read* is assumed. If the data store is not computerized, this notation may also signify removal of a form or document from the data store.
   (b) A data flow to a data store means that the process updates the data store. Updates may include any or all of the following:
      - *Adding or storing new records or forms in the data store* (This also includes making a new entry in a log.)
      - *Deleting or removing old records from the data store* (or deleting a log entry)
      - *Changing existing data records in the data store* (or changing a log entry)
3. Some processes both use and update data stores. For detailed level DFDs, use separate data flows for the use and the update. For more general DFDs, doubled-ended arrows may enhance readability.

Data Flow Names for Data Stores

ADD A NEW CUSTOMER

DELETE INACTIVE ACCOUNT

NEW STATUS

MODIFIED DEMOGRAPHIC DETAILS

REMOVE <name of any document>

USE <name of data retrieved>

<name of specific details used, e.g. CREDIT DETAILS>

Opinions on whether data flows to and from data stores should have unique names vary from one expert to another. Because data store usage and updates are usually numerous, we do not recommend unique names. However, it can be useful to give processlike names to these data flows to describe the nature of the use or up-

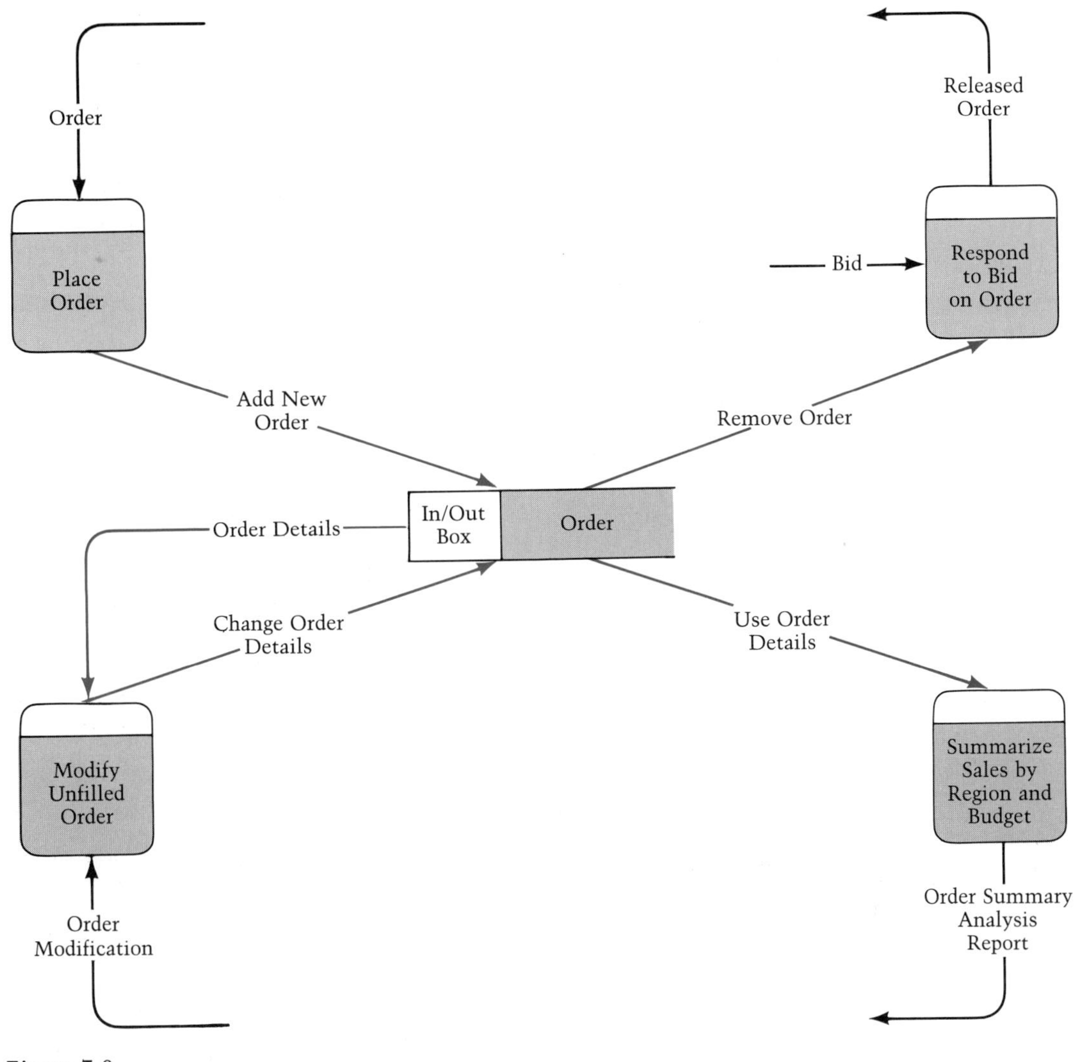

Figure 7.8

The significance of data flows to and from data stores. Be careful with data flows to and from data stores. The direction of the arrow may signify use of data, removal of data, creation of data, deletion of data, or modification of data. Read the guidelines carefully to make sure you know the difference. DFDs never show the reading of data for its own sake!

date. Sample names for data flows to and from data store are indicated in the margin on the previous page. You may find a better technique or even choose not to name such data flows.

The Documentation Value of Data Flow Diagrams

Before you try your hand at drawing DFDs, perhaps it will help if you appreciate exactly what DFDs can and cannot document. The documentation value of DFDs can be measured against your information system pyramid model—After all, it is the information system that we want to document. You may have already noticed that DFDs clearly depict all of the IPO components of the information system. The components of the information system (illustrated in the margin) correspond to the DFD symbols as follows:

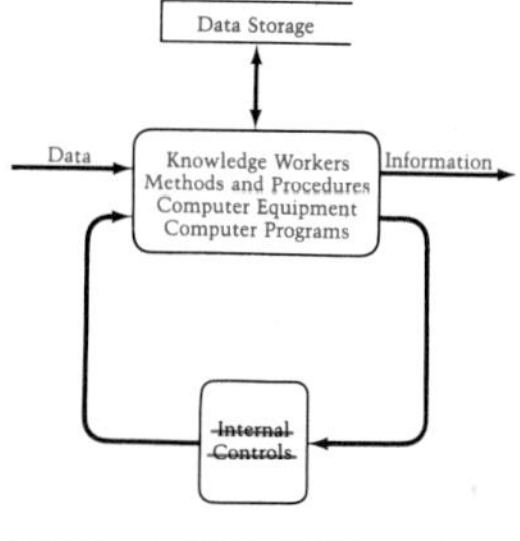

IPO Components of the Information System

IPO Component	*DFD Component*
Data (input)	Data flow
Information (output)	Data flow
Knowledge workers	External entity and process
Methods and procedures	Process
Data storage	Data store
Computer equipment	Process and data store
Computer programs	Process

Although DFDs depict all of the components of an information system, they do so without great detail. For example, the specific content of data flows and data stores and the exact policies and procedures implemented by processes are not shown on the DFD.

Additionally, DFDs can document all information system functions including transaction processing, management reporting, and decision support (part of the information system model is reproduced in the margin). This is demonstrated in Figure 7.9. Process 1 is processing a transaction (such as an employee time card) and updating a file (such as a payroll file). Process 2 is generating an output transaction (such as a paycheck) and a historical report (such as a payroll register). Processes 3 and 4 are generating management

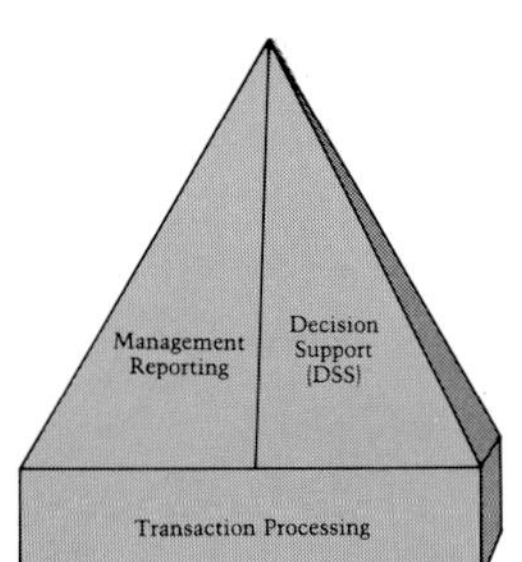

Information Systems Functions

Figure 7.9 ▶

A general model for a typical information system. This DFD demonstrates that the tool effectively models virtually any modern function of an information system. Most processing in real systems corresponds to one or more of the processes depicted here.

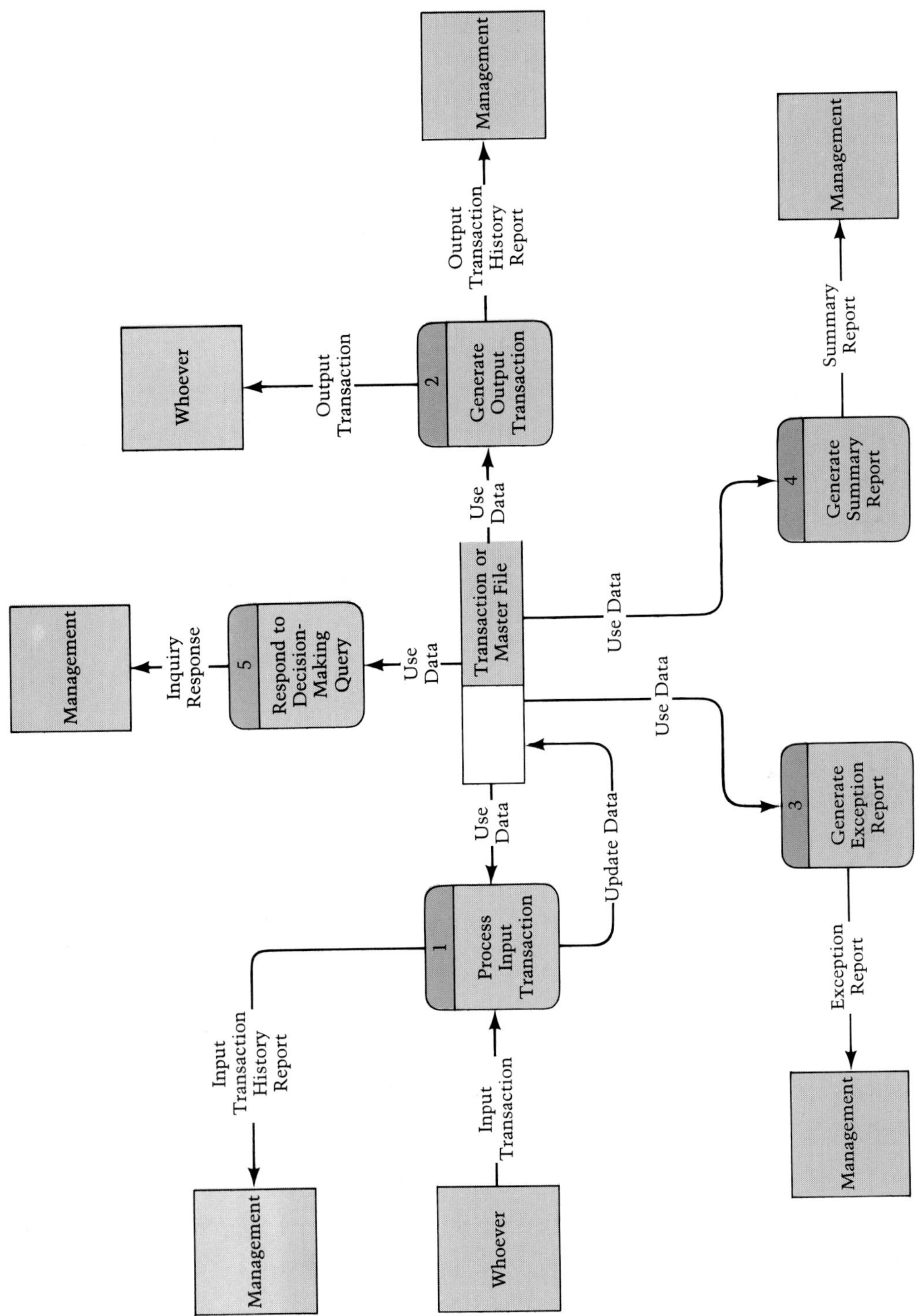
Management
Output Transaction History Report
Whoever
Output Transaction
2
Generate Output Transaction
Use Data
Management
Summary Report
4
Generate Summary Report
Use Data
Management
Inquiry Response
5
Respond to Decision-Making Query
Use Data
Transaction or Master File
Use Data
Use Data
Update Data
1
Process Input Transaction
3
Generate Exception Report
Exception Report
Management
Input Transaction History Report
Management
Input Transaction
Whoever

reports (such as a payroll-by-department summary and an overtime pay register). Finally, process 5 provides a query facility for decision support (such as an employee payroll query for the Personnel Department). This general DFD model will work, with some modification, for virtually any business application.

Now that we've learned the basic DFD conventions and values, let's learn when and how to draw DFDs for systems analysis.

USING DATA FLOW DIAGRAMS TO STUDY THE CURRENT SYSTEM

Let's begin our study of when and how to draw DFDs with the first *major* phase of our system development life cycle — Study the current system. During the study phase, we want to learn how the current system works. The best way to accomplish this task is to draw a picture of the system and then verify that picture with the users. Afterward, you will be able to identify and isolate problems, opportunities, and constraints using your DFDs.

Physical Data Flow Diagrams — What Are They?

Because the users see the system in terms of both *what* it currently does and *how* it works, we should draw a special kind of DFD that presents the system in these terms. A **physical data flow diagram** (PDFD) is just such a tool. The PDFD depicts those aspects of the current system that are dependent on *how* the processes, data flows, and data stores are implemented. Specifically, PDFDs should adhere to the following guidelines:

- Data flow names include implementation facts, such as form numbers, nicknames, and media (for example, *phone* or *form letter*). Data flow names may also explain timing (such as *end of the day*). In other words, names are sufficiently detailed to correspond with *how* the user knows the system to work.
- Data flows usually represent actual movements of data — the flow of forms, documents, reports, phone calls, correspondence, and so forth. A data flow that doesn't really flow may confuse the user and should not be shown.

- Data stores *may* include in/out boxes that serve only to buffer two sequential processes that operate at different rates of speed.
- Data store names identify their computer or manual implementation (for instance, ISAM File, IMS Database, Notebook, Clerk's Desk, or In/Out Box).
- Process names include the name of the *processor*—that is, the person, department, computer system, or computer program that actually executes the process.
- Processes shown should include trivial tasks. For instance, even if a secretary, clerk, or manager does nothing more than screen, route, or copy transactions, a process is shown for that action. Its absence may confuse the user.
- Finally, processes may include extraneous processes required because of any current data processing support. This may include processes such as data entry, input validation programs, file sorting and merging, job streams, and internal controls.
- PDFDs should only show normal, repetitive activities. Don't try to show all exceptional cases, *routine* file maintenance, backup and recovery, initializing the daily log, and the like.

Examples are forthcoming. But first, why show so much detail? A project is initiated because of problems, opportunities, or directives in the current system. The full extent of these may not be immediately apparent—even to the users! Detailed PDFDs get all the facts on the table so a true analysis of the system can be made. The physical implementation of the system may be the root cause of many problems. Therefore, the more implementation-oriented and realistic the PDFD, the better your chances of uncovering all problems, opportunities, and constraints.

The best way to appreciate PDFDs is to walk through the development of sample PDFDs. Our example is much smaller than a real project but representative of what we recommend for a student or training project. The example is large enough to demonstrate how you should deal with size and complexity. The case, based on a real business problem, is from the AAP order-processing project. You have little or no experience with real business applications; however, that is the case for most projects assigned to an analyst. Don't be overly concerned with the business problem. Focus on the strategy and techniques used to draw the PDFDs.

The Next Generation — *Graphics Support for Data Flow Diagrams*

Data flow diagrams, like program and systems flowcharts, can be tedious to draw and maintain. Users and analysts frequently find errors or make changes. Changes typically require several pages of diagrams to be redrawn. And redrawing any diagram carries with it the risk that you will make a copying error. Fortunately, data flow diagrams have become so popular that graphics software is now available for drawing and maintaining these diagrams. And even in those cases where it is not available, general purpose graphics software can be used to support data flow diagramming.

In the "Next Generation" feature in Chapter 6, we identified two microcomputer-based systems analyst productivity workstations, Index Technology's EXCELERATOR and Nastec's MTC 2000. These workstations support data flow diagramming as well as other diagramatic techniques. Although they cost several thousand dollars per workstation, they provide support for more than just data flow diagramming and graphics.

For the more restricted budget, there are graphics packages that do not include all of the sophisticated tools offered in the complete workstation. For example, Improved Systems Technology offers a data flow diagramming software package called DFD DRAW (for the IBM PC). Micrografx offers a general purpose diagramming software package, called PC-DRAW, that can be used to draw DFDs. These graphics-only packages typically retail for $500 or less. Finally, we should note that several of our students have developed their own DFD graphics tools using general purpose graphics software. For example, the DFD shown in Figure A was drawn by a student who used Apple's MACPAINT software on a MACINTOSH microcomputer.

The advantage of diagramming graphics software is clear once you have to start modifying a diagram. You can easily move symbols around on the chart. You can easily add, delete, and insert new symbols. (*Note:* This is not true of general purpose software, such as MACPAINT.) You can also change labels in or on any DFD symbol. The productivity improvements offered by these tools can be substantial. No longer do analysts have to live in fear of the statement, "This is pretty close, but I forgot to tell you about . . ." ■

Figure A ▶

A computer-generated data flow diagram.

Getting Started: Draw a Hierarchical Outline

A PDFD for a typical system, even a small to medium-sized system, could be very large — perhaps covering a wall in a good-sized room. Although physically impressive, such a diagram would be cumbersome to prepare, difficult to modify, and intimidating to your users.

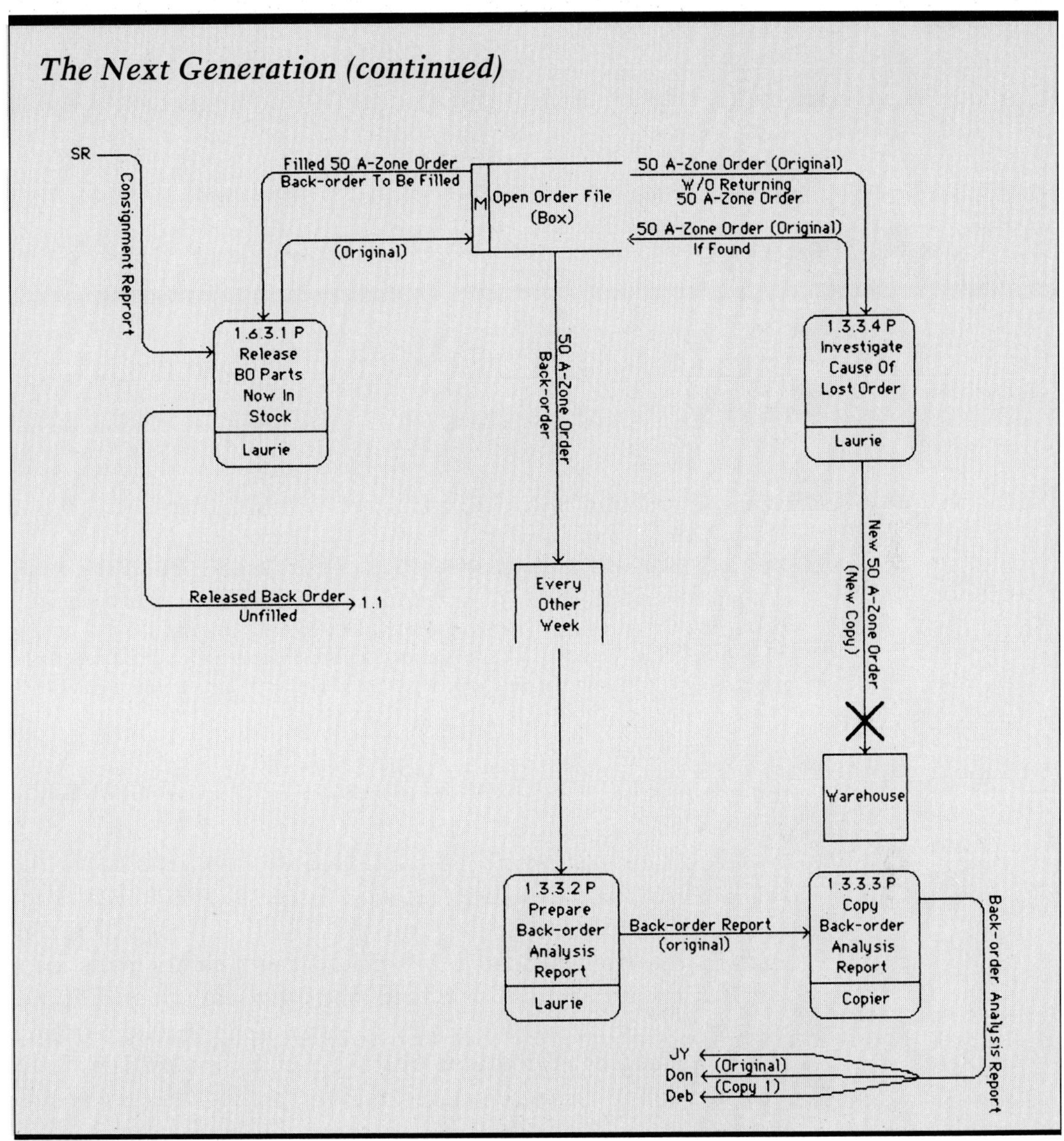

Let's learn how to model a system by drawing a series of interrelated, smaller PDFDs. These diagrams are easier to prepare, read, present, and modify.

Let's apply the same strategy we use to write a paper or code a large computer program: Divide and conquer. We will use an outline — a pictorial outline in this case. **Hierarchy charts** show the

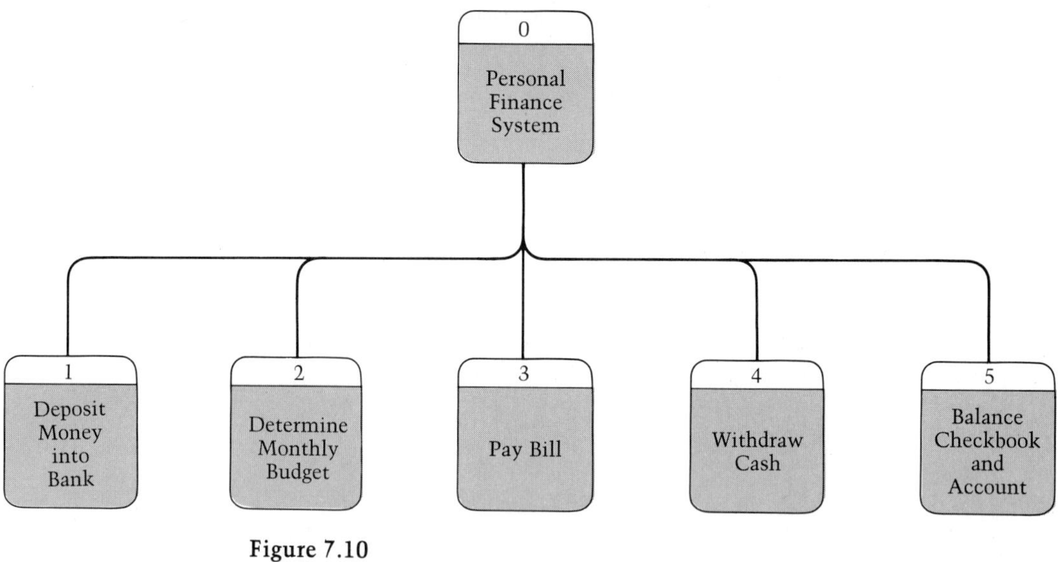

Figure 7.10

A simple hierarchy chart. This is a simple hierarchy chart that was used to outline the personal finance system prior to drawing the DFD you saw in Figure 7.1. Generally, there is a one-to-one correspondence between the processes on any level of the hierarchy chart and the same level of the DFD.

top-down structure of a system and give us an outline for drawing our PDFDs.

There is only one symbol used on the hierarchy chart; that is the rounded rectangle, which represents a process. The processes are connected to form a treelike structure. Figure 7.10 is a hierarchy chart for the personal finance system introduced earlier in the chapter. The top process, also called the *root,* represents all of the functions and activities we are calling *personal finance.* The root process is *factored* or *exploded* to greater detail at the next level of the tree. The connecting lines suggest that the personal finance system consists of five functions. If necessary, any or all of these functions could be exploded to even greater detail. Process names should conform to the naming guidelines described for DFDs.

When drawing *physical* DFDs, we suggest you begin with another hierarchy chart that may already be available—the company's organization chart. Our organization chart (actually, a subchart) is illustrated in Figure 7.11. The scope of our system project is drawn as a boundary on the chart. And Figure 7.12 is the hierarchy chart for our customer services system. Let's study this chart.

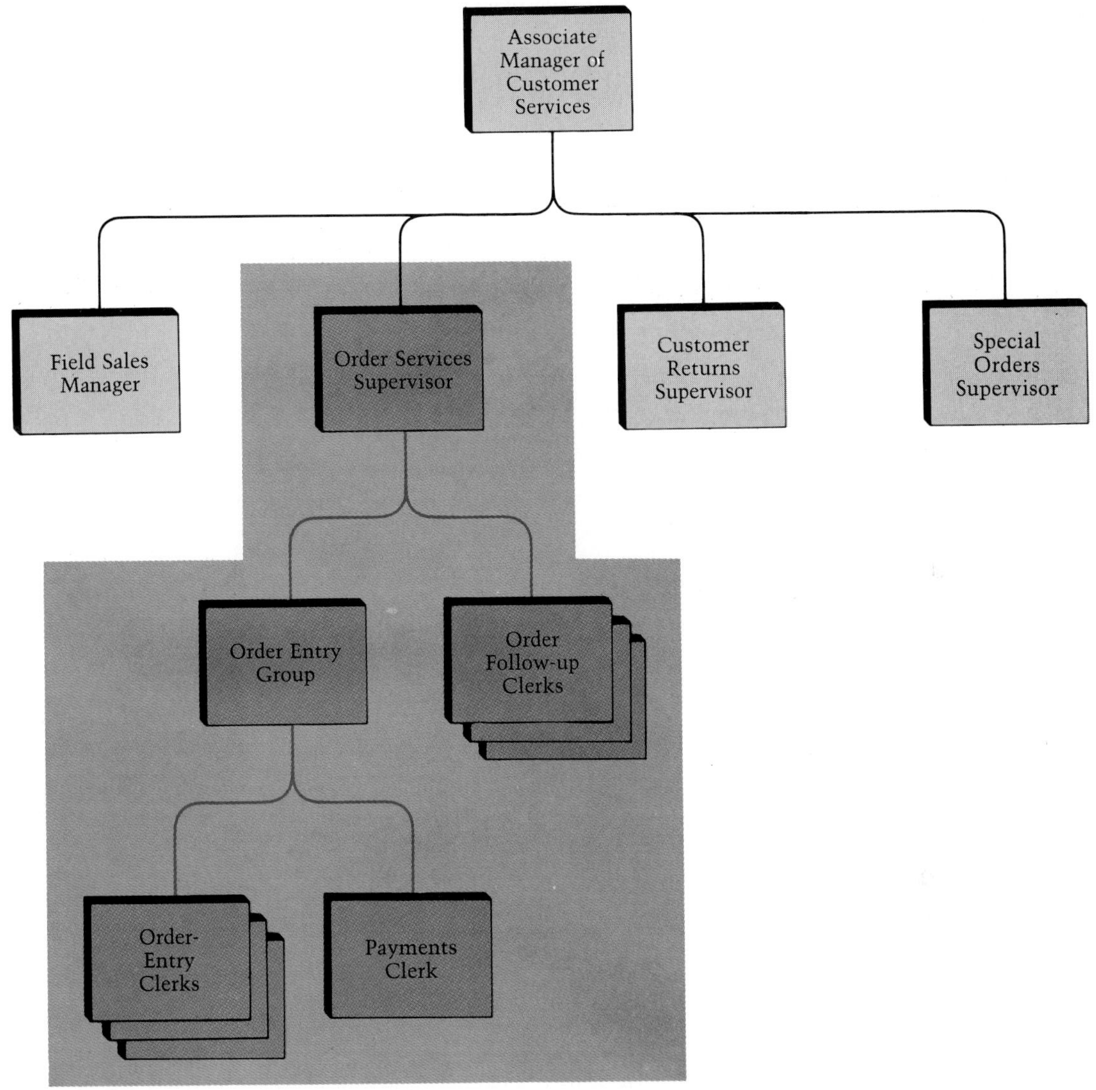

Figure 7.11

Organization chart for American Automotive Parts, Inc. The organization chart is a starting point for drawing hierarchy charts and physical data flow diagrams (PDFDs).

First we call your attention to the reference numbering scheme used in the chart depicted in Figure 7.12. We follow these guidelines for assigning reference numbers:

1. The root process is numbered 0.
2. The root process is factored into processes that are numbered consecutively, 1, 2, 3, and so on.
3. With subsequent factoring (also called leveling) of any process into subprocesses, each subprocess is numbered as a decimal of the parent process. For instance, process 1 is factored into processes 1.1, 1.2, 1.3, and so forth. Process 1.1 is factored into processes 1.1.1, 1.1.2, and so on. This strategy is repeated throughout the hierarchy charts.

The following is a step-by-step discussion of the development of the hierarchy chart depicted in Figure 7.12:

Ⓐ The root system process in the hierarchy chart corresponds to the highest-level organization unit within the scope of the system. We used names from the organization chart because the users recognize that physical structure. It should be noted that the scope of any project may change during any project.

Ⓑ The system is initially factored into subsystems that correspond to our organization chart. We recommend this strategy for PDFDs of current systems because the organization structure is familiar to the users. In our case, the Order Services Department is factored into the order-entry group and the order follow-up group.

Ⓒ To further factor the order-entry group process, we have to abandon our organization chart because it goes no further. (*Note:* The further factoring of the order follow-up group is used as an exercise at the end of the chapter.) After studying the order-processing tasks performed by the order-entry group, we learned that the tasks could be conveniently grouped into three functions: tasks performed to get an order ready for data processing, data processing tasks, and tasks performed after data processing.

Why didn't we just factor order entry straight into the *actual* tasks? Because there are too many of those tasks to place on a single data flow diagram (remember, PDFDs are our goal). Is there any limit to the number of subprocesses you can factor

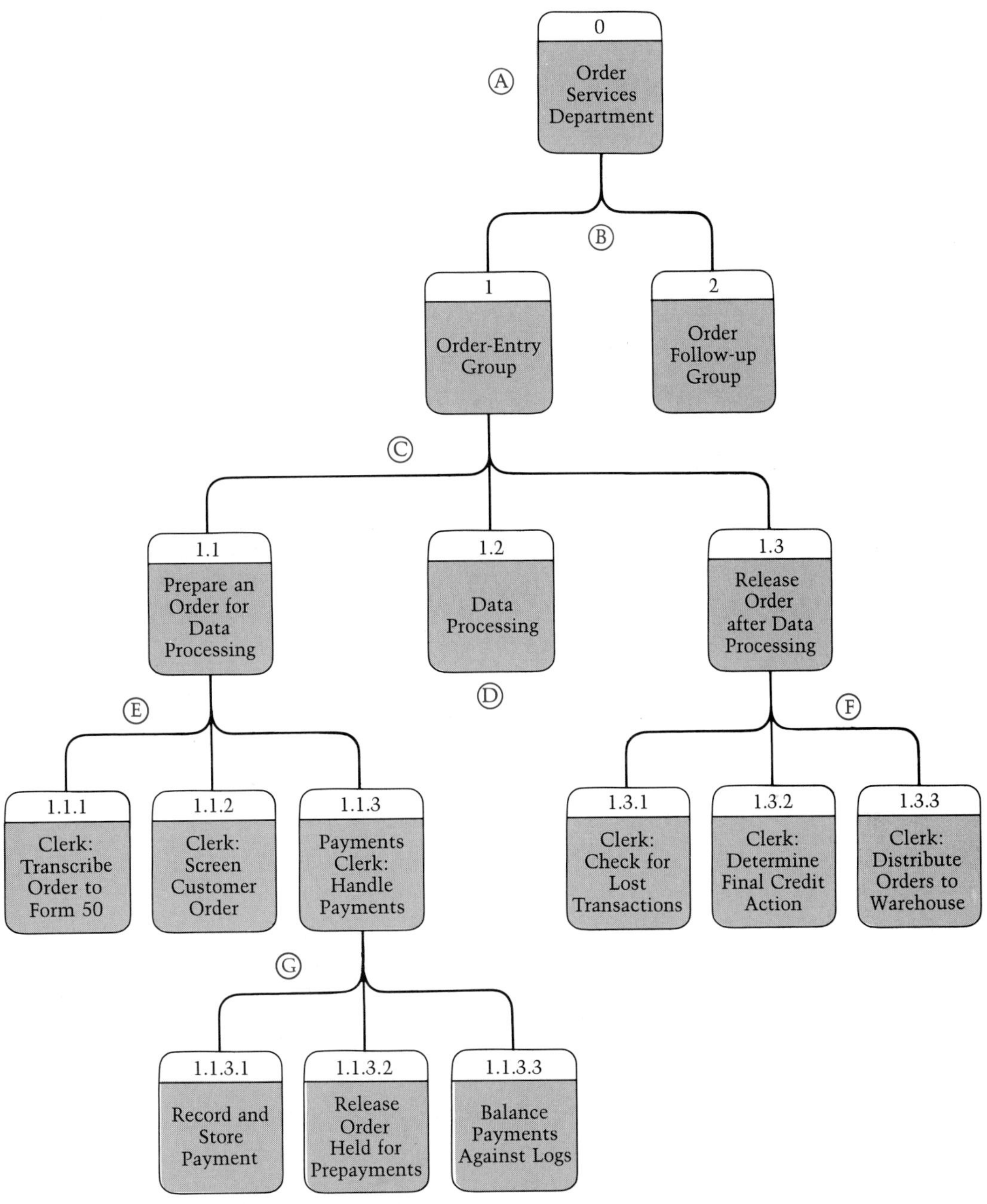

Figure 7.12

Hierarchy chart for AAP's customer services system. Circled letters correspond to letters assigned to points discussed in text.

a process into? Evidence suggests that a process should generally be factored into seven or fewer processes. This guideline will make DFDs much easier to draw by limiting to seven the number of processes that will appear on any given page. A process should never be factored into a single process — in such a case, no additional detail would be revealed.

Ⓓ Data Processing (DP) support should initially be introduced into the hierarchy charts as a single process. Why? Because DP is usually perceived by users as a single *black box*, the details of which are unfamiliar to them.

Ⓔ It was learned that between two and three clerks get involved in the processing of every order. Therefore, we factored process 1.1 into processes corresponding to those three clerks. We named these processes, as well as indicating who performed those tasks.

Ⓕ We also learned that process 1.3 could be exploded into three processes that correspond to the three key tasks and persons that may handle an order after Data Processing has processed the order.

How do you know when to stop factoring? We might have factored the SCREEN CUSTOMER ORDER process in this chart to indicate specific tasks. Why didn't we do it? Because all of the tasks for a single order are performed by one person; thus there is no physical flow of documents, forms, and the like — a clerk doesn't pass a document to himself or herself to do the next step! For *physical data flow* diagrams, we show only the *real* flow of data in the current system.

Ⓖ Why did we factor HANDLE PAYMENTS? The handling of payments involves the payments clerk and the Customer Services manager. But notice that the PAYMENTS CLERK has two subprocesses. If there is only one payments clerk, why two subprocesses? First, the subprocesses happen at entirely different times; they are not sequential. Second, the processes respond to different transactions.

That's about it for our hierarchy chart. A larger project would require more than one page to show the full hierarchy chart. Hierarchy charts can be continued to subsequent pages by duplicating a lower-level process from the first page as a root process on a subsequent page. Then you just continue the factoring. There is no need for connector symbols if you consistently use the reference numbering scheme.

Draw a Context Diagram

PDFDs are constructed in levels that correspond to the levels in our hierarchy chart. Figure 7.13 illustrates the general strategy to be applied. Because each page shows a greater level of detail, we sometimes call the collective DFDs a **leveled set of DFDs.** The first PDFD that is drawn (the top sheet in Figure 7.13) is called a *context diagram.* A context diagram always contains one and only one process —the root process from the hierarchy chart. That process represents the entire system that will be factored or exploded into more detailed PDFDs on the subsequent sheets. The **context diagram** depicts the inputs and outputs between the system (the process) and the rest of the business and outside world.

If we were to include all of the inputs and outputs between a system and the rest of the business and outside world, a typical context diagram might show as many as fifty or more data flows. Such a diagram would have little, if any, communication value. Therefore, we prefer to apply a different strategy, in the form of the context diagram: Only show those data flows that represent the *main objective* or *most common inputs and outputs* of the system. Defer all other data flows to lower-level PDFDs to be drawn later. This strategy is applied in Figure 7.14. The main purpose of our system (ORDER-ENTRY GROUP) is to process CUSTOMER ORDERS, to release them to the warehouse as ZONE ORDERS, and to respond to FILLED ZONE ORDERS by sending accounts receivable a NOTIFICATION TO BILL CUSTOMERS.

Explode Processes to Show Greater Detail

We can now explode the context diagram process into a more detailed picture of the system. And we can continue exploding processes (using the hierarchy chart outline) into more detailed PDFDs until we have a sufficient level of detail.

PDFD for the Customer Services Subsystem The context diagram process of Figure 7.14 is exploded into a more detailed PDFD in Figure 7.15. Note that some of the data flows are beginning to

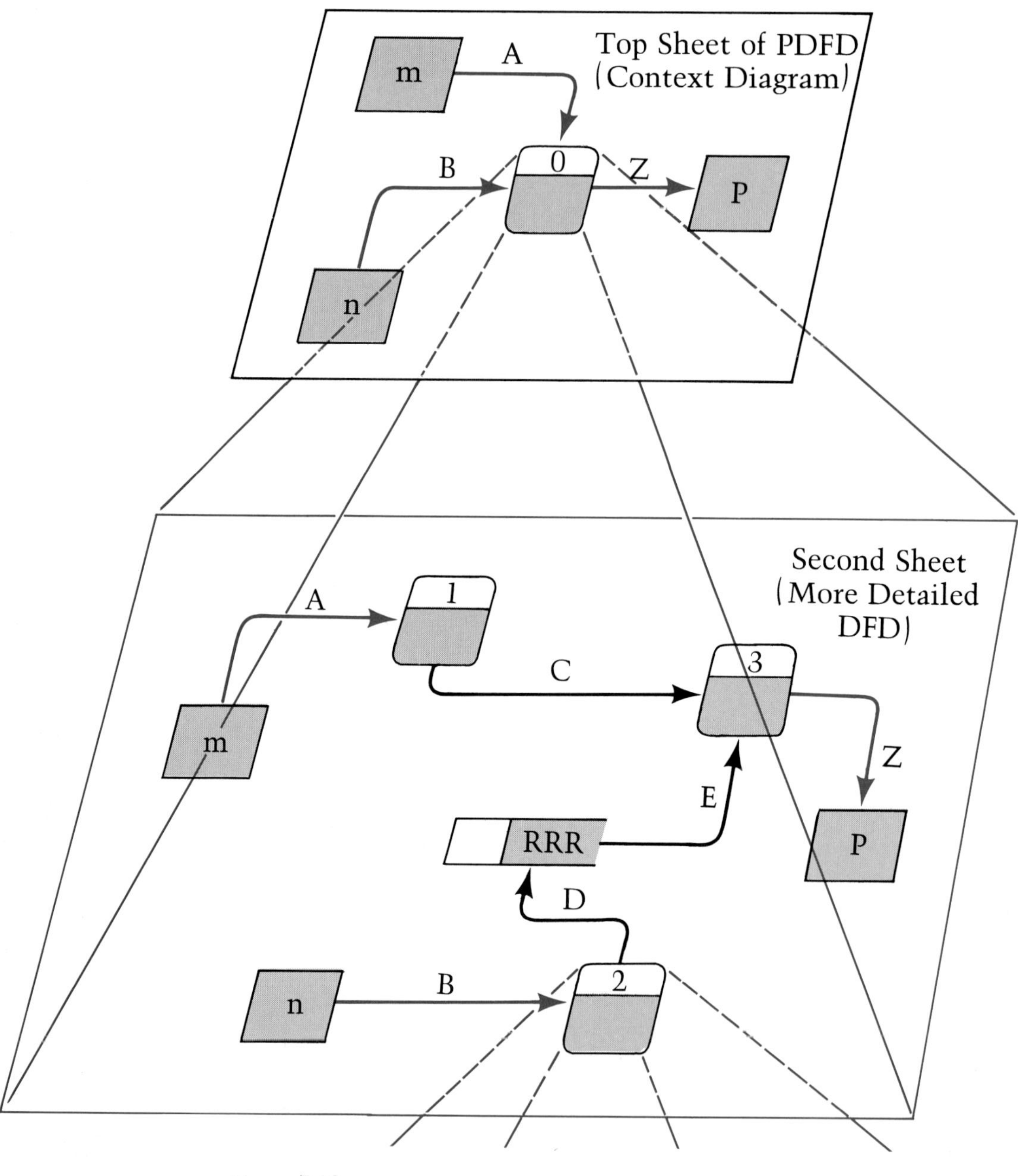

Figure 7.13

Leveled data flow diagrams. In order to deal with size and complexity, analysts should draw a series of data flow diagrams that progress from a very high-level, general view of the system to low-level, detailed views of subsystems.

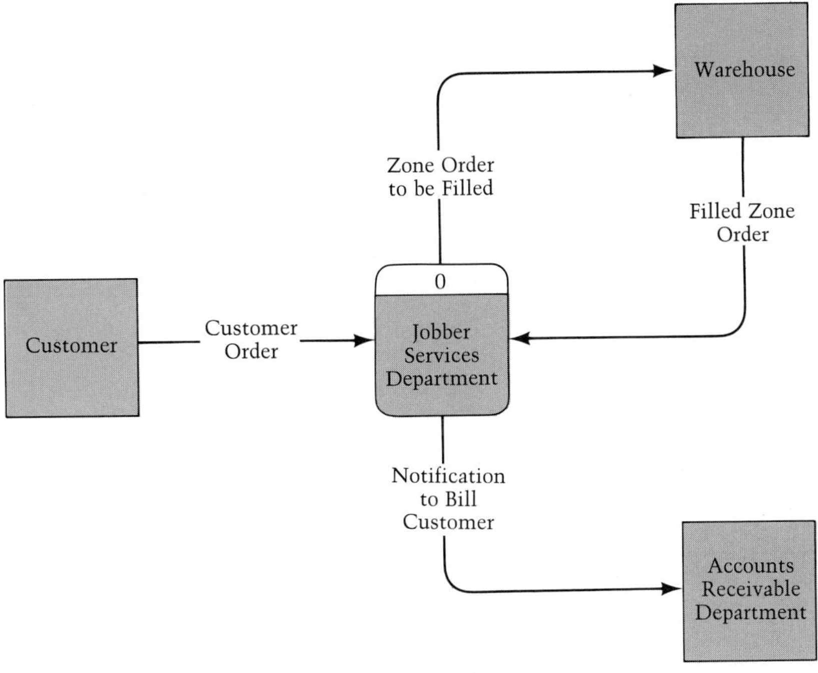

Figure 7.14

The context diagram. The context diagram is the most general picture of a system. The system is depicted as a single process. Its inputs and outputs convey the main purpose of the system.

show physical characteristics — for example CUSTOMER ORDER (PHONE). We also call your attention to the following items:

Ⓐ The data flows that appeared on the context diagram also appear on this diagram. This is done to maintain consistency with the previous diagram. In other books, you may find this called *balancing the diagrams.*

Ⓑ Some new data flows to and from external entities are introduced on this PDFD. They weren't considered common enough to include on the context diagram. These data flows have been marked with an "X" to tell the reader that they don't appear on the higher-level (context) diagram.

Ⓒ A PDFD should show all of the data flows that occur between the processes on the PDFD. Therefore, this PDFD documents all interfaces between the two order groups.

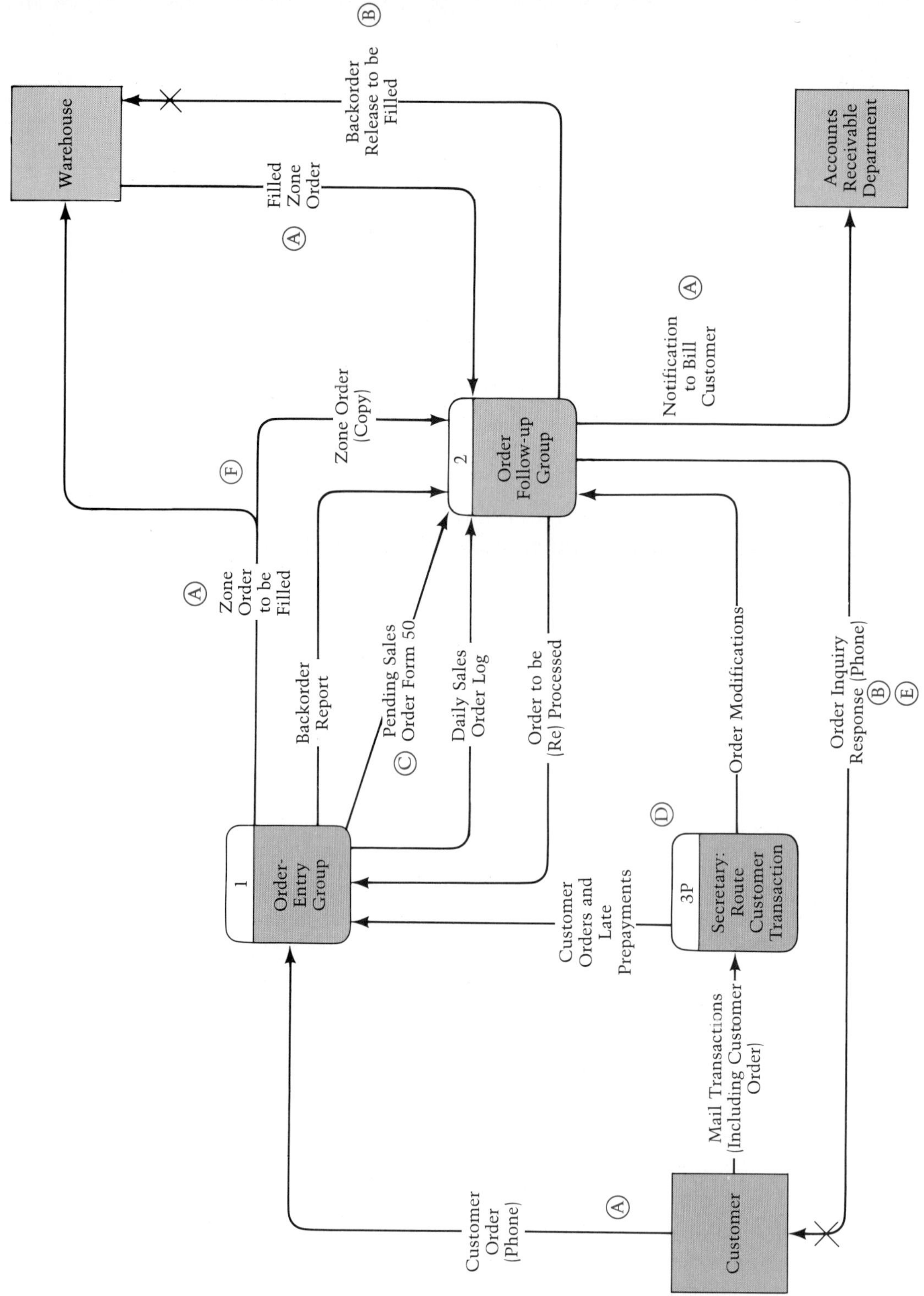
Warehouse
Accounts Receivable Department
Customer
1
Order-Entry Group
2
Order Follow-up Group
3P
Secretary: Route Customer Transaction
Filled Zone Order
Ⓐ
Backorder Release to be Filled
Ⓑ
Zone Order (Copy)
Ⓕ
Zone Order to be Filled
Ⓐ
Backorder Report
Pending Sales Order Form 50
Ⓒ
Daily Sales Order Log
Order to be (Re) Processed
Order Modifications
Ⓓ
Customer Orders and Late Prepayments
Notification to Bill Customer
Ⓐ
Order Inquiry Response (Phone)
Ⓑ
Ⓔ
Mail Transactions (Including Customer Order)
Customer Order (Phone)
Ⓐ

◀ **Figure 7.15**

Second-level PDFD for the customer services system. Circled letters correspond to letters assigned to points discussed in text.

Ⓓ Because we want a physical DFD to show *all* of the document flows as they actually occur, we have added the SECRETARY: ROUTE CUSTOMER TRANSACTION process to the diagram.

Ⓔ An inquiry is actually a two-way data flow. There is a question (input) and an answer (output). But to keep the DFD simple, we show only the *net* data flow, the output.

Ⓕ The diverging data flow, in this case, represents the routing of a five-part (carbon) ZONE ORDER form. Four parts are sent to the warehouse as a single, unburst packet. Only the original copy is burst off and routed to the order follow-up group.

This PDFD shows that the order-entry group is responsible for processing orders and then getting the resultant zone orders to the warehouse. The order follow-up group is responsible for initiating the billing of customers for filled orders and the eventual filling of back orders (orders that couldn't be filled the first time they were sent to the warehouse). To reveal more detail, we must explode each process on this diagram to its own PDFD. The remainder of our example here focuses on the activities of the order-entry group.

PDFD for the Order-Entry Group Now we can explode process 1, the ORDER-ENTRY GROUP, into the processes indicated on the hierarchy chart. Figure 7.16 shows the PDFD. Once again, we have carried all of the data flows to and from the parent process (shown on Figure 7.15) down to this diagram. And again, we have added new details at this level. As we have said, our strategy is to gradually unveil the details of the system. We call your attention to the following notes:

Ⓐ Data stores are first introduced on this diagram because this is the first level at which the data stores are actually *shared* by more than one process. Although it wouldn't have been wrong to show the data stores on the previous levels, their inclusion on such general DFDs would not have had any real communication value. Notice that the data stores on a PDFD include an

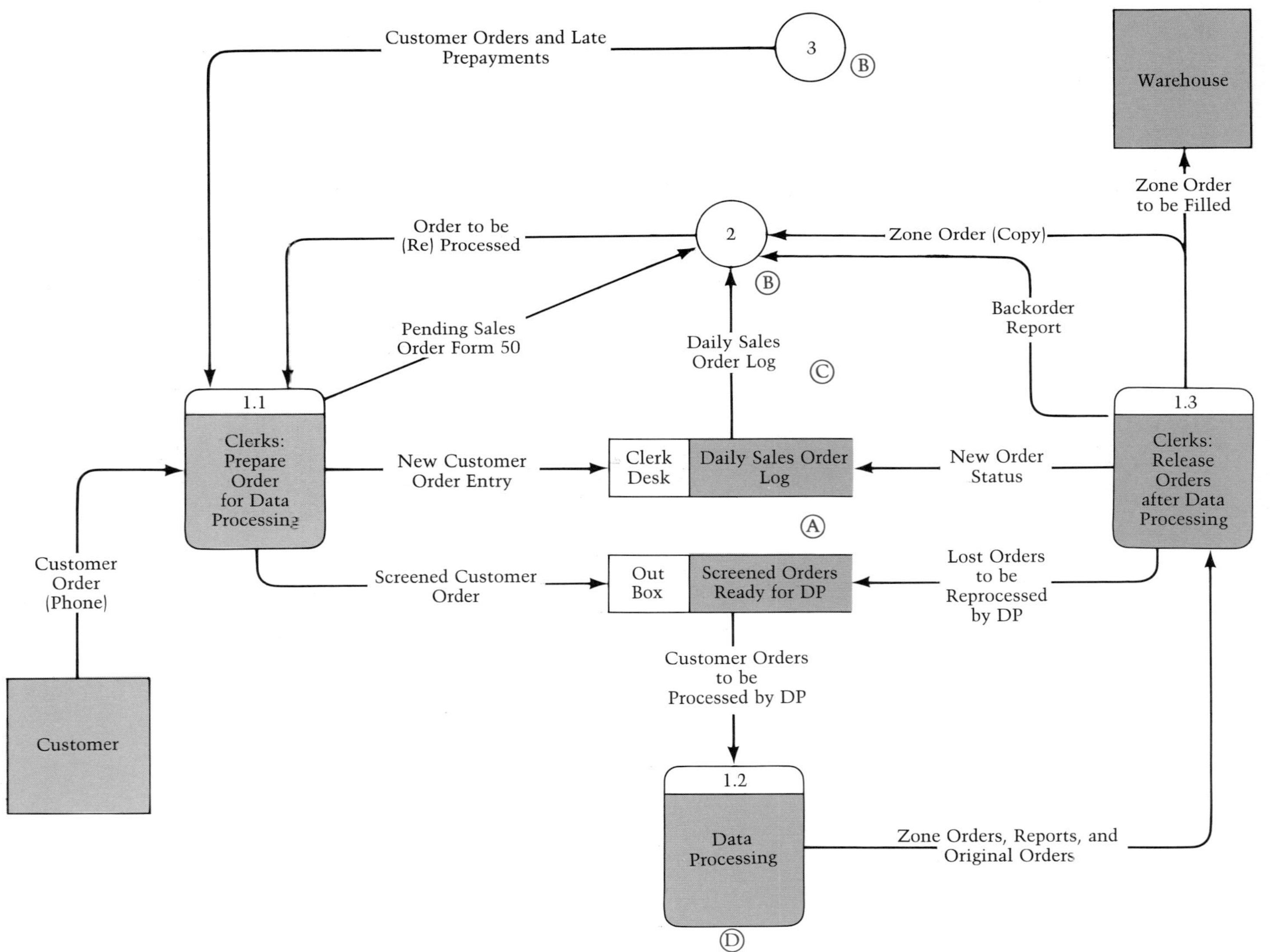

Customer Orders and Late Prepayments
3
B
Warehouse
Zone Order to be Filled
Order to be (Re) Processed
2
Zone Order (Copy)
B
Backorder Report
Pending Sales Order Form 50
Daily Sales Order Log
C
1.1
Clerks: Prepare Order for Data Processing
1.3
Clerks: Release Orders after Data Processing
New Customer Order Entry
Clerk Desk
Daily Sales Order Log
New Order Status
A
Customer Order (Phone)
Screened Customer Order
Out Box
Screened Orders Ready for DP
Lost Orders to be Reprocessed by DP
Customer Orders to be Processed by DP
Customer
1.2
Data Processing
D
Zone Orders, Reports, and Original Orders

◀ **Figure 7.16**

Third-level PDFD for the customer services system. Circled letters correspond to letters assigned to points discussed in text.

explanation of their implementation—in this case, a *clerk's desk* and an *out box.*

Ⓑ A circle with a number in it is a reference back to a process on an earlier (more general) PDFD. There are two such circles in Figure 7.16. In this case, we are referring back to the last PDFD we drew. A circled number is interpreted as follows: "This data flow is coming from [or going to, depending on the direction of the arrow] process #____ on a previous-level diagram. Refer to that diagram or its exploded, detailed diagrams for more information." This *on-page connector* helps you maintain consistency between levels of DFDs by describing the relationship between different pages in the leveled set of DFDs. An on-page connector always refers to a process reference number, never to an external entity.

Ⓒ Notice the data flow DAILY SALES ORDER LOG. At the end of the day, it is passed on to process 2, which we know from the previous PDFD is the ORDER-ENTRY GROUP. Why didn't we just show the data *store* DAILY SALES ORDER LOG on the previous PDFD (as a shared data store between ORDER ENTRY and ORDER FOLLOW-UP)? Because, on *physical* DFDs, the data store should be shown only on diagrams that correspond to its actual *location* in the business. The order follow-up group is not the location of this data store; therefore, the data store is not truly shared.

Ⓓ Note that data processing has been introduced as a single process at this level. Its output contains several reports and documents. However, because those documents are sent back to the order-entry group as a single packet, they are shown as a single data flow.

PDFD Depicting Preparation of an Order for Data Processing Next we explode process 1.1 on the diagram (Figure 7.16). Following our hierarchy chart outline, we introduce the PDFD as Figure 7.17. Again, this diagram is consistent with the input and output data flows of process 1.1 (its parent process) on the previous diagram.

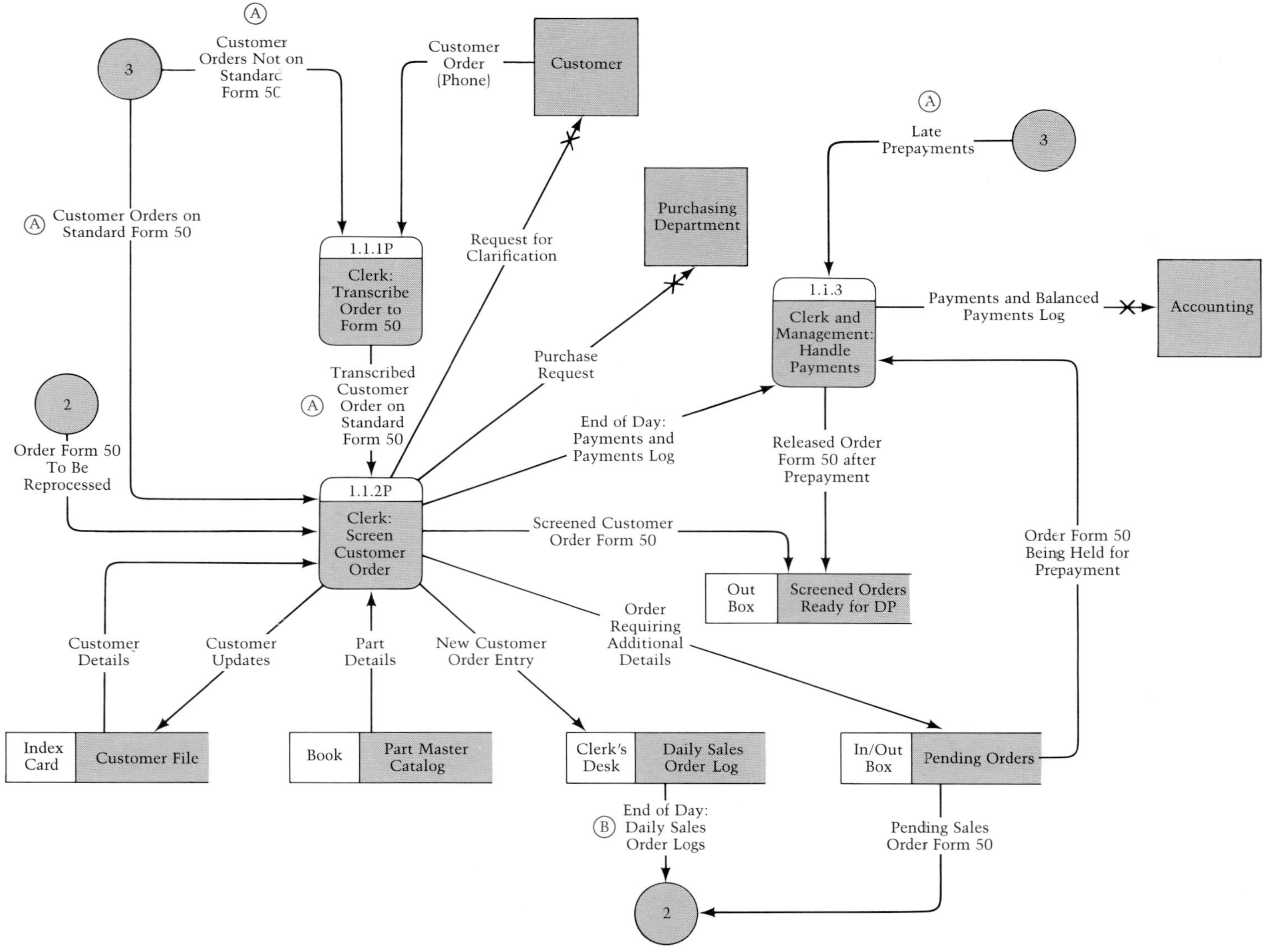

A
Customer Orders Not on Standarc Form 5C
3
Customer Order (Phone)
Customer
A
Late Prepayments
3
A Customer Orders on Standard Form 50
1.1.1P
Clerk: Transcribe Order to Form 50
Request for Clarification
Purchasing Department
1.i.3
Clerk and Management: Handle Payments
Payments and Balanced Payments Log
Accounting
Purchase Request
2
Order Form 50 To Be Reprocessed
A Transcribed Customer Order on Standard Form 50
End of Day: Payments and Payments Log
Released Order Form 50 after Prepayment
1.1.2P
Clerk: Screen Customer Order
Screened Customer Order Form 50
Order Form 50 Being Held for Prepayment
Out Box
Screened Orders Ready for DP
Order Requiring Additional Details
Customer Details
Customer Updates
Part Details
New Customer Order Entry
Index Card
Customer File
Book
Part Master Catalog
Clerk's Desk
Daily Sales Order Log
In/Out Box
Pending Orders
B End of Day: Daily Sales Order Logs
Pending Sales Order Form 50
2

◀ Figure 7.17

Fourth-level PDFD for the customer services system. Circled letters correspond to letters assigned to points discussed in text.

And once again, some new data flows and external entities have been unveiled to introduce some additional details. As you study Figure 7.17, note the following:

Ⓐ We've discussed the idea of exploding a process on a higher-level diagram to show a lower-level, more detailed PDFD for that process. Here we see that a data flow can also be exploded. The data flow CUSTOMER ORDERS AND LATE PREPAYMENTS on the previous PDFD (Figure 7.16) has been exploded into three data flows on this diagram. They are CUSTOMER ORDERS ON STANDARD FORM 50, CUSTOMER ORDERS NOT ON STANDARD FORM 50, and LATE PREPAYMENTS.

The reference numbers 1.1.1 and 1.1.2 have been annotated with the letter "P" meaning primitive. **Primitives** are processes that will not be further exploded. The absence of the "P" on process 1.1.3 tells the reader that a more detailed PDFD for this process is forthcoming.

The screening process (1.1.2P) looks fairly complicated, doesn't it? After discussing the work with the clerk, you might be tempted to level it into separate processes that perform the following tasks:

- Screen and update customer data.
- Screen part data for valid part numbers and request clarification where necessary.
- Initiate purchase requests for items not carried in inventory.
- Place successfully screened orders in the work out box for D.P.
- Log the order into the sales order log.

Why didn't we explode the process? Because there is no actual document or data flow between these tasks—they are performed by a single person.

Ⓑ The data flow from the SALES ORDER LOG on the CLERKS' DESKS indicates that, at the end of the day, the log sheets are sent to the order follow-up group.

As a general note about Figure 7.17, notice that we are using form numbers and media comments to a greater extent. This is because this PDFD represents the most detailed diagram for all but one process on the diagram.

Remainder of the PDFDs for the Order-Entry Group The rest of the PDFDs in our leveled set do not introduce new concepts or techniques. We provide them so you will have a complete example for your reference. Figure 7.18 is the explosion of the process HANDLE PAYMENTS from Figure 7.17. Notice that all of the processes are primitive and won't be further exploded.

Figure 7.19 is a little different. It is a PDFD for the tasks performed by data processing (the explosion of process 1.2 on Figure 7.16). We didn't include those on our initial hierarchy chart. Notice that data entry, data error correcting, all computer programs (including utilities, such as SORT), and all files (permanent and temporary) are illustrated. Alternatively, DP activities could be illustrated with system flowcharts, which are discussed in Chapter 15. Finally, Figure 7.20 depicts the explosion of process 1.3 on Figure 7.16. A leveled set of PDFDs similar to those in this example has proven easy for users to read and verify.

USING DATA FLOW DIAGRAMS TO DEFINE NEW SYSTEM REQUIREMENTS

Let's say that you've completed your study of the current system. You modeled the system with PDFDs. You analyzed the existing system's problems, opportunities, and constraints. And you determined that the potential benefits of eliminating the problems and exploiting the opportunities justify continuing the project. What next?

Figure 7.18 ►

The only fifth-level PDFD for the customer services system.

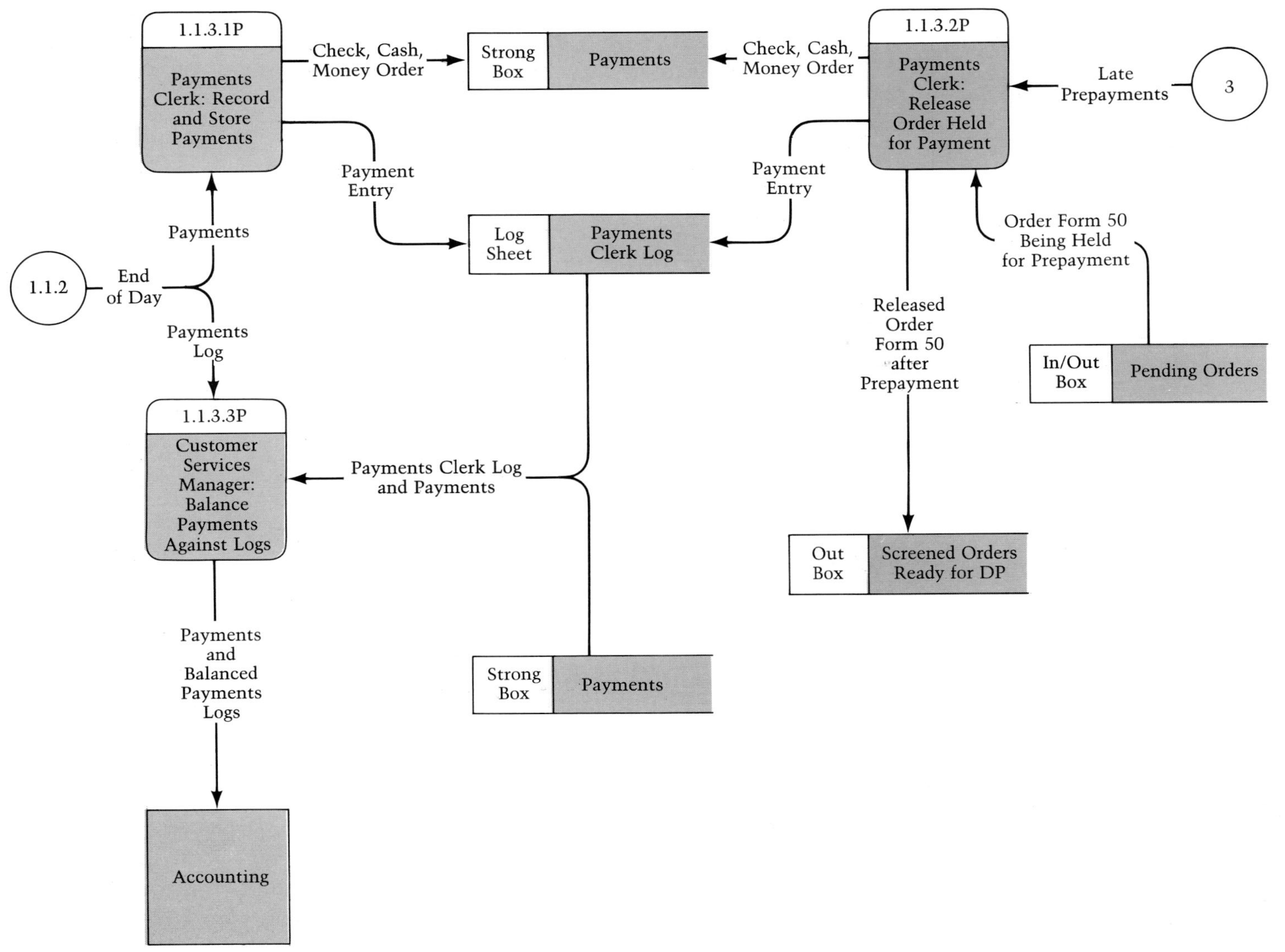
1.1.3.1P
Payments Clerk: Record and Store Payments
Check, Cash, Money Order
Strong Box
Payments
Check, Cash, Money Order
1.1.3.2P
Payments Clerk: Release Order Held for Payment
Late Prepayments
3
Payment Entry
Payment Entry
Log Sheet
Payments Clerk Log
Order Form 50 Being Held for Prepayment
Payments
1.1.2
End of Day
Payments Log
Released Order Form 50 after Prepayment
In/Out Box
Pending Orders
1.1.3.3P
Customer Services Manager: Balance Payments Against Logs
Payments Clerk Log and Payments
Out Box
Screened Orders Ready for DP
Payments and Balanced Payments Logs
Strong Box
Payments
Accounting

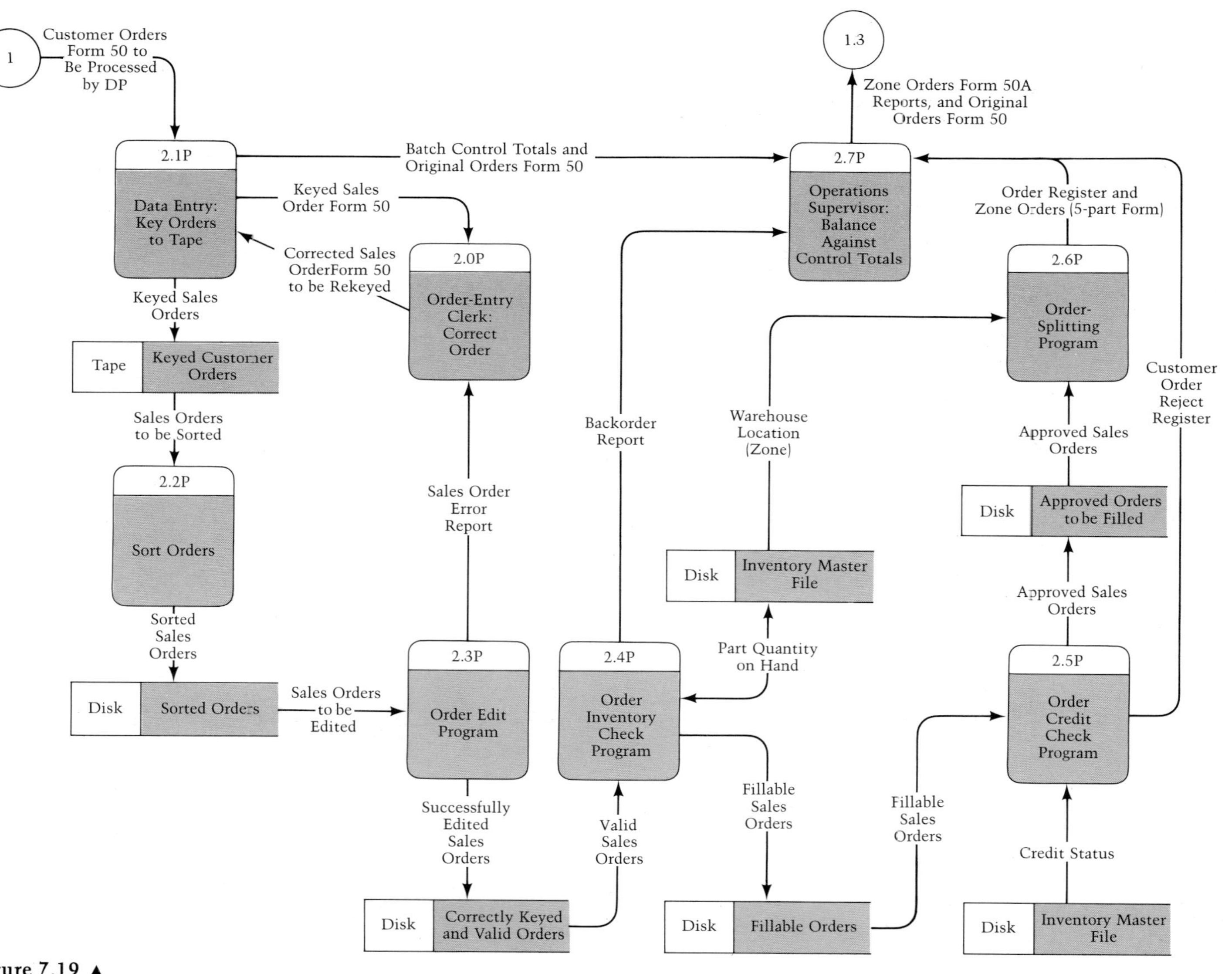

Figure 7.19 ▲

Another fourth-level PDFD for the customer services system. Even data processing activities can be documented with data flow diagrams.

Figure 7.20 ▼

The final PDFD for the customer services system.

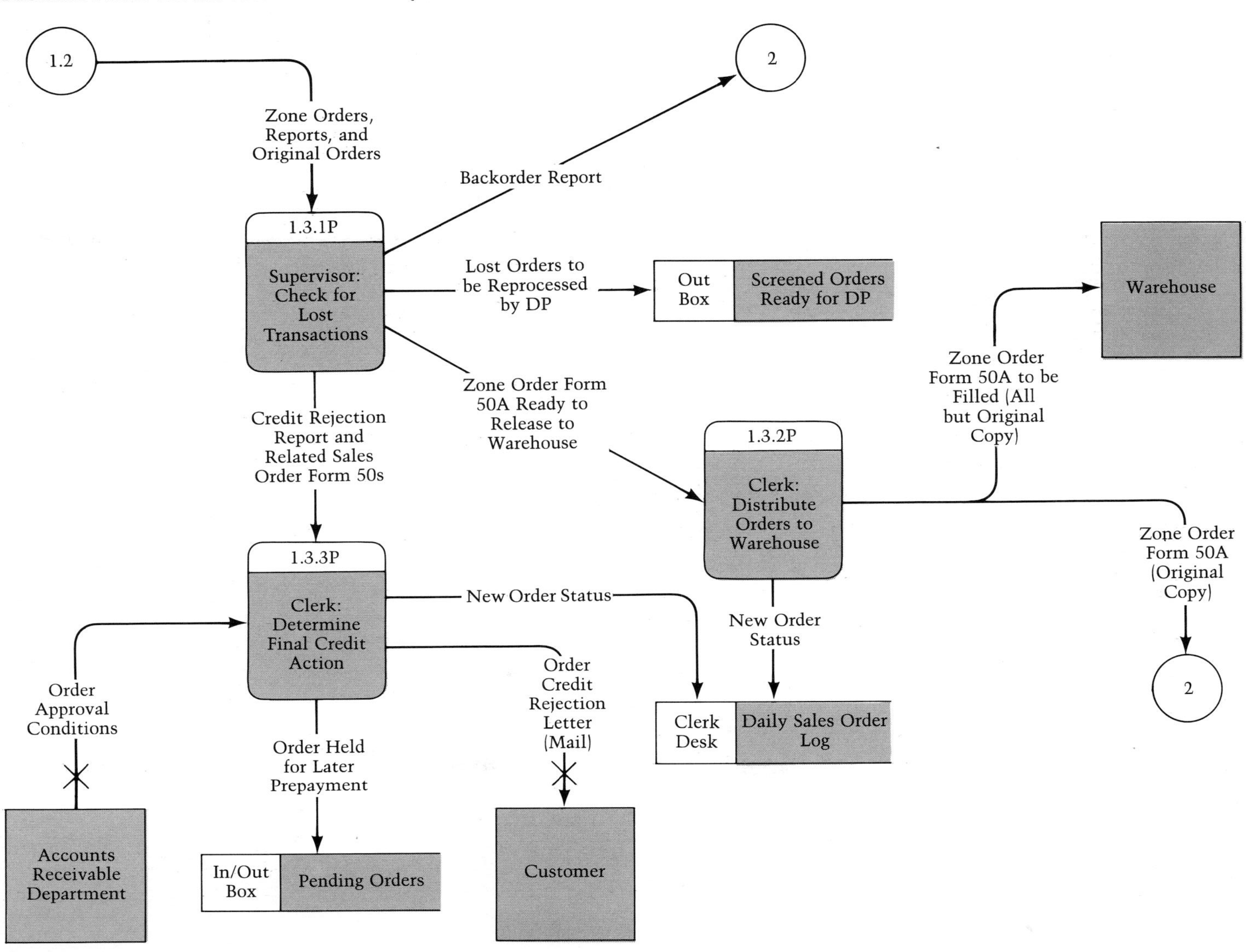

The next phase, definition, should identify and document the requirements for an improved information system. Ideally, these requirements should specify *what* the system will do rather than how the system will do it. Clearly, *physical* DFDs will not meet this objective because they show too much concern for implementation details. They must be modified.

Logical Data Flow Diagrams — What Are They?

An implementation-independent view of an information system is often called the *logical system.* Along those lines, analysts recommend **logical data flow diagrams** (LDFDs) be used to specify the logical system requirements. LDFDs show only the essential features of the system and avoid implementation concerns. Specifically, LDFDs adhere to the following guidelines:

1. Data flow and data store names do not describe implementation (such as medium, file organization, location, and timing). These names describe the data they contain rather than the form or document on which they reside. Process names describe the work done without any reference to who or what does the work (for instance, department, person, computer program).
2. Several processes that appear on the PDFD can be omitted from the LDFD because they are implementation-dependent. These include:
   (a) Processes that do not change the composition or nature of the incoming data flows (for instance, routing, forwarding, and copying processes)
   (b) Computer processes that would not be necessary if the system were implemented differently (for instance, data entry, data processing edit programs, computer sorting and merging)
   (c) Processes that are needed only because the world is imperfect (For instance, people who handle cash are usually required to maintain audit logs that must be balanced at the end of each day. These logs would be unnecessary in a perfect world — one in which embezzlement wasn't a possibility.)
3. Some processes are expanded into more detailed DFDs. PDFD processes often include multiple tasks performed by a single person without any real data flow. These complex processes can be factored into multiple individual tasks with data flows. Con-

sequently, the analyst will be encouraged to examine alternative ways to accomplish *each* task.

4. Many systems contain duplicate processes that can be consolidated into single processes on the LDFD.
5. Processes are frequently resequenced to take advantage of all parallel processing opportunities. Activities done in sequence in the current system may be overlapped if data flows are split. If processes are taken out of their current system sequence, data flows may have to split so that every process gets just enough data to its own job.
6. Data stores should be consolidated to minimize or reduce redundant data storage. Also, the physical location of data stores is irrelevant. They are shared by processes and subsystems to as great a degree as possible.

Examples are forthcoming. But first, because LDFDs present only the essential business requirements and do so in an implementation-independent fashion, they represent a better foundation on which to base the design of an improved system. Why? Because they eliminate both the bias of how things are done today and the bias of how somebody thinks things ought to be done. This clears the analyst's mind to creatively approach alternative solutions that will fulfill the essential requirements.

As was the case with PDFDs, the best way to learn LDFDs is to study a complete leveled set. In the next section of this chapter, we examine some of the fundamental differences between PDFDs and LDFDs by studying the LDFDs for the Customer Services system.

How to Draw Logical Data Flow Diagrams

If you've done PDFDs for the current system under consideration, it's not terribly difficult to move on to LDFDs for a new and improved system that meets user requirements. First we'll list the steps, and then we'll give examples. The steps are:

1. Transform the PDFDs for the current system into their LDFD equivalents. The LDFDs for the current system are a good foundation on which to base changes to the system.
2. Add, delete, and change features to accommodate management and user wishes.

3. Draw a new hierarchy chart that represents a sensible overall structure for the new system. Include all processes from the LDFDs constructed in steps 1 and 2.
4. Redraw the LDFDs according to the new hierarchy chart.

Let's perform these steps for the AAP case study.

Transforming PDFDs into Their LDFDs Figure 7.21 is the logical equivalent of the PDFD that was given in Figure 7.17. First, notice that, in transforming it into its logical equivalent, we eliminated the TRANSCRIBE ORDER TO FORM 50 process (process 1.1.1P) from the PDFD. It was entirely dependent on the current implementation—the fact that customers are allowed to submit orders on nonstandard forms (LDFDs won't force us to change this). Additionally, the process doesn't really change any data. It only copies data. So much for what we've eliminated from the PDFD. We now call your attention to the following features of Figure 7.21:

Ⓐ Orders are shown coming directly from the CUSTOMER. On the PDFD, those orders were coming from the secretary who routed the mail. That ROUTING process was eliminated because it didn't change data.

Ⓑ We expanded a complex process, called SCREEN CUSTOMER ORDER on the PDFD, into several less complex processes. This makes the LDFD easier to read and opens up the possibility that one or more of these simpler processes might be handled differently in the new system.

Ⓒ Notice that EDIT CUSTOMER DETAILS and EDIT ORDERED PARTS do not occur in sequence. We realized that the order in which these tasks are done is irrelevant. Each process receives only that portion of the ORDER data needed to do its own job. Why? What if each were a computer subroutine (a distinct possibility in the new system!)? You would want the subroutine to get only the data it needed because extra data

Figure 7.21 ▶

A PDFD transformed into its logical equivalent. Every PDFD that contains primitive processes should be transformed into a rough-draft LDFD. This is the LDFD for the PDFD of Figure 7.17. After the transformation is complete, the LDFD can be examined for changes, additions, and deletions of appropriate features.

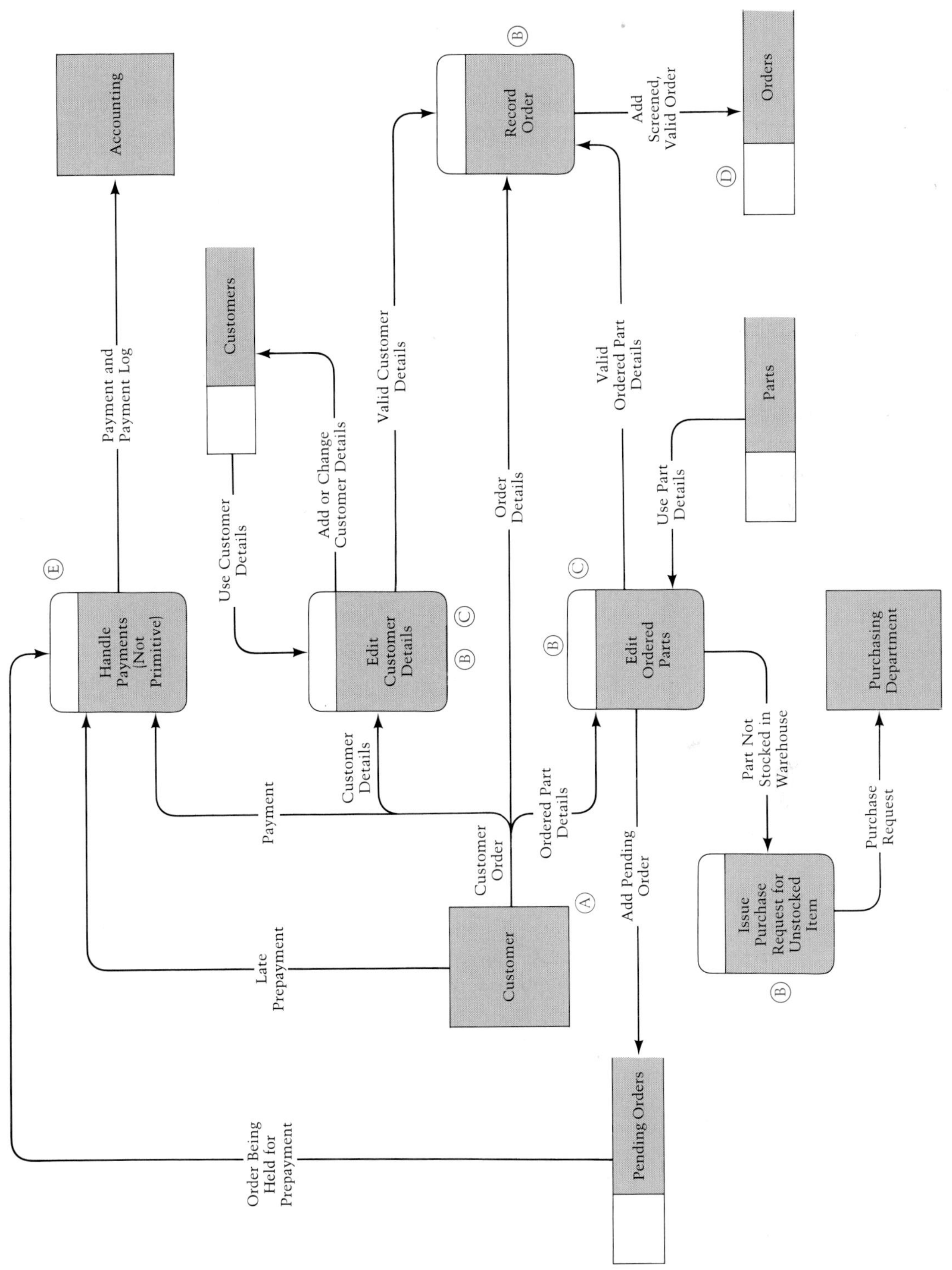
Accounting
Payment and Payment Log
Handle Payments (Not Primitive)
E
Customers
Use Customer Details
Add or Change Customer Details
Valid Customer Details
Edit Customer Details
B
C
Record Order
B
Add Screened, Valid Order
Orders
D
Order Details
Valid Ordered Part Details
Parts
Use Part Details
Edit Ordered Parts
B
C
Purchasing Department
Customer Details
Payment
Ordered Part Details
Customer Order
Customer
A
Late Prepayment
Add Pending Order
Part Not Stocked in Warehouse
Purchase Request
Issue Purchase Request for Unstocked Item
B
Pending Orders
Order Being Held for Prepayment

would make the subroutine too dependent on other subroutines.

Ⓓ The DAILY SALES ORDER LOG from the PDFD has become the ORDERS data store on this logical equivalent. Unlike the log on the PDFD, the data store doesn't have to be forwarded to the order follow-up group at the end of the day. The data store can be shared by the two subsystems. Furthermore, the PDFD data store, SCREENED ORDERS READY FOR DP has become part of the ORDERS data store. The orders aren't forwarded to DP because we don't know (or care) what DP's role in the new system will be (yet)!

Ⓔ The HANDLE PAYMENTS process from the PDFD wasn't primitive; therefore, we didn't transform it here. The primitive processes of the exploded HANDLE PAYMENTS process would go through a similar transformation to their logical equivalents — as would all primitive PDFDs.

Special Note: When transforming the PDFDs for data processing activities, retain only those processes that would have to be done regardless of whether DP were used to do them (for example, retain credit checking, checking for available inventory; eliminate data entry, sorting, editing, controls). Note also that all data flow, data store, and process names are simplified to eliminate any reference to implementation. There is no need to transform nonprimitive (higher-level) PDFDs to their logical equivalents because the overall structure of the new system may be radically different from the current system.

Add, Delete, and Change Features This step is simple. The LDFDs from step 1 usually represent the first draft of the transaction-processing requirements for the new system. Examine those DFDs to determine if there is a better way to do things. *Do not consider ways to implement the system, computer or otherwise!* Do look for opportunities to consolidate redundant processes and to do parallel processing. Some unnecessary processes might be eliminated. Finally, new processes might be added to accommodate management wishes to change transaction processing.

Many current systems offer little or no management reporting and decision support capabilities. First, compile a wish list of new reports and queries. The purpose of each report and query should be determined. This may reveal alternative reports or queries that would better meet management's needs. Then, using separate sheets of paper, draw new LDFDs to add management reporting and decision support features. Normally, this requires adding new processes that use data from the data stores created on the LDFDs during steps 1 and 2 of the four-step process of transforming PDFDs to LDFDs. The outputs normally flow to managers, shown as external entities in this case.

Draw a New Hierarchy Chart By this time, you have several pages of detailed-level LDFDs for the new system. The processes depicted on these LDFDs should be reorganized into a new, sensible structure for the target system. Determine this structure by drawing a new hierarchy chart. This hierarchy chart should not be dependent on organization structure (as was the hierarchy chart for the PDFDs). Instead, the system should be factored into systems, subsystems, and functions. Each function can eventually be factored into transaction-processing tasks, management-reporting tasks, and decision support tasks.

Figure 7.22 illustrates the structure for a new customer services information system for AAP. Compare this with the current system hierarchy chart in Figure 7.12. In our example, the new system is relatively small. There was no need to factor into subsystems, and there was only one function, order entry. A more complex system might have different functions for different types of orders (regular stock orders, emergency orders, interwarehouse orders, to name a few). In that case, each function may have its own transaction-processing, management-reporting, and decision support requirements. Also notice that the Order Follow-Up subsystem was eliminated from the project's scope (reflecting a change in priorities, which is not uncommon during the course of a project).

Redraw the LDFDs According to the Hierarchy Chart Following the same top-down procedure you learned for PDFDs, you now draw a leveled set of LDFDs. You begin with the context diagram and explode the processes to gradually reveal details. The only difference is that the diagrams conform to the guidelines for LDFDs — that is, they do not constrain your system to any implementation alternative. A complete set of LDFDs for the new customer services information system is presented in Figures 7.23 through 7.29. The LDFDs are self-explanatory. They introduce no new concepts. And they become the basis for every remaining systems analysis AND design task during the project — and throughout this book!

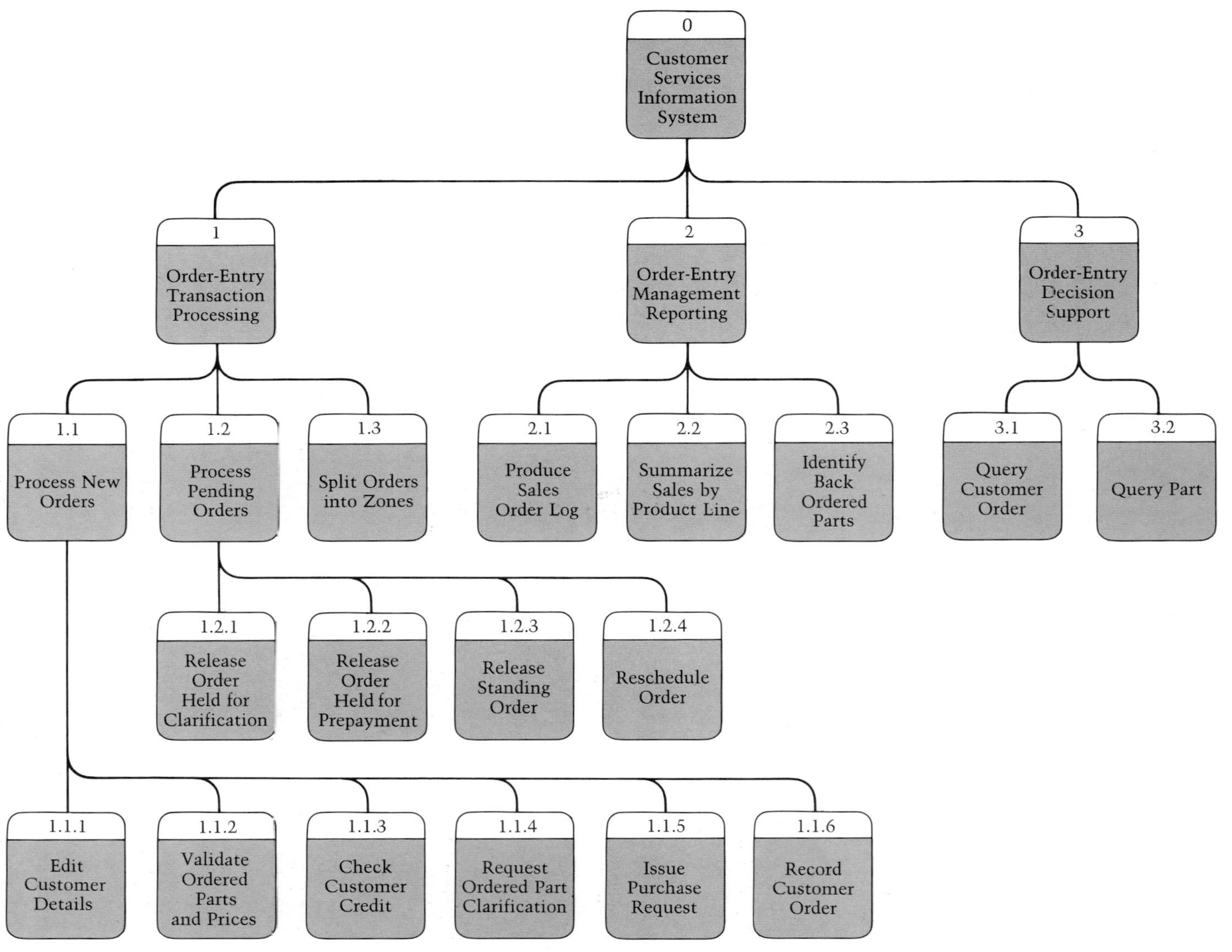
0
Customer Services Information System
1
Order-Entry Transaction Processing
2
Order-Entry Management Reporting
3
Order-Entry Decision Support
1.1
Process New Orders
1.2
Process Pending Orders
1.3
Split Orders into Zones
2.1
Produce Sales Order Log
2.2
Summarize Sales by Product Line
2.3
Identify Back Ordered Parts
3.1
Query Customer Order
3.2
Query Part
1.2.1
Release Order Held for Clarification
1.2.2
Release Order Held for Prepayment
1.2.3
Release Standing Order
1.2.4
Reschedule Order
1.1.1
Edit Customer Details
1.1.2
Validate Ordered Parts and Prices
1.1.3
Check Customer Credit
1.1.4
Request Ordered Part Clarification
1.1.5
Issue Purchase Request
1.1.6
Record Customer Order

◄ Figure 7.22

Hierarchy chart for a new customer services information system. The hierarchy chart for a new information system should not necessarily reflect the current organization structure. The processes in the hierarchy chart depict the *essential* requirements for a new customer services information system for AAP.

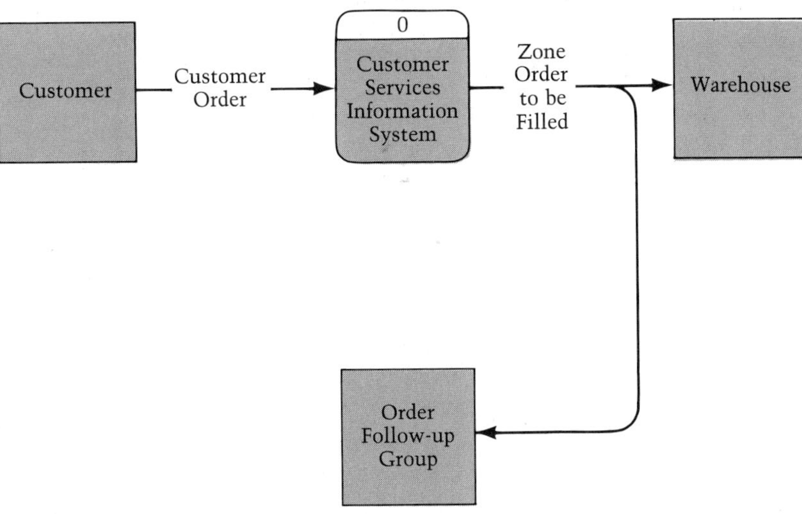

Figure 7.23 ▲

Context diagram for customer services information system. Notice that the order follow-up group has become an external entity in the new system. It was eliminated from the project's scope.

Figure 7.24 (overleaf) ►

LDFD for the order-entry function. Order entry is the only function supported in the new system. We conveniently factored it according to your information system functions model: transaction processing, management reporting, and decision support.

Figure 7.25 (overleaf) ►

LDFD for transaction processing. On the PDFD for order processing, we factored tasks according to whether they occurred before, during, or after data processing. LDFDs don't imply any data processing. For the logical system, we factored order processing into those tasks that deal with newly submitted orders and those that deal with orders that have already been processed once (pending orders). Both new and pending orders must be split into zone orders and released to the warehouse.

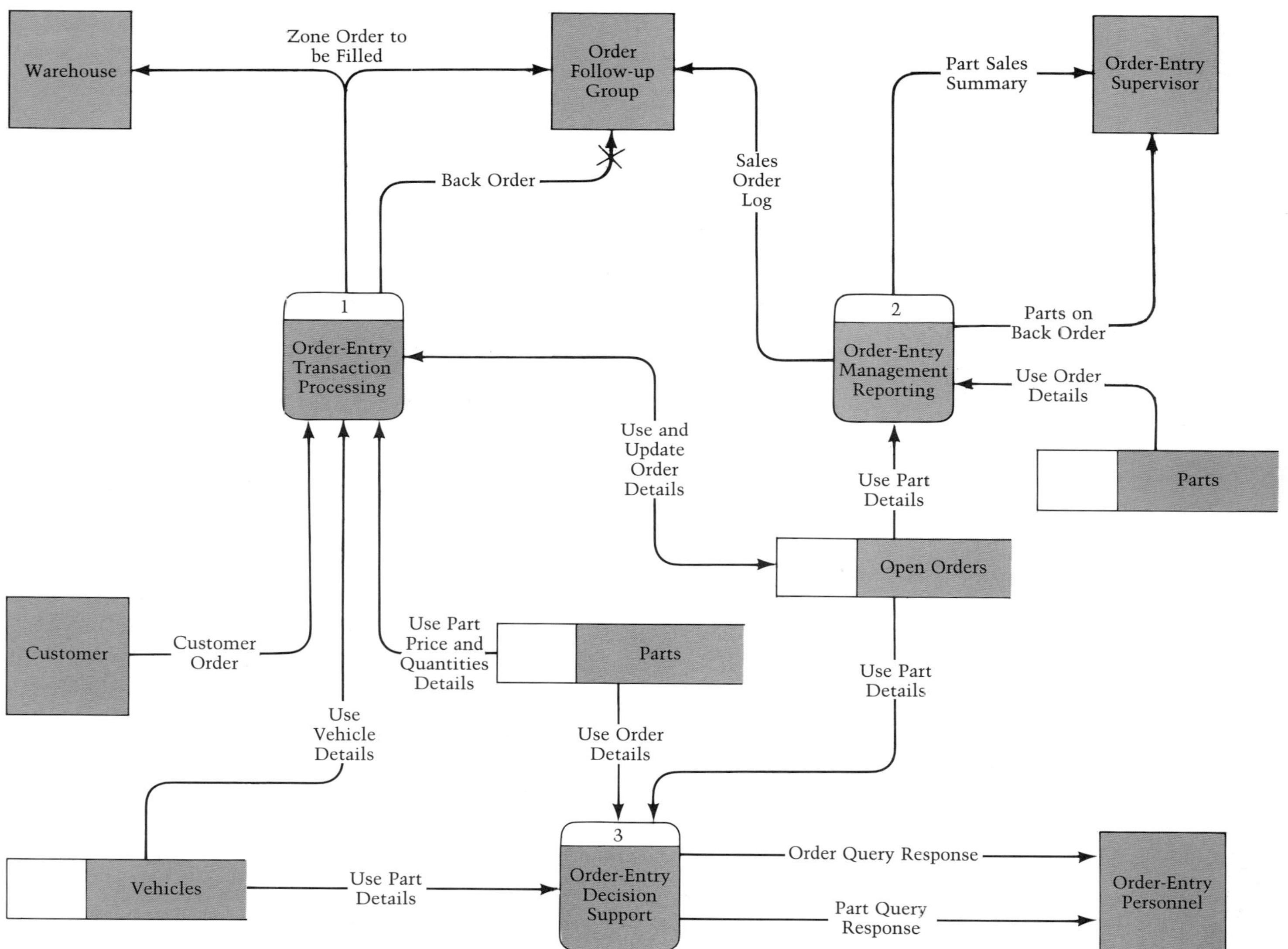

▲ **Figure 7.24** *(see p. 265 for caption)*

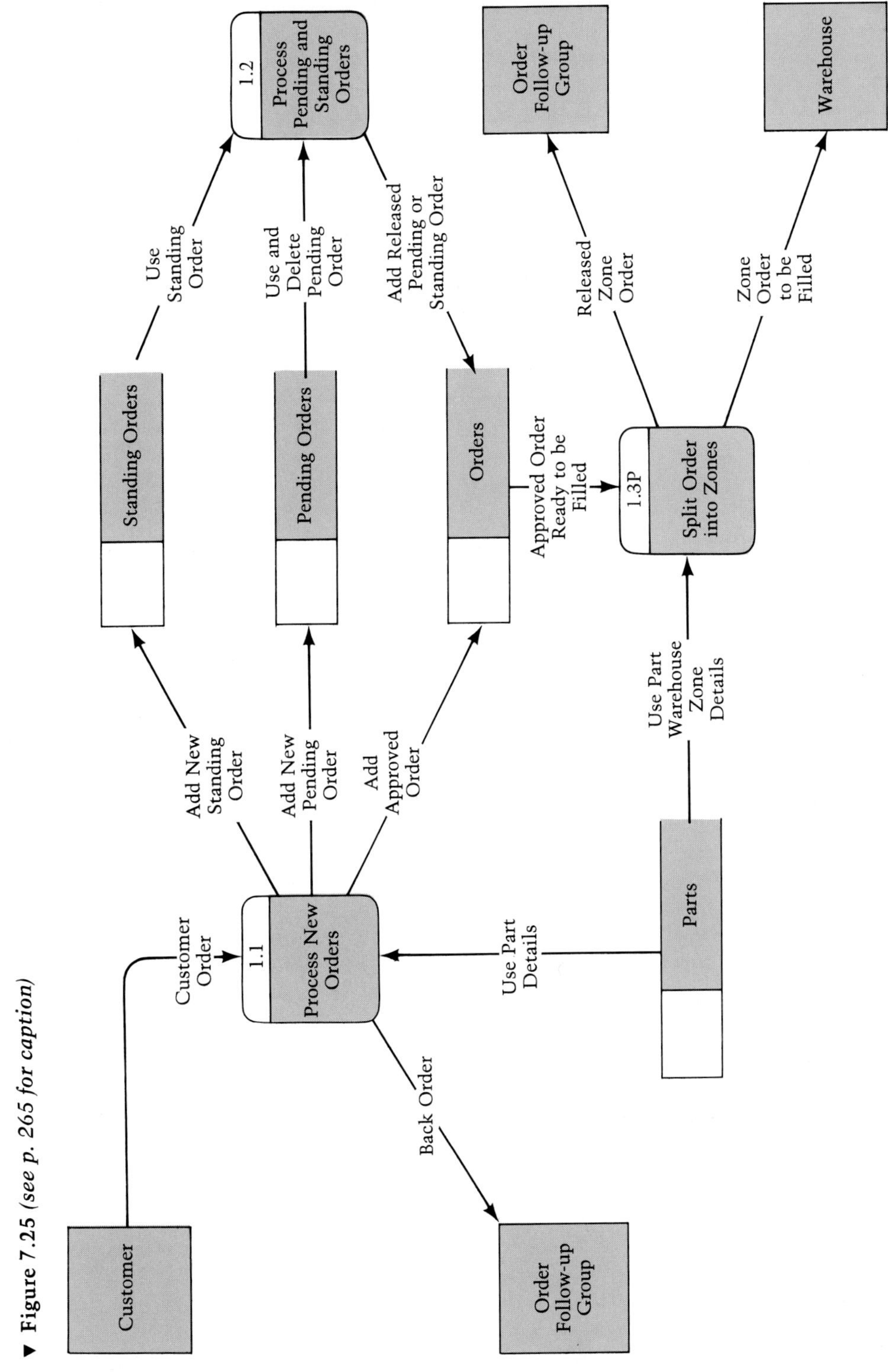

▸ **Figure 7.25** *(see p. 265 for caption)*

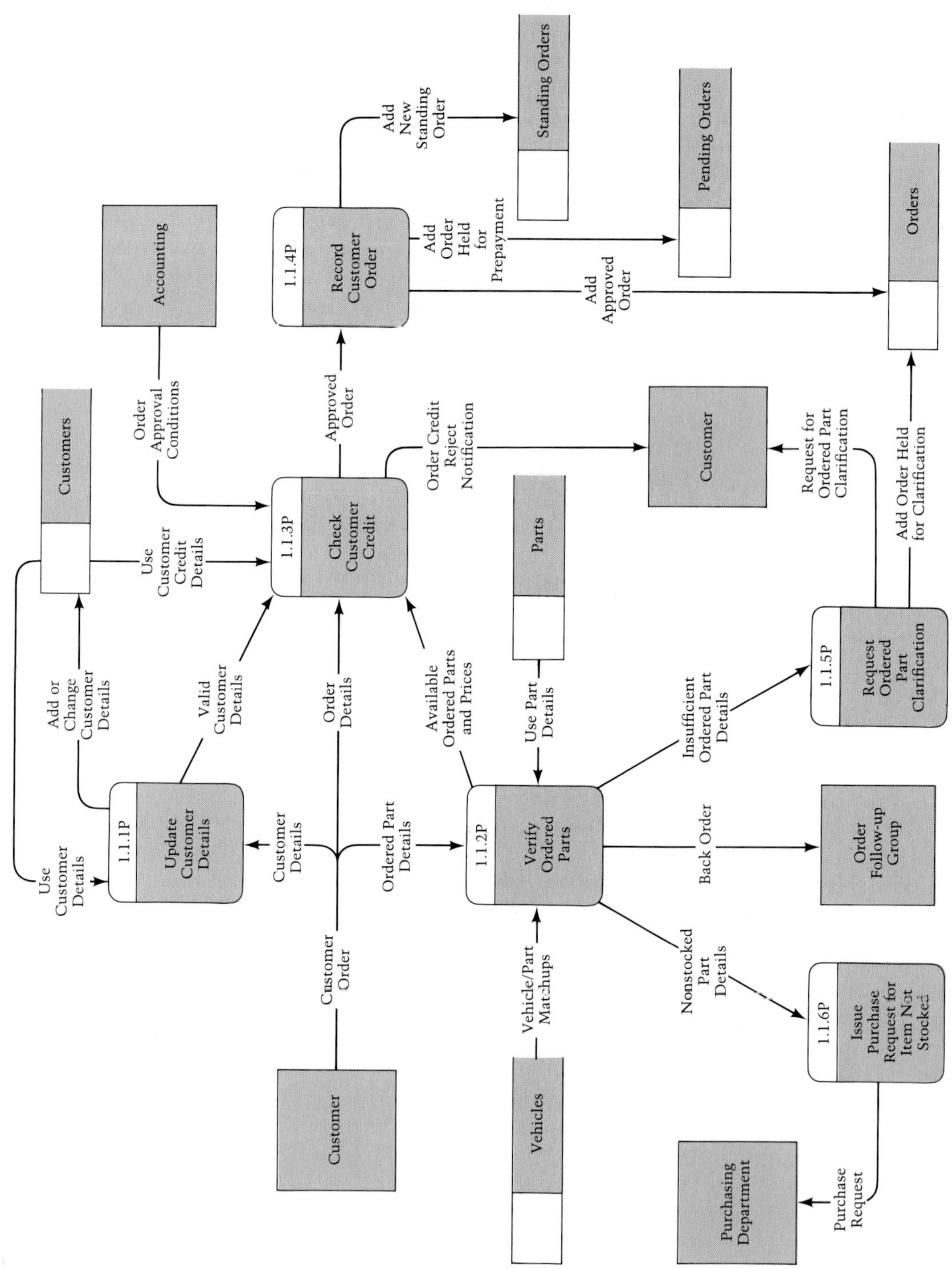

Customer
Customer Order
Customer Details
Ordered Part Details
Order Details
1.1.1P
Update Customer Details
Use Customer Details
Add or Change Customer Details
Valid Customer Details
Customers
Use Customer Credit Details
Accounting
Order Approval Conditions
1.1.3P
Check Customer Credit
Approved Order
Order Credit Reject Notification
Available Ordered Parts and Prices
1.1.4P
Record Customer Order
Add New Standing Order
Standing Orders
Add Order Held for Prepayment
Pending Orders
Add Approved Order
Orders
Vehicles
Vehicle/Part Matchups
Parts
Use Part Details
1.1.2P
Verify Ordered Parts
Insufficient Ordered Part Details
Back Order
Nonstocked Part Details
1.1.5P
Request Ordered Part Clarification
Request for Ordered Part Clarification
Add Order Held for Clarification
Customer
Order Follow-up Group
1.1.6P
Issue Purchase Request for Item Not Stocked
Purchase Request
Purchasing Department

◀ **Figure 7.26**

LDFD for processing new orders. For the most part, this DFD represents the combination of the logical equivalents of the screening and data processing tasks from the PDFDs.

Figure 7.27 ▼

LDFD for pending-order processing. For the most part, this LDFD represents capabilities that don't exist in the current system. For example, management wanted to shift responsibility for existing order clarification to the order entry system (currently it is in the order follow-up system). In addition, management decided to let customers establish standing orders (orders to be filled at the same time each month).

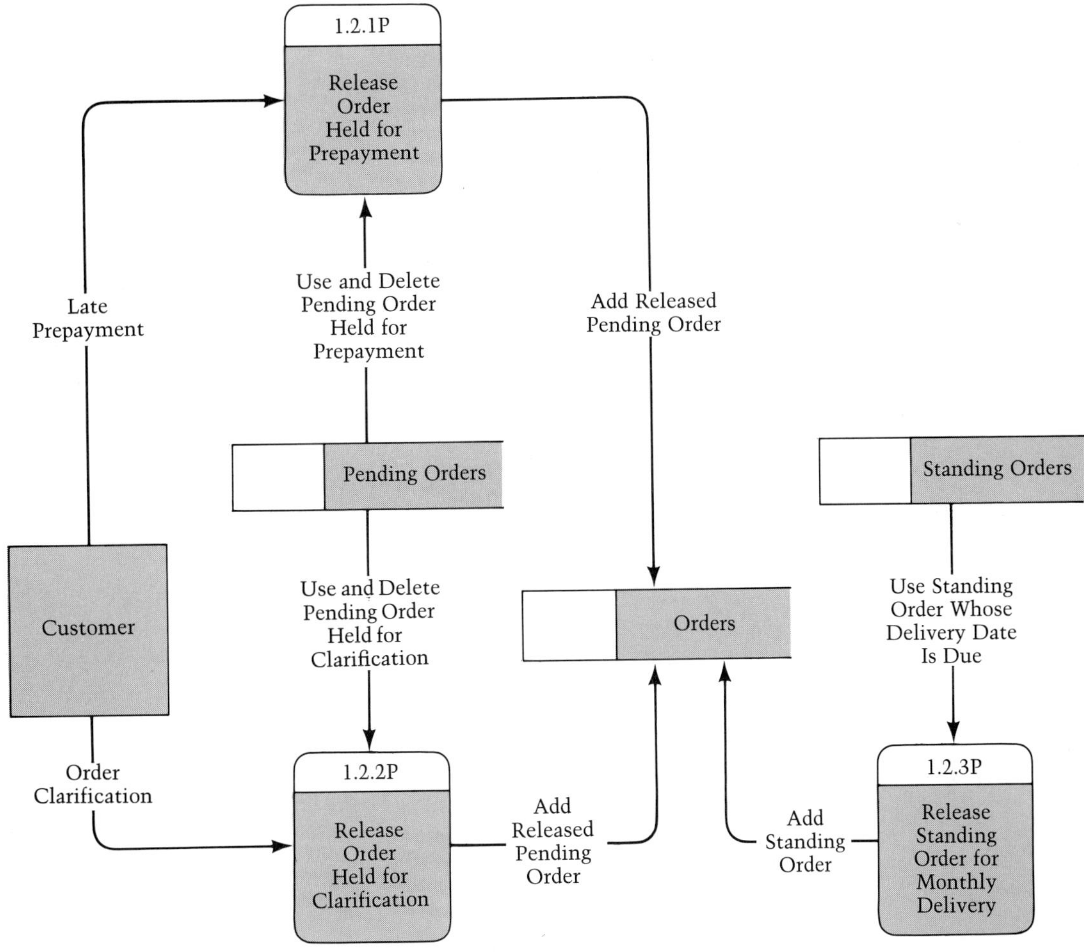

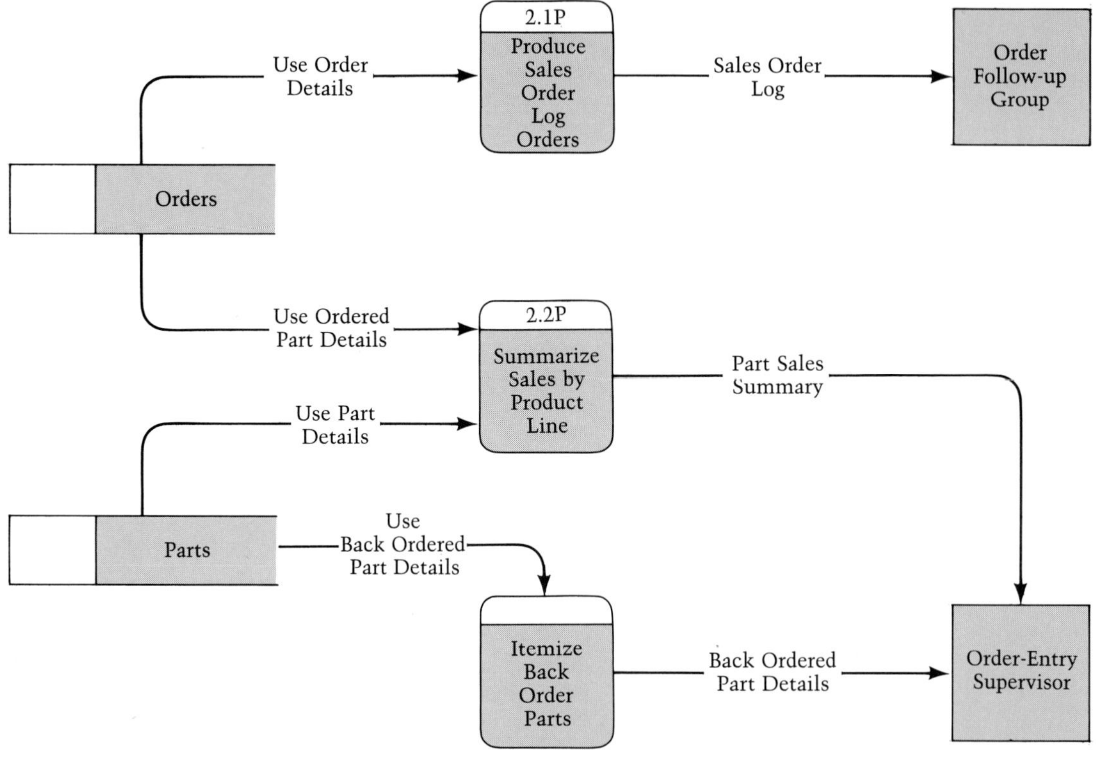

Figure 7.28

LDFD for management-reporting features. Management has requested several new reports. This LDFD depicts how those reports will be generated.

SUMMARY

A data flow diagram is a tool for drawing a picture of an information system. It illustrates the flow of data and work through a system. There are only four symbols that can appear on a data flow diagram: the process, the external entity, the data store, and the data flow. With these symbols, you can model virtually any business or information system. Data flow diagrams should not be confused with system flowcharts. The key difference is that data flow diagrams, unlike flowcharts, can show parallel processes — processes that can operate simultaneously.

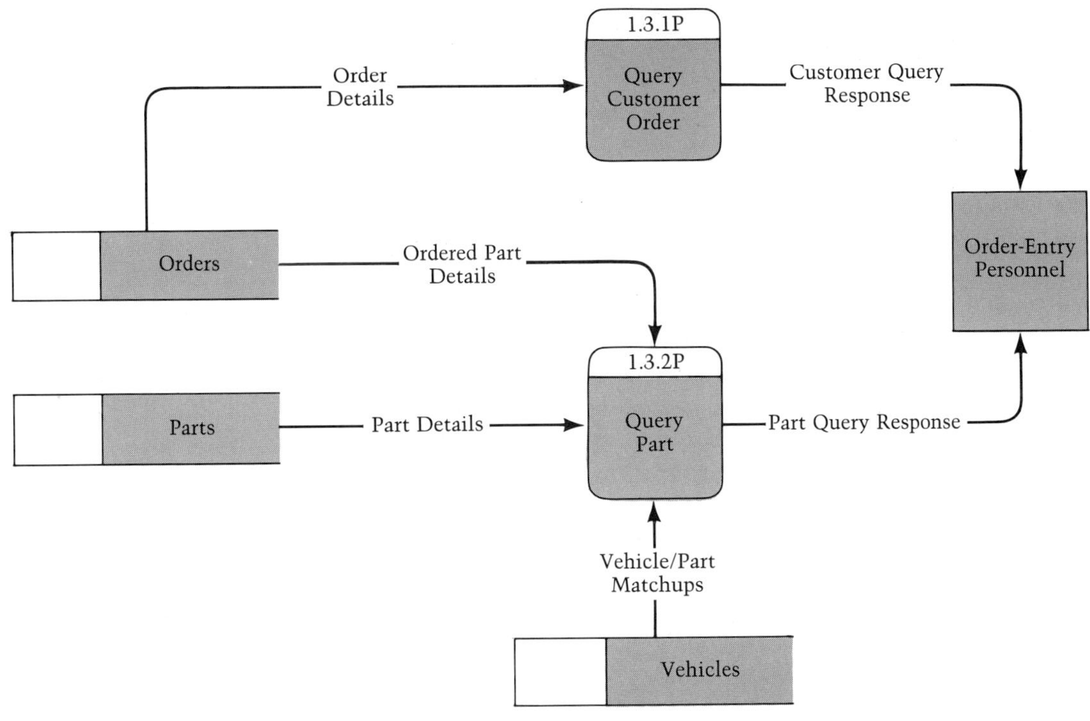

Figure 7.29

LDFD for decision support features. This LDFD illustrates new decision support features to be added to the target system.

A data flow diagram has no peer in its ability to document all aspects of a system including data, information, data storage, knowledge workers, methods and procedures, and computer equipment and programs. Additionally, data flow diagrams can effectively model all transaction processing, management reporting, and decision support functions in a system.

The first opportunity to use data flow diagrams occurs in the study phase of a project. Physical data flow diagrams are used during the study phase to document the systems analyst's understanding of what the current system does and how it does it. This understanding is a sound basis on which to analyze problems, opportunities, and constraints.

During the definition phase, the emphasis shifts away from how the current system works to what the new system should do, independent of how that might be accomplished. Logical data flow diagrams allow the analyst to document user requirements without concern for implementation alternatives or preferences.

PROBLEMS AND EXERCISES

1. A manager, who has noted your use of data flow diagrams to document an existing (or proposed) system, has expressed some concern because of prior, less-than-satisfying experience with such data processing tools as flowcharts. Defend your use of DFDs. Explain why they are useful and how they are superior to flowcharts. Concisely explain the symbology and how to read a DFD. (*Note:* The answer to this exercise should be a standard component in any report that will include DFDs. You cannot be certain that the person who reads the report will be familiar with the tool.)
2. Explain why you should include as many implementation details as possible when drawing a physical DFD.
3. Explain why a systems analyst might want to use data flow diagrams to document the automated portion of an existing information system rather than simply accepting the existing technical data processing documentation (such as systems flowcharts and program flowcharts).
4. Draw a physical data flow diagram for the Platters by Mail minicase that opened this chapter. How does your DFD compare with the picture you drew in response to the challenge that concluded that minicase?
5. Draw a physical data flow diagram to document the flow of documents and data in your school's course registration and scheduling system.
6. Draw a physical data flow diagram for some day-to-day "system" that you go through (for instance, your morning routine; making your favorite meal including appetizer, entree, side dishes, and desert; constructing something from scratch).
7. Explain why it is desirable to transform a physical DFD into a logical DFD. What could happen if you failed to define new system requirements with a logical DFD?

8. Transform your physical data flow diagram for problem 6 into a logical data flow diagram. Can you think of any improvements you would like to see in the system? If so, document those improvements.
9. Draw a data flow diagram for the manual inventory control system that Larry Dunam describes to John Becker in the Outland Engine/Hightech Electronics, Inc., minicase in Chapter 3.
10. Draw a data flow diagram for the new inventory control system that Larry Dunam might envision at the conclusion of his conversation with John Becker in the minicase in Chapter 3.
11. Given the following narrative description, draw a context data flow diagram and the next level data flow diagram.

The purpose of the Production Scheduling System is to respond to PRODUCTION REQUESTS by generating a daily PRODUCTION SCHEDULE (one copy each for the plant manager and the shop foreman), generating MATERIAL REQUESTS (sent to the STORES DEPARTMENT) for all production orders scheduled for the next day, and generating JOB TICKETS for the work to be completed at each workstation during the next day (sent to the SHOP FOREMAN). The work is described in the following paragraphs.

The Production Scheduling Problem can be conveniently broken down into three functions: routing, loading, and releasing. For each product on a PRODUCTION REQUEST, we must determine which workstations are needed, in what sequence the work must be done, and how much time should be necessary at each workstation to complete the work. These data are available from the PRODUCT ROUTE SHEETS, which are kept in loose-leaf binders. This process is referred to as ROUTING THE ORDER and results in a ROUTE TICKET.

Given a ROUTE TICKET (for a single product on the original PRODUCTION REQUEST), we then LOAD THE REQUEST. Loading is nothing more than "reserving" dates and times at specific workstations. The reservations that have already been made are recorded in another loose-leaf binder, labeled WORKSTATION LOAD SHEETS. Loading requires us to look for the earliest available time slot for each task — being careful to preserve the required sequence of tasks (determined from the ROUTE TICKET).

At the end of each day, the WORKSTATION LOAD SHEETS for each workstation are pulled from the binder. A PRODUCTION SCHEDULE is created from these worksheets. JOB TICKETS are prepared for each task at each workstation. The materials needed are determined from the BILL OF MATERIALS FILE (a notebook), and MATERIAL REQUESTS are generated for appropriate quantities.

12. Health Care Plus is a supplemental health insurance company that pays claims after their policyholders' primary insurance benefits (through their employer or another policy) have been exhausted. The following narrative partially describes their claim processing system. Draw a physical data flow diagram for the portion of the system activities described.

The policyholder must submit an Explanation of Health Care Benefits (EOHCB) form along with proof that their primary health care policy claim has been paid. All claims are mailed to the claim processing department.

All claims are initially sorted by the claims screening clerk. This clerk returns (with a form letter) all requests that do not include the EOHCB or EOHCB reference number. For those requests returned, a PENDING CLAIM TICKET is created, dated, and stored in a file cabinet (by date). Once each week, the clerk deletes all tickets that are more than forty-five days old and sends a form letter to the policyholders notifying them that their case has been closed. Requests that include the EOHCB are then sorted according to type of claim (any PENDING CLAIM TICKET is destroyed at this time). Requests that include an EOHCB reference number are matched up with the EOHCB form (pulled from the OPEN CLAIMS file cabinet). At the end of each day, all these claims are forwarded to the preprocessing department.

In the preprocessing department, clerks screen the EOHCB for missing data. The clerk completes the form if possible. Otherwise, a copy of the claim is returned to the policyholder with a letter requesting the missing data. The original EOHCB is placed in the OPEN CLAIMS file cabinet, and a PENDING CLAIM TICKET is sent to the claims screening clerk. Completed claims are assigned a claim number, and the claim is microfilmed and filed for archive purposes.

A different clerk checks to see if the proof of primary health care policy payment was included or is on file (PRIMARY PAYMENT file cabinet). If it is not available, the policyholder is sent a letter requesting the proof. The EOHCB is placed in a PENDING PROOF file cabinet. Claims are automatically purged if they remain in this file for more than fourteen days (a letter is sent to policyholders whose claims have been purged).

If proof is available, another clerk pulls the policyholder's policy record (from the POLICY file cabinet), records policy and action codes on the EOHCB, and refiles the policy record. At the end of the day, all preprocessed claims are forwarded to Data Processing.

13. The following narrative describes the order follow-up group's activities for the AAP case used in this chapter. Using this narrative, complete the hierarchy chart and physical data flow diagrams for the case. The high-level framework for the PDFDs has already been given in Figures 7.15 and 7.16. If there are situations that you don't understand or feel are incomplete, prepare a schedule of questions that you will ask the users in order to clarify the case.

The Order Follow-Up Group (OFU) works only with orders that have been fully or partially processed by the Order Entry Group (OEG). The OEG released fully processed orders, on ZONE ORDER Form 50A, to the warehouse for filling. The original copy of Form 50A was sent to OFU by the OEG. Partially processed orders arrive in one of the following ways: either in the BACK ORDER REPORT, which identifies specific parts on specific orders that have been identified by the computer as out-of-stock, or as PENDING SALES ORDERS on Form 50 (not to be confused with ZONE ORDERS, Form 50A) that require some clarification before processing can continue. The OEG also sends the previous day's DAILY SALES ORDER LOGS to the OFU at the beginning of each day.

The OFU Group is responsible for the following: initiating the billing function for filled ZONE ORDERS, initiating and filling back orders for ordered products that are out of stock, processing clarifications for orders delayed by inadequate data, and responding to customer inquiries.

Most orders are completely filled by the warehouse without any difficulty. Three times each day, the warehouse returns the billing and picking copies of filled ZONE ORDERS, to the OFU Group. An OFU clerk matches the returned copies with the corresponding original copy (which has been held in the OPEN ORDERS FILE, an in/out box, since being received from the OEG). If any of the parts were back ordered in the warehouse, the clerk fills out a new ZONE ORDER Form 50A for those parts, stamps the form "Back ordered," and places the form in the OPEN ORDERS FILE, an in/out box. It should be noted that these back orders were not anticipated by the computer — they were not discovered until the warehouse tried to fill the orders. Regardless of whether any items were back ordered, the clerk recombines the original and picking copies of the ZONE ORDER and places them in the CLOSED ORDER FILE, a file cabinet. At that time, an appropriate status entry is made in the DAILY SALES ORDER LOG. At the beginning of each day, a clerk goes through the OPEN ORDERS FILE to find any orders that are not stamped "Back order." These orders are presumed "lost." After determining the status by phoning the warehouse, any order that cannot be found must be rereleased to the warehouse. This requires a new ZONE ORDER Form 50A. The old order is stamped "Lost," attached to the original copy of the new ZONE ORDER, and placed back in the OPEN ORDERS FILE. The other copies (four carbons) are sent to the warehouse for filling.

Two clerks are permanently assigned to handle back orders. There are three standard back order activities. Each day, the OFU Group receives a BACK ORDER REPORT from the OEG. The BACK ORDER REPORT is sequenced by sales order number. The BACK ORDER REPORT identifies ordered parts that the computer knew could not be filled in the warehouse because the items were not in stock. For each listed sales order, the back ordered parts and quantities are listed. The clerk must initiate a ZONE ORDER FORM 50A for each sales order on the report. The 50A is stamped "Back order" and placed in the OPEN ORDERS FILE, and an appropriate entry is made in the DAILY SALES ORDER LOG. Each day, the OFU Group receives a RECEIVING REPORT from the shipping and receiving dock. This report lists all new stock that was received on the previous day. An OFU clerk checks these parts against the parts on ZONE ORDER Form 50As in the OPEN ORDERS FILE. If the back ordered parts match the part numbers received, the ZONE ORDER is sent to the warehouse via a courier. Once every other week, the OFG supervisor must prepare a BACK ORDER SUMMARY REPORT. This supervisor uses the data from the OPEN ORDERS FILE (only those ZONE ORDERS stamped "Back order") to generate a part-by-part back order summary.

The OFU Group supervisor handles all order inquiries. Given the sales order number, the supervisor determines the order status using the DAILY SALES ORDER LOGS. If further detail is necessary, the OPEN and CLOSED ORDER FILES contain the ZONE ORDERS for that sales order number.

SALES ORDERS that require clarification are received daily from the OEG (who have notified the customer of the problem). The order is placed in a PENDING ORDERS FILE (cabinet) until the customer responds. Clarifications are received from the customer via the secretary who sorts and routes the mail. An OFU clerk responds to the clarification by recording the proper data on the SALES ORDER Form 50 (from the PENDING ORDERS FILE). At the end of the day, these clarified orders are sent back to the OEG to be reprocessed into ZONE ORDERS.

ANNOTATED REFERENCES AND SUGGESTED READINGS

DeMarco, Tom. *Structured Analysis and System Specification.* Englewood Cliffs, N.J.: Prentice-Hall, 1979. This is the classic book on the structured systems analysis methodology, which is built heavily around the use of data flow diagrams. Tom is a gifted writer who expresses complex ideas with ease. He uses a slightly different symbology, but it is easy to grasp.

Gane, Chris, and Trish Sarson. *Structured Systems Analysis: Tools and Techniques.* Englewood Cliffs, N.J.: Prentice-Hall, 1979. An early structured analysis methodology book. Not as thorough as DeMarco but relatively easy to read and grasp. Their DFD symbology is identical to ours.

McMenamin, Stephen M., and John F. Palmer. *Essential Systems Analysis.* New York: Yourdan Press, 1984. The most thorough reference to date on logical data flow diagrams and the transformation of physical DFDs to logical DFDs, the specification of essential business requirements, and structure of the new system. We recommend that you read DeMarco before you read McMenamin and Palmer.

Analysts in Action

Requirements Analysis for the New System

When we left Cheryl and Doug, they had completed their study of the current order-entry system. Now they must define the business requirements for a new and improved system.

Episode 4

We begin this episode shortly after AAP's steering committee has approved Cheryl and Doug's study phase report. The committee agreed that the projected benefits of solving AAP's order-processing problems were worth the projected costs for continuing the project. Cheryl is on vacation. We join Doug during a meeting with Joey.

Objectives for the Target System

"Afternoon, Doug. Don't forget we're playing raquetball tomorrow. I hope you're ready to get beat this time. What's up for today?"

Doug took a seat. "Let's see. Today, I'd like to begin establishing some objectives for the new system. The objectives we come up with today shouldn't address the computer solutions or specific reports the system is to produce. Instead, we want to find a set of business criteria against which we can evaluate the alternative solutions. An example of such an objective might be 'we want to increase order throughput by 25 percent.' Do you have the idea?"

"Yeah, but I hope we'll eventually get to talk about the computer."

"Sure we will, Joey, but only at the proper time. Cheryl and I want the business problem to drive the computer solution, not vice versa. Believe me, before this is over you'll probably be tired of hearing us talk about the computer. But in the end, we think you'll appreciate that the solution supports your business needs. As a reminder of our last meeting, order follow-up support has been put on hold. The scope of the project was reduced so priority could be given to order entry, which is where most of your critical problems are occurring. Now, how about some business objectives?"

"Well, Doug, I think the top priority would be to decrease the amount of time it takes to process customer orders."

Doug replied, "I'd like to get a little more specific than that, Joey. Right now, you're capable of processing 125 phone and 255 mail orders per day. I assume you want to improve these figures. But, by how much?"

"I see where you're going. Okay, I'd like for the new system to be able to process at least twice that number of phone and mail orders."

"That's the kind of thing I need," said Doug.

"I've got the idea," Joey began to talk. "My boss has informed me that our company will start allowing customers to place standing orders. Many of our customers place orders for specific parts on a regular basis. Rather than require a ►

customer to continue to submit the order, I've been instructed to establish methods for creating standing orders that'll be filled on the same date, or thereabout, every month. He thinks the customers will really appreciate this service and we can be assured of an increase in customer orders."

"Okay! I think I've got an objective, Joey. How about stating that the system should identify any unfilled customer orders so you can track down an order at any stage during processing?"

"I never thought of that, Doug. It's a good idea because . . ."

[*We can leave this meeting now. The dialog will continue until all objectives have been defined.*]

The General Requirements for the New System

Two weeks have passed since the meeting that established objectives. Cheryl has returned from vacation and has been working with Doug on the business requirements statement for the new order-entry system. They have already determined the general system requirements and documented those requirements with logical data flow diagrams (see Chapter 7, Figures 7.22 through 7.29). We join Cheryl as she is leading a walkthrough of the general requirements. Doug, Joey, Madge, Karen, and Ted are in attendance.

Cheryl placed a diagram of the proposed system on the overhead projector (see Figure 1). "This is a detailed diagram of the order processing requirements for the new system. We want to bounce this proposal off you to see if it is agreeable."

"I notice you haven't indicated where the computer fits in, Cheryl," Madge remarked.

"That's right! What we want to do now, Madge, is to define *what* the system will do. In the next phase, we'll determine different alternative computer solutions. It's important to define the requirements independent of the solution."

"That makes sense," said Madge.

Cheryl continued, "Let's begin by tracing a new customer order. As you can see, orders are screened for valid parts. [See ① on Figure 1.] The part file is used to verify that the ordered part number corresponds to an AAP part number. The part file is also used to determine the price and availability of the part. So this process also identifies parts we don't carry in stock and must purchase, parts that are back ordered, incorrect order part numbers or part descriptions, and customer order part numbers that were correctly verified."

Karen interrupted, "Is that the Part Master Catalog or the Part Catalog Listing?"

"Neither, really," Cheryl answered. "You see, this picture is a *logical* diagram of the system. By *logical,* we mean that the medium or location of the file is not yet determined. You should think of the part file as a combination of what you know as the part master catalog and the part catalog listing. This file contains *all* the data about a part. When we design your new system, we may retain the original files that you know or combine the files into one computer file as indicated on this diagram."

Cheryl looked around the group to be sure everyone understood. Then she pointed at another process [② on Figure 1] on the picture and continued. "In addition to verifying the ordered parts, the new system must keep accurate records of all customers. Here we see that the customer's record is checked against the incoming order to identify any changes that must be made. If there is no record for a new customer, then a record is to be created."

Pointing at another process on the picture [③ on Figure 1], Cheryl continued, "Most of your orders request credit and must be approved. As you can see, the customer's credit status is obtained from the cus- ▶

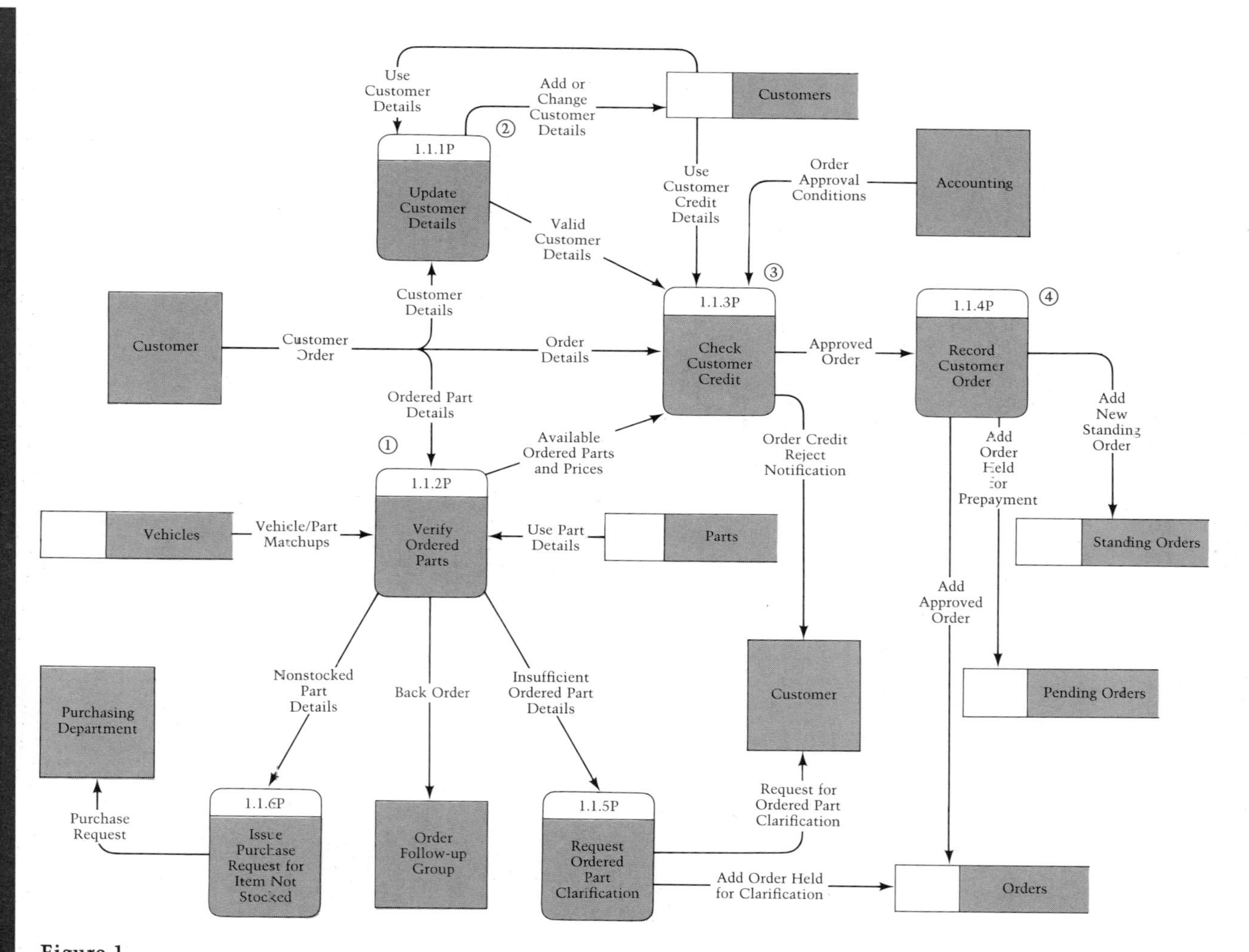

Figure 1

Order-processing picture for the new system.

tomer file and compared against the amount of credit required for the order. Both accounting and the customer would be notified when the credit is not granted."

She pointed at another process on the picture [④ on Figure 1]. "This process records the customer's order for future purposes. Orders may be placed in the pending order file if that order is to be held for a particular condition, such as until prepayment or part clarification is received. Other orders are placed in the regular order or standing order files. The standing order file is to contain those orders that customers would want filled on a regular basis. As you'll see later, we'll be able to monitor these orders and release them to be filled on the appropriate dates."

[*As the conversation continues, we leave the room.*]

An APPROVED ORDER is an output that describes a customer order that has gone through a credit check.

An occurrence of APPROVED ORDER is uniquely identified by the data element SALES ORDER NUMBER.

An APPROVED ORDER consists of the following data elements:

- SALES ORDER NUMBER
- CUSTOMER NUMBER
- ORDER DATE
- PREPAYMENT AMOUNT
- CREDITED AMOUNT
- ORDER TYPE

and one or more occurrences of the following data elements:

  - PART NUMBER
  - PART DESCRIPTION
  - UNIT OF MEASURE
  - QUANTITY ORDERED
  - QUANTITY BACK ORDERED
  - UNIT PRICE

NUMBER OF ORDERED PARTS

Figure 2

Contents of a typical data flow.

The Detailed Requirements for the Target System

Two weeks later, Cheryl and Doug had completed their general requirements and logical data flow diagrams for the new system. Cheryl was starting to work on defining and evaluating alternative computer-based solutions [the topic of the next episode]. Meanwhile, Doug was working on the detailed system requirements. We join Doug as he discusses some of those requirements with Karen.

"Well, that takes care of the procedures for the CHECK CUSTOMER CREDIT process. Can we work on the RECORD CUSTOMER ORDER process now? If you have to get back to work, we can discuss that procedure later."

"No," said Karen. "Let's do it now; I have a few minutes."

Doug continued, "Let's get these data flows defined first. We just defined the APPROVED ORDER data flow. Now where did I put that definition? Here it is! [see Figure 2]. We just defined APPROVED ORDER as the output of the CHECK CUSTOMER CREDIT process, but it's also the input to this RECORD CUSTOMER ORDER process. ►

You can see from our diagram [Figure 1] that the outputs of this procedure are updates to the STANDING ORDER, PENDING ORDER, and ORDER data stores. Can we define those data stores?

Karen replied, "Yes. Essentially these files consist of exactly the same elements as APPROVED ORDER except that the ORDER file will include an ORDER STATUS field."

Doug interrupted, "Just a second." He took a minute and wrote all that out [see Figure 3]. "Okay. Now can we discuss the procedure itself?"

Karen replied, "I'm starting to get the hang of this! Let's see, you should check to see if the APPROVED ORDER is a standard or regular customer order. If the order is a standard order, you place the APPROVED ORDER in the STANDING ORDER file. Otherwise, you place the APPROVED ORDER in the REGULAR ORDER file."

"Is that all there is to it?" asked Doug.

"Not quite!" answered Karen. "If the APPROVED ORDER was rejected for credit purposes, it's placed in the PENDING ORDER file until prepayment is received. By the way, why don't we have the STANDING ORDER also going into the ORDER file?"

"It will eventually, but not until it has been scheduled to be filled in the warehouse," responded Doug. "Remember, that's a whole different procedure. We'll be getting around to documenting the procedures for that task very shortly."

Doug paused to write a RECORD CUSTOMER ORDER procedure description (Figure 4). He then showed the description to Karen who verified its correctness. ►

An ORDER is a data store that describes a customer order that is to be filled.

An occurrence of an ORDER is uniquely identified by the data element SALES ORDER NUMBER.

The data store ORDER consists on the average of 265 customer orders.

An occurrence of an ORDER exists until that order is filled.

An ORDER consists of the following data elements:

- SALES ORDER NUMBER
- CUSTOMER NUMBER
- ORDER DATE
- PREPAYMENT AMOUNT
- CREDITED AMOUNT
- ORDER TYPE
- ORDER STATUS
- and one or more occurrences of the following data elements:
    - PART NUMBER
    - PART DESCRIPTION
    - UNIT OF MEASURE
    - QUANTITY ORDERED
    - QUANTITY BACK ORDERED
    - UNIT PRICE
- NUMBER OF ORDERED PARTS

Figure 3

Typical contents of a data flow.

"Well, that'd better be it for today. I have to go back to work now," said Karen.

"Thanks for your help," replied Doug.

Where Do We Go from Here?

This episode reinforced the use of data flow diagrams, (discussed in Chapter 7) for outlining the *general* requirements for a new information system. But the case previewed two tools used to specify the detailed requirements for the system, a data dictionary and Structured English. Both of these tools have become popular for specifying detailed system requirements.

Chapter 8 introduces you to the concept, use, and implementation of a project data dictionary. The data dictionary is used to document the *contents* of data flows and data stores depicted on the data flow diagram. Chapter 9 introduces you to tools and techniques for documenting policies and procedures—specifically, to structured English and decision tables. These tools specify the details about how the processes on a data flow diagram accomplish their work.

This episode also reinforced the need for analysts to develop sound communication skills. Doug and Cheryl are spending considerable time talking with their users. As a systems analyst, you don't have to worry about becoming deskbound. Once again, we direct you to Part IV, Module C, "Communications Skills for the Systems Analyst" to learn more about how to make presentations and conduct walkthroughs. ■

For each APPROVED ORDER do the following:

  If the ORDER TYPE is "standard" then:

    Record the APPROVED ORDER in the STANDING ORDER file.

  Otherwise (ORDER TYPE is "regular") then:

    For each ordered part do the following:

      Calculate the TOTAL EXTENDED PRICE using the following formula:

        TOTAL EXTENDED PRICE = TOTAL EXTENDED PRICE + (UNIT PRICE × QUANTITY ORDERED)

    If the PREPAYMENT AMOUNT is less than the TOTAL EXTENDED PRICE then:

      If the CREDITED AMOUNT is less than the TOTAL EXTENDED PRICE do the following:

        Record the APPROVED ORDER in the PENDING ORDER file.

      Otherwise (CREDITED AMOUNT is equal to or greater than the TOTAL EXTENDED PRICE) then:

        Record the APPROVED ORDER in the ORDER file.

    Otherwise (PREPAYMENT AMOUNT is equal to or greater than the TOTAL EXTENDED PRICE) then:

      Record the APPROVED ORDER in the ORDER file.

Figure 4

Typical procedure description.

8 Defining Data and Information Requirements in a Data Dictionary

Minicase: Americana Plastics

Angela was thoroughly confused! A part number is a part number is a part number — isn't it? Why then, is management so confused over the definition of a part number? Or maybe Angela's wrong! As the lead analyst on the cost accounting information system project, Angela had seemingly uncovered a terminology problem in the system.

Americana Plastics is a manufacturer of custom-engineered plastic products that become components of their customers' product lines. Each part is carefully engineered to the customer's specifications of size, shape, durability, temperature resistance, and the like. Because Americana products are custom built for individual customers and are subject to that customer's demand, parts are manufactured and shipped only after they have been ordered.

The cost accounting project had been designed to serve two groups of users: the manufacturing group and the accounting group. While working with the accounting group, Angela had learned that all parts sold by Americana were uniquely identified by a six-character part number. She had designed the entire new system using the six-character code as defined by the accounting group. After defining a number of manufacturing cost control analysis reports, she encountered a problem.

"No!" insisted the manufacturing group. "What they are calling a part number, although unique, is actually a mold number. Mold numbers identify the basic molds used to manufacture parts. We identify the actual part by a combination of the mold number and two process codes, the part process method code and the insert code. The part process method code is a one-letter code that tells us whether the plastic parts are to be formed using heat (H), cold (C), or pressure (P). The insert codes identify slugs that can be inserted into the basic mold to form slightly modified versions of the plastic part to be manufactured."

"Is this really a problem?" Angela asked. "After all, the six character basic code is unique, so can't we go ahead and use that code for all reports? I'll even design two sets of reports, one set using the heading 'Part Number' and the other set using 'Mold Number'."

"No," the manufacturing group countered. "We need those additional codes to determine which processing methods and insert requirements are responsible for cost overruns or inefficiencies. How will we be able to use the information to effect changes to our manufacturing methods without the extra codes? In fact, we'd like to suggest alternative structures for the manufacturing reports to make them more useful for pinpointing detailed problems. We'd like to see alternative report structures organized around the different processing methods and inserts as well as the basic molds."

Angela was perplexed! How will she be able to keep track of details when the terminology is not consistent? Each report will have to be redefined to use the terminology of a specific user. But, a part number is a part number is a part number . . .

Discussion

1. How would you suggest an analyst keep track of the special terminology characteristic of most business applications?

2. Could Angela have done something to avoid wasting the time she spent designing the reports?
3. What would you have done differently? If you would have tried to establish terminology and content before format, how would you have communicated your understanding (or lack thereof) back to the two user groups?

WHAT WILL YOU LEARN IN THIS CHAPTER?

In this chapter, you learn how to define the contents of data flows (inputs and outputs) and data stores (files and databases) in a systems data dictionary. You will know that you have mastered the use of the data dictionary as a systems analysis tool when you can:

1. Describe the need for a systems data dictionary, its contents, and its value as a documentation tool.
2. Define the contents of data flows and data stores in terms of restricted data structures that consist of data elements.
3. Create complete data dictionary entries for data flows and data stores. These entries should include pertinent facts about terminology, properties, and content.
4. Create complete data dictionary entries for data elements. These entries should include pertinent facts about terminology, properties, and values (ranges).
5. Analyze and define a code for a data element.
6. Organize, implement, and present a systems data dictionary.

Suppose you are reviewing the logical data flow diagrams (LDFDs) for a new information system. These LDFDs describe the essential business requirements for the new system, but only in general terms. Details still have to be defined. Questions may arise such as:

> What data are we putting in that invoice file?
>
> Just exactly what information is needed on that overtime analysis report?

Did we remember to include the new disputed amount field in the customer statement?

These are questions that can easily be answered from a systems data dictionary. In this chapter, we examine the systems data dictionary and its purpose, content, and use.

WHAT IS A SYSTEMS DATA DICTIONARY AND WHY DO WE NEED IT?

A **systems data dictionary** is a catalog of facts about the data and information requirements for a new information system. A sample entry in a dictionary is shown in Figure 8.1. The tool helps the systems analyst keep track of the enormous volume of details that are part of every system, even small ones. Using a data dictionary, the analyst minimizes the chance of becoming overwhelmed by these details. What facts are recorded in the data dictionary? How is the data dictionary organized? When is the data dictionary used?

Why Do You Need a Systems Data Dictionary?

During the definition phase, the analyst is defining the transaction-processing, management-reporting, and decision support needs for the new information system. No matter what your methods are, you will likely generate a wish list of

- Transactions to be processed by the system
- Reports to be generated by the system
- Decision support inquiries to be answered by the system
- Files (or databases) to be used and maintained by the system.

If you drew a logical data flow diagram of the system, all of these items would appear on that diagram as either data flows or data stores.

A systems data dictionary expands on the definitions of the data flows and data stores. Given a data flow, let's say COURSE REQUEST, we need to define the content of a typical COURSE REQUEST. Given a data store, such as COURSE MASTER FILE, we need to define the content of a record in that file. The data dictionary provides a vehicle for recording these definitions.

Figure 8.1

A sample entry in a systems data dictionary. This is a sample of one complete entry in a systems data dictionary. As you can see, the entry describes pertinent details about a data flow (from a data flow diagram).

DATA DICTIONARY ENTRY
DATA FLOW

DATA FLOW NAME: STUDENT SCHEDULE

DESCRIPTION: A student's schedule of classes for any given term.

ALIASES: FEE RECEIPT

TIMING: Generated once per week beginning four weeks before classes begin and once per day for two weeks after classes begin.

VOLUME: Average volume is 2,500 per week before classes begin (peak is 7,500 for the same period). Average volume is 100 per day after classes begin (peak is 250 for the same period).

COMPOSITION:

A STUDENT SCHEDULE consists of the following data elements:

- DATE THAT SCHEDULE WAS RUN OR REVISED
- STUDENT IDENTIFICATION NUMBER
- STUDENT NAME
- STUDENT CLASSIFICATION
- STUDENT MAJOR
- STUDENT MINOR
- STUDENT MAILING ADDRESS
- STUDENT FEES DUE

One to fifteen of each of the following data elements:

- SUBJECT
- COURSE NUMBER
- COURSE TITLE
- CREDIT
- DIVISION ASSIGNED
- DAYS OF WEEK THAT CLASS MEETS
- TIME OF DAY THAT CLASS MEETS

What Do You Record in the Systems Data Dictionary?

Every transaction, report, inquiry response, and file consists of data elements. You may know data elements by one or more of the following synonyms: *field, attribute, data item,* or *variable.* We'll use the term *data element* throughout this book. A **data element** is the smallest unit of data or information that has any meaning to a user. Examples of data elements are listed in the margin.

By themselves, data elements have little value. However, data elements combine to form data structures that do have meaning—to users, management, and data processing professionals. A **data structure** is a specific arrangement of data elements that define one occurrence of a data flow or one record in a data store. Thus, the arrangement of data elements on a report or document or in a file is a data structure. The sample data structure (a sequence of elements) in the margin describes a STUDENT—possibly a data flow or a data store on a DFD.

Figure 8.2 suggests a model for a systems data dictionary. Data flows and data stores are defined in the dictionary. Each definition will consist of the aforementioned data structures (which, as you can see, consist of data elements). Additionally, you should note that a single definition may also contain the following:

- Terminology and explanations that clarify the data flow or data store to the reader
- Properties of the data flow or data store (such as how often it occurs and number of occurrences)
- Value ranges and properties of data elements (codes for easily identifying products, valid numeric ranges for a wage rate, and the like)

Data Elements

CUSTOMER NUMBER
ORDER DATE
QUANTITY ORDERED
PRODUCT DESCRIPTION
UNIT OF MEASURE
CREDIT RATING
ACCOUNT BALANCE

STUDENT Data Elements

STUDENT ID NUMBER
STUDENT NAME
STUDENT ADDRESS
STUDENT PHONE NUMBER
MAJOR
MINOR
CREDIT HOURS EARNED
GRADE POINT AVERAGE

What Is the Documentation Value of the Systems Data Dictionary?

What is the specific documentation value of the systems data dictionary? Using your information system pyramid model (reproduced in the margin on the next page) as a reference, the systems data dictionary does not document as many of the IPO components as data flow diagrams did. In fact, the dictionary documents only the data, information, and data storage components. On the other hand, the systems data dictionary documents those components in considerably more detail than the data flow diagram. Actually, the two tools complement one another nicely. The data flow diagram presents the "big picture" of the system. The systems data dictionary defines the details about the data flows and data stores.

Figure 8.2

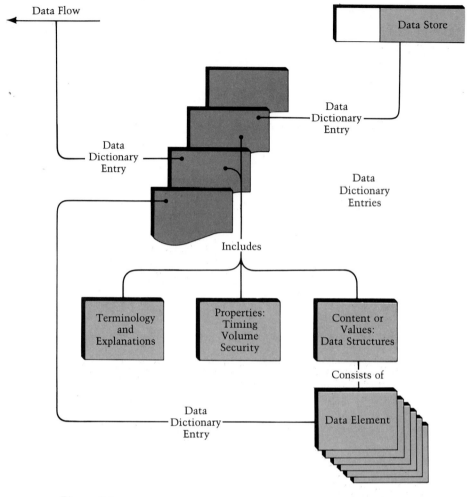

Model for a data dictionary. The entries in a data dictionary correspond to data flows and data stores (on a DFD) and the data elements that make up the data flows and stores. This model shows what types of details are recorded in the data dictionary.

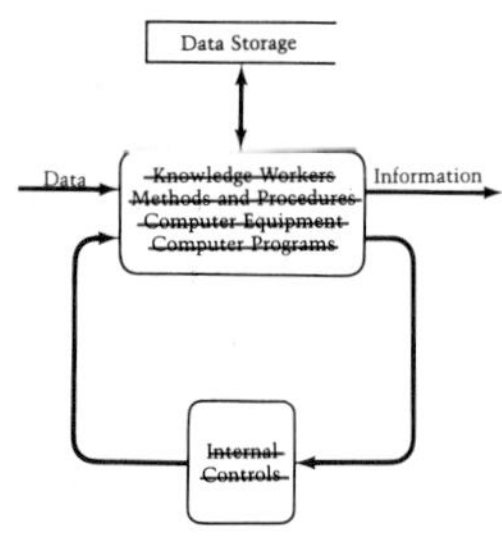

Information System IPO Components

When Is the Systems Data Dictionary Created and Used?

A systems data dictionary (hereafter called *data dictionary*) is usually created during the definition phase of the systems development project. You can initiate data flow and data store definitions either while you are drawing the corresponding data flow diagrams or after you have completed those diagrams. The data dictionary is a living document. This means that it is constantly used for reference and subject to change throughout the remaining phases of the system development life cycle.

When you get into Part III, the system design chapters, you will see the data dictionary expand to record details about how data flows and data stores will be implemented (as forms, computer inputs, computer outputs, terminal displays, computer files, and the like). Therefore, it is important for you to learn how to make systems analysis entries into a data dictionary.

DEFINING DATA STRUCTURES IN A DATA DICTIONARY

In the last section you learned that any data flow or data store is defined by a data structure or arrangement of data elements. When defining a new system, we need to find a way to document this data structure.

Now, you might be thinking, why not just take the current form, document, or report to the user and ask which elements to keep, delete, and add? Assuming such a form, document, or report exists, this approach presents a potential problem. When you look at the document, you (and your user) often become prematurely concerned with changing the format of the document—in other words, you start to think about how it looks or should look. When you do this, you frequently miss fundamental content issues that can be expensive or impossible to correct for at a later date.

So what *should* you do? If a document exists for your data flow or data store, describe its contents using the data structure that we discuss in the following pages. The suggested notation presents the contents only in terms of *what* data elements are on the form, not in terms of *how* they are currently formatted. Once this description has been completed, you can sit down with the users and discuss that content objectively. Data flows and data stores can be defined in terms of the following types of data structures:

1. A sequence of data elements or group of data elements that occur one after the other
2. The selection of one or more data elements from a set of data elements

3. The repetition of a group of data elements

The notation suggested in the following discussion has been chosen because it can be easily understood by people who haven't ever read a data dictionary.

The definition of the data structure for any data flow or data store should begin with a statement such as

> A WAGE AND TAX STATEMENT consists of the following data elements:

The Sequence Data Structure

The sequence of data elements that define a data flow or data store are listed as follows:

> A WAGE AND TAX STATEMENT consists of the following data elements:
>
> SOCIAL SECURITY NUMBER
>
> EMPLOYEE NAME
>
> EMPLOYEE ADDRESS
>
> EMPLOYER NAME
>
> EMPLOYER ADDRESS
>
> WAGES, TIPS, COMPENSATION
>
> FEDERAL TAX WITHHELD
>
> STATE TAX WITHHELD
>
> FICA TAX WITHHELD

Notice that we indented the data element names to improve readability. Each of the preceding data elements is *required* to assume a value for every occurrence of WAGE AND TAX STATEMENT.

The Selection Data Structure

The selection construct allows you to show situations where given any occurrence of a data flow or data store, one of the following is true:

- *One and only one* data element from a list of data elements will assume a value.
- One or more data elements in a list will assume a value.

There must be at least two data elements in the list from which you choose. Otherwise, you would not be able to select anything. Some examples will make the selection construct clear.

Suppose an order can be placed either by an individual or by a company. The following data structure is defined:

An ORDER consists of the following data elements:

  ORDER DATE

  and one and only one of the following elements:

    SOCIAL SECURITY NUMBER

    CUSTOMER ACCOUNT NUMBER

Any given occurrence of an order will consist of either an ORDER DATE plus a SOCIAL SECURITY NUMBER *or* an ORDER DATE plus a CUSTOMER ACCOUNT NUMBER.

The following data structure suggests a different selection construct:

TRAVEL EXPENSE consists of the following data elements:

  EMPLOYEE ID NUMBER

  EMPLOYEE NAME

  DATE TRIP STARTED

  DATE TRIP COMPLETED

  PURPOSE OF TRIP

  MILES TRAVELED

  MILEAGE CHARGE

  One or more of the following elements:

    AIR TRAVEL EXPENSE

    TAXI FARE EXPENSE

    REGISTRATION FEES

    LODGING EXPENSES

    MEAL EXPENSES

  TOTAL EXPENSES

The preceding data structure states that a TRAVEL EXPENSE consists of *one or more* of the listed expenses. TOTAL EXPENSES always occurs because it is not indented as part of the sublist.

The following definition is *incorrect:*

A STUDENT consists of the following elements:

STUDENT ID NUMBER

STUDENT NAME

One of the following CLASSES:

FRESHMAN

SOPHOMORE

JUNIOR

SENIOR

This does not work because CLASS is a data element whereas FRESHMAN, SOPHOMORE, JUNIOR, SENIOR are values of the data element CLASS, not data elements themselves: The correct data structure would be

A STUDENT consists of the following data elements:

STUDENT ID NUMBER

STUDENT NAME

STUDENT CLASS

Later in this chapter, you'll learn where to record values and value ranges in the data dictionary.

The Repetition Data Structure

The repetition construct is used to set off a data element or group of data elements that will repeat a specified number of times for a single occurrence of the data flow or data store. The construct is documented as follows:

M to *N* occurrences of each of the following elements:

where *M* is the minimum number of occurrences of the repeating group and *N* is the maximum number of occurrences of the data structure. The notation suggests that the entire group of data elements repeats as a group. If the number of repetitions is indefinite, you may write:

One or more occurrences of each of the following elements:

The list that follows the colon may consist of a sequence of data elements, a selection construct or constructs, or even additional repetition constructs. Let's expand on our ORDER example to demonstrate the repetition construct:

> An ORDER consists of the following data elements:
>
> ORDER NUMBER
>
> ORDER DATE
>
> One of the following elements:
>
> > SOCIAL SECURITY NUMBER
> >
> > CUSTOMER ACCOUNT NUMBER
>
> SHIPPING ADDRESS
>
> 1 to 20 occurrences of each of the following:
>
> > PRODUCT NUMBER
> >
> > PRODUCT DESCRIPTION
> >
> > QUANTITY ORDERED
> >
> > PRODUCT PRICE
> >
> > EXTENDED PRICE
>
> TOTAL ORDER COST

Notice that a sequence of related data elements was defined as the repeating group. Let's look at one more example:

> A TIME CARD consists of the following data elements:
>
> EMPLOYEE IDENTIFICATION NUMBER
>
> EMPLOYEE NAME
>
> 1 to 4 occurrences of each of the following:
>
> > FIRST DAY OF PAY WEEK
> >
> > LAST DAY OF PAY WEEK
> >
> > 1 to 7 occurrences of each of the following:
> >
> > > HOURS WORKED

There are four weeks in a pay period. That explains the first repeating group. For each (or any) of those weeks, an employee will have from one to seven values of hours worked — one value for each day worked. This is a **nested repeating group,** meaning one repeating group inside another.

A Notation for Optional Data Elements

Sometimes, certain data elements or groups of data elements optionally take on values for occurrences of data flows. Consider, for a moment, the following data structure:

A CLAIM consists of the following data elements:
- POLICY NUMBER
- POLICYHOLDER NAME
- POLICYHOLDER ADDRESS
- SPOUSE NAME (optional)

For any occurrence of CLAIM, the element SPOUSE NAME may or may not take on a value. Let's expand the example to show you how to indicate optional repeating groups:

A CLAIM consists of the following data elements:
- POLICY NUMBER
- POLICYHOLDER NAME
- POLICYHOLDER ADDRESS
- SPOUSE NAME (optional)
- 0 to 15 occurrences of each of the following:
  - DEPENDENT NAME
  - DEPENDENT RELATIONSHIP
- CLAIMANT NAME
- OVER AGE DEPENDENT RELATIONSHIP (optional)
- OVER AGE DEPENDENT AGE (optional)
- 1 or more of the following:
  - EXPENSE DESCRIPTION
  - SERVICE PROVIDED BY
  - TOTAL CHARGE

Note that we still used the repeating construct for the optional group of data elements. But we only have to provide dependent relationship and age if the claim is for a dependent over a certain age. We also provided a mandatory repeating group to reinforce the nonoptional repeating group concept. Let's consider the difference between

optionally, the following:

OVER AGE DEPENDENT AGE

OVER AGE DEPENDENT RELATIONSHIP

and

OVER AGE DEPENDENT AGE (optional)

OVER AGE DEPENDENT RELATIONSHIP (optional)

The former suggests that both elements occur together or neither element occurs. It's all or nothing. The second suggests that either element may occur independent of the other.

Groups of Elements

Groups of data elements that always occur together, such as the elements in a street address, can be set off as follows:

A WAGE AND TAX STATEMENT consists of the following data elements:

SOCIAL SECURITY NUMBER

EMPLOYEE NAME

EMPLOYEE ADDRESS, which consists of:

One or both of the following elements:

STREET ADDRESS

POST OFFICE BOX NUMBER

CITY

STATE

ZIP CODE

EMPLOYER NAME

EMPLOYER ADDRESS, which consists of:

One or both of the following elements:

STREET ADDRESS

POST OFFICE BOX NUMBER

CITY

STATE

ZIP CODE

WAGES, TIPS, COMPENSATION

FEDERAL TAX WITHHELD

STATE TAX WITHHELD

FICA TAX WITHHELD

This is technically correct. However, as a shorthand notation, you might try the following:

A WAGE AND TAX STATEMENT consists of the following data elements:

SOCIAL SECURITY NUMBER

EMPLOYEE NAME

EMPLOYEE ADDRESS, which is the same as ADDRESS (as follows)

EMPLOYER NAME

EMPLOYER ADDRESS, which is the same as ADDRESS (as follows)

.
.
.

The group ADDRESS consists of the following data elements:

One or both of the following elements:

STREET ADDRESS

POST OFFICE BOX NUMBER

CITY

STATE

ZIP CODE

What we did was to define both addresses to be equivalent to a single group called ADDRESS. That group is defined immediately following the original data structure. This way, the reader does not have to go looking for it!

Before we leave the subject of data structure notation we call your attention to the shorthand, algebraic notation in Figure 8.3. This notation, or something similar, is suggested in several books. Although the notation is easy for the analyst to learn and write, it can be cryptic to the user. We offer it only as an alternative and so that you will recognize it when you see it.

NOTATION	MEANING
=	is COMPOSED OF or CONSISTS OF
+	AND (which implements *sequence*)
[. . .]	*select* one of the data elements inside the brackets
< . . . >	*select* one or more of the data elements inside the brackets
N{ . . . }M	the data elements or data structure inside the braces occurs or *repeats* a minimum of N times and may occur or repeat up to M times
(. . .)	the data elements or data structures inside the parentheses are *optional*
*	allows *comments* to be inserted into the definition
:	is defined elsewhere in the data dictionary

Figure 8.3

Shorthand notation for data structures. This table shows a mathematics-like shorthand notation for documenting data flows and data stores. This notation is popular in many books. Although it is easy for the analyst to learn and apply, the notation is not very easy for users to read and verify.

ENTRIES IN A TYPICAL DATA DICTIONARY

We've learned how data dictionaries can be used to define different data structures. Our goal is to define all important facts about the data flows and data stores that appear on primitive levels of a logical data flow diagram. In this section, you will learn how to write complete data dictionaries entries.

Data Flow Entries in a Data Dictionary

A complete data flow entry should contain the following:

- *Data flow name* Names should be chosen carefully. Do not use abbreviations or acronyms even if the form from which you took the name uses such abbreviations.
- *Data flow description* What is the data flow? What is its purpose? Do not describe its current implementation because that implementation may change.

- *Aliases* Is the data flow known by any other names? In this case, we might recognize abbreviations and acronyms; however, we should still avoid aliases that imply how the data flow is or will be implemented.
- *Timing and volume* How often does the data flow happen? Daily? Monthly? Any time? How many occurrences of the data flow happen in a given time period? Are there peak or valley periods?
- *Data structure* What is the content of the data flow? Use the restricted data structures to define the elements that make up the data flow.

For example, one of the management-reporting requirements of the customer services system for AAP is the generation of PART SALES SUMMARY. The summary will provide management with information concerning part sales over a daily, weekly, and monthly basis. Furthermore, the information is to be segregated by warehouse zones and product lines, with summary totals for each zone and product line. The data dictionary for this output follows (*Note:* an asterisk indicates a supplementary comment.):

> The data flow PART SALES SUMMARY is an output that describes sales volume over a daily, weekly, and monthly period.
>
>> The PART SALES SUMMARY is to be provided between 8 A.M. and 10 P.M. on the last working day of each week.
>>
>> The data flow PART SALES SUMMARY consists of the following data elements:
>>
>>> DATE * of report
>>>
>>> 1 to 5 occurrences of the following:
>>>
>>>> ZONE
>>>>
>>>>> 1 to 35 occurrences of the following:
>>>>>
>>>>>> PRODUCT LINE
>>>>>>
>>>>>>> 1 to 200 occurrences of the following:
>>>>>>>
>>>>>>>> PART NUMBER
>>>>>>>>
>>>>>>>> PART DESCRIPTION
>>>>>>>>
>>>>>>>> UNIT SALES PAST DAY

UNIT SALES
PAST WEEK

UNIT SALES
PAST MONTH

PAST DAY UNIT SALES
LINE

PAST WEEK UNIT SALES
LINE

PAST MONTH UNIT SALES
LINE

PAST DAY UNIT SALES ZONE

PAST WEEK UNIT SALES ZONE

PAST MONTH UNIT SALES ZONE

Notice that our complete definition includes all of the pertinent facts described in our list. Programmers will recognize the data structure as a multilevel control break report. Notice how indentation was used to help maintain readability.

Another interesting and challenging data flow in the customer services system is the decision support output PART QUERY RESPONSE. This data flow is a general purpose query response output for the customer services system. Management has suggested the need for information regarding general part data, part-to-vehicle matchups, and part back order analysis. Pay particular attention to the data structure. We chose this data structure because a three-option part query has been requested.

The data flow PART QUERY RESPONSE is an output that describes ordered parts, back ordered parts, or part-to-vehicle matchups.

PART QUERY RESPONSE will be requested approximately 50 times per day (approximately 65 percent of the requests will occur during the hours from 8 A.M. to 11:30 A.M.).

A PART QUERY RESPONSE consists of the following data elements:

PART NUMBER

PART DESCRIPTION

and one and only one of the following data groups:

PART ORDER RESPONSE (as follows)

PART-VEHICLE MATCH RESPONSE (as follows)

PART BACK ORDER RESPONSE (as follows)

PART ORDER RESPONSE consists of the following elements:

WHOLESALE PRICE

RETAIL BASE PRICE

FRANCHISE DISCOUNT RATE

QUANTITY REQUIRED FOR VOLUME DISCOUNT

VOLUME DISCOUNT RATE

QUANTITY ON HAND

QUANTITY BACK ORDERED

QUANTITY ON ORDER

PART-VEHICLE MATCH RESPONSE consists of the following elements:

VEHICLE MAKE

VEHICLE MODEL

MODEL YEAR

and one or more occurrences of the following element:

PART RESTRICTIONS

PART BACK ORDER RESPONSE consists of the following elements:

QUANTITY ON HAND

QUANTITY ON ORDER

TOTAL QUANTITY BACK ORDERED

and one or more occurrences of the following elements:

SALES ORDER NUMBER

SALES ORDER DATE
CUSTOMER NUMBER
QUANTITY BACK ORDERED

Users can now evaluate the requirement for completeness. Notice that, rather than combine the data dictionary entries for each data structure that composed the PART QUERY RESPONSE data flow, we treated each data structure (query response option) as a group of elements defined elsewhere in data dictionary notation. The group data structures should immediately follow their initial reference so the reader doesn't have to search for them.

Data Store Entries in a Data Dictionary

Data stores are also easy to describe using a data dictionary. A complete data store entry should contain the following:

- *Data store name* Again, names should be meaningful—avoid abbreviations and acronyms.
- *Data store description*
- *Aliases*
- *Identifier elements* Are there any data elements (key) in the data store whose values determine one and only one occurrence (record) in the data store?
- *Volume* How many occurrences (records) will be stored? Will this grow in the future?
- *Security* Are there any restrictions governing who can see, change, or use the data?
- *Data structure* What is the content of *one* occurrence (record) in the data store? Use the restricted data structure notation suggested in this chapter to document the content.

For example, an appropriate data dictionary for AAP's CUSTOMER file would be

The data store CUSTOMER is a collection of records that describe customer accounts.

An occurrence of CUSTOMER is uniquely identified by the element CUSTOMER NUMBER.

The CUSTOMER data store contains 600 occurrences of CUSTOMER with an anticipated growth of 3 to 5 percent per year.

A CUSTOMER consists of the following data elements:

- CUSTOMER NUMBER
- CUSTOMER NAME
- BILLING ADDRESS which consists of:
  - One or both of the following elements:
    - STREET ADDRESS
    - POST OFFICE BOX NUMBER
  - CITY
  - STATE
  - ZIP CODE
- BILLING PHONE
- CUSTOMER TYPE
- CREDIT RATING *
- CREDIT CEILING *
- CURRENT BALANCE DUE *
- BALANCE PAST DUE *

The elements marked by an asterisk may only be updated by the Accounts Receivable Department.

Data Element Entries in a Data Dictionary

Preparing data dictionaries to describe data elements is just as important as preparing data dictionaries to describe data flows and data stores. Why? Data elements are not composed of data structures or other data elements. But data elements are assigned values, and it is very important that we learn the legitimate values for data elements so we can design controls in information systems to guarantee that occurrences of data elements are valid. We can use data dictionaries to describe the data elements and to verify our understanding of the data element with the user. A complete data element entry in the dictionary should include the following:

- *Data element name* Again, meaningful and without abbreviations or acronyms.
- *Data element description*
- *Aliases* We refer you back to the problems encountered in the Americana Plastics case that started this chapter. List all aliases for the data element.
- *Values and defaults* What values or range of values can the element assume? Is there a default value that should be assigned if the user fails to assign a value?

Data values can be classified into three categories; indefinite values, value ranges, and finite values. Each category requires some explanation.

Many data elements can assume a virtually unlimited number of values. Examples include STUDENT NAME and STUDENT ADDRESS. The data dictionary entry for such an element might look like this:

> The element STUDENT NAME is the name that will appear on all official correspondence and reports.
>
> > The format should be last name, first name, middle name. Nicknames should be avoided.

Notice that we only placed format limitations and recommendations on the values of STUDENT NAME.

Some data elements are restricted to a *range* of element values. Most of these elements are numeric in nature, and the limits or the legal range may vary from time to time. The legal value range for any element should be defined by the analyst when the *business* is studied or defined. For example:

> The element PAY RATE is the hourly rate of pay for a nonsalaried employee.
>
> > Also known as WAGE RATE and HOURLY RATE.
> >
> > Values must fall between $3.35 and $12.50 according to the current union contract. Rates are subject to changes in minimum wage laws and future union contracts.

Finally, many data elements can only assume a limited set of well-defined values. Consider the following example:

The element ORDER NUMBER is a number that uniquely identifies a customer order.

ORDER NUMBER is a nine-digit element that can be interpreted as follows:

digits 1–6	date on which order was submitted
digits 7–9	unique sequence number for orders submitted on the date (001 up to 999)

ORDER NUMBER is a *code*. The subject of codes and coding techniques is very important to the systems analyst.

Business Codes and Coding Techniques

A **code** is a group of characters and/or digits that identify and describe something in the business system. Codes are frequently used to describe customers, products, materials, or events. The use of codes is popular for several reasons. First, codes can often be used for quick and easy identification of people, objects, and events. For instance, a product coded A-57-G may mean "product number 57, gallon can, in warehouse zone A." Second, codes usually condense numerous facts into concise format. And finally, the concise format usually reduces data storage space requirements.

Systems analysts are frequently charged with analyzing and defining coding schemes for information systems. Codes are entered into the data dictionary as part of a data element entry. Let's examine some of the more common coding schemes.

Sequential and Serial Codes Sequential and serial codes are quite similar. Both number items with consecutive numbers — for example, 1,2,3 . . . *n*. Sequential numbers are typically assigned to a set of items (such as customers) that have been previously ordered (alphabetically, for example). Although the scheme is simple, new items cannot be easily inserted without disrupting the original ordering or changing many assigned numbers.

Serial numbers are assigned according to *when* new items are first identified. The first item identified is numbered 1, the second item is numbered 2, and so forth. Although serial coding also offers simplicity and a nearly infinite number of occurrences, the code has little information value.

Sequential and serial coding are frequently used as components in the more complicated coding schemas described in the following sections.

Block Codes Block coding is a variation on sequential coding. A set of sequential or serial codes is divided into *blocks* that classify items into specific classes. For instance, a block code could be defined for customers as follows:

1000 through 4999	Franchise Customers
5000 through 6999	Nonfranchise Customer Chains
7000 through 7999	Nonfranchise Independent Customers
8000 through 9999	Casual Customers

Every customer would be assigned a serial or sequential number within its proper block classification. The number for any given customer identifies the customer type.

Alphabetic Codes Alphabetic codes use different combinations of letters and/or numbers to describe items. Alphabetic codes have greater information value than any of the previously described codes. Many such codes have been standardized—for example, the two-letter abbreviations for states of the union in which TX = Texas. Most alphabetic codes are abbreviations; therefore, with a little practice, such codes can easily be interpreted.

Group Codes Group codes are the most powerful of the coding schemes because they convey much more information content than the other coding schemes (which they frequently utilize). Each position or group of positions in the code describes some pertinent characteristic of the item being coded. Thus, the code number tells the reader a great deal about the item itself. There are two common types of group codes: significant digit codes and hierarchical codes.

For **significant digit codes,** each digit or group of digits describes a measurable or identifiable characteristic of the item. Significant digit codes are frequently used to code inventory items. For example, the following code might be defined for paint and stain inventory items:

First Digit	Product Classification: P = Paint S = Stain

Second Through Fourth Digits	Base Color Block 100 – 199 Browns 200 – 299 Greens 300 – 399 Blues 400 – 499 Whites 500 – 599 Reds 600 – 699 Blacks 700 – 799 Walnut 800 – 899 Oak 900 – 999 Rosewood
Fifth Digit	Tint (tenths per gallon)
Sixth Digit	Base Type 0 = Not Relevant 1 = Lacquer 2 = Water 3 = Oil
Seventh Digit	Unit of Measure P = Pint Q = Quart G = Gallon D = Drum (5 gallons)

Once again, with a little practice, users can easily code and decode inventory items. As was the case with alphabetic codes, significant digit codes are frequently standardized for some industries (zip codes, light bulb codes, tire codes).

Hierarchical codes provide a top-down interpretation for an item. Every item coded is factored into groups, subgroups, and so forth. Each group and subgroup can be coded such that the codes identify specific groups and subgroups. For instance, we could code (or partially code) all inventory items by warehouse location as follows:

first digit	Warehouse Zone (A,B,C,D,or E)
second digit	Section in Zone (1 – 5)
third and fourth digits	Aisle in Section (1 – 20)
fifth digit	Shelf Number (A – M)

Coding Guidelines The five coding schemes discussed can be combined in any arrangement desired to achieve business goals. Codes are intended to make the handling of data easier. Whenever you encounter a data element, which can only assume a finite set of values, a coding scheme may have to be studied, defined, or expanded. Codes are, first and foremost, a business tool. Therefore, you should consider the following business issues when analyzing or proposing codes:

1. *Codes should be expandable.* To accommodate natural growth, a code should allow for additional entries.
2. *Codes should be unique.* Each occurrence should define one, and only one, occurrence of data.
3. *Size of codes is important.* A code should be large enough to describe relevant characteristics but small enough to be easily read and interpreted by people.
4. *Codes should be convenient.* A new occurrence of a code should be easy to construct and interpret. A computer should *not* be required.

ORGANIZING AND IMPLEMENTING THE SYSTEMS DATA DICTIONARY

In this section, we examine how to organize, implement, and use a data dictionary. Several alternatives are presented for your consideration.

Data Dictionary Organization

A data dictionary should be organized to allow easy reference to definitions that you or the user need. Furthermore, the data dictionary can be keyed to the names and terms originally documented on some sort of system model or picture. The DFDs from Chapter 7 provide an outstanding framework for your data dictionary. Each data flow and data store should be named and defined in the dictionary.

All data dictionary entries should be organized alphabetically by name. Do not organize the dictionary by type (such as *data flows* or *data stores*). When was the last time you saw a conventional dictionary organized into separate sections for nouns, verbs, adverbs, and so forth? It doesn't make sense because it would require the reader to know which section(s) to go to.

Data Dictionary Implementation

There are several ways to implement a data dictionary. One of the more popular options is to print special forms for data flow, data store, and data element entries. For instance, a data flow form might look something like Figure 8.4. The advantage of forms is that the analyst is provided with standards for what to include in the dictionary.

Another popular option is to record data dictionary entries on simple index cards. The cards can easily be shuffled, reorganized, and stored. And a still more powerful and relatively simple strategy is to implement a simple computerized data dictionary using the local line editor on your computer system. The line editor (which you have probably used to write computer programs and test data files) is used to create, insert, move, and delete data dictionary entries. Some editors even allow you to create blank form files that can be read into the dictionary and then filled in. The disadvantage of simple line editor data dictionaries is that it can be difficult to get listings of subsets of the dictionary — it's all or nothing.

There are a number of data dictionary software packages that allow you to create and maintain sophisticated data dictionaries on the computer. The packages, usually associated with database management system software, allow you to examine your data dictionary in many different ways. See the "Next Generation" feature in this chapter for more on this powerful tool.

Using the Data Dictionary

A data dictionary for any project, even a small one, can get very large. And size is frequently cited as a major disadvantage of the data dictionary. Some analysts find this disadvantage sufficient reason to ignore the tool. These analysts frequently make two errors in judgment. First, they *dump* a large data dictionary into the laps of their users and request verification. Nobody's going to read an epic novel! When you want the user to verify a data dictionary, you should present it in pieces. Often, you extract the desired dictionary definitions and format them so the reader doesn't have to shuffle back and forth through the pages (even if it means a little duplication).

Second, many analysts include redundant data in their data dictionaries. For instance, some data dictionaries duplicate pieces of the data flow diagrams to which they are keyed. Other data diction-

DATA FLOW DEFINITION

NAME ______________________________

DATE CREATED ______________ BY ______________

LAST DATE UPDATED ______________ BY ______________

ALIASES ______________________________

****

BRIEF DESCRIPTION:

TIMING: ______________________________

VOLUME: ______________________________ (AVG)

PEAK VOLUME ______________ OCCURS (when) ______________

____

****

COMPOSITION (data structures)

Figure 8.4

Sample form for a data dictionary. Some analysts prefer to use forms to implement their data dictionary. Forms impose standards on the documentation. This form would be used to document data flows. Similar forms could be developed for data stores and data elements.

aries include entries that describe the source and destination of data flows and the processes that use a data store. In all these cases, the entries are redundant because we have a data flow diagram to refer

The Next Generation

Integrated Data Dictionaries: An Idea Whose Time Has Come

In many businesses, data has become their most precious rcsourcc — and thcir most uncontrolled resource! As data files and databases proliferate, data administration (or the lack thereof) becomes a serious problem. Just how serious can the problem get? Consider a law that mandates a nine-digit zip code (or larger). Do you have any idea how difficult it is to find every computer program and file that has a zip code field in it? Why so difficult? Over the years, programmers and analysts came and went. Each introduced a bit of *uniqueness* into the systems and computer program library. How many unique field names exist for zip code? Let's see — there's ZIPCODE, ZIP.CODE, ZIP, ZP, Z, ZC, ZCODE, ZCOD, ZIPCD well, you get the idea. Where do you look for the fields? How do you look for them? Clearly, there's got to be a better way of keeping track.

And there is! A formal data administration function has developed in some businesses. That's *data administration* — not *database administration.* The idea is to create and maintain a data dictionary for the business as a whole. That dictionary keeps track of where data elements are used and stored — every file, database, computer program, report, document, and so forth. The aliases, descriptions, formats, limitations, and properties of every data element are recorded in a centralized data dictionary. As new systems are developed and old systems are maintained, analysts and programmers are urged to use the dictionary to curb the proliferation of aliases and to minimize the creation of new data elements. In other words, we are taking the project data dictionary concept and increasing its perspective to include the business as a whole!

The only way to implement an enterprise-wide data dictionary is to use one of the commercially available data dictionary software packages. Automated data dictionaries aren't new. They've been with us almost since the advent of database ▶

to. The additional entries in the dictionary, although useful, can require considerable extra effort — which we don't recommend!

SUMMARY

A project data dictionary is a catalog of details for a new information system's data and information requirements. The principle purpose of the dictionary is to record details about essential data flows (inputs and outputs) and data stores (files). Data flows and data stores consist of data elements, the smallest unit of data or information that has any meaning to a user. Data elements are

The Next Generation (continued)

management systems software. In fact, you usually get a data dictionary package when you buy a database management system (database-independent products are also available). These automated data dictionaries were originally conceived to help the database professionals keep track of the data elements and records in databases. But they are being increasingly used to catalog all the data flows, stores, and elements in a business.

What can an automated data dictionary do for you? Data dictionaries may allow you to do the following:

- Get full listings of all known facts about all or specific subsets (such as a group of related applications, a single related application, and/or a single program) of data flows, stores, elements, and so forth.
- Get partial listings (such as name and description only) for data flows, stores, elements, and so forth.
- Reorganize facts into a convenient format. For example, give full facts for all data elements that are part of specific data flows.
- Find all data flows, data stores, or data elements that share a certain property (such as the same unit of measure or the same length).
- Answer queries about data. For instance, LIST ALL KNOWN ALIASES FOR ZIP CODE. And then, LIST ALL FILES IN WHICH ZIP CODE (including its aliases) IS STORED. And finally, LIST ALL PROGRAMS THAT USE THE FIELD ZIP CODE (again, including all its aliases).

Where does the systems analyst fit into this picture? The analyst's system data dictionary can be a subset of the business data dictionary. Thus, the systems analyst of the future may not have to worry about proliferating the creation of duplicate data elements and data stores. Indeed, the future systems analyst may not be allowed to operate in isolation from other analysts and information systems! ■

arranged in specific patterns, called data structures, that describe a single occurrence of a data flow or data store. These data structures, along with terminology, properties, and value ranges, are recorded in the dictionary. A data dictionary is normally initiated during the definition phase of the system development life cycle. It remains the principle source of facts throughout the remainder of the life cycle.

The content of any occurrence of a data flow or data store can be documented as combinations of three restricted data structures: a *sequence* of data elements, the *selection* from a list of data elements, and the *repetition* of one or more data elements. The notation presented in this chapter is easy to write and even easier to read (important to users!). The notation also provides for the specification of optional data elements and common groups of data elements.

Every data dictionary entry should include a descriptive name, brief narrative description, and aliases for the name. Data flow entries should also include facts about timing, volume, and content. Content is always defined in terms of the aforementioned data structures. Data store entries should include facts about identifier elements, number of occurrences, security restrictions, and content. Finally, data elements should include facts about values, value ranges, and defaults. Many data elements use business codes, which are groups of characters or digits that identify and describe business entities. There are a number of useful coding schemes.

Data dictionaries should be organized alphabetically without regard to object type. There are many ways to implement data dictionaries including forms, index cards, line editors, and commercial data dictionary software.

PROBLEMS AND EXERCISES

1. Why is a data dictionary a valuable systems analysis tool? What are the possible consequences of not creating a data dictionary during systems analysis?
2. Can you think of any specific times that a data dictionary might have been helpful when you were writing a computer program? Can you think of a situation in which you misinterpreted a computer program requirement because you didn't know something that could have been recorded in a data dictionary?
3. Dig out your last computer program. Prepare data dictionary entries for the following:
   (a) Inputs (data flows)
   (b) Outputs (data flows)
   (c) Files or database (data store)
   (d) All variables or fields (data elements)
4. Using the data structure notation in this chapter, create a data dictionary entry for each of the following:
   (a) Your driver's license
   (b) Your course registration form
   (c) Your class schedule

(d) IRS Form 1040 (any version)
(e) An account statement and invoice for a credit card
(f) Your telephone, electric, or gas bill
(g) An order form in a catalog
(h) An application for anything (for example, insurance, housing)
(i) A retail store catalog
(j) A typical real estate listing
(k) A computer printout from a business office or computer course
(l) A catalog that describes the classes to be offered next semester
(m) Your checkbook
(n) Your bank statement

5. Select one of the data dictionaries you developed in problem 4 and complete a set of data element dictionary entries for each element appearing in the data dictionary.

6. During the study phase of systems analysis, the analyst must gather facts concerning both the manual and automated portions of the system. Why would it be desirable for a systems analyst to obtain samples of the existing computer files and computer-generated outputs? What value would data dictionary entries for computer files and computer-generated outputs be during systems analysis?

7. Visit a local business (or school) office. Ask them for samples of five business forms, logsheets, or regular reports. Prepare complete data dictionary entries for each sample. If possible, review your entries with the users. Did they find your entries easy to read and understand? Can they think of additional data elements that would make their job easier? Add these elements to your data dictionary entries.

8. Find an example of a business code (possibly on the forms from problem 7). Make a data element data dictionary entry for that code. Analyze that code according to the guidelines presented in this chapter. Can you suggest a better coding scheme?

9. Create forms, similar to that in Figure 8.4, to standardize the definitions of data stores and data elements in a data dictionary.

10. Create a simple data dictionary using your local line editor. Try to implement standard forms that can be read into the diction-

ary (to initiate new data flows, data stores, and data elements entries).

11. Research (through data processing trade journals) a commercial data dictionary package. Evaluate that package's potential value as a *project* data dictionary.
12. The sales manager for Holster Supplies Company has requested an improved sales analysis report. He envisions a new report that might appear as follows:

05/07/86 HOLSTER SUPPLIES CO. PAGE 1

SALES ANALYSIS REPORT

REGION NUMBER	DISTRICT NUMBER	SALESPERSON NUMBER	CUSTOMER NUMBER	SALES AMOUNT
14	141	14101	10001	1,219.95
			12202	765.92
			13210	32.00
	TOTAL SALES FOR SALESPERSON		14101	2,017.87
		14101	11022	976.45
	TOTAL SALES FOR SALESPERSON		14102	976.45
	TOTAL SALES IN DISTRICT 141			2,994.32
	142	14201	11231	1,423.99
	TOTAL SALES FOR SALESPERSON		14201	1,423.99
	TOTAL SALES IN DISTRICT 142			1,423.99
	TOTAL SALES IN REGION 14			4,418.31
15	151	15101	20110	3,300.00
			20121	1,020.00
	TOTAL SALES FOR SALESPERSON		15101	4,320.00
	TOTAL SALES IN DISTRICT 151			4,320.00
	TOTAL SALES IN REGION 15			4,320.00
	TOTAL COMPANY SALES			8,738.31

Note that Holster Supplies' sales territory covers four regions, each divided into two to four districts. There are forty-five salespersons, and each salesperson is assigned to one and only one district. Prepare a data dictionary entry to describe the content of the envisioned sales analysis report. Why would developing a data dictionary be beneficial even though the manager has already got an idea of what he wants? What additional information concerning this report should be included in the data dictionary before the layout of the final report is designed?

ANNOTATED REFERENCES AND SUGGESTED READINGS

DeMarco, Tom. *Structured Analysis and System Specification.* Englewood Cliffs, N.J.: Prentice-Hall, 1979. Chapters 11 through 14 present the most comprehensive treatment of the systems data dictionary that we've seen so far. DeMarco uses the algebraic notation we depicted in Figure 8.3.

Gane, Chris, and Trish Sarson. *Structured Systems Analysis: Tools and Techniques.* Englewood Cliffs, N.J.: Prentice-Hall, 1979. Another classic reference on the systems data dictionary (Chapter 4 covers automated data dictionaries in greater depth).

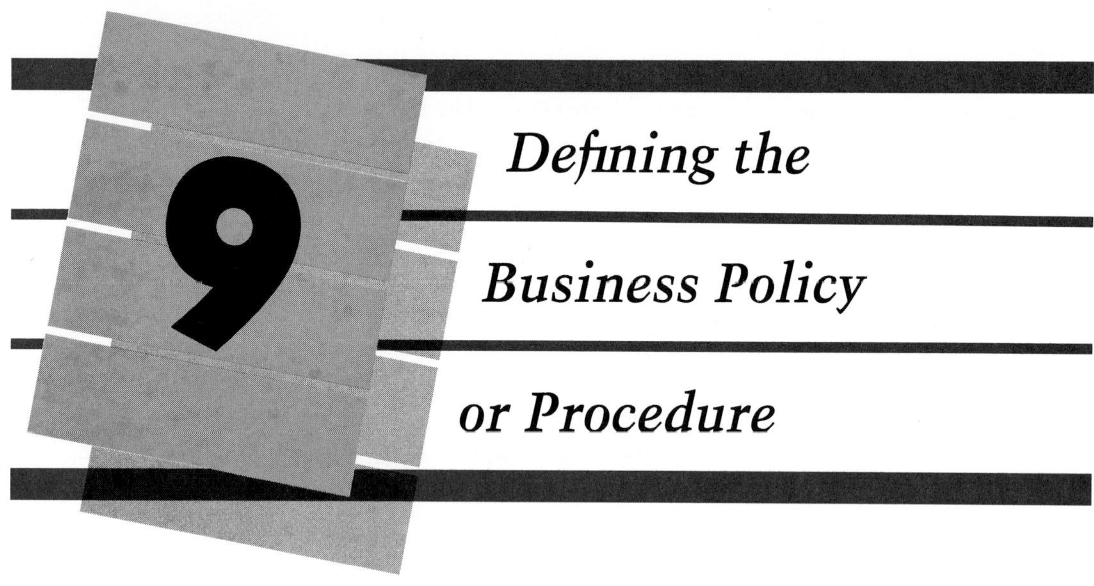

9 Defining the Business Policy or Procedure

Minicase: Winner Take All

The three business partners who owned BUMER Computers, Inc., were in dire financial straits. They didn't have enough money to meet their next payroll. They were $250,000 short and could not get a bank loan because of their poor credit rating. Between them, they could only collect $50,000.

They decided on a drastic and risky solution to their problem. They would go to Las Vegas and try to gamble their $50,000 into enough money to cover their payroll and save the company. There was only one problem. They were lousy gamblers! Within one short hour, they had lost the entire $50,000. As the partners exited the casino, they ran into the president of their fiercest competitor. He had been trying, unsuccessfully, to buy BUMER for several months.

The business trio offered BUMER to their greedy competitor for a ridiculously low price. However, their rival sensed the impending ruin of his archrivals and greedily offered the trio an opportunity to either save their business or lose it with no financial gain. He stated his proposition: "I have five poker chips in my pocket: three white chips and two red. I'm going to blindfold each of you and then give you each a chip. One by one, I'm going to remove your blindfolds. You will be permitted to see the chip in your colleagues' hands, however, you must keep your own chip concealed in your closed palm. If any one of you can tell me the color of your own chip, I will give you $1,000,000 cash, which should be more than enough to ensure the financial future of your business. Each of you has the option of guessing or not guessing. However, if any one of you guesses wrong, you must give me your company, free and clear. Is it a deal?"

The business trio, who had little choice and no other reasonable hope, accepted the challenge. The competitor then showed them the five chips — three white and two red — and chuckled as he placed the blindfolds in place and gave each person one chip. He returned the two unused chips to his pocket.

The blindfold was removed from the eldest businessman first. He looked at his partners' chips but could not determine the color of his own chip. He responded, "I just cannot give an answer. It's too risky."

The blindfold was removed from the second businessman, a graduate from a prestigious business school. After looking at the chips of his two partners, he too was unable to guess the color of his own chip.

The competitor smothered a grin as he started to remove the blindfold from the third partner, a businesswoman. You see, this man refused to believe that any woman could have the savy or intelligence to come up with the right answer. "One last chance," he offered. "I'll buy your company for $5,000,000. Yes, it's worth three times that much. But do you really want to risk losing it for nothing?"

The woman interrupted softly and confidently, "You can leave my blindfold on. How about double or nothing!" The competitor laughed aloud, "It's your funeral!"

The businesswoman replied, "I'll take that $2,000,000! I know from the answers of my colleagues that my chip is ___________." She was correct and the winnings saved BUMER from financial ruin.

Discussion

What color was the businesswoman's chip? Prove your answer! Are you willing to gamble your course grade on that answer?

Assumptions

1. None of the partners cheated.
2. All of the partners were intelligent. Accordingly, if either of the first two partners had seen two red chips, he would have known his own chip was white.

WHAT WILL YOU LEARN IN THIS CHAPTER?

In this chapter, you will learn about tools and techniques for specifying business policies and procedures that govern computerized and manual tasks. You will know that you have mastered policy and procedure specification techniques when you can:

1. Differentiate between a policy and a procedure.
2. Describe some of the typical problems encountered in documenting procedures, and explain the ambiguities of ordinary English as a policy and procedure specification tool.
3. Construct a decision table to describe a policy in terms of conditions and actions to be taken under various combinations of conditions.
4. Use Structured English to write procedure specifications.
5. Explain why decision tables and Structured English documentation are useful in performing systems analysis.

As a new information system evolves, many policies and procedures must be communicated to computer programmers for implementation. Other policies and procedures, although they will be performed manually, must be documented for the knowledge workers. The preparation of clear, accurate, and concise specifications of policy and procedure becomes an important skill to be mastered by the systems analyst.

In this chapter, we will study two tools for specifying business policies and procedures: decision tables and Structured English. These tools provide us with an alternative that avoids the natural ambiguity of the English language. We will examine the best situations for using each tool as well as opportunities for combining the tools to describe a single policy or procedure. Finally, we will learn how the tools can be used in performing systems analysis.

UNDERSTANDING THE BUSINESS POLICY AND PROCEDURE

Processes on DFDs represent tasks performed by the system. These tasks are performed according to business policies and procedures. The policies and procedures of the information system are (or will become) the basis for computer programs and manual procedures, two of our information system components. What are policies and procedures? How can they be specified? Why are policies and procedures difficult to specify?

What Is the Business Policy or Procedure?

A **policy** is a set of rules that govern some task or function in the business. In most firms, policies are the basis for decision making. For instance, most companies have a credit policy for determining whether to accept or reject an order. A credit card company must bill cardholders according to policies that adhere to restrictions placed upon them by state and federal governments (for instance, maximum interest rates, minimum payments). Policies consist of rules, and because of this, they can often be translated into computer programs, *if* the systems analyst can accurately convey those rules to the computer programmer. You may recall that policies were one of the components of the business mission dimension of our pyramid model (see the illustration in the margin).

What are procedures? To the programmer, **procedures** may represent the executable instructions in a computer program. But to the knowledge worker, **procedures** are step-by-step instructions for accomplishing a task or tasks. And in many businesses, well-defined procedures are sorely missed by the knowledge workers.

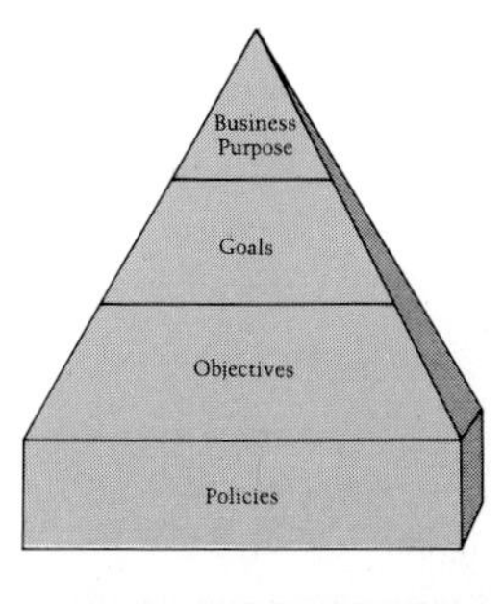

Business Mission

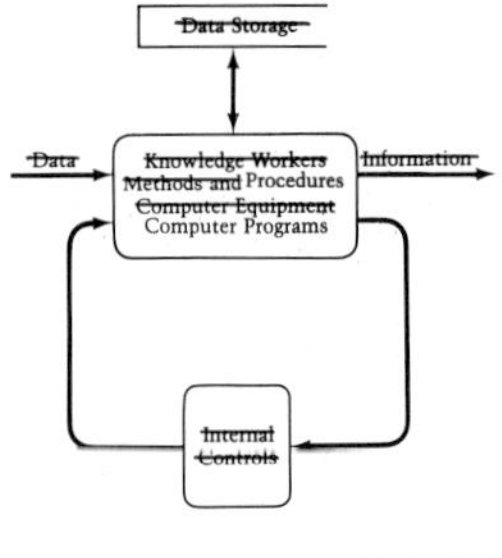

IPO Components

Do not confuse policies and procedures. Recall that policies and procedures are part of the business mission to be supported by the information system (see margin illustration). Policies represent management decisions. Procedures put those policies into action. For instance, most companies have a policy on vacations, leaves, sick days, and the like. Those policies are implemented by procedures that define how to call in sick, request and approve vacations, and so forth. The procedures typically indicate how policies are to be documented. Thus, policies and procedures complement one another.

Most policies are documented, albeit poorly. However, most procedures are *not* documented (unless you consider forms containing instructions to be documentation). And documentation for most procedures is frequently outdated or incomplete. Why? Because procedures are easier to do than they are to describe. Think about it! Take out a scratch paper and write a description of how to ride a bicycle. Not too easy, is it? You probably learned by watching and trying, correct? We are people who do things, not describe things.

Most of you have come from a programming course or background. As computer programmers, your job is to translate business requirements into syntactically correct code. Unfortunately, the language and idiosyncrasies of the business world and the programming world are vastly different. The language of computer programming is extremely precise, much more so than natural English. Many programmers spend more time debugging the business requirements than they do debugging their computer programs! We would like to suggest that the programmer should not have to interpret or clarify business requirements. That is the analyst's job!

Why study, document, or design procedures? You have learned that computer equipment and programs are only a subset of the entire information system—a system that also includes people, methods, and manual procedures. The computer system affects the way manual tasks are performed. Therefore, documenting the manual tasks is just as important as specifying the computerized tasks. But documenting policies and procedures isn't easy.

The Problems with Procedures

When was the last time you received a programming assignment you didn't have to spend class or office time to clarify? In defense of analysts and teachers, the English language has effectively sabotaged the smooth transition from the business policy and procedure to the computer program. Manual procedures are no easier to write. Indeed, you may have experienced frustration in completing your tax return. Why? The manual procedures that describe the process are difficult to communicate. Let's examine some of the problems associated with policy and procedure specification. Hopefully, we can learn from our past mistakes as we prepare to study tools for improving policy and procedure specification.

General Criticisms of Procedures Leslie Matthies is a systems analyst with some unique opinions on the often ignored art of procedure writing. In his book *The New Playscript Procedure* (1977) he described several problems encountered with typical procedures. We'd like to paraphrase a few of those problems that are pertinent to this chapter.

1. Most of us are *too* educated! The average college graduate (which includes most analysts) has a working vocabulary of between ten and twenty thousand words. On the other hand, the average non-college graduate has a working vocabulary of around five thousand words. Many of our procedures violate the first law of good writing—*know your audience*—know what they can read and understand. A procedure has little value if it cannot be interpreted by those who will perform it.
2. A related problem deals with jargon. Too often, we allow the jargon of computing to control our procedures. The computer industry has demonstrated an inclination for inventing terms and acronyms to describe their products and discipline.
3. One of the most frustrating problems with procedures is their variability. They are frequently written with several different tools and styles. Workers find it frustrating to deal with multiple procedure specification tools and formats.
4. Writing a procedure does not necessarily communicate that procedure. Most of us do not write well. And unfortunately, most of us don't question our writing abilities. Although this *is* a problem, even the best writers are handicapped by the ambiguity of the English language.

Problems with Ordinary English Problems arise when the English language is used as a procedure specification tool. Let's examine some of the problems associated with the use of the English language.

1. One problem is determining the scope of the statements in the procedure. How would you carry out the following procedure, described to you by your new employer? "If customers walk in the door and they do not want to withdraw money from their account or deposit money to their account or make a loan payment, send them to the trust department." Does this mean that the only time you should not send the customer to the trust department is when they wish to do all three of the transactions? Or does it mean that if a customer does not wish to withdraw money from an account, and does not wish to deposit money to the account, and does not wish make a loan payment (that is, the customer does not wish to do *any* of these things), that customer should be sent to the trust department? The scope of each statement in a procedure should be clear.

2. Compound sentences (two complete sentences connected by *and, but,* or some other similar word such as *yet*) are another serious problem. Consider the following example — a procedure describing how to replace an electrical outlet. "Remove the screws that hold the outlet cover to the wall. Remove the outlet cover. Disconnect each wire from the plug, but first make sure the power to the outlet has been turned off." Did you catch the compound sentence structure in the last instruction? An unwary person might try to disconnect the wires prior to turning off the power. We use compound sentences to make our writing more interesting. But procedures are not supposed to entertain users!

3. Another problem is the multiple definitions associated with many words. An example of this problem was seen in the Americana Plastics case that began Chapter 8 — part number did not mean the same thing to each of the users!

4. Another problem with the English language is the use of undefined adjectives. Each semester, we receive several "Good Student Driver" discount forms from our students. These forms are quite amusing. What is a student in *good* standing? The descriptions provided vary significantly and are often difficult to interpret. What does "upper 10 percent of his/her class" mean? Ten percent of what? The entire university's class? The class of students classified as Computer Information Systems majors? And *good* is an example of an undefined adjective that frequently leaves room for considerable interpretation!

5. Another problem with English is use of conditional instructions. **Conditional instructions** occur when specific conditions determine whether certain steps are performed. The statement of the conditions can be part of the problem. Many conditions involve ranges of values, and we tend to be careless with such ranges. If we state that "all applicants under the age of nineteen must secure parental permission," do we mean less than nineteen or less than or equal to nineteen years of age? Although programmers are familiar with this problem, users and analysts frequently forget to carefully specify value ranges.

   This problem is further complicated by multiple combinations of conditions. For example, credit approval may be a function of several conditions: credit rating, credit ceiling, annual dollar sales for that customer, and payment history. Different combinations of these factors result in different decisions (such as accept order on credit, reject order on credit and require full prepayment, reject order until down payment is received). As the number of conditions and possible combinations increase, the procedure becomes more and more tedious and difficult to write.

There is a current trend toward the use of nonprocedural languages. This technology is presumably progressing to a point where we will be able to program in natural English. But if natural English is so vague, you could argue that the computer may misinterpret our instructions in much the same manner as we humans do! For another viewpoint, see the "Next Generation" feature in this chapter.

Fortunately, there are ways to formalize the specification of policies and procedures. These techniques may not be perfect, but they do address the problems we've stated.

When Do You Define Policies and Procedures?

During the definition phase of systems analysis, it is essential that all policies and procedure requirements be documented. Each process for the new system should be documented in detail as a policy and/or procedure. You should define the detailed processing requirements for the new system without premature concern about which processes will be computerized and which will be performed manually.

The Next Generation — *Will Policy and Procedural Specification Become Obsolete?*

Much time and effort has gone into the study of systems analysis tools and techniques for defining the policy and procedure requirements for an information system. The benefits of these studies include a number of effective tools for describing and verifying policy and procedure requirements. But tools alone won't do the job. The policy and procedure specifications still must be clearly communicated between users, analysts, and programmers. This communication process is difficult— even with such tools as decision tables and Structured English. Obviously, it would be much nicer if this line of communication were not necessary. In other words, what if the systems analyst didn't have to define the policies or procedures at all? Perhaps that day isn't too far off!

Think about the technology that's here today. We are starting to see a number of software packages that are more user-friendly. These software packages, called *natural language query processors,* include the capability to allow users to define and log the data elements to be stored (an automated version of a data dictionary). In addition, report-generation or query facilities for accessing the stored data are made available to the users through the database. The dialogue for these facilities is very close to actual English. For example, when performing an inquiry, a user may have entered the command WHAT CUSTOMER ACCOUNTS HAVE A BALANCE MORE THAN 300? Obviously, the user wishes to see all those customer accounts that have a current balance over $300. The command is very similar to the way we might request the information from another individual.

The ability for the user to make requests in unrestricted English, is dependent on the intelligence of the software. Most software requires the user to enter explicit commands that can be interpreted precisely. For example, the verb must be one of the verbs reserved for use by the software, object names such as CUSTOMER ACCOUNTS must have been memorized or be known by the user, and adjectives must have been defined in the software. This is the nature of languages such as COBOL, FORTRAN, BASIC, and PASCAL. Although this does place some constraints on the formulation of the user's command, many software packages allow the user more flexibility and less formality. For example, it would be nice if the user could have substituted the word RECORDS for the word ACCOUNTS without jeopardizing the query.

Indeed, there are some very powerful natural-language query processors available today, and user inquiries that cannot be directly interpreted by the software are commonly handled as in the following query dialogue:

User	WHERE CAN WE GET 3/4 INCH LUG NUTS?
Terminal	I'M NOT FAMILIAR WITH THE ▶

During the design phase, the systems analyst will need to communicate those policy and procedure specifications that are to be implemented as computer programs by the programmer. There-

The Next Generation (continued)

	TERM 3/4 INCH LUG NUTS. HOW MANY TERMS IS IT?
User	TWO
Terminal	ENTER THE TWO TERMS SEPARATED BY A COMMA.
User	3/4 INCH, LUG NUTS
Terminal	IS 3/4 INCH STORED IN THE DATABASE?
User	YES
Terminal	WHAT FIELD IS 3/4 INCH STORED IN?
User	SIZE
Terminal	THE FIELD SIZE IS STORED IN 2 PLACES IN THE DATABASE. ARE YOU REFERRING TO "PRODUCT" SIZE OR "VENDOR PART" SIZE?
User	VENDOR PART
Terminal	IS LUG NUTS STORED IN THE DATABASE?
User	YES
Terminal	WHAT FIELD IS LUG NUTS STORED IN?
User	PART DESCRIPTION
Terminal	THE FIELD PART DESCRIPTION IS STORED IN 2 PLACES IN THE DATABASE. ARE YOU REFERRING TO "PART" PART DESCRIPTION OR "VENDOR PART" PART DESCRIPTION?
User	VENDOR PART
Terminal	ARE YOU REQUESTING THOSE VENDORS FOR WHICH SIZE = 3/4 INCH AND PART DESCRIPTION = LUG NUTS?
User	YES
Terminal	WHAT FIELDS DO YOU WISH TO SEE FOR VENDOR?
User	NAME, ADDRESS, PART NUMBER, PRICE, DISCOUNT TERMS . . .

Scary, isn't it?! So, what impact does this have on specification of policies and procedures? Policies and procedures can become very complex and make it difficult for the user to communicate clearly. Wouldn't it be nice if the user could bypass the systems analyst and describe the policies and procedures to the computer, which could then implement the policies and procedures as a program? Clearly the ability to do so would require software that is more intelligent than that just described. The user would have to have the ability to enter a series of commands or instructions in a manner that is even more English-like in interpretation. The software — instead of the analyst! — would address the ambiguity problems of the English language. Are we dreaming? We suggest you research a Cullinet product called *ON-LINE ENGLISH.* ■

fore, the specifications should be modified to include additional technical details that describe physical implementation characteristics (such as hashing algorithms and sort functions).

DECISION TABLES AS A POLICY SPECIFICATION TOOL

Decision tables, unfortunately, don't get enough respect! People who are unfamiliar with the tool tend to avoid them. But decision tables are very useful for specifying complex business policies and decision-making rules. Figure 9.1 illustrates the components of a standard decision table. The decision table is divided into three sections:

1. **Condition stubs** describe the conditions or factors that will affect the decision or policy.
2. **Action stubs** describe, in the form of statements, the possible policy actions or decisions.
3. **Rules** describe which actions are to be taken under a specific combination of conditions. A rule consists of values for each condition stub plus actions to be taken, given that set of condition values.

Figure 9.1(a) represents a description of the check-cashing policy that appears on the back of a check-cashing identification card for a grocery store. In Figure 9.1(b), this same policy has been defined with a decision table. Three factors or conditions affecting the check-cashing decision include the type of check (1 = Personal, 2 = Payroll), whether the amount of the check exceeds the maximum limit (Y = Yes, N = No), and whether the company is accredited by the store (Y = Yes, N = No). The actions or decisions are either to cash the check or to refuse to cash the check. Notice that each combination of conditions defines a rule that results in the proper action, denoted by an X. Finally, notice that rules 1, 3, and 5 contain a "–" entry for certain conditions. This means that the condition is irrelevant for these rules.

Decision tables offer a number of advantages over ordinary English. They use a standard format and handle combinations of conditions in a very concise manner. The English equivalent for a decision table would be much more difficult to read and write because each combination of conditions would have to be described. Decision tables also provide techniques for identifying policy incompleteness and contradictions. In other words, if a rule (combination of conditions) has no actions, it is a potential hole in the policy. Let's

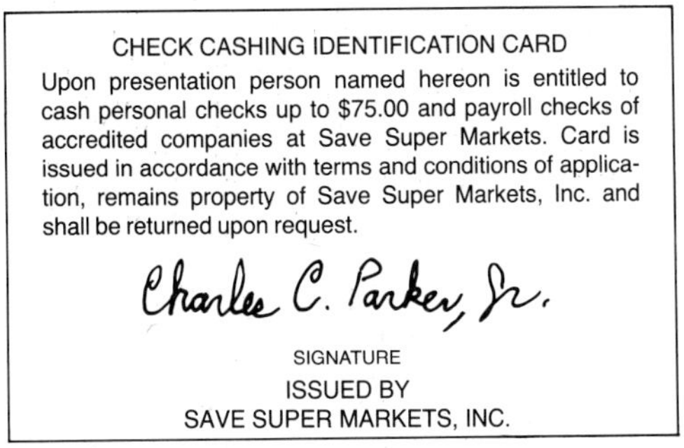

CHECK CASHING IDENTIFICATION CARD

Upon presentation person named hereon is entitled to cash personal checks up to $75.00 and payroll checks of accredited companies at Save Super Markets. Card is issued in accordance with terms and conditions of application, remains property of Save Super Markets, Inc. and shall be returned upon request.

Charles C. Parker, Jr.

SIGNATURE

ISSUED BY
SAVE SUPER MARKETS, INC.

(a)

	Check Cashing Policy	Rules 1	2	3	4	5
Conditions	Type of Check	1	2	1	2	2
	Check Amount Less Than or Equal to $75	Y	Y	N	N	–
	Company Accredited by Store	–	Y	–	Y	N
Actions	Cash Check	X	X			
	Refuse Check			X	X	X

(b)

Figure 9.1

A decision table for specifying a store's check-cashing policy. Decision tables offer a number of advantages over ordinary English. Although the narrative equivalent of the decision table in 9.1(a) is also short and concise, the decision table clearly assures that the policy described on the check-cashing identification card in 9.1(b) is complete and without contradictions.

learn how to construct decision tables. But first, let's end the suspense! What color chip did the businesswoman have?

Solving the Poker Chip Problem in our Minicase

Figure 9.2 sets up a decision table for solving our poker chip problem. All possible combinations of poker chips are recorded as rules. The actions represent possible outcomes of the problem. Note that the first rule results in the action "Impossible" because we know that there were only two red chips. We can also eliminate rules 3 and 5 because, if either businessman had seen two red chips, he would have known his own chip was white. That didn't happen. We cannot eliminate rule 2 because the businesswoman requested that her blindfold not be removed.

Examine the remaining rules for the third condition stub carefully. Do you see that only one of the remaining rules (rule 7) results in the businesswoman having a red chip? She solved the problem by concluding from her colleagues responses that she didn't have a red

Process Name		Rules 1	2	3	4	5	6	7	8
Conditions	Businessman 1	R	R	R	R	W	W	W	W
	Businessman 2	R	R	W	W	R	R	W	W
	Businesswoman	R	W	R	W	R	W	R	W
Actions	Impossible—Only Two Red Chips	X							
	Businessman 1 Would Have Guessed					X			
	Businessman 2 Would Have Guessed								

Figure 9.2

A decision table for solving the poker chip problem.

chip. Before you read the next paragraph, try to eliminate rule 7 on your own.

Here's how to eliminate rule 7. If rule 7 had been true, person 2 would have known that his chip was white, and the business would have been saved *before* the businesswoman was asked to guess. Why? Because person 1 couldn't answer, person 2 knew that person 1 did not see two red chips. Person 1 had to see either two white chips or a red chip and a white chip. Now, remove the blindfold from person 2 *and* assume that rule 7 is true. If rule 7 is true, then person 2 is looking at a red chip in person 3's hand. Therefore, his own chip could not possibly be red because, if person 1 had seen a red chip in both other people's hands, he would have known that his was white. Thus, we can eliminate rule 7 because person 2, as an intelligent person, would have known his chip was white.

Looking at the completed decision table in Figure 9.3, we see that all the remaining rules result in the businesswoman's chip being white. Therefore, she didn't need to see her colleagues' chips. She didn't need to pinpoint which rule represented the actual combination. All she was required to do was recognize that her chip was

	Process Name	1	2	3	4	5	6	7	8
Conditions	Businessman 1	R	R	R	R	W	W	W	W
	Businessman 2	R	R	W	W	R	R	W	W
	Businesswoman	R	(W)	R	(W)	R	(W)	R	(W)
Actions	Impossible—Only Two Red Chips	X							
	Businessman 1 Would Have Guessed					X			
	Businessman 2 Would Have Guessed			X					
	Businesswoman Knows Her Chip Is White		↑		↑		↑		↑

Figure 9.3

The final solution to the poker chip problem.

white — and all rules resulting in a red chip had been eliminated by her colleagues' answers!

Building a Decision Table

Let's begin with a policy statement. A local credit union offers two types of savings accounts, regular rate and split rate. The regular rate account pays dividends on the amount on deposit at the end of each quarter. Funds withdrawn during the quarter have no earnings. There is no minimum balance on the regular rate account. Regular rate accounts may be insured. Insured accounts pay 5.75 percent annual interest. Uninsured regular rate accounts pay 6.00 percent annual interest. There is no insurance on split rate accounts. For split rate accounts, dividends are paid monthly on the average daily balance even if funds were deposited and withdrawn during the month. No dividends are paid for any month during which the closing balance drops below $25. The average daily balance is determined by adding each day's closing balance for the month and dividing this sum by the number of days in the month. If the average daily balance is less than $25, then no dividend is paid. Otherwise, if the average daily balance is $25 or more, 6 percent per annum is paid on the first $500, 6.5 percent on the next $1,500, and 7 percent on funds over $2,000.

We will demonstrate the construction of a decision table using this credit union example. Recall the simple decision table presented in Figure 9.1. That table is called a **limited-entry decision table** because its condition stubs can only assume one of two values. Many conditions have more than two possible states. For instance, if MARITAL STATUS were a condition, the possible condition values include *never married, married, separated, divorced,* and *widowed.* **Extended-entry decision tables** permit condition stubs that can assume any number of values. The rules for constructing limited- and extended-entry decision tables are identical. Let's look at the procedure.

Step 1: Identify the Conditions and Values Identify the data element each condition tests and all of the values that these data elements can assume. For our example:

Data Elements or Conditions	*Values (or ranges)*
Account Type	R = Regular S = Split Rate
Insurance?	Y = Yes N = No
Balance Dropped Below $25 During Month	Y = Yes N = No
Average Daily Balance	1 = 0.00 – 24.99 2 = 25.00 – 500.00 3 = 500.01 – 2,000.00 4 = more than 2,000.00

Notice that we have yes and no conditions as well as multivalue conditions.

Step 2: Determine the Maximum Number of Rules The maximum number of rules in a decision table is calculated by multiplying the number of values for each condition data element by each other. For example:

Condition 1 offers two values	2
Condition 2 offers two values	x 2
Condition 3 offers two values	x 2
Condition 4 offers four values	x 4
Number of rules in decision table (calculated as $2 \times 2 = 4 \times 2 = 8 \times 4 = 32$)	32

Step 3: Identify the Possible Actions Identify each independent action to be taken for the decision or policy. For our example:

Pay no dividend

5.750% ÷ 4 quarterly dividend on entire balance

6.000% ÷ 4 quarterly dividend on entire balance

6.000% ÷ 12 monthly dividend on balance up to $500

6.500% ÷ 12 monthly dividend on balance between $500.01 and $2,000

7.000% ÷ 12 monthly dividend on balance over $2,000.01

Step 4: Enter All Possible Rules Record the conditions and actions in their respective places in the decision table (see Figure 9.4). All possible rules can easily be identified by completing the following steps:

ⓐ For the first condition, alternate its possible values.

ⓑ Note the size of the pattern that repeats in step ⓐ (in our example, two values). Cover each pattern of two values in the previous condition with the values of the second condition, repeating as necessary until the row is filled.

ⓒ Again, note the size of the pattern that repeats in the second condition (this time, four values). Cover each pattern of four values with the values of the next condition, repeating as necessary until the row is filled.

ⓓ Once again, note the size of the pattern that repeats in the third condition (this time, eight values). Cover each pattern of eight

	Process Name: Dividend Rate	Rules																															
		1	2	3	4	5	6	7	8	9	10	11	12	13	14	15	16	17	18	19	20	21	22	23	24	25	26	27	28	29	30	31	32	
Conditions	Account Type	R	S	R	S	R	S	R	S	R	S	R	S	R	S	R	S	R	S	R	S	R	S	R	S	R	S	R	S	R	S	R	S	(a)
	Insurance	Y	Y	N	N	Y	Y	N	N	Y	Y	N	N	Y	Y	N	N	Y	Y	N	N	Y	Y	N	N	Y	Y	N	N	Y	Y	N	N	(b)
	Balance Dropped Below $25 During Month	Y	Y	Y	Y	N	N	N	N	Y	Y	Y	Y	N	N	N	N	Y	Y	Y	Y	N	N	N	N	Y	Y	Y	Y	N	N	N	N	(c)
	Average Daily Balance	1	1	1	1	1	1	1	1	2	2	2	2	2	2	2	2	3	3	3	3	3	3	3	3	4	4	4	4	4	4	4	4	(d)
Actions	Pay No Dividend																																	
	5.750% ÷ 4 Quarterly Div. on Entire Balance																																	
	6.000% ÷ 4 Quarterly Div. on Entire Balance																																	
	6.000% ÷ 12 Monthly Div. on Balance up to $500																																	
	6.500% ÷ 12 Monthly Div. on Balance Between $500.01 and $2000																																	
	7.000% ÷ 12 Monthly Div. on Balance over $2000																																	

Figure 9.4

Entering all possible rules into a decision table. This decision table identifies all possible rules for which actions will have to be identified. Note that all of the rules could also have been identified by applying step (a) to the fourth condition, step (b) to the third condition, step (c) to the second condition, and step (d) to the first condition.

values with the values of the next condition, repeating as necessary until the row is filled.

This simple process defines all possible combinations of conditions for any decision table. We could have continued the process for any number of conditions.

Step 5: Define the Actions for Each Rule Determine which action or actions are appropriate for each rule and mark them with an X. In the event that certain rules are impossible (cannot happen), then add an action stub labeled *Impossible* and mark the rules with an X. A question mark is used when the action for a rule is unknown. It reminds you to check with your users to learn how this rule should be handled. Figure 9.5 illustrates the actions for our rules.

Step 6: Verify the Policy Decision tables have been unfairly criticized as poor communication tools. They are really quite easy to read after you explain them to your user. Your completed decision table should be reviewed with your users. Resolve any rules for which the actions have not been specified. Verify that rules specified as *impossible* cannot occur. Resolve apparent contradictions (such as one rule with two possible interest rates covering a single balance). Finally, verify that each rule's actions are correct.

Step 7: Simplify the Decision Table At this point, our decision table is both complete and correct. Still, thirty-two rules can be a bit overwhelming. We can simplify the decision table by eliminating and consolidating certain rules. The technique is described as follows:

a. Eliminate impossible rules.
b. Look for indifferent conditions. An **indifferent condition** is a condition whose values do not affect the decision and always result in the same action. These rules can be consolidated into a single rule. The technique is described as follows:
   1. Find a *set* (pair, trio, etc.) of rules for which:
      - The actions are *identical.*
      - The condition values are the same except for *one and only one* condition or factor.
      - *All* possible values of an entry for a given condition must become indifferent before the rules can be collapsed. (This is important, especially in extended entry tables.)

	Process Name: Dividend Rate	Rules 1	2	3	4	5	6	7	8	9	10	11	12	13	14	15	16	17	18	19	20	21	22	23	24	25	26	27	28	29	30	31	32
Conditions	Account Type	R	S	R	S	R	S	R	S	R	S	R	S	R	S	R	S	R	S	R	S	R	S	R	S	R	S	R	S	R	S	R	S
	Insurance	Y	Y	N	N	Y	Y	N	N	Y	Y	N	N	Y	Y	N	N	Y	Y	N	N	Y	Y	N	N	Y	Y	N	N	Y	Y	N	N
	Balance Dropped Below $25 During Month	Y	Y	Y	Y	N	N	N	N	Y	Y	Y	Y	N	N	N	N	Y	Y	Y	Y	N	N	N	N	Y	Y	Y	Y	N	N	N	N
	Average Daily Balance	1	1	1	1	1	1	1	1	2	2	2	2	2	2	2	2	3	3	3	3	3	3	3	3	4	4	4	4	4	4	4	4
Actions	Pay No Dividend				X				X				X								X								X				
	5.750% ÷ 4 Quarterly Div. on Entire Balance	X				X				X				X				X				X				X				X			
	6.000% ÷ 4 Quarterly Div. on Entire Balance			X				X				X				X				X				X				X				X	
	6.000% ÷ 12 Monthly Div. on Balance up to $500																X								X								X
	6.500% ÷ 12 Monthly Div. on Balance Between $500.01 and $2000																								X								X
	7.000% ÷ 12 Monthly Div. on Balance over $2000																																X
	Impossible (No Insurance for Split Rate)		?				?				?				?				?				?				?				?		

Figure 9.5

Defining the actions for each rule in a decision table. This decision table resulted in the identification of some rules that were determined to be impossible (the combination of condition values could not happen). Therefore an appropriate entry was added to the action portion of the decision table and an "X" was entered for those rules.

2. Consolidate that set of rules into a single rule, replacing the value of the indifferent condition with a minus sign, also called the *indifference symbol.*

This technique should be repeated as often as sets of rules satisfy the criteria in step b. *But be careful! You cannot consolidate rules based on conditions that have already been identified as indifferent!* In other words, a set of rules cannot be said to have identical condition values just because one condition is indifferent for each rule in the set.

Before we simplify our dividend table, let's look at an easier example. In Figure 9.6(a) notice that rules 1, 5, and 9 result in the same action. Also note that all condition values for the three rules are the same except for the third condition. Also note that the three rules cover all possible values for the third condition. Do you see that the third condition's value does not affect the action? That condition is indifferent. We can consolidate the three rules into a single rule as in Figure 9.6(b). We recorded the original rule numbers above the consolidated rules for your clarification. Also note that we consolidated rules 11 and 12 based on indifference for the first condition stub. You may have been tempted to consolidate rules 3 and 7. But notice that the third condition hasn't been satisfied: only two (L and M) of the three values (L, M, and H) of the alleged indifferent condition are covered! Therefore, that condition is not indifferent.

Returning to our dividend example, Figure 9.7 demonstrates the simplified decision table for the credit union's dividend policy. Note that *both* conditions three and four are indifferent to regular accounts.

STRUCTURED ENGLISH AS A PROCEDURE SPECIFICATION TOOL

Whereas decision tables are particularly effective for describing policies, Structured English is a tool for describing procedures. The tool is called *Structured English,* primarily because it is based on the principles of structured programming.

Figure 9.8 illustrates a procedure for which Structured English has been used. This procedure may be a process on a DFD. You may have already noticed some similarity between Structured English

		1	2	3	4	5	6	7	8	9	10	11	12
Conditions	Condition 1	Y	N	Y	N	Y	N	Y	N	Y	N	Y	N
	Condition 2	Y	Y	N	N	Y	Y	N	N	Y	Y	N	N
	Condition 3	L	L	L	L	M	M	M	M	H	H	H	H
Actions	Action 1	X				X				X			
	Action 2		X						X		X	X	X
	Action 3				X		X						
	Action 4			X				X					

(a)

		1, 5, 9	2	3	4	6	7	8	10	11, 12			
Conditions	Condition 1	Y	N	Y	N	N	Y	N	N	–			
	Condition 2	Y	Y	N	N	Y	N	N	Y	N			
	Condition 3	–	L	L	L	M	M	M	M	H			
Actions	Action 1	X											
	Action 2		X					X	X	X			
	Action 3				X	X							
	Action 4			X			X						

(b)

Figure 9.6

Simplifying a decision table. Most decision tables can be reduced in size and complexity. Simplified decision tables are much less intimidating to users and therefore more easily verified. 9.6(b) is a simplified version of 9.6(a).

and computer program pseudocode. **Pseudocode** is a tool to define detailed program algorithms or logic prior to coding. But pseudocode often tends to take on a programming accent that makes it unsuitable for nonprogrammers. For instance, array and variable

Process Name		Dividend Rate	Rules						
			1	2	3	4	5	6	7
Conditions	Account Type		R	R	S	S	S	S	S
	Insurance		Y	N	-	-	N	N	N
	Balance Dropped Below $25 During Month		-	-	Y	N	N	N	N
	Average Daily Balance		-	-	-	1	2	3	4
Actions	Pay No Dividend				X	X			
	5.750% ÷ 4 Quarterly Div. on Entire Balance		X						
	6.000% ÷ 4 Quarterly Div. on Entire Balance			X					
	6.000% ÷ 12 Monthly Div. on Balance up to $500						X	X	X
	6.500% ÷ 12 Monthly Div. on Balance Between $500.01 and $2000							X	X
	7.000% ÷ 12 Monthly Div. on Balance over $2000								X

Account Type: R = Regular
S = Split Rate

Insurance: Y = Yes
N = No

Balance Dropped Below
$25 During Months: Y = Yes
N = No

Average Daily Balance: 1 = Daily balance of 0.00–24.99
2 = Daily balance of 25.00–500.00
3 = Daily balance of 500.01–2000.00
4 = Daily balance more than 2,000.00

Figure 9.7

Simplified decision table for the credit union's dividend policy.

initialization, opening and closing files, and read/write operations are often included in pseudocode. Also, most programmers tend to accent their pseudocode with the syntax of a computer programming language (for example, BASIC, COBOL, FORTRAN), usually the first such language they learned. Otherwise, the two tools are essentially equivalent.

Structured English borrows the logical constructs of structured pseudocode but restricts the use of nouns, verbs, adjectives, ad-

For each LOAN ACCOUNT NUMBER in the LOAN ACCOUNT FILE do the following steps:

 If the AMOUNT PAST DUE is greater than $0.00 then:

  While there are LOAN ACCOUNT NUMBERs for the CUSTOMER NAME do the following steps:

   Sum the OUTSTANDING LOAN BALANCEs.

   Sum the MINIMUM PAYMENTs.

   Sum the PAST DUE AMOUNTs.

 Report the CUSTOMER NAME, LOAN ACCOUNTs on OVERDUE CUSTOMER LOAN ANALYSIS.

Figure 9.8

A sample Structured English description of a business policy.

verbs, and computer jargon to make the specification easier to read for knowledge workers. Let's learn how to prepare Structured English.

Structured English Syntax

Structured English is the marriage of the English language with the syntax of structured programming. The term *structured* is appropriate because the following restrictions are placed on the use of English:

1. Only strong, imperative verbs may be used.
2. Only nouns and terms defined in the data dictionary may be used. Note the integrated use of the data dictionary with Structured English.
3. Compound sentences should be avoided. We discussed the problems inherent in compound sentences earlier in this chapter.
4. Undefined adjectives and adverbs (*good,* for instance) are not permitted unless defined in the data dictionary.
5. Footnotes are discouraged because they interrupt the flow of the procedure.
6. A limited set of logic or flow constructs must be used. These

constructs are familiar to those who practice structured programming. The three valid constructs are:

(a) A sequence of single declarative statements
(b) The selection of one or more declarative statements based on a decision (the IF-THEN-ELSE or decision construct)
(c) The repetition of one or more declarative statements (the looping construct)

The best way to learn Structured English is to study some examples. We won't have to explain the policies involved because, if that were required, the value of Structured English would be highly questionable.

Sequential Instructions Sequential instructions are simple, declarative statements that follow one another. These instructions do not include branching or looping. Each declarative statement should begin with a strong action verb that describes exactly what should be done in that step of the procedure. Avoid vague, meaningless verbs, such as *process, handle,* and *perform.* Also avoid computer programming language verbs such as *move* or *open ____ file.*

Many declarative statements are arithmetic. They specify how to calculate data elements such as GROSS PAY, FEDERAL TAX WITHHELD, and NET PAY. We suggest the following format:

Calculate < insert data element > using the formula:
< insert formula >

All of the formula data elements should be defined in the data dictionary. Many business calculations involve summation and running totals. In this situation, we suggest you simplify the calculation as follows:

Sum < data element > giving < data element >

You will likely develop your own Structured English style. We try to write simple but complete sentences. To as great an extent as possible, we want to eliminate the rigid style of computer programming while maintaining the syntax. The procedure specification should focus on how the incoming data flows for a DFD process are transformed into the outgoing data flows on the DFD process. The following statements are valid sequential instructions:

Find the MEMBER ACCOUNT using the MEMBER ACCOUNT NUMBER.

Compute the new ACCOUNT BALANCE using formula:
ACCOUNT BALANCE = ACCOUNT BALANCE +
ADJUSTMENT AMOUNT.

Record the new ACCOUNT BALANCE in the MEMBER ACCOUNT file.

Write the new ACCOUNT BALANCE on the CUSTOMER STATEMENT.

Notice that each sentence ends with a period and can be more than one line long. Also notice that we have capitalized the names of data flows, data stores, and data elements. This is our technique for indicating that these nouns are recorded in the data dictionary.

The Decision Construct The decision construct of Structured English allows you to place branching instructions into the procedure specification. The following formats for the decision construct are permitted:

- If < insert condition > then:
  < insert instruction(s) >
  Otherwise: (not condition)
  < insert instruction(s) >.
- If < insert condition > then:
  < insert instruction(s) >.
- Select the appropriate case:
  Case 1: < insert condition value 1 >
  < insert instruction(s) >
  Case 2: < insert condition value 2 >
  < insert instruction(s) >
  .
  .
  .
  Case n: < insert condition value n >
  < insert instruction(s) >

Use the first format for conditions that can only assume two values (for example, *yes* and *no, male* and *female*). Use the second format whenever the condition can assume more than two values (for example, *freshman, sophomore, junior,* and *senior*). The instructions within the decision construct include one or more statements.

Figure 9.9 demonstrates the **If-then-Otherwise construct.** Note that the construct is **nested,** that is, one *If-then-Otherwise* construct lies within another. To enhance readability, we line up the *If* with its

Find the MEMBER ACCOUNT using MEMBER ACCOUNT NUMBER.

If the MEMBER ACCOUNT STATUS is not FROZEN then:

> If the TRANSFER AMOUNT is less than or equal to the ACCOUNT BALANCE then:
>
> > Record the TRANSFER TRANSACTION on the FUNDS TRANSFER.
> >
> > Calculate new ACCOUNT BALANCE for debit MEMBER ACCOUNT TYPE using the formula:
> >
> > > ACCOUNT BALANCE = ACCOUNT BALANCE + TRANSFER AMOUNT
> >
> > Calculate the new ACCOUNT BALANCE for the credit MEMBER ACCOUNT TYPE using the formula:
> >
> > > ACCOUNT BALANCE = ACCOUNT BALANCE − TRANSFER AMOUNT
> >
> > Record the new ACCOUNT BALANCES and the TRANSFER TRANSACTION in the MEMBER ACCOUNT file.
> >
> > Record the TELLER TRANSFER TRANSACTION in the TELLER AUDIT file.
>
> Otherwise (if TRANSFER AMOUNT is greater than the ACCOUNT BALANCE)
>
> > Record ACCOUNT BALANCE on the TRANSFER TRANSACTION.
> >
> > Reject the TRANSFER TRANSACTION.

Otherwise (if MEMBER ACCOUNT STATUS is FROZEN) then:

> Reject the TRANSFER TRANSACTION.

Figure 9.9

The If-then-Otherwise decision construct of Structured English.

associated *Otherwise.* Also notice how we *indent* and *block* the instructions to be performed as a result of the *If-then* and the *Otherwise.* All of this improves readability for the knowledge worker and nonprogrammer. We also recorded the negative of the condition in parentheses with the *Otherwise* statements, again to enhance readability. And notice that we have tried to avoid the use of arithmetic signs (such as, =, <, >) except in calculations.

Figure 9.10 demonstrates the *Case* format. The *Case* format is initiated by the declarative statement *Select the appropriate case.* The instructions for each case are *indented* and *blocked* for read-

Find the MATERIAL NUMBER in the INVENTORY FILE.

Select the appropriate case:

    Case 1: MATERIAL CLASS = 'stock,' then:

        If the QUANTITY ON HAND is greater than or equal to the QUANTITY REQUISITIONED then:

            Calculate new QUANTITY ON HAND using the formula:

                QUANTITY ON HAND − QUANTITY REQUISITIONED.

            Record QUANTITY ON HAND in the INVENTORY FILE.

            Issue a STORES TICKET.

        Otherwise (QUANTITY ON HAND is not greater than the QUANTITY REQUISITIONED) then:

            Issue a STORES STOCKOUT TICKET.

    Case 2: MATERIAL CLASS = 'seasonal,' then:

        Calculate QUANTITY NEEDED using the formula:

            REQUISITION QUANTITY × SEASONAL ADJUST RATE.

        Issue a PURCHASE REQUISITION.

    Case 3: MATERIAL CLASS = 'requisition,' then:

        Issue a PURCHASE REQUISITION.

Figure 9.10

The case decision construct of Structured English.

ability. The condition value that causes the instructions to be executed is written beside the *Case:* statement. We also included the use of an *If-then-Otherwise* construct within the *case* statement.

The Repetition or Looping Construct The repetition or looping construct allows us to specify that a sequence of instructions is to be repeated until some condition or desired result is satisfied. The following formats are permitted:

- Do the following < insert some number > times:
    < insert instruction(s) >.
- Repeat the following steps:
    < insert instruction(s) >
  Until < insert condition > is satisfied.

- While < insert condition >, do the following steps:
  < insert instruction(s) >.
- For < insert condition >, do the following steps:
  < insert instruction(s) >.

The first format allows you to specify that certain steps be performed a specific number of times. Do you see the difference between the second and third formats? The second format requires that the instructions be executed at least one time. The third format specifies that the instructions might not be executed at all (if the condition is not initially satisfied).

Repetition constructs are frequently the first statement in a procedure specification because they *drive* the specification. For instance, a procedure that generates a monthly account statement for each customer might begin as follows:

> For each CUSTOMER ACCOUNT NUMBER in the CUSTOMER FILE, do the following steps:
> < appropriate instructions >.

Figure 9.11 demonstrates the repetition construct for the procedure that produces a consolidated bank statement for each customer. The first repetition construct, *For each* . . . , drives the entire procedure. Because a customer can have numerous accounts but must have at least one account, we use the *Repeat-Until* construct for an inner loop of the procedure. Also notice that the block of statements for the loop can include decision constructs.

Guidelines for Writing Structured English Procedures

Structured English looks more formal and difficult than it is. However, you will have to practice the tool to become comfortable with it. We offer the following guidelines and suggestions for writing procedure descriptions using Structured English:

1. Name each procedure to match the DFD process names.
2. Write one procedure specification (also called a **mini spec**) for each primitive process on your data flow diagram.
3. Limit the length of any one procedure to a single eight-and-a-half- by eleven-inch sheet of paper.
4. Do not use *go to, perform,* or *do* statements. They destroy the natural flow of the procedure and give it a programming flavor.

For each CUSTOMER NUMBER in the CUSTOMER ACCOUNT file, do the following:

    Repeat the following steps for each ACCOUNT NUMBER:

        For each ACCOUNT TRANSACTION for the ACCOUNT NUMBER, do the following:

            Report each ACCOUNT TRANSACTION.

            Sum the following account totals:

                NUMBER OF DEBIT TRANSACTIONS

                NUMBER OF CREDIT TRANSACTIONS

                TOTAL OF DEBIT TRANSACTIONS

                TOTAL OF CREDIT TRANSACTIONS

                ACCOUNT EXPENSES

        Report the account totals for the ACCOUNT NUMBER.

    Until there are no more ACCOUNT NUMBERs for the CUSTOMER NUMBER.

Figure 9.11

The repetition construct of Structured English.

Decision Table or Structured English?

This is the first chapter in which we've offered two tools for specifying one DFD component, the process. We need to address the question of when to use each tool. Some experts believe you should choose one tool and use it exclusively. We disagree! The situation should *always* dictate the choice of tool.

Decision tables should be used whenever different combinations of two or more conditions determine different actions. This is particularly common in policy statements. Structured English is preferred whenever the procedure involves looping or limited numbers of decision constructs. It should not surprise you that decision tables and Structured English can complement one another to describe a single process. Let's discuss how!

Recall that procedures often implement policies. Why then, can't we describe all procedures using Structured English and reference appropriate decision tables to describe any policies implemented by the procedures? We can demonstrate this idea while

For each VALID ORDER, do the following steps:

If PREPAYMENT AMOUNT is less than the TOTAL ORDER COST then:

(1) Search the CUSTOMER file for the CUSTOMER ACCOUNT using the CUSTOMER ACCOUNT NUMBER.

(2) If the CUSTOMER ACCOUNT is not found then:

(a) Set the CREDIT HISTORY equal to none.

(b) Set the AMOUNT OF BUSINESS equal to none.

(c) Set the CREDIT CEILING to $5,000.

(d) Set the CURRENT BALANCE to zero.

(e) Record the CREDIT DETAILS in the CUSTOMER file.

(3) Calculate the PROPOSED BALANCE using the formula:

PROPOSED BALANCE = CURRENT BALANCE + TOTAL ORDER COST − PREPAYMENT AMOUNT.

(4) Select the CREDIT ACTION using the CREDIT DETAILS and CREDIT decision table.

(5) If the action is "approve credit" then:

Report the APPROVED ORDER details.

Otherwise (the action selected was a prepayment request)

Report the CREDIT REJECTED ORDER.

Figure 9.12

Procedures for CHECK CUSTOMER CREDIT transaction process (Structured English). Structured English may include numbers and letters beside specific procedure entries. This allows users to make easy reference to particular instructions. Many users feel that this tends to take away the programming flavor or appearance of many procedure descriptions.

documenting some of the policies and procedures for some typical primitive-level processes appearing on the logical DFD that we drew for AAP.

Transaction Policy and Procedure First, we will examine a transaction processing process description, CHECK CUSTOMER CREDIT from AAP's logical DFD. The CHECK CUSTOMER CREDIT process will be performed for each order that was not completely prepaid (payment accompanying the order). The mini spec for the CHECK CUSTOMER CREDIT process is illustrated in Figures 9.12 and 9.13. Notice that the Structured English in Figure

Process Name		Credit								Rules							
		1	2	3	4	5	6	7	8	9	10	11	12	13	14	15	16
Conditions	Type of Customer	-	-	-	-	-	-	-	-	2	1	1	2	1	2	1	2
	Credit History	A	B	D	B	A	B	C	D	C	C	A	A	C	C	D	D
	Amount of Business	-	-	-	H	L	L	L	L	-	-	H	H	H	H	H	H
	Proposed Balance ≤ Credit Ceiling	Y	Y	Y	N	N	N	N	N	Y	Y	N	N	N	N	N	N
Actions	Approve Credit	X	X									X					
	Request 10% Prepayment			X	X	X	X				X		X			X	
	Request 25% Prepayment								X	X				X			X
	Request 100% Prepayment							X							X		

Type of Customer: 1 = Franchise Jobber
2 = Nonfranchise Jobber

Credit History: A = Good
B = Average
C = Poor
D = None

Amount of Business: H = Less Than or Equal to $100,000
L = Less Than $100,000

Proposed Balance Less Than or Equal to Credit Ceiling: Y = Yes
N = No

Figure 9.13

Policies for CHECK CUSTOMER CREDIT transaction process (a decision table). Simplified decision tables should include a legend for users to refer to when verifying the decision table policy.

9.12 *references* the decision table of Figure 9.13. The decision table does a clear, concise job of specifying the policies for granting credit for customer orders. Most procedures don't require decision tables. Think about the implications of writing the entire policy and procedure using only Structured English. Study the mini spec for the CHECK CUSTOMER CREDIT process. No further explanation of the process is necessary. This is a tribute to the effectiveness of

1. For each record in the ORDER file:
   a. Report the contents of the record.
   b. Sum the following sales totals:
      TOTAL NUMBER OF ORDERS
      TOTAL COST OF ORDERS
2. Report the sales totals.

Figure 9.14

Procedures for PRODUCE SALES ORDER LOG management reporting process.

using Structured English and decision tables as communication tools!

Management Reporting Procedure The logical DFD for AAP also included primitive-level processes that fulfill management reporting requirements. Let's examine how the procedures for two of the management-reporting processes are defined using Structured English.

The PRODUCE SALES ORDER LOG process obtains data from the ORDER file and produces a detailed report called SALES ORDER LOG. This report informs the order-entry supervisor of the status of each customer order. The mini spec for this process is presented in Figure 9.14. The simplicity of this mini spec is typical of management-reporting processes. Computer programs for such processes are also relatively simple, particularly when report-writing languages are used.

A second primitive-level DFD process that supports management reporting for AAP is SUMMARIZE SALES BY PRODUCT LINE. The mini spec for this process is depicted in Figure 9.15. It's certainly not as simple as the procedure description for the previous process. But then again, the PART SALES SUMMARY report is more complex than the SALES ORDER REGISTER. Let's study this mini spec in greater detail.

The procedure requires four loops. The two innermost loops, step 1, include instructions for calculating the sales totals for a particular part for the previous day, week, and month. These inner

I. For each WAREHOUSE ZONE do the following:
   A. For each PRODUCT LINE for that WAREHOUSE ZONE do the following:
      1. For each PART NUMBER for that PRODUCT LINE do the following:

         For each PART record for that PART NUMBER, do the following:

            If the ORDER DATE is yesterday's date

               Sum TOTAL ORDER COST giving the UNIT SALES PAST DAY.

            If the ORDER DATE is past week's date

               Sum TOTAL ORDER COST giving the UNIT SALES PAST WEEK.

            If the ORDER DATE is past month's date

               Sum TOTAL ORDER COST giving the UNIT SALES PAST MONTH.
      2. Report the above sales totals for that PART NUMBER.
      3. Sum UNIT SALES PAST DAY giving the PAST DAY UNIT SALES LINE.
      4. Sum UNIT SALES PAST WEEK giving the PAST WEEK UNIT SALES LINE.
      5. Sum UNIT SALES PAST MONTH giving the PAST MONTH UNIT SALES LINE.
   B. Report the above sales totals for that PRODUCT LINE.
   C. Sum PAST DAY UNIT SALES LINE giving the PAST DAY UNIT SALES ZONE.
   D. Sum PAST WEEK UNIT SALES LINE giving the PAST WEEK UNIT SALES ZONE.
   E. Sum PAST MONTH UNIT SALES LINE giving the PAST MONTH UNIT SALES ZONE.
II. Report the above sales totals for that ZONE.

Figure 9.15

Procedures for SUMMARIZE SALES BY PRODUCT LINE management reporting process.

loops are included within a third loop, *A*, that sums and reports the sales information for each part within a particular product line. Finally, the outermost loop, step I, sums and reports the sales for a

Select the appropriate case for the user chosen query option:

Case 1: (user chose option for general part data)

Given a PART NUMBER or PART DESCRIPTION supplied by the user:

Find the general part data in PART CATALOG using the PART NUMBER.

Report the general part data for that PART NUMBER or PART DESCRIPTION.

Case 2: (user chose option for part-to-vehicle matchups)

Given a VEHICLE NUMBER and a PART DESCRIPTION by the user:

Find the PART NUMBER for that VEHICLE NUMBER and PART DESCRIPTION using the PART file.

Report the PART RESTRICTIONS for that PART NUMBER.

Case 3: (user chose option for part back order analysis)

Given a PART NUMBER or PART DESCRIPTION by the user:

Report the back order status for that PART NUMBER or PART DESCRIPTION, using the PART file.

Figure 9.16

Procedures for QUERY PART decision support process.

product line and calculates the sales over the past day, week, and month for a warehouse zone. This type of procedure should look familiar to those of you who have written computer programs with multiple control breaks.

Decision Support Procedure Structured English can also describe the primitive-level DFD processes that represent decision support requirements. One of the decision support processes on the logical DFD for AAP is QUERY PART. This process allows the user to obtain general part data, identify part and vehicle matchups, and analyze back ordered parts. Let's examine the mini spec for QUERY PART to determine how these inquiries are fulfilled.

The mini spec for QUERY PART is presented in Figure 9.16. Notice that the *case* construct was used to clearly separate the instructions for providing each type of part inquiry. Also notice how we demonstrated the query input, *Given PART NUMBER*.

Well, that's enough examples. We have demonstrated that decision tables and Structured English can be used to reference data dictionaries and define any process on a data flow diagram. This completes our study of systems analysis. In Part III we'll study how tools used in the analysis process can complement and support the tools and techniques used by the systems analyst in performing systems design.

SUMMARY

Systems analysts must give special concern to the specification of policies and procedures. Policies specify management decisions and rules. Procedures execute those policies as well as the tasks that support day-to-day business operations and management. Although most existing procedures are specified in ordinary English, we have learned that most such procedures are often unclear and incomplete. Fortunately, we learned two tools that can help better specify policies and procedures. Decision tables are particularly effective for policies and for procedures that contain complex combinations of decisions. Structured English is a procedure specification tool that overcomes many of the limitations and ambiguities of ordinary English. Together, these two tools complement data flow diagrams and data dictionaries. Furthermore, these tools help us effectively communicate business requirements to computer programmers and knowledge workers alike!

This chapter concludes Part II. It is important for you to realize that the tools presented in Part II have their greatest value in the systems analysis phases. However, we have seen that these tools are also useful during the design and implementation phases. In Part III, "Systems Design and Implementation Tools and Techniques," we will demonstrate some of these uses and emphasize how the tools used in the analysis phases can complement and support the tools used in the design phases.

PROBLEMS AND EXERCISES

1. Explain the difference between a policy and a procedure. Give an example of a policy and the procedure to implement or administer that policy.
2. Obtain a formal statement of a policy and procedure from a local company (or from home, such as a policy for a credit card). Evaluate the policy and procedure statement in terms of the common specification problems identified earlier in this chapter.
3. Reconstruct the policy and procedure used in exercise 2 with the tools you learned in this chapter.
4. Simplify the following decision table.

	Rules											
	1	2	3	4	5	6	7	8	9	10	11	12
condition 1	Y	N	Y	N	Y	N	Y	N	Y	N	Y	N
condition 2	Y	Y	N	N	Y	Y	N	N	Y	Y	N	N
condition 3	A	A	A	A	B	B	B	B	C	C	C	C
action 1	X				X				X			
action 2			X				X				X	
action 3		X				X						
action 4				X				X		X		X

5. Were you able to combine rules 2 and 6 in problem 4? Why?
6. Obtain a copy of your last programming assignment. Using Structured English, write procedure specifications to clearly communicate the procedures that you were asked to implement. Did you avoid unnecessary details? Does your Structured English take on an unnecessary programming accent? Does your Structured English accurately communicate the processing procedures that are to be implemented as a computer program? Did you avoid programming-dependent statements (such as OPEN, and PERFORM)? Would you have appreciated such a description when you were originally given the assignment?
7. Prepare a decision table that accurately reflects the following course grading policy:

   A student may receive a final course grade of "A," "B," "C," "D," or "F." In deriving the student's final course grade, the instructor first determines an *initial* or tentative grade for the student. The initial course grade is determined in the following manner.

A student who has scored a total of no lower than 90 percent on the first three assignments and exams and received a score no lower than 70 percent on the fourth assignment will receive an initial grade "A" for the course. A student who has scored a total lower than 90 percent but no lower than 80 percent on the first three assignments and exams and received a score no lower than 70 percent on the fourth assignment will receive an initial grade "B" for the course. A student who has scored a total lower than 80 percent but no lower than 70 percent on the first three assignments and exams and received a score no lower than 70 percent on the fourth assignment will receive an initial grade "C" for the course. A student who has scored a total lower than 70 percent but no lower than 60 percent on the first three assignments and exams and received a score no lower than 70 percent on the fourth assignment will receive an initial grade "D" for the course. A student who has scored a total lower than 60 percent on the first three assignments and exams, *or* received a score lower than 70 percent on the fourth assignment will receive an initial and final grade "F" for the course. Once the instructor has determined the initial course grade for the student, the *final* course grade will be determined. The student's final course grade will be the same as their initial course grade if they missed no more than three class periods during the semester. Otherwise, the student's final course grade will be one letter grade lower than their initial course grade (for example, an "A" will become a "B").

Are there any rules for which there was no action specified for the instructor to take? If so, what would you do to correct the problem? Can your decision table be simplified? If so, simplify it.

8. Write a mini spec (Structured English) for balancing your checkbook.

9. Produce a mini spec to describe how to prepare your favorite recipe, tune a car, or perform some other familiar task. Ask a novice to perform the task working from your specification.

ANNOTATED REFERENCES AND SUGGESTED READINGS

Copi, I. R. *Introduction To Logic.* New York: Macmillan, 1972. Copi provides a number of problem-solving illustrations and exercises that aid in the study of logic. The poker chip problem in our chapter case was adapted from one of Copi's reasoning exercises.

Demarco, Tom. *Structured Analysis and System Specification.* Englewood Cliffs, N.J.: Prentice-Hall, 1979.

Gane, Chris, and Trish Sarson. *Structured Systems Analysis: Tools and Techniques.* Englewood Cliffs, N.J.: Prentice-Hall, 1979. Gane and Sarson include an entire chapter on defining process logic. In addition to decision tables and Structured English, this chapter explains how the tools decision trees and pseudocode can be used to define process logic.

Gildersleeve, T. R. *Successful Data Processing Systems Analysis.* Englewood Cliffs, N.J.: Prentice-Hall, 1978. This book includes an entire chapter on the construction of decision tables. Gildersleeve does an excellent job of demonstrating how narrative process descriptions can be translated into condition and action entries in decision tables.

Matthies, L. H. *The New Playscript Procedure.* Stamford, Conn.: Office Publications, 1977.

PART THREE Systems Design and Implementation Tools and Techniques

We suspect that some of you are wondering when we will finally start discussing the information system's computer elements in greater detail. We all know that the computer elements of the system must be specified sooner or later, right? Systems design is the process during which the computer elements of a new information system take shape! The basis for a good system design is a good systems analysis — the specification of a feasible, computer-based solution for a business problem, opportunity, or directive.

Like systems analysis, systems design is an essential activity in the system development life cycle. Although systems design is usually performed with somewhat greater rigor and standards than systems analysis, systems design is still often shortchanged. The fault does not lie entirely with the systems analyst. Indeed, many users become impatient with both the analysis and design activities. The prevalent attitude is, "You are a computer person. Computer people program. If you aren't programming, you aren't doing your job!" The result? The project moves into the construction phase prematurely. The net result? The system takes longer to implement, costs more to implement, and is more difficult for the users to work with. The system is then doomed to a lifetime of criticism, limited usefulness, and costly modifications!

We are partially responsible for the problem. For years, we have spoon-fed our technical terminology and documentation to the users. Like castor oil, it's left a bad taste! For some time now, we've had good tools, but we've abused them. We've drawn too many cryptic flowcharts and printer spacing charts. We've worried too much about the computer and not enough about the person who will use the computer. The result? Many users no longer want our help. And they don't want to help us design good systems. Meanwhile, the tools and techniques of systems design are unfairly criticized and often abandoned.

Enough preaching! The purpose of this unit is to introduce you to the systems design process and to useful tools and techniques for performing that process. Eight chapters make up the unit. The first chapter introduces the systems design process. The next five chapters develop systems design skills including output design, file design, input design, on-line terminal dialogue design, design of data processing methods and procedures, and program design. We will focus as much attention on human engineering as on the design techniques themselves. The last chapter (Chapter 17) presents the systems implementation process.

In addition to design tools and techniques, you may elect to skim, read, or review a few of the applicable modules in Part IV. These modules survey skills that are not restrictive to the systems design and implementation processes but are important to effective systems design and implementation. Modules that survey relevant skills include Module A (project management), Module C (presentations and other communications skills), Module D (cost/benefit analysis), and Module E (the database alternative and its design implications).

10 How to Perform a Systems Design

Minicase: Transport Pipe Company (revisited)

In Chapter 6, we sat in on a job performance review with Ken Hayes, the MIS manager at Transport Pipe Company, and Tim Stallard, one of Ken's programmers. Six months have passed since that meeting. Tim has been performing entry-level systems design tasks under the supervision of a senior systems analyst. It's time for another job performance review so let's listen in.

"Well, Tim, do you still want to be a systems analyst?" asked Ken.

"More than ever," answered Tim. "Now that I've had a taste of systems work, I know it's right for me. I assume this meeting will determine whether I keep moving in this direction. Have I done well enough?"

"I discussed your performance on the MRP Project with both your supervisor and your client," Ken replied. "Your design specification document was quite impressive. But I have to ask you, where did you learn to complete such thorough specifications? We certainly didn't teach you. Your document is much better than our minimum standards, and the implementation appears to be moving along much smoother than average."

"I did a lot of reading in systems analysis and design textbooks at the college library. But to be honest, I really was embarrassed by the Bill of Materials project that you gave me right after my last job performance review."

Ken interrupted, "I don't understand. It was a little behind schedule, but that's the only problem I recall."

Tim replied, "Well, it was a little more complicated than that. Bill was supervising me since it was my first experience with systems design [Bill had done the analysis]. But Bill had to be called off the project to fix a major flaw in another system. I kept working on the design and passed the design document to Debbie [a programmer]. Then lightning struck for a second time. Debbie had to go into the hospital and I had to assume her programming responsibilities. It was the first time that I ever had to cut code from my own specifications. There were so many details, and I hadn't documented all of them. Unfortunately, I couldn't remember all of them either."

"But I eventually got the system up and running — only to find out that some of the reports produced were not acceptable to my users. I had taken certain liberties with format, and they didn't agree. I fulfilled all of the requirements that Bill had documented, but I guess the formats weren't ideally suited to the way the reports would be used. I guess I just didn't appreciate the importance of working with the user during output design. I figured Bill's analysis had taken care of all the user issues. Since then, Bill has explained to me that the analysis phase identifies outputs and content but not format.

"And then, the Audit Department got ahold of my design specification. And they didn't like it at all! Not enough internal controls for their taste. By that time, I had half the programs written, and I had to go back and redesign parts of the system and rewrite those programs. To make a long story short, I didn't ever want that to happen again. So I went to the library and checked out several systems analysis and design books. And unlike college, this time I read them carefully and I learned."

Ken smiled. "And you still wanted to be an analyst? After that?"

"Yes. Despite the problems, I found the work to be so much

more interesting than anything I had done before. I knew it wasn't going to be easy. But it was fun!"

"Well," said Ken, "we've talked about the good things you've done. And there have been no catastrophes in the MRP project. But we do need to work on a few things. First, as you know, most of our older batch systems are being converted to on-line applications. And all new development projects are going on-line. I don't know if you've heard, but the Bill of Materials users aren't exactly jumping for joy about the terminal dialogue design you did for that system. Second, you really need to work on your writing and speaking skills. The report you did to sell the MRP system to management wasn't well organized, was too wordy, and contained numerous spelling and grammar errors. You were lucky that Bill got hold of it and cleaned it up before your client saw it. And the presentation you made to management should have gone smoother. You seemed unconfident about what you were selling. You had a good design, Tim. If you don't seem confident about your design, how will management be confident. We got it through though. But your communications skills must improve before you can advance much further."

"I understand," responded Tim. "I guess I never really took my college English courses too seriously. I guess I'll have to enroll in some continuing education courses at the college. I'm sure not going to let poor communications skills get in the way of my future."

Ken leaned back in his chair and pondered for a moment. "Let's get to the bottom line, Tim. You've shown tremendous promise as an analyst. And that's why, effective first of next month, you're being promoted to programmer/analyst. You'll continue to learn new skills. Now, let's talk about that impressive design specification document you did for the MRP project. Do you think you could teach other analysts how to do that? We could sure use some standards that measure up to what you did . . ."

Discussion

1. Thinking back to your programming courses (or experiences), what are some of the problems you've had responding to your programming assignments (which are the classroom equivalent of a systems design)?

2. What did Tim learn about design by working from his own specifications?
3. As a systems analyst performing a systems design, what other types of people did Tim have to communicate with? Why does communication become tougher during systems design than during systems analysis?

WHAT WILL YOU LEARN IN THIS CHAPTER?

In this chapter, you will learn more about two phases in the systems development life cycle: *design* and *selection* — collectively referred to as the **systems design process.** You will know that you understand the systems design process when you can:

1. Define systems design and relate the term to the design and selection phases of the life cycle.
2. Describe the design and selection phases in terms of:
   (a) Purpose and objectives.
   (b) Tasks and activities that must or may be performed.
   (c) Skills you must master to perform the phase properly.
3. Describe the continued importance of cost/benefit analysis during the systems design phases.
4. Explain how the time spent on systems design can be managed.

What is *systems design?* Let's approach the question the same way we did *systems analysis* in Chapter 6. You already know what a system is, so the key term here is *design.* Webster's New World Dictionary of the American Language offers us the following:

> **de·sign:** . . . 1. to make preliminary sketches of; . . . 2. to plan or carry out, esp. by artistic arrangement or in a skillful way . . . (From *Webster's New World Dictionary of the American Language, Second College Edition,* Simon & Schuster, a Divison of Gulf & Western Corporation, 1980. Used with permission.)

For our purposes, design is the skillful planning of the computer elements for an improved information system. In this chapter, we will examine two systems design phases: the selection of computer equipment and programs for a new information system and the design of computer specifications for a new information system. Figure 10.1 illustrates these phases as part of the system development life cycle. For each phase, we will study *purpose* and *objectives, tasks* that should be performed, and important *skills* to be mastered. And we will address the continuing issues of cost/benefit and feasibility analysis. For comparison purposes, this chapter is organized in the same manner as Chapter 6, the systems analysis overview.

Now you might be thinking, "Weren't we designing a new system during the definition and evaluation phases of systems analysis (Chapter 6)?" The answer is, "Sort of." Some people refer to the definition of user requirements as the *logical design.* The logical design specifies the essential features of the new system, independent of how those features might be implemented. During the evaluation phase, we looked at alternative ways to implement the essential features, and we selected one of those alternatives. In this chapter, we'll study *physical design.* Physical design results in the purchase of computer equipment and software, the specification of programs for computer programmers, or both.

HOW TO SELECT COMPUTER EQUIPMENT AND PROGRAMS FOR A NEW INFORMATION SYSTEM

The selection of new computer equipment (hardware) and programs (software) for information systems is not necessary for *all* new systems. On the other hand, when new computer equipment or software is needed, the selection of appropriate products is often difficult. The decision to purchase a specific product is wrought with technical, economic, and political considerations. And the decision can become a nightmare if the wrong technology is selected. The systems analyst is becoming increasingly involved in the selection of computer technology to support specific applications being developed—particularly in the selection of microcomputers, peripherals, and software packages.

Figure 10.1 ▶

The systems design process. The systems design process is defined as the selection and design phases of the system development life cycle.

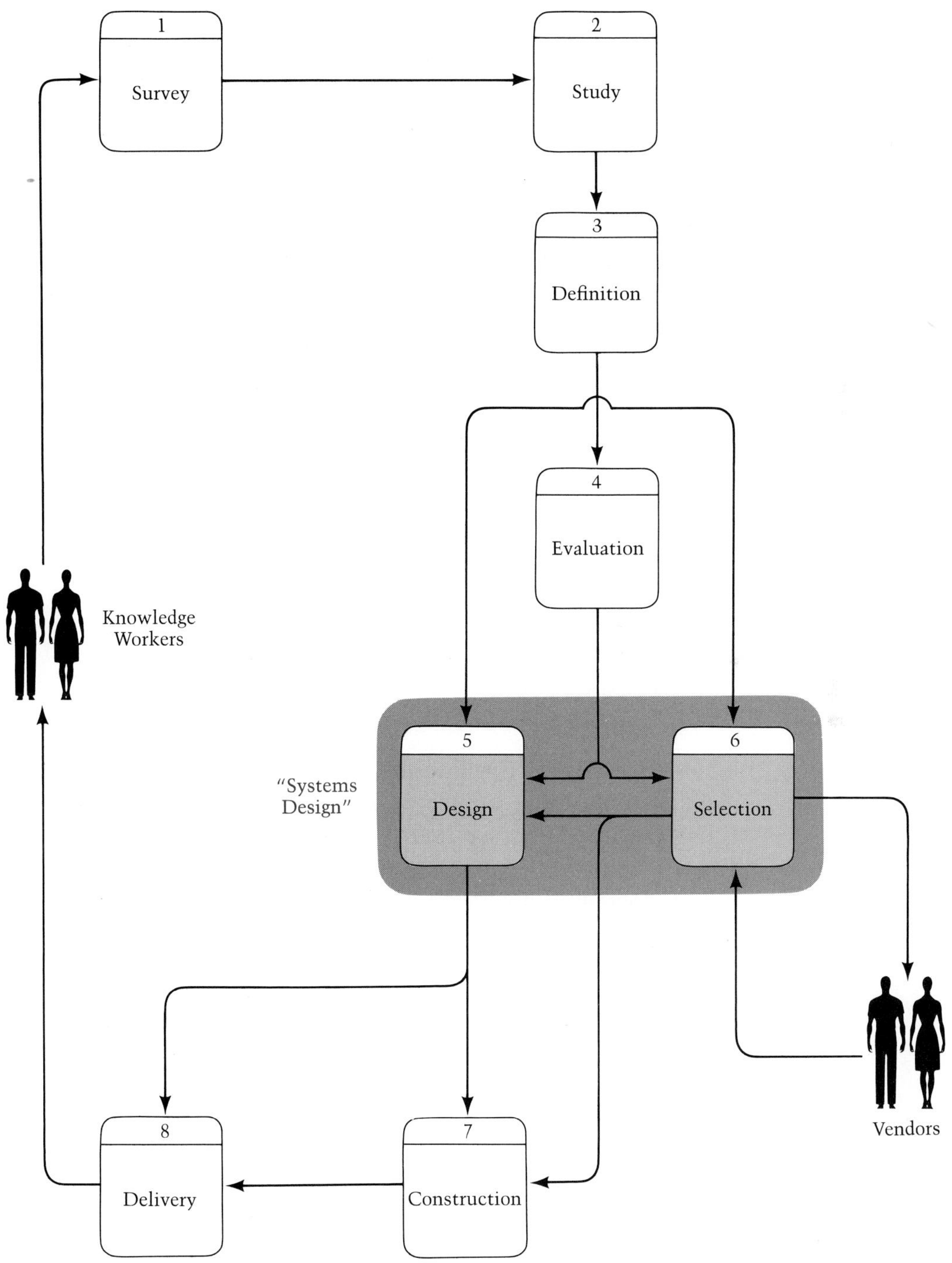
1
Survey
2
Study
3
Definition
4
Evaluation
Knowledge
Workers
"Systems
Design"
5
Design
6
Selection
Vendors
8
Delivery
7
Construction

Purpose and Objectives of the Selection Phase

The purpose of the selection phase is twofold. First, we need to determine whether new or additional hardware and software will be needed for the proposed system. In many cases, the technology we already own or have access to will support the new information system. If so, the selection phase can be bypassed. But if not, we come to our second purpose, which is to choose the *specific* technology to support the proposed information system. To achieve the second goal, we must accomplish the following objectives:

- Identify and select technology that the knowledge workers will feel comfortable using and that can be cost-justified to management.
- Establish, for the desired technology, technical and functional requirements that are consistent with the business mission.
- Identify and evaluate alternative products that provide the capabilities desired of the new information system.
- Select hardware and software components that complement the other components of the new information system.

These objectives are related to the four dimensions of our information system pyramid model. Let's examine each objective in greater detail.

Knowledge-Worker Involvement in the Selection Phase In our not too distant past, the knowledge workers (depicted in the margin) seldom wanted to be involved in the selection phase. But times have changed. Knowledge workers are becoming more computer literate. Most college graduates have been exposed to computers and their potential. Also, microcomputers and intelligent terminals have found their way into many business offices. Consequently, users and management have become more interested in this technology.

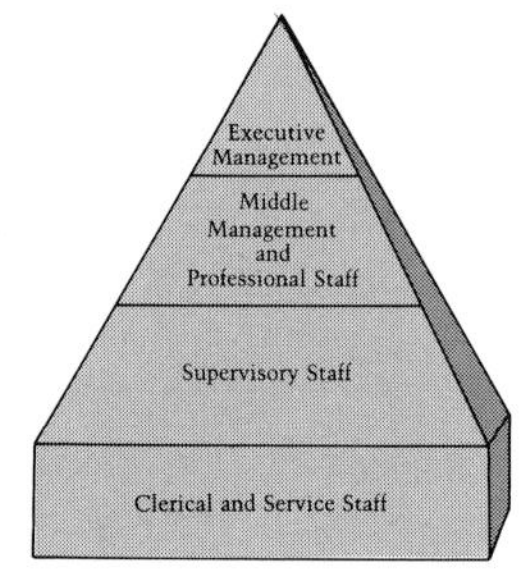

Knowledge Workers

But our concern for the knowledge worker (stressed throughout this book) goes beyond their increased interest in the technology. Issues such as ergonomics and human engineering have become important factors that only the knowledge workers can address. **Ergonomics** refers to the physical orientation of the person/machine environment. For instance, the tilt of a terminal screen, color and glare of a display, and slope and layout of a keyboard are all ergonomic issues. **Human engineering** refers to the friendliness and ease of use of a software package, manual, computer dialogue, or report.

Finally, most selection decisions involve sizable capital outlays that must be approved by knowledge workers. Management typically defers the research and recommendations to data processing professionals, but the final decision is economic and is, therefore, made by management.

Importance of the Business Mission to the Selection Phase The business mission (see margin) should drive the technology-selection decision, not vice versa. It is the analyst's responsibility to ensure that the organization's purpose, goals, objectives, and policies are best served by the technology that is selected. Thus the business mission perspective of the information system is again reinforced.

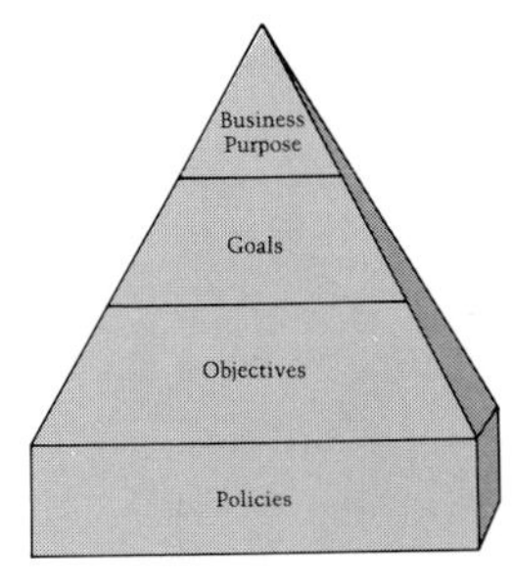

Business Mission

Unfortunately, computer professionals must innoculate themselves against "Bell and Whistles" disease. We must confess our infatuation with the marvelous technology that becomes available with each passing day. But we must also force ourselves to recognize as frivolous any technology that does not cost-effectively address the purpose, goals, objectives, and policies of the business and its information systems. To this end, we need to be wary of technical specifications and features. They *are* important, but we must always be cognizant of the business requirements to be fulfilled.

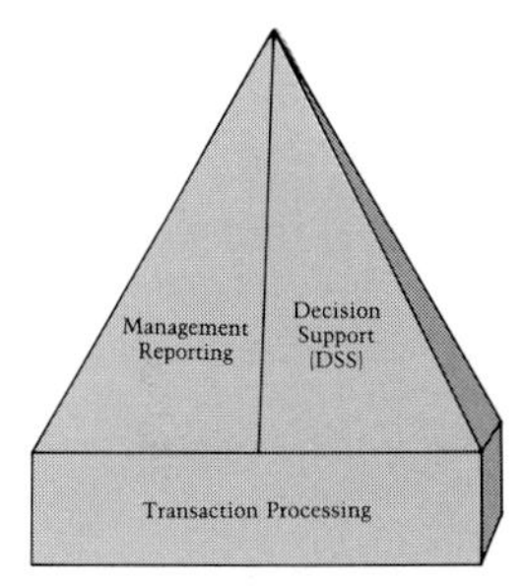

Information Systems Functions

Implications of the Information System Functions for the Selection Phase Some consultants believe most software should be purchased, not built. They argue that most industries and applications have access to a wealth of packaged software that will more than adequately meet their *basic* requirements. The *make-versus-buy* decision is often difficult. Arguments for both options are listed in the margin on the next page. Normally, the make-versus-buy decision will be made during the evaluation phase when the detailed cost/benefit analysis is performed. Understanding the fundamental information system functions and requirements is critical to the selection of the best software packages for the business.

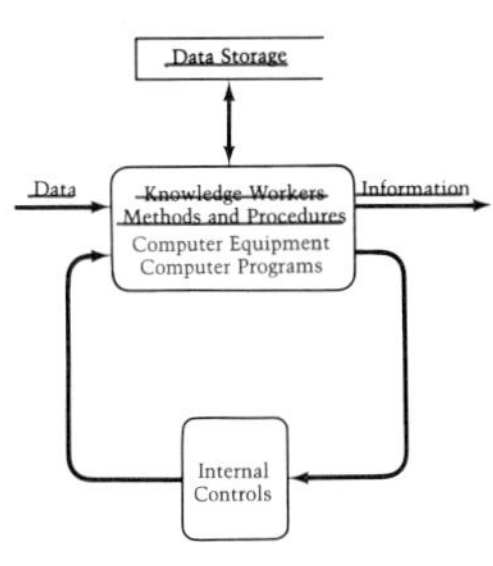

IPO Components

Selection of Information System Components The selection phase is primarily concerned with the computer equipment and software components of your IPO model (see margin). The analyst must evaluate how well alternative products complement the other components in the model. For instance, a specific software package will dictate specific methods and procedures, affect people who will use the system, and store data in predetermined formats. Is that hardware and software configuration suitable to the other components in the model?

Arguments for Making Software

1. It's designed to meet your exact requirements.
2. It's reliable—you built it yourself.
3. You control quality of documentation.
4. It's more easily modified (often difficult or impossible with purchased software).

How to Complete the Selection Phase

Now that you know *what* we want to accomplish in the selection phase, let's discuss *how* you do that phase. Specifically, let's study the tasks, documentation, and skills required. Figure 10.2 illustrates the selection-phase tasks and documentation. Many of the systems analysis skills from Part II are also useful during the selection phase. Although there is no way to guarantee that the best hardware or software will be selected, there are ways to minimize the probability of making a bad decision.

Task 1: Determine Technical Requirements and Evaluate Need The first task is to determine the technical requirements and evaluate the need for new technology. This task responds to the requirements statement (from the definition phase) and the approved hardware/software requirements (from the evaluation phase). These requirements may request specific features and capabilities that are needed to support the recommended (feasible) solution. They should also specify the critical performance parameters for the system (for instance, throughput, minimum acceptable response time, amount of data to be stored, security constraints).

The task will analyze the features, capabilities, and parameters to determine whether the existing computer system will be able to support this new information system.

Arguments for Buying Software

1. Why reinvent the wheel?
2. System is implemented sooner.
3. May be cheaper (development cost is spread out over all the customers who purchased the software).
4. Assured documentation (although it isn't always good).
5. Frees programmers and analysts to work on other projects.
6. Meets most requirements.

Task 2: Research Technical Criteria and Options If new or additional technology is needed, the next task is to research technical alternatives. This task helps identify the specifications that are important to the hardware and/or software that is to be selected.

When researching specifications for any hardware and software purchases, you must do your homework. Do not get your education from a salesperson! Remember, that salesperson's principal goal is the sale. We aren't suggesting that vendor sales representatives are dishonest, but we need not remind you that the number one rule of

Figure 10.2

Selection phase tasks. The selection phase can be broken down into the tasks suggested on this diagram. The arrows depict important documentation.

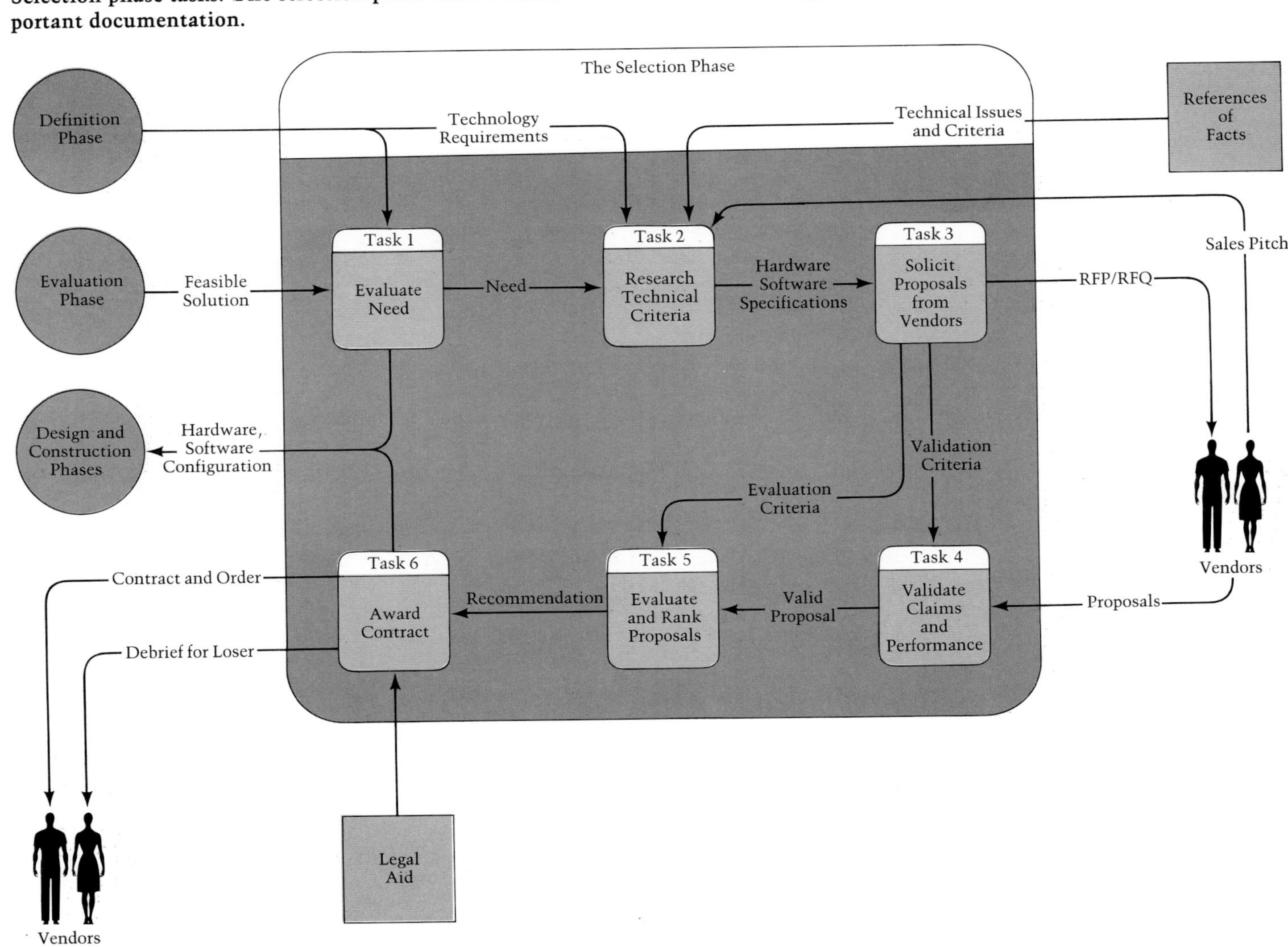

salesmanship is to emphasize your product's strengths and deemphasize its weaknesses.

Research identifies those technical and business issues and specifications that will become important to the selection decision. These may include the following:

- *Internal memory size.* The computer system's main memory must be large enough to hold the computer's operating system, support software that you want to use (for example, spreadsheet software, database software, telecommunications software), and application programs.
- *Processor speed.* The computer system must provide adequate throughput and response time, as defined by your users.
- *Storage capacity.* The disk, diskette, and tape files must be able to store your databases, files, operating system and utilities, support software, and application programs.
- *Input/output units.* The number of peripheral input, output, and communications devices is limited by the hardware.
- *Input/output volume.* Peripherals must be able to handle the volume of work that will be added by the new information system.
- *Features and capabilities.* Research also helps you identify the latest features and capabilities of the technology and determine which features and capabilities are important and how they affect performance.

You will compile a list of the requirements and features for the technology to be selected. Then you need to determine whether each requirement or feature is absolutely essential, desirable (could be acquired through a third-party vendor or built in-house), or just nice to have (you could live without it).

Information Services

Data Pro
EDP Auerbach
International Computer Programs
The Source

There are a number of useful sources of information for your research, including the following:

- *Information services* are primarily intended to constantly survey the marketplace for new products and advise prospective buyers on what specifications to consider. They also provide information on a number of installations and general customer satisfaction with the products. Some information services are listed in the margin.

- *Trade newspapers and periodicals* offer articles and experiences on various types of hardware and software that you may be considering. Some examples of these are listed in the margin. Many can be found in school and company libraries. Subscriptions (sometimes free) are also available.
- *Trade associations* offer you the opportunity to interact with data processing professionals who may be able to offer you advice. Examples include the Data Processing Management Association (DPMA), Association of Small Computer Users, Association for Systems Management (ASM), Society for Information Management, and product user groups.

Trade Publications

Computerworld (weekly)
Datamation (monthly)
Computer Decisions (monthly)
Infosystems (monthly)
Byte (monthly)

These resources can also help us identify potential vendors that supply the types of hardware and software we desire. After you've done your homework, initiate contact with these vendors. You will be better equipped to deal with vendor sales pitches after doing your research!

Task 3: Solicit Proposals (and Quotes) from Vendors Given the hardware/software specifications, your next task is to solicit proposals from vendors. If your company is committed to buying from a single source (IBM, for example), the task is quite informal. You simply contact your supplier and request price quotations.

On the other hand, many (if not most) decisions offer multiple alternatives. This is especially true of peripheral equipment (such as terminals and printers), microcomputers, communications equipment, and software packages. In this situation, good business sense dictates that you use the competitive marketplace to your advantage.

The solicitation task prepares one of two documents: a request for proposals (RFP) or a request for quotations (RFQ). The **request for quotations** is used when you have already decided on the vendor or product you want, but that product can be acquired from several distributors. This is often the case with peripheral computer equipment, such as terminals and printers.

The **request for proposals** is used when several different vendors and products appear as candidates and you want to provide the vendors with greater flexibility to configure equipment and software to meet your needs. The RFP presents both technical and business requirements to the vendors. We'll address the RFP for the remainder of this task description.

Because the quality of the RFP will significantly impact the quality and completeness of the resulting proposals,the RFP is the most important document for the selection phase. A suggested outline for an RFP is presented in Figure 10.3. An actual RFP is too lengthy to include in this book. Obviously, your ability to write clearly will affect the quality of proposals you get in response to your RFP. Furthermore, you can expect that any RFP will raise additional questions that you will address in meetings and other communications with prospective vendors. Therefore, verbal communication skills will also be tested in this task.

The primary purpose of the RFP is to communicate your requirements to the prospective vendor. Many of the skills you developed in Part II, such as data flow diagrams and data dictionaries, can be very useful for communicating requirements in the RFP. We have found vendors are very receptive to these tools because they find it easier to match products and options and package a proposal that is directed toward your needs. Everybody benefits from clear and complete requirements.

Task 4: Validate Vendor Claims and Performance Soon after the RFPs are sent to prospective vendors, you will begin receiving proposals. Proposals cannot and should not be taken at face value. An important philosophy during the selection phase should be *caveate emptor!* This is a Latin term meaning Let the buyer beware! Therefore, we validate vendor claims and performance. It is very important to note that this task is performed *independently* for each proposal. Proposals are not compared with one another at this point.

During this task, you should eliminate any proposal that does not meet *all* of your essential requirements. Care should be taken to first determine why the vendor's proposal does not meet all the essential requirements. The vendor's proposal may be inadequate because essential requirements were not clearly specified in the RFP. However, if you clearly specified your requirements, no vendor should have submitted such a proposal. You must also validate vendor claims and promises. Claims (about essential, desirable, and nice-to-have requirements) can be validated by completed questionnaires and checklists (included in the RFP) with appropriate vendor-supplied references to user and technical manuals. Promises can be validated by ensuring that they are written into the contract.

Performance is best validated by a demonstration. This is particularly important when evaluating software packages. Demonstra-

REQUEST FOR PROPOSALS

I. Introduction
   A. Purpose of the document
   B. Background leading to this document
   C. Brief summary of request
   D. Narrative explanation of document structure
II. Standards and instructions
   A. Schedule for selection phase
   B. Rules that will govern the selection procedure
   C. How the proposals will be evaluated
   D. Bidding instructions
III. Bid specifications (requirements)
   A. Computer equipment
      1. Mandatory requirements
      2. Desirable requirements
   B. Software
      1. Mandatory requirements
      2. Desirable requirements
   C. Miscellaneous requirements
IV. Technical questionnaires to be completed
V. Conclusion

Figure 10.3

Request for proposals. This is an outline for a typical Request for Proposals. The outline for a Request for Quotations would be similar; however, the RFQ's requirements are more technical and don't allow the vendor as much flexibility to tailor alternatives to the customer's business.

tions allow you to confirm capabilities, features, and ease of use. For equipment, you might consider a more formal demonstration, called a *benchmark*. A **benchmark** executes a small sample of programs or files (preferably from your own environment) on each vendor's proposed computer equipment. The benchmark performance gives you some indication of how well the system will perform when presented with your entire workload.

With the exception of confirming that essential requirements have been filled, the purpose of the validation task is not to eliminate proposals from consideration. Instead, we want to adjust the proposals so the claims and promises they contain can be evaluated fairly when we begin comparing them.

Task 5: Evaluate and Rank Vendor Proposals The validated proposals can now be compared with one another—that is, we evaluate and rank the vendor proposals. It is highly recommended that the evaluation criteria and scoring system be established *before* the actual evaluation takes place. Why? Because we don't want to bias the criteria and scoring to subconsciously favor any one proposal.

Some methods suggest that requirements be weighted on a point scale. The best scoring systems use dollars and cents! Monetary systems are easier to defend to management than *points.* One technique is to evaluate the proposals on the basis of hard and soft dollars. One popular approach, requirements costing, suggests this hard-dollar/soft-dollar evaluation. Hard-dollar costs are the costs you will have to pay to the selected vendor for the equipment or software. Soft-dollar costs are additional costs you will incur if you select a particular vendor (for instance, if you select vendor A, you may incur an additional expense to vendor B in order to overcome a shortcoming of vendor A's proposed system). This approach awards the contract to the vendor who fulfills all essential requirements while offering the lowest total hard-dollar plus soft-dollar penalties for desired features not provided (for a detailed explanation of this method see Joslin, 1977).

The evaluation and ranking task is, in reality, another cost/benefit analysis performed during systems development. Instead of evaluating and ranking information system alternatives, you are evaluating and ranking technology alternatives (specific vendor products). The techniques suggested in Part IV, Module D are applicable to this task.

Task 6: Award Contract and Debrief Losing Vendors Having ranked the proposals, your recommendations are usually presented to management for final approval. Once again, communications skills, especially salesmanship, will be important to your ability to persuade management to follow the recommendations.

Once the final decision has been made, a contract must be negotiated with the winning vendor. Certain special conditions and terms may have to be written into the standard contract. No computer contract should be signed without the advice of a qualified lawyer. Along the same lines, no final decision should be approved without the consent of a qualified accountant. Purchasing, leasing, or leasing with a purchase option involve complex tax considerations.

It is considered ethical to debrief the losing vendors. The debriefing involves contacting these vendors and explaining why they didn't get the contract. If you've handled the selection fairly and impartially, this won't be difficult. There are two benefits to be realized from this procedure. First, you maintain goodwill with these vendors which can be useful in future selection decisions. Second, both you and the vendors can learn from any mistakes made.

HOW TO DESIGN A COMPUTER-BASED INFORMATION SYSTEM

Now we come to a more traditional phase of the systems development life cycle, the design of computer specifications for a new information system. Let's set the stage. From the definition phase we have a requirements statement. From the evaluation phase, we have a feasible target solution that specifies which aspects of the system to computerize and how they should be automated (for instance, batch, on-line, centralized, distributed). Given this target solution, we must specify the detailed computer specifications that the computer programmers and technicians will need to implement that solution.

Purpose and Objectives of the Design Phase

The purpose or goal of the design phase is twofold. First and foremost, the analyst seeks to design a system that both fulfills requirements and will be friendly to its users. Human engineering will play a pivotal role during design. Second and still very important, the analyst seeks to present clear and complete specifications to the computer programmers and technicians. To achieve these two goals, we must accomplish the following objectives:

- Design a system the knowledge workers will find useful, easy to learn, and easy to use. This means that data must be captured easily, methods must be easy to apply, and information must be presented in such a way that it is easy both to understand and to use.

- Design a system that supports the business mission defined during systems analysis.
- Design a system that efficiently and effectively supports transaction processing, management reporting, and decision support—including those tasks *not* performed by the computer.
- Prepare detailed specifications for each of the following information system components: data and information, data storage, methods, procedures, people, hardware, software, and internal controls.

As usual, we have geared our objectives to your information system pyramid model, a copy of which appears in the margin.

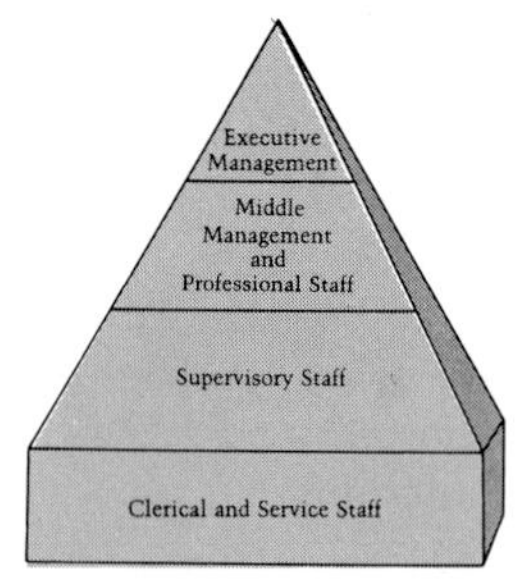

Knowledge Workers

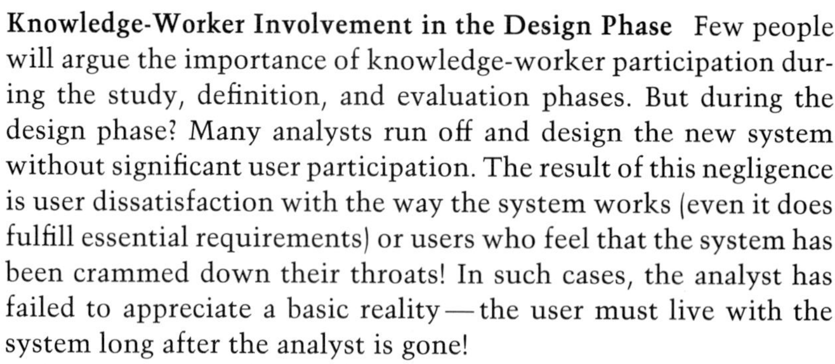

Knowledge-Worker Involvement in the Design Phase Few people will argue the importance of knowledge-worker participation during the study, definition, and evaluation phases. But during the design phase? Many analysts run off and design the new system without significant user participation. The result of this negligence is user dissatisfaction with the way the system works (even it does fulfill essential requirements) or users who feel that the system has been crammed down their throats! In such cases, the analyst has failed to appreciate a basic reality—the user must live with the system long after the analyst is gone!

It is quite possible (and common) for a system to fulfill user requirements but be so difficult for the knowledge worker to use that the system fails. For this reason, knowledge workers should be intimately involved in the design phase. As requirements are transformed into computer inputs, outputs, files, and program specifications, the user should at least review key components. Ideally, the users, themselves, should assist in the design tasks.

For instance, users should review the layout of all reports and terminal screens. They should also evaluate the conversational flow of terminal dialogue at the CRT terminal workstation. And they should evaluate their proposed role in the capture of data, processing of that data, and distribution of information. In other words, you need to bring your knowledge workers along with you. Unless they accept it, the best-designed technical system will be in trouble.

The Business Mission and the Design Phase The purpose, goals, objectives, and policies for both the business and the information system (see margin) were established during the definition phase. The analyst's principle concern during the design phase is to ensure that the subsequent design remains consistent with the business mission. Many goals are performance-, control-, or security-oriented. These goals are achieved (or missed!) during the design and implementation phases.

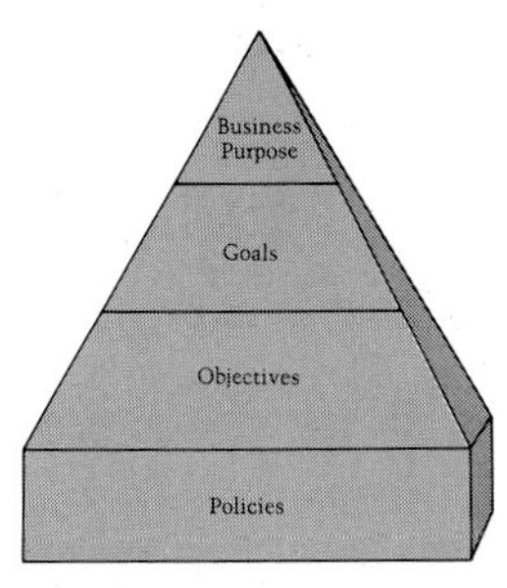

Business Mission

Information System Functions and the Design Phase The systems analyst should have defined all required information system functions long before system design. The analyst should now ensure that the design fulfills those requirements. More importantly, this phase determines *how* those requirements are fulfilled. Additional requirements may be introduced during system design because a computer is used. For instance, edit reports for input data and audit trails for transactions are typically added to the basic user-defined requirements to ensure the proper operation of a *computer-based* system.

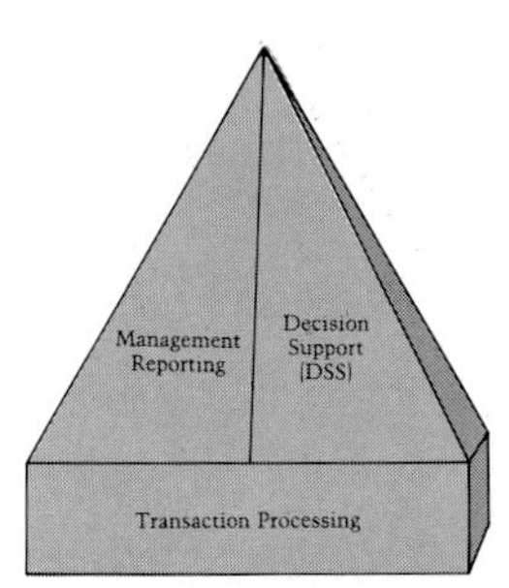

Information Systems Functions

Information System Components to Be Designed For the design phase, the information-components dimension is the most visible dimension. We design each of the following components (illustrated in the margin):

- *Data and information.* We specified the content of each data and information flow during the definition phase. We specified the media during the evaluation phase. Now we need to design the style, organization, and format of all inputs and outputs.
- *Data stores.* Once again, content and media have already been defined. During design, we must specify format, organization, and access methods for all files and databases to be used in the computer-based system.
- *Knowledge workers.* The roles people must play in the new system must be specified. For instance, when and how will data be input, and when will data be edited, verified, and corrected?
- *Methods and procedures.* During design, the sequence of steps and flow of control through the new system must be specified. The processing methods and intermediate manual procedures must also be clearly documented.

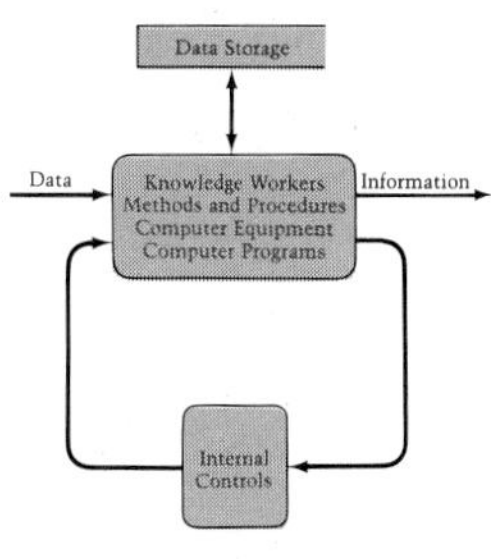

IPO Components

- *Computer equipment.* Although hardware is not selected or designed during the design phase, the hardware does constrain the system. The specific hardware configuration specified during the selection phase must be considered as various other components are designed.
- *Computer programs.* Complete programming specifications must be prepared for every program that must be written or modified.

As you might guess from the preceding discussion, the design phase gets into considerably greater detail than any of the previous phases of the life cycle.

How to Complete the Design Phase

Now we can discuss the specific tasks and documentation for the design phase. Figure 10.4 depicts the design-phase tasks and documentation. Each task represents a unique set of skills that you must learn and master in the forthcoming chapters and modules. One set of skills is common to the entire system design phase—communications skills! As an analyst, you will be conducting meetings and walkthroughs during or upon completion of each task. Some of these meetings and walkthroughs are with users. Others are with technical specialists. You need to learn how to communicate with each audience on its own level. No other phase of system development places the analysts in contact with such diverse audiences.

One issue that reoccurs during the design phase tasks is the importance of internal controls. The complexity of modern computer-based systems, many of which use sophisticated database, data communications, and on-line technology, makes businesses more vulnerable to mistakes, security violations, and disasters. For this reason, internal controls are designed into the system. Some internal controls prevent mistakes, violations, and disasters. Other internal controls respond to and recover from mistakes, violations, and disasters. In this section, we'll only mention the tasks during which the controls are designed. In all of the subsequent chapters, you'll learn how to design specific controls. We adopted this strategy because design of internal controls should never be thought of as an afterthought of the design phase—it is integral to each design phase task.

Figure 10.4

Design phase tasks. The design phase can be broken down into the tasks illustrated in this diagram. The named arrows depict documentation flow between the tasks. The half-moon symbol is not a task; it illustrates both • the routing of subsets of the requirements statement and feasible solution to the various tasks.

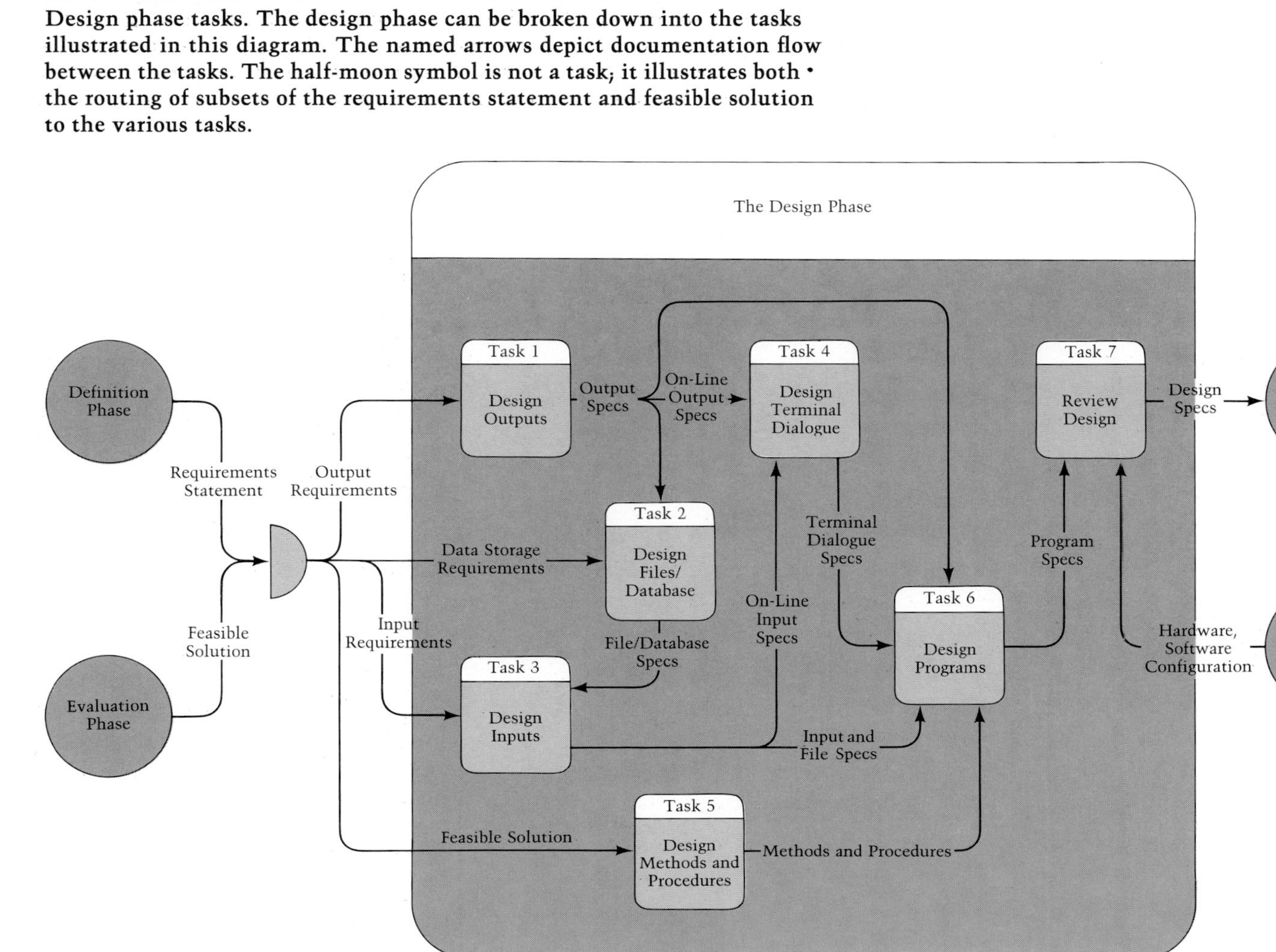

As we go through these tasks, keep in mind that we are only discussing *what* the analyst does. In the next several chapters we'll discuss how to do these tasks and demonstrate specific tools and techniques with which to accomplish them.

Task 1: Design Computer Outputs During the definition phase, we specified the required content and timing for the output data flows. In this task, we must format each of those outputs. Transaction outputs will frequently be designed as preprinted forms onto which transaction details will be printed. Management reports and decision support outputs are usually printed directly onto paper or displayed on a terminal screen. In any event, the precise format and layout of the outputs must be specified.

Because users and managers will have to work with these outputs, we must be careful to solicit their ideas and suggestions, especially regarding format. Management involvement is also necessary because management must approve expenditures on all outputs. Finally, internal controls must be specified to ensure that the outputs are not lost, misrouted, misused, or incomplete.

Task 2: Design Computer Files and/or Databases Given the data store requirements from the definition phase, we must design the corresponding computer files. The output design from the previous phase is also required because subtle changes or additions to the required data elements may have occurred during the output-design task. The design of files goes far beyond the simple layout of records. Files are a shared resource. Many programs will typically use the various files and databases. We must analyze how each program will access the data and then structure the files for optimal performance (you may be familiar with some of these data structures from your programming courses; they include ISAM, VSAM, and relative).

A significant trend, noted in Chapter 3, is the use of integrated databases instead of files. Recall that databases encourage the consolidation of numerous files (usually containing considerable redundant data) into a single, nonredundant data structure that supports numerous applications. Database design is a subject that can only receive adequate coverage in its own book. Database design frequently involves specialists, usually called *database administrators* or *database analysts,* whose expertise and experience can significantly aid in the task.

Some of the issues to be addressed during both file and database design include record size and file organization or structure. Because files and databases are shared resources, we must also design internal controls to ensure proper security and disaster recovery techniques (in case data are lost or destroyed).

Task 3: Design Computer Inputs The design of computer inputs naturally follows file and database design because the files and databases are maintained through the timely and accurate input of data. In addition to file/database specifications, the input-design task uses input requirements that were specified during the definition phase of systems analysis. The design of computer inputs can be a more complex process than you might imagine.

It is crucial to design the data capture methods for inputs. For instance, you may design a form on which data to be input will be initially recorded. "Easy," you say? Think about it! You want to make it easy for the data to be recorded on the form, but you also want to simplify the entry of the data from the form into the computer or onto a computer-readable medium. This is particularly true if the data are to be input by people who are not familiar with the business application (keypunch operators, for example). The layout of the input record as it will be presented to the computer must also be designed.

And that brings us to a second complication. Any time you input data to the system, you can make mistakes. We need to define editing controls to ensure the accuracy of input data. (Have you noticed that the design of internal controls is common to all of our design tasks?) Normally, we will be forced to define additional outputs (called *edit reports* or *edit screens*) to identify input errors. As an additional control to ensure against lost or erroneous inputs, you usually design historical reports that commit input transaction processing to paper where they can be audited and confirmed (this concept was first introduced in Chapter 3).

Task 4: Design Terminal Dialogues This is a task that is omitted from many design plans. It has become important because of the trend toward on-line and microcomputer-based systems. It's not really input design, even though it uses the on-line input design specifications from Task 3. And it's not really output design, although it uses the on-line output design specifications from Task 1. But for on-line systems, the design of terminal dialogue (the dialogue between the user and the computer) may well be the most critical design task! Too many on-line systems are difficult to learn and use because they contain poor human engineering.

The idea behind terminal dialogue design is to build an easy-to-learn-and-use dialogue around the on-line inputs and outputs. This dialogue must take into consideration such factors as terminal familiarity, possible errors and misunderstandings that the user may have or encounter, the need for additional instructions or help at certain points in timc, and screen content and layout. Essentially, you are trying to anticipate every little error or keystroke that a user might make — no matter how silly or improbable. Furthermore, we are trying to make it easy for the user to understand what the screen is displaying at any given time. Appropriate attention to this task can save many a late-night wake-up call — "We just crashed your system. We need you to come in and fix it right way!"

Task 5: Design Methods and Procedures The general procedures to be used in the new system were approved during the evaluation phase. For example, we should already know whether the system is on-line or batch, centralized or distributed, and so forth. In this task, we specify exactly *how* the new system will work, answering these questions: Who does what? When? Where? What comes next?

The internal controls from the previous tasks must be integrated into the new system work flow. This is particularly important for batch systems because data entry, data editing, and processing tasks must be executed in a specific sequence. The timing of scheduled reports and transaction processing must be clearly specified. Internal controls to ensure that the system cannot be deliberately or accidentally abused must be installed. For on-line systems, how will access be controlled? How will transactions be monitored and controlled? For all systems, when will files and databases be backed up? These are all issues to be addressed during the design of methods and procedures.

Task 6: Design Computer Program Specifications This task packages the input, output, file, database, terminal dialogue, and methods and procedures specifications into computer program specifications that will guide the computer programmer's activities during the construction phase of the system development life cycle. But there is more to this task than packaging.

How much more depends on where you draw the line between

the systems analyst's and computer programmer's responsibilities. (This may be a moot point if the analyst and programmer are one and the same person.) In addition to packaging, you need to determine the overall program structure. There are numerous strategies for top-down, modular decomposition. They will be surveyed in Chapter 16. The purpose of the modular-design subtask is to factor the program specifications into independent programming assignments. The modules must be designed so they can be reassembled into working final programs.

Task 7: Present and Review the Design This is a much more elaborate task than the name indicates. Before the design can be presented, you need to prepare three more components:

- *An implementation plan* that presents a proposed schedule for the construction and delivery phases (detailed in Chapter 17).
- *A final cost/benefit analysis* that determines if the design is still feasible. Given the design specifications and implementation plan, you should be able to make much more refined estimates for the remaining costs!
- *A system test,* which is a set of sample data for test inputs, files, and databases that will be used as the final test to ensure that the system is functioning properly.

The final system design specifications are typically organized into a workbook or technical report. An outline of this report is provided in Figure 10.5. Notice how the individual programs are packaged so they can be removed and distributed to the computer programmers.

The system design should be reviewed with all appropriate audiences, which may include the following:

- *Users.* Users have already seen and approved the outputs, inputs, and terminal dialogue. The overall work and data flow for the new system should get a final walkthrough and approval.
- *Management.* Management should get a final chance to question the project's feasibility (given the latest cost/benefit estimates).
- *Technical support staff.* Computer center operations management and staff should get a final chance to review the technical specifications to be sure that nothing has been forgotten and so

DESIGN SPECIFICATIONS

I. Introduction
   A. Purpose of report or workbook
   B. Background leading to report
   C. Scope of project
   D. Narrative explanation of report structure
II. Standards and specifications
   A. Standards followed or tools used
   B. Brief summary of user requirements
III. Design specifications
   A. System overview (with DFDs and system flowcharts)
   B. Shared files and database specifications
      1. File and database layouts
      2. Backup and recovery procedures (with system flowcharts)
   C. Program specifications
      1. Program 1
         a. Output specifications
         b. Local file specifications
         c. Input specifications
         d. Processing specifications

      .
      .
      .

      n. Program *n*

      .
      .
      .

IV. Implementation plan
V. Conclusion

Figure 10.5

Format of the design specifications. This is one possible format for organizing the system design specifications into a single document. Notice that the output, file, input, and processing specifications (from tasks 1–4 in Figure 10.4) have been reorganized into subunits corresponding to computer programs that must be written.

they can commit computer time to the construction and delivery phases of the project.

- *Audit staff.* Many firms have full-time audit staffs whose job it is to pass judgement on the internal controls in a new system.

As you probably guessed, the results of any of these reviews may necessitate a return to previous tasks in the design phase.

This concludes our overview of the design phase. The design phase leads directly into the computer programming activities (construction phase) with which you are likely familiar. Did you have any idea that this many activities preceded programming?

HOW TO MANAGE THE TIME SPENT ON SYSTEMS DESIGN

We'll conclude our survey of the systems design process with a discussion of project management implications for the two phases. The first issue to be addressed is the amount of time to be spent on systems design. We will then discuss the sequencing and overlapping opportunities for both the design tasks and the analysis process tasks that were introduced in Chapter 6. You might want to quickly review the analysis phases and their associated tasks before reading this discussion.

How Much Time Should Be Spent on Systems Design?

The amount of time that should be allocated to the design and selection phases might be a function of the following factors:

- The size of the project (as was the case with the analysis phases)
- The quality and completeness of the definition phase

The second factor is particularly important. If the detailed requirements were not specified in the definition phase (as is often the case with the more classical approach to analysis), then those details will have to be specified during the design phase. You can think of it as a pay me now or pay me later proposition.

Estimates vary significantly. Given a good set of user requirements, the design and selection phases should consume no more than 25 percent of the entire project schedule. If the requirements

The Next Generation

Prototyping: The Design Strategy for the Next Decade?

The sequencing of the system design phase tasks as presented in this chapter represents a classical, tried and proven strategy for system design. But to be perfectly honest, the approach hasn't proven perfect. It takes a lot of time. The resulting design specification document is usually quite sizable. And there are numerous opportunities for errors and omissions, some of which are not identified until the system is being implemented. And finally, the output is a *paper design* (a set of specifications on paper). Users can become very impatient during the generation of this paper design. They can also lose sleep wondering whether the actual system will live up to the paper design. But there is an alternative.

The design-by-prototyping strategy is being used by a rapidly increasing number of businesses. **Design by prototyping** consolidates the definition, design, and (at least partially) construction phases of your system development life cycle. Because users and managers frequently have difficulty specifying both the requirements and the best way to fulfill those requirements, the prototyping approach can prove useful. After the study phase and the specification of some general objectives or requirements, the prototype approach is initiated. A prototype, which is a *working* system or subsystem, is quickly developed. The prototype system is reviewed by users and management, who then make recommendations about requirements, methods, and formats. The prototype is then corrected, enhanced, or refined to reflect the new requirements. This process continues until the prototype evolves into the final system.

The trend toward prototyping has been fueled by the availability of special purpose software called application generators, program code generators, and fourth-generation languages. Examples include Cullinet's *ADS On-line*, Information Builder's *FOCUS*, and Mathematica's *RAMIS*. All of these languages allow the analyst to define and load databases, develop input records, define terminal screens, develop terminal dialogues, and write reports —all within a matter of hours or days instead of the usual weeks and months associated with languages such as BASIC, COBOL, and PL/I. It should be noted that many of these tools are now available for use on microcomputers. This means that prototyping doesn't have to have an adverse effect on the central computers!

Because many of these new packages *currently* generate inefficient systems when using full-sized files and transaction volumes (compared with traditional languages and database management systems), the final prototype system may have to be rewritten in a tradi- ▶

are incomplete, too general, or erroneous, you may increase that percentage of the total effort to as much as 35 to 40 percent. Some of that additional time would, of course, come from a lesser time requirement for the definition phase. However, generally speaking,

The Next Generation (continued)

tional language. But the prototype was developed much more rapidly than normal requirements and paper designs. And the prototype serves as the design specification for the system to be rewritten. In the future, we anticipate that most prototypes won't have to be rewritten—rather, the prototype generators are likely to improve!

How does prototyping affect the system design phase? There is a slight modification to the design approach. Let's review the procedure:

1. *Design the database.* Instead of beginning with output design, prototyping normally begins with database design (most application generators have a self-contained database management system). The data requirements for this database should have been defined during systems analysis. (Prototyping shouldn't take shortcuts around systems analysis.)
2. *Load a prototype database.* The database is loaded with a representative set of data. The total database is only a fraction of the size of the anticipated final database. It will be used for testing the prototypes.
3. *Design outputs.* This is not a paper design! You get a general feel for the requirements (perhaps using the data dictionary notation you learned in Chapter 8) and use the application generator to generate one or more sample formats using the prototype database prepared in step 2. Repeat this step until the users have approved the outputs.
4. *Design inputs and dialogues.* Again, not a paper design. This step is similar to step 3. Input validation should not be added until the basic input screens have been approved. On-line dialogues can actually be tested by having the user work on the prototype system. New paper forms for recording data may still have to be designed by the analyst.
5. *Design methods and procedures.* Prototyping cannot do everything for you. Even after the prototype programs have been approved, you will have to redefine the user's work and data flow for the new system. This step is frequently forgotten by those who advocate prototyping. Also, internal controls for such things as backup and recovery of databases and audit trails may have to be defined. Thus we see that prototyping doesn't totally eliminate paper design tasks!

Many forecasters predict that this technique will eventually replace traditional system design. Oh well, we're already committed to rewriting this book *eventually!* ■

the better the definition, the less time required to complete the design. There is a trend toward a new, time-saving design methodology called design by prototyping. This strategy is highlighted in the "Next Generation" feature for this chapter.

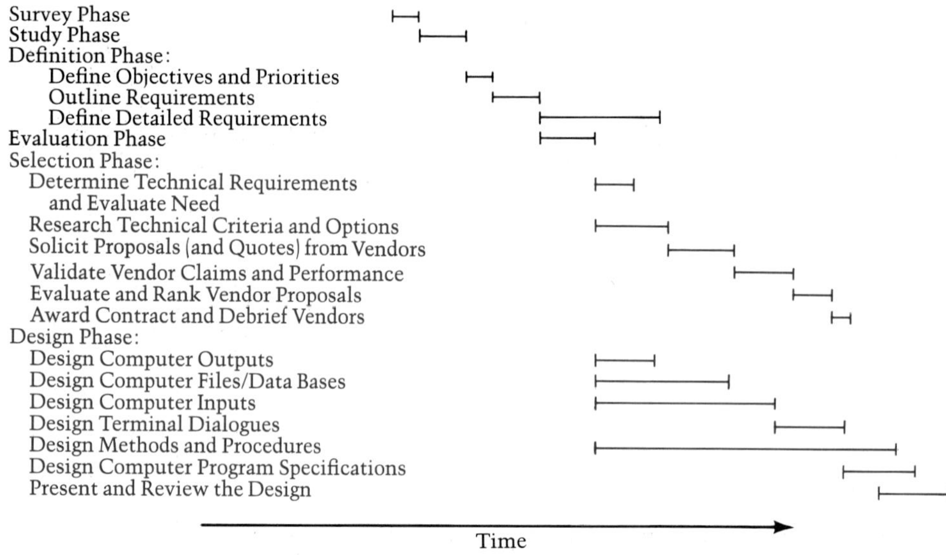

Figure 10.6

Overlapping the design and selection tasks. This Gantt chart depicts the possibility for overlapping the design and selection phases—both with one another and with the analysis phases (Chapter 6). Notice that both the selection and design phases are dependent on the completion of the evaluation phase and a commitment to a feasible solution.

To What Degree Can the Phases and Tasks Be Overlapped?

The selection and design tasks are essentially completed in parallel. You should note that this differs from the analysis phases, which were generally completed in sequence. Why are selection and design parallel phases? The selection phase requires some lead time for the necessary equipment and software to be delivered and installed. Ideally, you want that technology delivered and installed by the time the design is completed. Parallel scheduling of the selection and design phases is illustrated on the Gantt chart in Figure 10.6.

Notice that both the selection and design phases can be started only after the evaluation phase of systems analysis has been completed. The evaluation phase resulted in the feasible target to be input to both the selection and design phases.

The tasks that make up the selection and design phases can also be overlapped. We remind you that the selection phase should be concluded with sufficient lead time for delivery and installation of the technology. Thus, the design phase will typically continue as we await delivery and installation. The Gantt chart in Figure 10.6 depicts the optimal sequencing and overlap opportunities for the selection and design tasks. Vertical lines show the dependence of starting one task only after another is complete. The parallel bars illustrate overlapping tasks.

SUMMARY

Systems design is the process whereby the users' requirements are transformed into specifications for a computer-based information system. Systems design consists of two phases that can be successfully completed through a series of well-defined tasks that are common to all projects.

The purpose of the selection phase is to determine whether the new information system requires the acquisition of new computer equipment or software. If so, the phase also includes the selection of specific vendor products and the execution of the hardware/software order and contract for those products. The products of this phase include the final hardware/software configuration for the new system and any necessary hardware/software orders and contracts. But the most important document of the phase is the request for proposals or request for quotations. These documents communicate our needs to prospective vendors who will respond with formal proposals.

The most detailed phase of systems development is the design phase. The purpose of this phase is to generate detailed specifications for the computer elements of the new information system. These design specifications will be passed on to the computer programmers for implementation. Obviously, the degree to which computer programmers will be able to construct the system without further assistance is dependent on the completeness and clarity of the design specifications. Although the ultimate goal of systems design is to communicate specifications to programmers for implementation, the importance of user participation cannot be overstressed. Systems design is the phase in which the outputs, inputs,

Figure 10.7 ►

System-design-task/skill-cross-reference chart. This table identifies which of the chapters and modules in this book will help you develop the various skills needed to perform systems design tasks.

and on-line dialogues take form. An understanding of the importance of human engineering and user acceptance is crucial to overall project success. Finally, the completion of the system design presents management with one last chance to see the cost/benefit feasibility of the new system — before resources are committed to the expensive implementation phases.

There are two notable project management implications for the design process. First, the selection and design activities usually occur in parallel. This results from our need to execute any necessary hardware/software orders to provide sufficient delivery lead time so that the hardware and software will be delivered and available when the design is complete. Second, there are numerous opportunities for overlapping the analysis and design phases so long as the evaluation phase (which established the feasible target) has been completed.

In the following chapters, you will be introduced to tools and techniques for accomplishing the systems design tasks presented in this chapter. You may find Figure 10.7 to be a useful cross reference guide for chapters and modules that develop the design skills for the design tasks you learned in this chapter. Furthermore, you may, at your option, proceed to Chapter 17, *How to Perform a Systems Implementation.* That chapter may give you further insight into implications for the system design process.

PROBLEMS AND EXERCISES

1. How can a successful and thorough systems analysis be ruined by a poor system design? Answer the question relative to:
   (a) The impact on the subsequent implementation (in other words, the construction and delivery phases. You studied those two phases in Chapter 5).
   (b) The lifetime of the system after it is placed into operation.
   (c) The impact on future projects.

How the Chapters and Modules Assist in the Systems Design Process	Mod. E Systems Analysis and Design for Data Base	Mod. D Cost Benefit Analysis	Mod C Written Presentations	Mod. C Oral Presentations	Mod. B Fact Finding Techniques	Mod. A Project Management Tools and Techniques	Ch. 16 Program Design and Packaging	Ch. 15 Design of Methods and Procedures (includes System Flowcharting)	Ch. 14 Terminal Dialogue Design	Ch. 13 Input Design	Ch. 12 File/Data Base Design	Ch. 11 Output Design	Ch. 9 Structured English and Decision Tables	Ch. 8 Data Dictionary	Ch. 7 Data Flow Diagrams	Ch. 17 An Overview of Systems Implementation Process
Learn How To Select Technology			X			X										X
Determine Technical Requirements and Evaluate Need					X			X							X	
Research Technical Criteria and Options					X											
Solicit Proposals (and Quotes) from Vendors			X	X												
Validate Vendor Claims and Performance					X											
Evaluate and Rank Vendor Proposals		X														
Award Contract and Debrief Vendors				X												
Learn How To Design a Computer-Based Information System			X			X										X
Design Computer Outputs				X	X							X		X	X	
Design Computer Files/Data Bases	X			X	X						X			X	X	
Design Computer Intputs				X	X					X				X	X	
Design Terminal Dialogues				X	X				X	X		X				
Design Methods and Procedures				X	X			X							X	
Design Computer Program Specifications				X	X		X						X	X	X	
Present and Review the Design		X	X	X		X									X	X

2. What skills are important during systems design? Create an itemized list of these skills. Identify other computer, business, and general education courses that would help you develop or improve your skills. Prepare a plan and schedule for taking the courses. (If you are not in school, prepare a plan for using available corporate training resources, reading appropriate books, enrolling in seminars or continuing education courses, and so on.) Review your plan with your counselor, advisor, or instructor.
3. How does your information system pyramid model aid in systems design?
4. What by-products of the systems analysis phases are used in the system design phases? Why are they important? How are they used? What would happen if they were incomplete or inaccurate?
5. What are the end products of the design and selection phases? What is the content of each end product?
6. A client has approached you for help in selecting a microcomputer system for her office. Write a letter of proposal that suggests a disciplined approach to selecting an appropriate hardware/software system. Assume that your client is inclined to ignore a disciplined approach and would prefer to go to the local computer store and just buy something. In other words, defend your approach.
7. Differentiate between *validation* and *evaluation* as the terms apply to the selection of computer equipment and software.
8. What would you do if a vendor refused to respond to an RFP or RFQ using the following argument?

   "These things are not useful to you or me. They rarely tell me what you really want or need. I can do a better job by visiting your business and configuring a system to meet your needs. Also, it takes too long for me to answer all the questions in an RFP. And even if I do, you may not fully understand or appreciate the answers and their implications."
9. A programming assignment in the classroom is a subset of a system design. Obtain a copy of a programming assignment from a current course. Evaluate the design from the perspective of the system design phase tasks and the completeness of the design specification.

10. Write a letter of proposal for your last (or favorite) programming instructor. Suggest a disciplined approach to developing a system specification to guide the programming assignments for the next term. Your goal should be system (of programming) specifications that will eliminate or drastically reduce the need for students to request clarification from the systems analyst (played by the instructor). Defend your approach.
11. Obtain a copy of a computer programming assignment. Assume that the assignment is to be implemented on a microcomputer that has not been acquired. Estimate the costs necessary to complete the project (hardware, programming, and so forth). State your assumptions about salaries, supplies, and whatever else seems relevant.
12. Explain how the time spent on system design can best be managed.

ANNOTATED REFERENCES AND SUGGESTED READINGS

Isshiki, Koichiro R. *Small Business Computers: A Guide to Evaluation and Selection.* Englewood Cliffs, N.J.: Prentice-Hall, 1982. Although it is oriented to small computers, this book surveys most of the better-known strategies and methods for validating and evaluating vendor proposals. It also surveys most of the steps of the selection process, although they are not placed into the perspective of the entire systems development life cycle.

Joslin, Edward O. *Computer Selection* (Augmented Edition). Fairfax Station, Va.: Technology Press, 1977. Although somewhat dated, the concepts and selection methodology originally suggested in this classic book are still applicable. The book provides keen insights into vendor, customer, and user relations.

Analysts in Action

Output and File Design for the New System

Cheryl and Doug have completed their requirements statement for the new order-entry system and have selected what appears to be the most feasible solution. Now they must design the computer-generated outputs and computer files for the new system.

Episode 5

Two weeks have passed since the feasibility report was completed. The Data Processing Steering Committee has approved the report. Meanwhile, Cheryl and Doug have begun working on the design. Because the requirements statement had thoroughly defined all data flows and data stores for the new system, Cheryl and Doug were able to work independently—Cheryl on the design of computer files and Doug on design of computer outputs. To maintain consistency, they will cross-check their final specifications.

Doug has completed the first-draft design specifications for some of the reports to be produced by the new system. Doug, Joey, and Madge are reviewing the proposed reports in Joey's office.

Output Specifications for the New System

"You look tired, Joey!" said Doug. "Did the storm keep you up last night?"

"Yeah! My kids were scared to death. We're trying to get them not to come running into our room everytime they hear something, but that storm was pretty bad for them. Have you ever tried to sleep four to a queen-size water bed?"

"Can't say as I have. Well, we'll try to keep this meeting brief. I'd like to review some proposed reports with the two of you."

Madge's eyes lit up. "Oh good! You mean we're finally talking about the new system and exactly what it will do for us! I'm all ears."

Doug grinned. "Let's start with the Zone Order form. Based on your requirements statement, I've sketched this picture of what the form might look like (see Figure 1). Do you mind if I verify a few facts before we review the form?"

Not hearing any objections, Doug continued. "These forms will be printed in DP. But I need to know approximately how many forms would need to be printed in a single day."

"I'd say no more than a hundred a day," answered Joey.

"I suppose if you consider our expected growth in business, you'd better make that two hundred," countered Madge. "The new directive that requires us to start accepting standing orders from customers will likely cause an increase in business."

Madge was looking at the ▶

Figure 1

Sketch of the new ZONE ORDER form.

A A P, INC

AMERICAN AUTOMOTIVE PARTS, INC
P.O. BOX 4576
AIRPORT EXPRESSWAY
CINCINNATI, OH 45208

FORM 17

SALES ORDER

ORDER DATE:	CUSTOMER NO:	CUSTOMER ORDER NO.
SHIP TO:		SOLD TO:

#	PART NUMBER	DESCRIPTION	QUANTITY	UNIT MEASURE	DISCOUNT RATE	DISCOUNT	UNIT PRICE	EXT. PRICE
1								
2								
3								
4								
5								
6								
7								
8								
9								
10								

FOR OFFICE USE ONLY
DATE RECEIVED
CLERK
PREPAYMENT AMOUNT $_____

ALL SALES SUBJECT TO THE TERMS AND CONDITIONS ON REVERSE SIDE

SIGNATURE OF CUSTOMER OR REPRESENTATIVE

SUB TOTAL	
SALES TAX	
TOTAL	
PAID	
BALANCE	

ORIGINAL COPY TO SALES DEPARTMENT

form Doug was recording their answers on (see Figure 2). "Doug, what's that form you're using?"

"It's a list of output specifications I'm writing for the data processing people. I'm trying to help them anticipate the impact of your outputs on their facilities. I also want them to be able to select the best printer for your needs," answered Doug. "Which leads to my next question. Do you still need four carbons for each form?"

Madge nodded. "Absolutely! But do they have to be carbons? I hate getting that mess all over myself."

Doug smiled and responded, "No. Let me just note that you want chemical carbons. Chemical carbons are safe and clean, and no actual carbon paper is used. The paper is treated with a chemical that darkens under the pressure of your pen. Okay, now, let's look at that sketch. What do you think about the design?"

"It looks pretty good. What is that number in the upper right-hand corner?"

Doug looked over Joey's shoulder and answered, "It's a form's sequence number. It identifies the sequence number of the form. It's entirely for data processing control purposes. Don't confuse it with ORDER NUMBER. ORDER NUMBER will be printed according to the coding scheme you're used to."

"Will we have to print that ▶

Figure 2

Typical output specifications.

Data Dictionary: Output

Name of Output ZONE ORDER

(MASTER, PICKING, PACKING, SHIPPING)

Ref.	Data Element Name	Type	Size	Edit Mask	Seq.	Source
1	ZONE ORDER NUMBER	A/N	7	X (7)		FIRST 6 DIGITS = SALES ORDER NUMBER OF APPROVED ORDER, 7TH DIGIT = ZONE OF INVENTORY
2	ZONE ORDER DATE	A/N	8	MM-DD-YYYY XX-XX-XXXX		APPROVED ORDER
3	CUSTOMER NUMBER	A/N	4	X(4)		APPROVED ORDER
4	SHIPPING ADDRESS					APPROVED ORDER
5	SHIP TO STREET ADDRESS	A/N	15	X (15)		
6	SHIP TO POST OFFICE BOX NO.	A/N	10	X (10)		
7	SHIP TO CITY	A/N	15	X (20)		
8	SHIP TO STATE	A/N	2	STANDARD CODE XX		
9	SHIP TO ZIPCODE	A/N	9	X(9)		
10	BILLING ADDRESS					APPROVED ORDER
11	BILL TO STREET ADDRESS	A/N	15	X(15)		
12	BILL TO POST OFFICE BOX NO.	A/N	10	X (10)		
13	BILL TO CITY	A/N	20	X (20)		
14	BILL TO STATE	A/N	2	STANDARD CODE XX		
15	BILL TO ZIPCODE	A/N	9	X(9)		
16	PART NUMBER	A/N	9	X(9)	1	APPROVED ORDER
17	PART DESCRIPTION	A/N	20	X(20)		APPROVED ORDER

ORDER NUMBER?" asked Madge.

"No," answered Doug. "The system will do it."

"Could you reverse the SHIP TO and SOLD TO addresses?" asked Madge. "They're reversed from the way they're located on the current form. You can be sure that will cause confusion."

"Oops! I had no idea I had reversed them. Now you know why I asked you to look these over." Doug made some corrections on a new form (see Figure 3).

Madge continued. "I hate to ▶

Figure 3

Typical printer spacing chart.

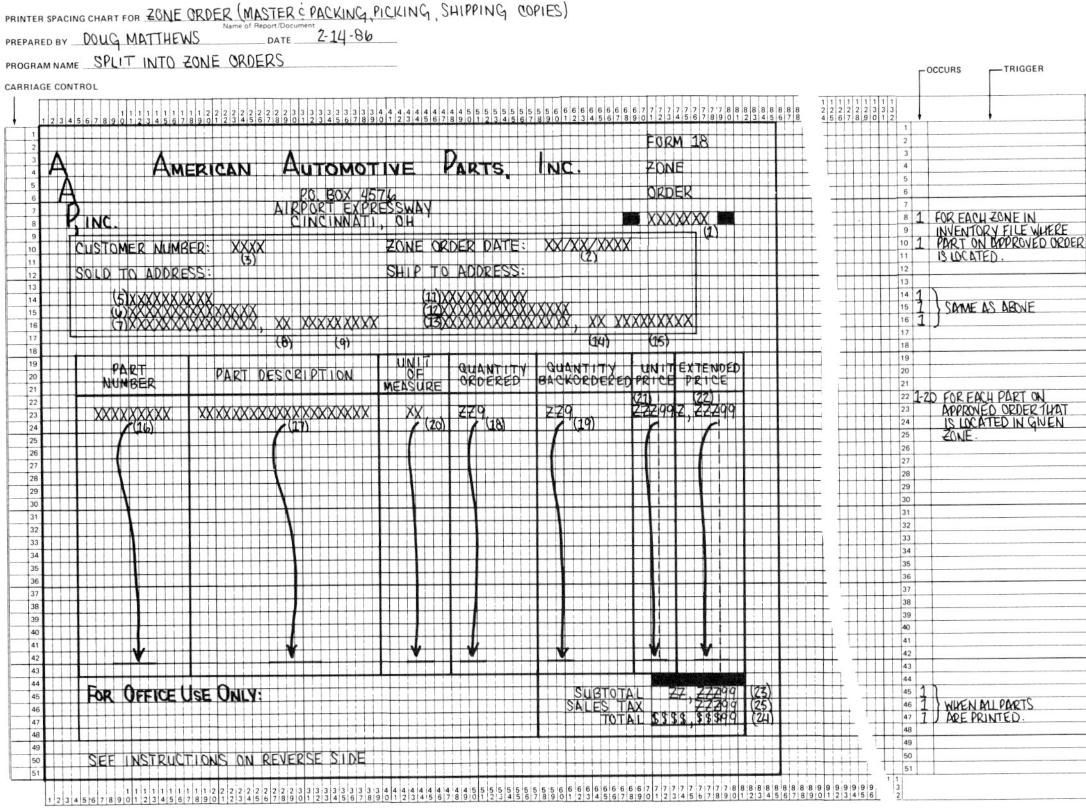

sound nosy, but what's that form you just marked on? I hope I don't have to read that one. It looks terribly confusing."

Doug smiled. "Fear not! This is a Printer Spacing Chart. I use it to communicate the final layout to the computer programmers. Well, back to the form — is there anything else? Let's look at the columns . . ."

The walkthrough continued in this manner. Doug eventually completed the specifications for all the outputs. After reviewing the first outputs with the users, Doug requested that they sketch the first draft of several other outputs. This generated user interest and amplified their sense of ownership in the system. Doug walked through their designs and carefully resolved inconsistencies with the original requirements statement. As re- ▶

Figure 4

Typical record layout chart.

RECORD LAYOUT CHART FOR ORDERS FILE
name of file
PREPARED BY: CHERYL MASON
DATE PREPARED: MARCH 12, 1986

Field Name	SALES ORDER NUMBER	CUSTOMER NUMBER	PREPAYMENT AMOUNT	ORDER DATE	ORDER TYPE	ORDER STATUS	NUMBER OF ORDERED PARTS
Characteristics*	Z	Z	P	Z	Z	Z	P
Position**	0-6	7-10	11-14	15-22	23	24	25-26

PART NUMBER	PART DESCRIPTION	QUANTITY BACKORDERED	UNIT PRICE	
Z	Z	P	P	OCCURS 1 TO 40 TIMES

port sketches were finalized, Doug prepared the more formal design specifications and layout charts.

File Specifications for the New System

Meanwhile, Cheryl has been working on the design of the new system's computer files. She chose not to directly involve users because file design is very technical to the users. We join Cheryl as she is finalizing her file design documentation.

Doug enters Cheryl's office. "Hi, Cheryl. Aha! Do I detect Record Layout Charts?" Doug had noticed the charts (see the sample in Figure 4) on Cheryl's desk.

"Yes, I'm just about done with these files. How are you coming with the outputs?" Cheryl looked relieved.

"All done!"

Cheryl continued, "Good! Have you got a few minutes to spare? I'd like you to review these files. Then we can go to lunch together. OK?"

"You bet," said Doug.

"These layout charts aren't too complicated. Just your basic fixed- and variable-length record files. During your output design walkthroughs, did you discover any new file requirements?"

Doug responded, "None that I haven't already told you about. We did a good job on those requirements. And I've kept you up to date on all changes as they occurred."

"Good. I'd like to review some more technical aspects of the file designs with you. Here are the specifications for the ORDERS file. Most of this is pretty straightforward. I was considering hashing the file because all of the programs require direct access."

Doug interrupted. "Hey, wait a minute. Where's the PRODUCE SALES ORDER LOG program? And what about the SUMMARIZE SALES BY PRODUCT LINE program? They both require the ORDERS file."

Cheryl answered, "*That's* where I blew it. Because those two programs access nearly all the records in the file, I should change the organization to indexed. I think I owe you lunch! Let's take these specifications and finish this discussion over a Chef salad." ▶

Where Do We Go from Here?

This episode previewed two tasks that are accomplished during systems design—the design of computer-generated outputs and the design of computer files. Cheryl and Doug may have used some terminology you aren't too familiar with. Furthermore, you saw some documentation that you may not have seen before. In the following two chapters, you will learn about the design issues and tools introduced in this episode. You will learn how to design computer-generated outputs in Chapter 11. In Chapter 12, you will learn how to design computer files.

This episode also reinforced the need to develop good communication skills. Doug, especially, spent considerable time conducting walkthroughs with users. To learn more about how to make presentations and conduct walkthroughs, we suggest you read Part IV, Module C, "Communication Skills for the Systems Analyst." ■

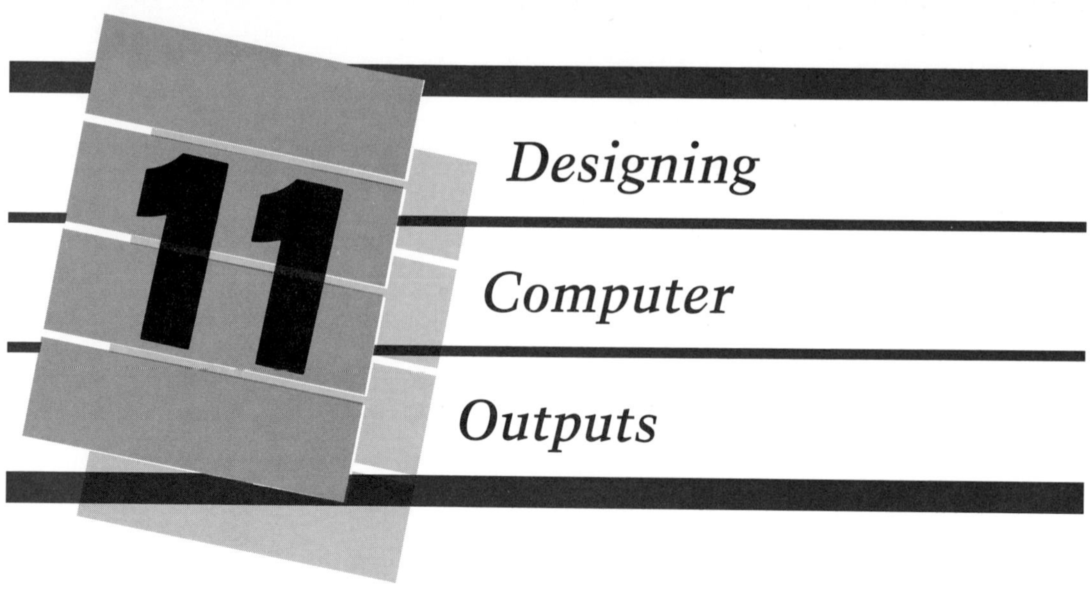

11 Designing Computer Outputs

Minicase:
New Wave Fashions, Inc.

John Weaver had a nine o'clock appointment with Mike Hayes, the Accounts Receivable manager. John was the systems analyst responsible for the accounts receivable system implemented last fall. Mike had requested the meeting to voice his displeasure with the new system. The conversation began as follows:

Mike John, I'm having a little trouble with this new accounts receivable system. I was told the information I would receive from the new system would make my job much easier, and it just doesn't.

John What isn't working for you, Mike? We included all the fields you requested. Aren't you getting the reports on time?

Mike That's not the problem. It's just that I find the report difficult to use. For example, this report doesn't tell me what I need to know. I spend most of my time trying to interpret it.

John Why don't you tell me how you use the report?

Mike Well, first I read down the report, line by line, and attempt to count and classify the number of customer accounts that are less than ten days past due, the number that are twenty to thirty days past due, and the number that are more than thirty days past due. You see, I have this graph here that shows the totals for each category over the past twelve months. I compare the new totals from this report with the totals on the graph to identify any significant trends in our ability to collect on accounts. I also use the report to identify any customer accounts that have been repeatedly overdue. To do this, I choose the particular customer account off the report and look up that customer's account record on this previous copy of the report. If the record shows that the customer has had previous overdue account balances, I instruct my subordinates to take proper action.

John Hmmm, we did a data dictionary entry for this report. I assumed I understood what information you were requesting. Sounds as if there're some additional data that should appear on the report. You're wasting a lot of time looking for information.

Mike That's right. And I hope you can do something about it. I'm pretty frustrated with that report.

John I'm sure I can have it fixed in no time. I'm really sorry. I guess I just didn't understand what information you wanted and how you would be using it.

Mike Now, let's talk about this other report. I'm getting some flack about this report I asked you to produce for my subordinates. It was supposed to list those customer accounts that owe us money. Anyhow, they claim the report is too cluttered and is difficult to use. All they really needed to know was the customer's account number, current balance due, and the balance past due. As you can see, there are a number of unnecessary fields, and the report lists two customer accounts on the same line. Could you clean this report up too?

John No problem. I'm sorry I was so off-target on those reports.

Discussion

1. What type of report was Mike receiving?
2. What type of report(s) does Mike really need?
3. What did John do wrong? What erroneous assumption did John make regarding data requirements for the reports?
4. Why do you suppose the report for Mike's subordinates was inappropriate? Who's to blame, Mike or John?

WHAT WILL YOU LEARN IN THIS CHAPTER?

In this chapter, you will learn how to design and document computer outputs using two new tools, the printer spacing chart and the display layout chart. You will know that you have mastered the tools and techniques of output design when you can:

1. Define the appropriate format and media for a computer output.
2. Differentiate between internal, external, and turnaround outputs.
3. Apply human factors to the design of computer outputs.
4. Design internal controls into computer outputs.
5. Identify data flows on the DFD that must be designed as computer outputs.
6. Define output design requirements, and record those requirements in an expanded data dictionary format.
7. Use printer spacing charts and display layout charts to format internal and external computer outputs.

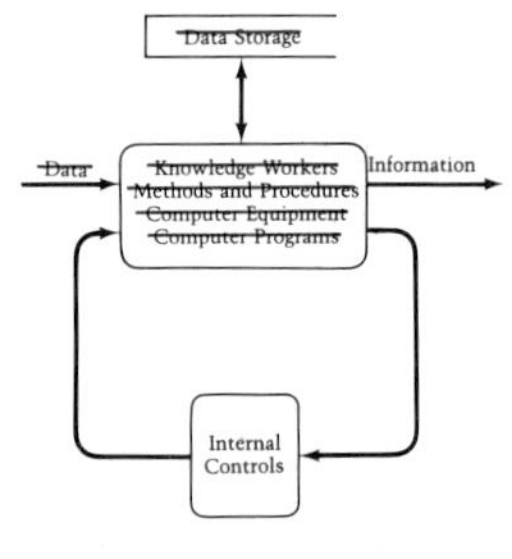

IPO Components

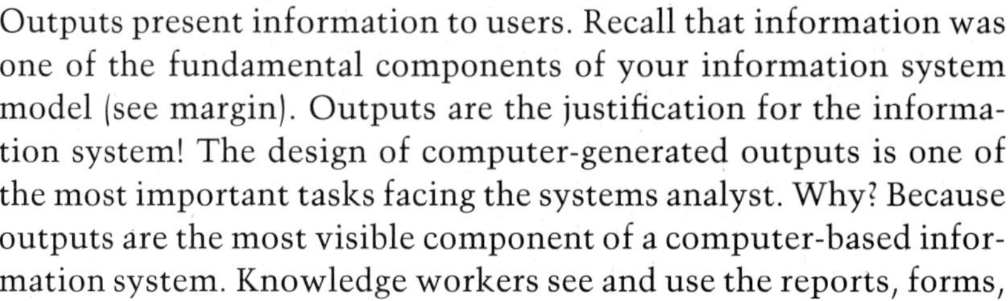
Outputs present information to users. Recall that information was one of the fundamental components of your information system model (see margin). Outputs are the justification for the information system! The design of computer-generated outputs is one of the most important tasks facing the systems analyst. Why? Because outputs are the most visible component of a computer-based information system. Knowledge workers see and use the reports, forms,

and queries. During systems analysis, you identified the need for outputs but you didn't design those outputs. Output design is usually the first systems design task because output designs will determine many of the requirements for input, file, and program design. In this chapter, you will learn how to design effective outputs.

OUTPUTS ARE FOR PEOPLE

So we're going to learn how to design computer outputs. All we need are a few printer spacing charts and we can begin, right? If that's your initial impression, you're mistaken! There is much more to output design than printer spacing charts. You may have designed reports for a computer programming class assignment. But you probably never had to justify your design to users—except, perhaps, your instructor who may have played the role of user. There are many output issues that must be addressed *before* the output is designed. And most of them are people-oriented.

Human Factor Issues for Output Design

It is particularly important to consider human factors when designing computer outputs. Knowledge workers must find such outputs easy to use and useful to their jobs. The following factors are pertinent:

1. *Computer outputs should be simple to read and interpret.* Computer jargon and computer error messages should not be included in the output. Titles, column headings, section headings, and legends should be provided to help the user read the output. Spacing and page breaks should be employed to enhance readability. On many computer outputs, these factors are ignored, and consequently, they appear cluttered and disorganized, making them difficult or impossible to use.
2. *The timing of computer outputs is important.* Outputs must be received by their recipients while the information is pertinent to transactions or decisions.
3. *The distribution of computer outputs must be sufficient to assist all relevant knowledge workers.*

4. *The computer outputs must be acceptable to the knowledge workers who will receive them.* An output design may fulfill the information requirements and still not be acceptable to the user. To avoid this, the systems analyst must understand how the recipient plans to use the output. This appeared to be the problem Mike was experiencing with his reports in the New Wave Fashions minicase.

Computer-Generated Ouputs: Media, Formats, and Classes

We assume you are familiar with different output devices, such as printers, plotters, computer output on microfilm (COM), and cathode ray tube (CRT) displays and terminals. These are standard topics in any introductory Data Processing course. In this chapter, we are more concerned with the actual output than with the device. A good systems analyst will consider all available options for implementing an output, especially medium and format options. A **medium** is what the output information is recorded on (for example, paper). The **format** is the way the information is displayed on that medium (for instance, columns of numbers). To select an appropriate medium and format for an output, consider the human factors we discussed earlier, paying particular attention to how the output will be used and when it is needed.

Alternative Media for Presenting Information The most common medium for computer outputs is paper; such outputs are called printed output. Currently, paper is the cheapest of the three media we will survey. Although paper is plentiful, it is also bulky. Storage of paper reports and documents has become a major problem for many firms.

To overcome the paper storage problem, many businesses have turned to the use of film as an output medium. There are two film formats: microfilm and microfiche. **Microfilm** is a roll of photographic film that is used to record information in a reduced size. **Microfiche** is a single sheet of film that is capable of storing many pages of reduced output. The use of film does present its own problems — microfiche and microfilm can only be produced and read by expensive special equipment.

The fastest growing medium for computer outputs is video, the display of information on a visual display device, such as a CRT terminal. Although this medium provides convenient user access to the desired information, the information is only temporary. When the image leaves the screen, that information is lost unless it is redisplayed. If a permanent copy of the information is required, paper and film are superior media.

Alternative Formats for Presenting Information There are several formats you can consider for communicating information on a medium. The **table** is the most common format for computer-generated information. The tabular format presents information as columns or designated areas of information. Most transaction documents and management reports use such a format. And most of the computer programs you've written generated tabular information on paper.

Graphic output is becoming an increasingly popular alternative format for information. To the knowledge worker, a picture can be more valuable than words. Bar charts, pie charts, line charts, step charts, histograms, and other graphs can help knowledge workers see trends and data relationships that cannot be easily seen in tabular reports. The popularity of graphics output has been stimulated by the availability of low-cost, easy-to-use graphics printers and software.

Another current trend is the increased use of the narrative format. In this type of format, words replace or supplement numbers and pictures. Word processing technology has exploited the narrative format for reports, business letters, and personalized form letters. You may already be familiar with mail that begins with, "Congratulations, *Jeff Whitten!* You may have already won $500,000 in our SO YOU'VE NEVER WON ANYTHING sweepstakes."

Classes of Reports and Documents There are two basic classes of computer outputs — external outputs and internal outputs. **External outputs** leave the system to trigger actions on the part of the recipients or confirm actions to the recipient. A customer invoice is an example of an external output. Invoices are sent to customers (outside the system) to prompt (trigger) them to make a payment (action). Most transaction outputs are external outputs. Examples of external outputs are listed in the margin. Most external outputs are designed as preprinted forms that are loaded onto the printer and then completed by an appropriate computer program. Many preprinted forms are specially designed to be burst, folded, or mailed.

External Outputs

- Invoices
- Paychecks
- Course Schedules
- Customer Receipts
- Airline Tickets
- Telephone Bills

Some external outputs are designed as **turnaround documents.** These documents are designed in such a way that all or part of the form reenters the system as a transaction input at a later date. Thus the document is both an output and an input of the system. The revolving charge account invoice depicted in Figure 11.1 is a typical external and turnaround document. Half of this output is the customer's account statement and is retained by the customer. The other half is returned with the customer's payment and input to the system.

Internal outputs are intended to support management planning, control, and decision-making activities. They stay inside the system to support the system. These outputs include all of the detailed reports, summary reports, exception reports, and decision support inquiries you learned about in Chapter 3. Sample internal outputs are shown in Figure 11.2.

Internal Controls for Information **Internal controls** are a requirement in all computer-based systems. They ensure that the computer-based system is protected against accidental and intentional errors and use, including fraud. In this book, we will cover classes of controls for each task in system design. Output controls ensure the reliability and distribution of the outputs generated by the computer. The following are some guidelines for establishing output controls:

- *The timing and volume of each output must be precisely specified.* You cannot simply state that a report is needed daily. When daily? 8:00 A.M.? 10:30 A.M.? 2:00 P.M.? Computer facilities offer limited resources, and the systems analyst must discuss an appropriate schedule with the computer operations staff.
- *The distribution of all outputs must be specified.* For each output, the recipients of all copies must be determined. Additionally, a distribution log is frequently established. This log provides an audit trail for the outputs. The dates, output titles, and recipients of all copies are logged. Occasionally, the initials of the recipient are also entered.
- *Access controls are used to control accessibility of video outputs.* For example, a password may be required to display a certain output on a CRT terminal.
- *Control totals should be incorporated into all reports.* These controls can be compared with the input controls that will be

5574831011 0044445 96486803829900055

ACCOUNT NUMBER	CLOSING DATE	NEW BALANCE	MINIMUM PAYMENT DUE
55-748-3101-1	03-05-86	88.80	88.80

PAYMENT IS DUE UPON RECEIPT OF STATEMENT. PAY EITHER AMOUNT.

PLEASE INDICATE AMOUNT PAID

DOLLARS	CENTS

MAKE CHECK PAYABLE TO WESTERN OIL CO.
RETURN THIS PORTION WITH CHECK.
INDICATE ACCOUNT NUMBER ON CHECK.

P. O. BOX 3576
SAN FRANCISCO, CA
94123-2300

MICHAEL WINTERS
1414 LINDBERGH DRIVE
MEDFORD, OR 97504

NEW ADDRESS

PLEASE PRINT STREET

CITY STATE ZIP CODE

ACCOUNT NUMBER 55-748-3101-1 CLOSING DATE 03-05-86

PLEASE PLACE YOUR ON ALL CORRESPONDENCE AND INDICATE THE DATE AND REFERENCE NUMBER SHOWN BELOW, IF APPLICABLE

SEND INQUIRIES TO: WESTERN OIL CO.
P.O. BOX 4400
DENVER, CO 80203
(303) 550-2600

TRAN. DATE		REFERENCE NUMBER	PRODUCT CODE	TRANSACTION LOCATION/DESCRIPTION	AMOUNT (CR=CREDIT)
02	05	045762212662	1	534COUNTRY FMRD MEDFORD OR	11.20

PREVIOUS BALANCE	PAYMENTS/CREDITS	CHARGES	FINANCE CHARGE	NEW BALANCE
76.45		11.20	1.15	88.80

TO AVOID ADDITIONAL FINANCE CHARGE PAYMENT OF NEW BALANCE MUST BE RECEIVED BY 03-30-86

MINIMUM PAYMENT DUE 88.80

SCHEDULE OF FINANCE CHARGES

BALANCE RANGE	PERIODIC RATE (MONTHLY)	ANNUAL PERCENTAGE RATE
TO $ / OVER $ 000	1.50 %	18.00 %

BALANCE SUBJECT TO FINANCE CHARGE SEE REVERSE SIDE	
76.45	A

NOTICE: SEE REVERSE SIDE FOR IMPORTANT INFORMATION.

PLEASE KEEP THIS PORTION FOR YOUR RECORDS

DO 54495-B

Figure 11.1

Sample external turnaround document. This output is *external* because it initiates a transaction (payment). It is also a turnaround output because a portion of the output is returned, with payment, as input.

PAGE 01

SUMMARY OF MONTHLY
BANK MACHINE TRANSACTIONS
FOR THE PERIOD 03/01/86 TO 03/31/86

MACHINE NUMBER	BRANCH NUMBER	NUMBER OF DEPOSITS	AMOUNT OF DEPOSITS	NUMBER OF WITHDRAWALS	AMOUNT OF WITHDRAWALS	NUMBER OF TRANSFERS	AMOUNT OF TRANSFERS	NUMBER OF LOAN PAYMENTS	AMOUNT OF LOAN PAYMENTS
01	01	192	57,600.32	672	31,213.50	140	14,025.33	23	1,725.86
02	03	134	43,756.45	478	23,144.75	63	6,192.88	11	1,545.38
03	05	112	47,650.44	462	24,897.26	43	5,023.61	13	1,195.76
05	07	155	49,864.04	567	27,875.00	97	11,729.58	15	2,304.42
06	08	234	61,768.34	748	37,563.73	153	17,688.93	26	2,112.45

TOTAL DOLLARS DEPOSITED	$260,639.59
TOTAL DOLLARS WITHDRAWN	$144,694.24
TOTAL DOLLARS PAID ON LOANS	$ 8,883.87
TOTAL DOLLARS TRANSFERRED	$ 54,660.33

10/02/86 INTERNATIONAL MANUFACTURING COMPANY PAGE 1

BONUS REPORT

CLOCK NUMBER	SHIFT	CLOCK HOURS	INCENTIVE HOURS	DOWN TIME	BONUS PERCENT	BONUS HOURS
1000	1	35.5	30.0	05.5	150	15.0
1010	1	40.0	32.0	08.0	110	03.2
1020	2	40.0	31.5	08.5	142	13.2
1030	2	36.5	20.3	16.2	113	02.6
1040	3	09.4	08.2	01.2	144	03.6
1050	3	10.2	02.8	07.4	107	00.2
2000	1	55.0	45.3	09.7	134	15.4
2010	1	50.0	33.2	16.8	139	12.9
2020	3	12.1	03.4	08.7	132	01.1
2030	2	20.4	17.9	02.5	125	04.5
3000	1	16.8	12.6	04.2	127	03.4
3010	2	40.5	30.1	10.4	104	01.2
3020	3	40.0	29.0	11.0	143	12.5
3040	3	32.0	29.5	02.5	147	13.9
3050	1	07.0	03.8	03.2	141	01.6
4000	2	60.2	47.8	12.4	150	23.9
4010	1	61.4	50.3	11.1	117	08.6
4020	3	14.7	08.5	06.2	121	01.8
5000	1	50.0	44.1	05.9	100	00.0
5010	1	52.5	40.0	12.5	133	13.2
TOTALS:		684.2	520.3	163.9		151.8

◀ **Figure 11.2**

Sample internal outputs. Internal outputs include the detail reports, summary reports, and exception reports you've studied throughout this textbook. They are intended primarily for use by managers.

discussed in Chapter 13. The number of records input should equal the number of records output. These control totals are compared before the outputs are distributed. If a discrepancy is found, the outputs are retained until the cause has been determined and corrected.

We'll apply these controls later in this chapter.

HOW TO DESIGN FORMS, REPORTS, AND SCREENS

In this section, we'll discuss both an output design process and the issues that need to be addressed in that process. We'll introduce some special purpose tools for documenting output design, and we'll also be applying the concepts you learned in the last section.

Identify the Output Requirements of the New System

Many output design requirements have already been addressed during systems analysis. A good starting point for output design is the data flow diagram. Look at the DFD in Figure 11.3. How is this DFD different from those you have already encountered? The difference is the **person-machine boundary** that has been added to the DFD. This bounded data flow diagram is normally drawn during the evaluation phase of systems analysis. It represents an alternative solution that was evaluated for feasibility during that phase.

Every data flow that travels across the boundary of the DFD, from the machine side to the person side, is an output that must be designed. We have noted all outputs with shaded bullets on the boundary in Figure 11.3. The bounded DFD also indicates preliminary medium and design decisions (such as the four-part form notation on the figure).

We can also learn more about these computer-generated output data flows by reviewing their associated data dictionary entries. These entries are typically generated during the definition phase of systems analysis. The data dictionary outlines the basic content of

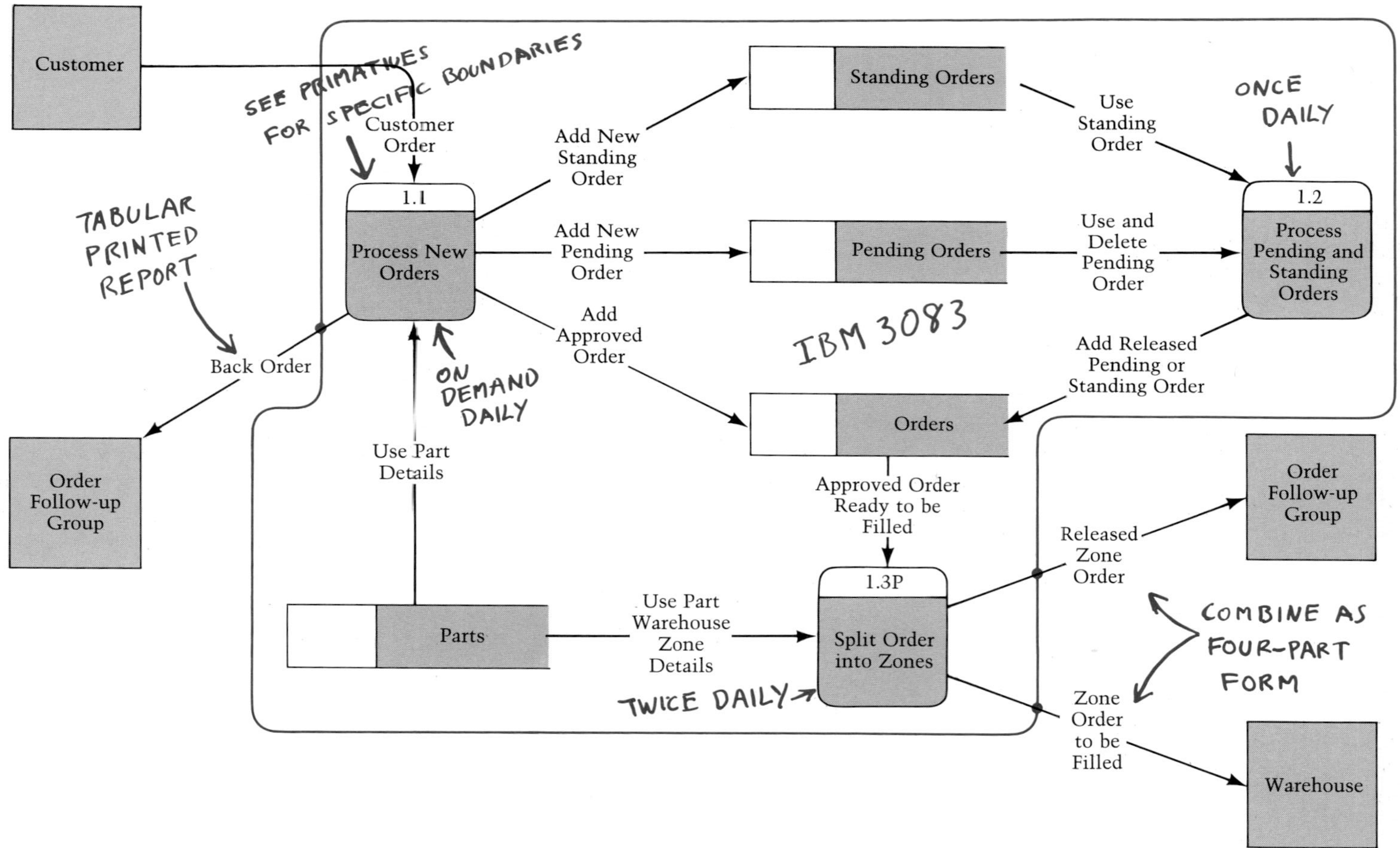

Figure 11.3

A bounded data flow diagram for AAP. When evaluating alternative solutions, the systems analyst will add the person-machine boundary to a logical data flow diagram. The systems analysts may also annotate the DFD with specific implementation requirements.

the outputs. During systems design, we will expand our understanding of each output by addressing numerous design issues. As we'll see later, we will want to include additional details about an output in the data dictionary.

Make Detailed Output Design Decisions

An output design must be communicated to the user, forms manufacturers, computer operators, and computer programmers. Failure to address important design issues with any of these individuals will have a negative impact on the success of the new system. The prerequisite to output design is to understand the type and purpose of the output. Is the output an internal or external report? If it's an internal report, is it a historical, detailed, summary, or exception report? If it's an external report, is the form a turnaround document? After assuring yourself that you understand what type of report the output is and how it will be used, you need to address the following design issues:

1. *What medium would best serve the output?* Alternative media were discussed earlier in the chapter. You will have to understand the purpose or use of the output to determine the proper medium. You can select more than one medium (for instance, video with optional paper). All of these decisions are best addressed with the users.

2. *What would be the best format for the report?* Tabular? Graphic? Words? Some combination of these? After establishing the format, you can determine what type of form or paper will be used. Standard stock fan-fold paper comes in three standard sizes: eight and a half by eleven, eleven by fourteen, and eight by fourteen inches. Many printers can easily compress 132 columns of print into an eight-inch width.

   If a preprinted form is to be used, requirements for that form must be specified. Should the form be designed for mailing? What should be the size of the form? Is the form to be perforated so it can be burst into several sections (recall Figure 11.1)? Are special instructions to be printed on the reverse side of the form? What colors are the various copies of the form? Incidentally, form images can be stored and printed with modern laser printers, thereby eliminating the need for preprinted forms in some businesses.

   All of these issues should be addressed to the users.

3. *How frequently is the output generated?* On demand? Hourly? Daily? Monthly? For scheduled outputs, when do users need the report? Scheduled reports have to be worked into the data processing operations schedule. For instance, a report the user needs by 9:00 A.M. on Thursday, may have to be scheduled for 5:30 A.M. Thursday. No other time may be available.
4. *How many pages of output will be generated for a single copy of a report?* How many special forms will be printed in a single run of a program? These data are necessary to accurately plan paper consumption, form ordering, and printer schedules.
5. *Does the output require multiple copies?* For reports, there are several copying alternatives:

   - Photocopy (doesn't tie up printer)
   - Carbon copies (most printers can make no more than six legible carbons)
   - Duplicate printing (requires the most printer time, although laser printers are changing this situation)

   For external documents, there are also several alternatives:

   - Carbon and chemical carbon are the most common duplicating techniques. Use of either of these must be arranged with the forms manufacturer.
   - Selective (partial) carbon is a variation on the previous technique. Selective carbon allows certain fields on the master form *not to be printed* on one or more of the carbon copies. The fields to be omitted must be communicated to the forms manufacturer.
   - Two-up printing is a technique whereby two sets of forms (possibly including carbons) are printed side by side on the printer.
6. For printed outputs, distribution controls should be finalized. For on-line outputs, access controls should be determined.

Lay Out the Output Format

The format or layout of an output directly affects the user's ability to read and interpret it. The format of an output is also one of the more difficult design requirements to complete and communicate to computer programmers. The format of a printed or displayed output includes title, headings, data elements, spacing, page breaks, and other details of importance to the computer programmer who must implement the report. Two tools available for describing the format of outputs are the printer spacing chart and the display layout chart. Let's see how these tools are used to design outputs.

Using Printer Spacing Charts to Document the Format of Printed Outputs **Printer spacing charts** should be used to describe the format of printed outputs. A sample printer spacing chart is provided in Figure 11.4. Don't worry about understanding the report — concentrate on the tool. The form has been annotated with circled numbers that are explained in the following guidelines:

① PRINTING GRID The printing grid indicates the print positions by row and column. Vertical and horizontal lines should be drawn to indicate the size and shape of the form or paper to be used. The grid chart is not necessarily to scale. Dot matrix printers can often print 132 columns on an 8.5-inch-wide form.

② CARRIAGE CONTROL Carriage controls identify the first and last print lines on a form. For most printers, carriage controls are stored in a small memory buffer in the printer. The computer programmer can specify spacing (for example, new page, double space) by using the carriage controls within their programs. The carriage controls for most standard stock paper sizes are preprogrammed into the printer's memory. But what about special preprinted forms?

For special forms, the systems analyst must specify the carriage controls to be loaded into the printer whenever that form is mounted on the printer. Depending on the printer used, up to twelve channels can be defined for a form. Each channel is given a number that forces the printer to skip to the line indicated on the printer spacing chart. Two channels are normally reserved:

1 first line *to be printed*
12 last line *to be printed*

The remaining channels, 2 through 11, can be defined by the analyst. Normally, they are used to skip several lines for which nothing is to be printed so the printer doesn't have to single space through those lines.

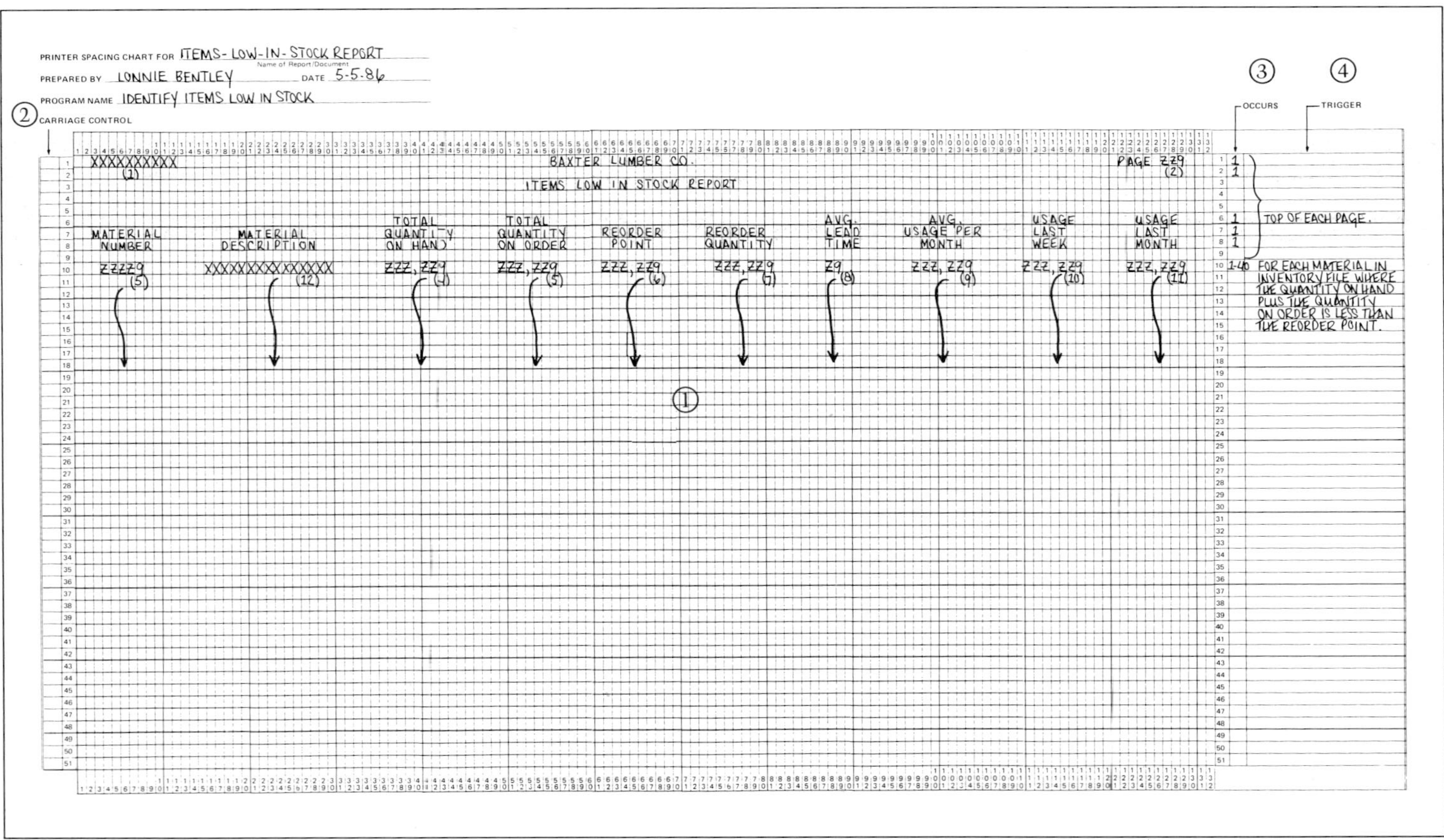

Figure 11.4

Sample printer spacing chart. This printer spacing chart communicates the format of the internal exception report ITEMS-LOW-IN-STOCK. Printer spacing charts are best used to communicate the format of printed outputs to computer programmers.

③ OCCURS For the corresponding line on the printer spacing chart this item specifies the number of times that line may be printed *on one page* of the report or document.

④ TRIGGER This column describes the conditions for printing the corresponding lines on the printer spacing chart. For example, some of the lines recorded on the chart might only be printed at the top or bottom of each page or whenever a control break occurs. A concise description of the trigger should be recorded for each line to be printed by the printer.

The trigger column can also be used to record any miscellaneous comments that should be communicated to the computer programmer.

The printing grid is used to formally specify the layout of both constant and variable information for the report or document. We'll discuss this later in the chapter.

Caution! Printer spacing charts are not intended for user verification. Users tend to be somewhat put off by the editing symbols and conventions. The best way to verify outputs is to sketch or, better still, generate a sample of the report or document. Show that sketch or prototype to the user, get feedback, and make modifications to the sample. Use realistic or reasonable data, and demonstrate all control breaks. After the user has approved the format, finalize that format as a formal printer spacing chart with which to communicate the final design to the programmer!

Using Display Layout Charts to Document the Format of Visual Outputs The guidelines for documenting video or display output are similar to those for preparing printed output. The only difference is that the size of the display screen limits the amount of data that can be displayed at one time. Furthermore, the user must page or scroll through the information being presented. Terminal screen **display layout charts** are used to document typical screens (80-column limit). For screens wider than 80 columns, printer spacing charts can be used.

A sample display layout chart for describing a video version of an items-low-in-stock report is illustrated in Figure 11.5. Again, don't bother trying to understand the report. Familiarize yourself with the form. The circled numbers call your attention to the following guidelines *(text continues on page 417):*

TERMINAL SCREEN DISPLAY LAYOUT FORM

APPLICATION IDENTIFY ITEMS LOW IN STOCK

SCREEN NO. ________ SEQUENCE ________

☐ INPUT ________

☒ OUTPUT ITEMS LOW IN STOCK

COLUMN

```
01                                    ITEMS LOW IN STOCK
02                                    AS OF XX/XX/XXXX
03                        (3)                (1)
04 MATERIAL NUMBER: ZZZZ9
05 DESCRIPTION:           XXXXXXXXXXXXXXX
06                                (12)
07  TOTAL      TOTAL                                    AVG.      AVG.        USAGE      USAGE
08 QUANTITY   QUANTITY  REORDER   REORDER    LEAD  USAGE PER     LAST       LAST
09 ON HAND    ON ORDER    POINT    QUANTITY   TIME     MONTH        WEEK      MONTH
10
11 ZZZ,ZZ9   ZZZ,ZZ9   ZZZ,ZZ9   ZZZ,ZZ9   Z9    ZZZ,ZZ9   ZZZ,ZZ9   ZZZ,ZZ9
12     (4)       (5)       (6)       (7)   480 (8)   (9)       (10)      (11)   1960
13
14                         ZZZZ9
15                         XXXXXXXXXXXXXXX
16
17 ZZZ,ZZ9   ZZZ,ZZ9   ZZZ,ZZ9   ZZZ,ZZ9   Z9    ZZZ,ZZ9   ZZZ,ZZ9   ZZZ,ZZ9
18
19
20                         ZZZZ9
21                         XXXXXXXXXXXXXXX
22
23 ZZZ,ZZ9   ZZZ,ZZ9   ZZZ,ZZ9   ZZZ,ZZ9   Z9    ZZZ,ZZ9   ZZZ,ZZ9   ZZZ,ZZ9
24 PRESS 'F1' FOR ADDITIONAL INFO.   PRESS 'F2' TO SEE PREVIOUS SCREEN OF INFO.  1920
                                        ①
42
43                                                                          3440
```

FUNCTION KEY ASSIGNMENTS

PF1	PAGE FORWARD	PF9		PF17	
PF2	PAGE BACKWARD	PF10		PF18	
PF3		PF11	②	PF19	
PF4		PF12		PF20	
PF5		PF13		PF21	
PF6		PF14		PF22	
PF7		PF15		PF23	
PF8		PF16		PF24	

Figure 11.5

Sample terminal screen display layout chart. Terminal screen display layout charts are used to communicate the format of video or display outputs to computer programmers. The example describes the format of the ITEMS-LOW-IN-STOCK output using video as an alternative medium.

① DISPLAY GRID This section is used in exactly the same way as the way we specified for the printing grid in the printer spacing charts. You may have noticed that the number of lines (43) is greater than the number of lines that can be displayed on most screens (24). Why? The additional space allows you to indicate additional information that can be scrolled up as the user *pages* through the output.

② FUNCTION KEY ASSIGNMENTS Function key assignments, available in most CRT terminals and microcomputers, can be made. Function keys can be assigned to perform a number of tasks at the stroke of a single key. If the keyboard does not have predefined keys for *paging forward* and *paging backward* through the output, the analyst can request that such a function be programmed and assigned to a specified function key. Two common function keys for a report are *display first page of output* and *display last page of output.*

As was the case with printer spacing charts, you should not use display layout charts when seeking approval of on-line output formats from users. The editing symbols and conventions are too foreign to noncomputer personnel. Instead, sketch or program some sample screens with sample information, and walk through the screens with your users. Be sure to simulate paging and function keys. When the format has been approved, finalize the design on the display layout charts for your computer programmers.

Now that we've covered the output design process, let's study some sample output designs.

SAMPLE OUTPUT DESIGNS

Output design is so critical to the success of the information system that we want to walk through some sample designs. Although many outputs could have been presented, we have chosen one example for each of the most common outputs: a preprinted form (external output), a printed report (internal output), and a video display inquiry response. Most outputs will be easy to design if you understand these three examples.

The Next Generation

Report Writers: Output Design and Implementation Without Programmers

A significant theme in several of these "Next Generation" features has been the emergence of *prototyping* as a systems design methodology. Output design by prototyping is particularly significant because the ultimate product of any information system is *information.* Few systems analysts have avoided the frustration of carefully designing new outputs only to discover that the implementation wasn't as well received as the design. Why? There's something about seeing a working example of the final product that gets users really thinking about the usefulness and format of a new computer output. Unfortunately, writing COBOL programs to produce prototypes can be time-consuming. And modifying those programs when users make their inevitable suggestions can be a nightmare. However, a new breed of software tools has recently become a popular alternative to traditional output design and programming. We'll call them **report writers.**

In reality, report writers have been available for some time. RPG, *Report Program Generator,* was an early example of a *nonprocedural* language that made writing reports easier. By *nonprocedural* we mean that the programmer does not have to specify logic to as great an extent as in more traditional languages. Instead, at the risk of oversimplification, the programmer specifies *what* is wanted, and the built-in logic of the report writer language takes care of the logic. COBOL also offers a report writing feature in some compilers. But both RPG and COBOL are still very much oriented to the computer programmer who works from traditional output design specifications.

Modern report writers are usually incorporated into what are popularly called *fourth-generation programming languages* (4GLs). Examples of 4GLs with report writers include Information Builder's *FOCUS,* Mathematica's *RAMIS,* and Userware's *USER-11.* They provide either an easy-to-learn, English-like, concise syntax or a question and answer dialogue for prototyping new reports against an existing file or database. For instance, the *USER-11* dialogue displayed in Figure A was used by an analyst to prototype a course enrollment report — the entire report program was written in less than two minutes! If the user isn't satisfied with the report, it can be changed in less than 2 minutes! That is a significant productivity improvement over COBOL and RPG.

These 4GL report writers are becoming quite sophisticated. For instance, *FOCUS* offers a feature called *TableTalk.* This product writes *FOCUS* report writer programs for you — in other words, you don't even have to learn the *FOCUS* language (which is easier to learn than COBOL, BASIC, and other traditional languages). When you invoke *TableTalk,* you are directed through a series of windows that appear on the terminal screen. These windows display a number of report-writing options, such as the selection of files, data elements, selection criteria, sorting, control breaks, titles, headings, and format. You select the desired option by moving the cursor within the window. Meanwhile, the *FOCUS* program code is generated in a window at the bottom of the screen. Sophisticated reports can be created quickly. Another trend in 4GLs is easy-to-learn graphics. With simple com- ▶

Figure A

USER-11 dialogue.

```
4-APR-85        R E P O R T   I N S T R U C T I O N S                HEADER PAGE

DATABASE--> course/instruct/explain
DETAIL LINE SPACING <SINGLE>--> single
SPACES BETWEEN EACH COLUMN (0-20) <1>--> 5
COL#1     POS:1     FIELD--> dept.cod/break
COL#2     POS:6     FIELD--> course.no
COL#3     POS:10    FIELD--> course.nam/heading:NAME OF COURSE
COL#4     POS:31    FIELD--> dept.nam
COL#5     POS:52    FIELD--> credit.hrs/mask
  EDIT MASK--> @.@@
COL#6     POS:57    FIELD--> number.enr/total
  FIELD LENGTH <3>--> 4
  EDIT MASK--> @@@@
COL#7     POS:62    FIELD--> enroll.lmt/total
  FIELD LENGTH <3>--> 4
  EDIT MASK--> @@@@
COL#8     POS:67    FIELD--> no more fields
LINES PER PAGE <55>--> 55
LEVEL BREAKS <0>--> 1
  LEVEL 1...FIELD--> dept.cod
    TOP OF PAGE AFTER LEVEL BREAK--> no
REPORT DATE (DD-MON-YY) <SYSTEM>--> default
HEADING 1)--> COURSE ENROLLMENT REPORT
HEADING 2)--> none
NUMBER OF COPIES <1>--> 1
REPORT NAME (6 CHARACTERS MAX) <COURS>--> enroll

Note:    USER-11 prompts are capitalized.  Defaults are in brackets, "<  >".
         User responses are in upper/lower case.
```

mands or function keys, a tabular report can be converted to a bar chart, pie chart, line chart, or similar picture. Graphics will likely become the preferred management summary report of the next decade.

What impact will these new technologies have on systems design? We're already seeing reports designed and implemented by analysts using 4GLs. In many cases, the need for rewriting these programs in such traditional languages as COBOL is entirely unnecessary! But consider this possibility. If reports are so easy to design and implement with 4GLs, why not restrict the analysts' and programmers' activities to transaction processing and file and database design, loading, and maintenance? Let the users generate their own reports. An interesting shift in strategy, don't you agree? ■

Design of a Printed Form

The data flow diagram in Figure 11.3 identified that the transaction outputs RELEASED ZONE ORDER and ZONE ORDER TO BE FILLED are to be designed as a single four-part form. The different parts include the master and the picking, packing, and shipping copies. To fulfill this requirement, we will design a preprinted form with carbon copies. Today, most carbons are produced using chemically coated paper rather than messy ink carbons.

The design specifications for ZONE ORDER are presented in Figures 11.6 through 11.8. Figures 11.6 and 11.7 make up an expanded data dictionary used to record our design decisions. Figure 11.6 presents the design criteria for the output. Take a moment to scan through the entries on this form . . .

The entries are relatively self-explanatory, don't you agree? They address the issues presented earlier in this chapter. These design criteria were developed with the cooperation of the users. Notice that the content of the output is expressed using the data structure notation you learned in Chapter 8. The data structure does not include title, column headings, or other constant information.

There are also a number of design considerations for data elements that are included in an output. We record these design decisions in a data element dictionary similar to the one in Figure 11.7. Note the following items on the figure:

Ⓐ The names of the data elements were indented under the group name, similar to a COBOL data division entry. It is important to clearly indicate groups of data elements to the programmer.

Ⓑ For each data element, we specified the data type as follows:

- Numeric (N)—a data element that can be involved in arithmetic operations.
- Alphanumeric (A/N)—a data element that contains any combination of alphabetic letters, nonarithmetic numbers, and special characters.

We recommend that nonarithmetic data elements consisting only of numbers be specified as alphanumeric, instead of numeric (for example, PRODUCT NUMBER, CUSTOMER NUMBER, ZIP CODE). Why? By specifying the element as alphanumeric, we discourage the computer programmer from

```
D A T A  D I C T I O N A R Y :  O U T P U T (Page 1)

DEFINITION

- NAME OF OUTPUT:  ZONE ORDER (Master, Picking, Packing, Shipping)
- PREPARED BY:  Doug Matthews (Feb. 14, 1986)
- DESCRIPTION:  A four-part document containing that portion of a sales order
      fillable by goods located in a particular warehouse zone.
- ALIASES:  Form 18        • MEDIUM:  Paper        - OUTPUT TYPE:  External/Form
  OUTPUT CHARACTERISTICS:  Preprinted 8 1/2" X 8 1/2",  designed for mailing.
         There  are to be three copies of the zone order.   The copies should
         have different colors:
              Original/Master = White      Picking Copy       = Yellow
              Packing Copy    = Pink       Shipping Copy      = Green
  FREQUENCY PREPARED:  Daily at 8:00 A.M. and 1:00 P.M.
  VOLUME:  5,000 per day    NUMBER OF COPIES:  3
  COPYING METHOD:  Selective Carbon
  OUTPUT  RECIPIENT(S):   All copies of ZONE ORDER will be picked up by Order
                          Entry.
  SPECIAL  INSTRUCTIONS:   The data elements  PRICE,  EXTENDED  PRICE,  TOTAL
        EXTENDED PRICE, TOTAL ORDER COST,  and SALES TAX should appear on the
        Picking and Shipping  copies  of the  ZONE ORDER.  The  data elements
        QUANTITY ORDERED and QUANTITY BACKORDERED  are to be  hand entered on
        the Picking and Shipping copies.   SHIPPING ADDRESS  must be  located
        such that it will appear in the window of an envelope.

OUTPUT COMPOSITION

     A ZONE ORDER consists of the following data elements:
          ZONE ORDER NUMBER
          ZONE ORDER DATE
          CUSTOMER NUMBER
          SHIPPING ADDRESS, which is the same as ADDRESS (see below)
          BILLING ADDRESS, which is the same as ADDRESS (see below)
          1 to 20 occurrences of the following:
               PART NUMBER
               PART DESCRIPTION
               QUANTITY ORDERED
               QUANTITY BACKORDERED
               UNIT OF MEASURE
               PRICE
               EXTENDED PRICE
          TOTAL EXTENDED PRICE
          TOTAL ORDER COST
          SALES TAX

     The group ADDRESS consists of the following data elements:
          One or both of the following elements:
               STREET ADDRESS
               POST OFFICE BOX NUMBER
          CITY
          STATE
          ZIP CODE
```

Figure 11.6

The expanded data dictionary for ZONE ORDER (Page 1). An expanded data dictionary should be developed to record the details of an output. Notice that the author's forms (see also, Figure 11.7) contain appropriate entries for addressing the design issues discussed earlier in this chapter.

establishing the variable as numeric and *accidentally* performing arithmetic on that variable.

© For each data element, we specified size without including special editing symbols, such as hyphens, commas, decimal points, and slashes. The size "6.2" can be interpreted as "an 8-digit, real number with two digits to the right of the decimal point."

Figure 11.7

The expanded data dictionary for ZONE ORDER (Page 2). The expanded data dictionary also contains details about data elements to be included in the output.

```
D A T A  D I C T I O N A R Y :  O U T P U T (Page 2)

NAME OF OUTPUT:  ZONE ORDER (Master, Picking, Packing, Shipping)
PREPARED BY:  Doug Matthews (Feb. 14, 1986)

REF.   DATA ELEMENT NAME        TYPE    SIZE   EDIT MASK     SOURCE

1.     ZONE ORDER NUMBER        A/N       7       X(7)     First 6 digits =
                                                           SALES ORDER NUMBER
                                                           of approved order,
                                 (B)     (C)      (D)      7th digit  =  ZONE
                                                           of INVENTORY.
2.     ZONE ORDER DATE          A/N       8    XX-XX-XXXX     ORDERS
3.     CUSTOMER NUMBER          A/N       4       X(4)        ORDERS
4.     SHIPPING ADDRESS                                       ORDERS
5.       STREET ADDRESS         A/N      15       X(15)
6.       POST OFFICE BOX        A/N      10       X(10)
         NUMBER
7.       CITY                   A/N      15       X(15)        (E)
8.       STATE                  A/N       2    standard code
                                                  X(2)
9.       ZIP CODE               A/N       9       X(9)
10.    BILLING ADDRESS                                        ORDERS
11.      STREET ADDRESS         A/N      15       X(15)
12.      POST OFFICE BOX        A/N      10       X(10)
         NUMBER
13.      CITY                   A/N      15       X(15)
14.      STATE                  A/N       2    standard code
                                                  X(2)
15.      ZIP CODE               A/N       9       X(9)
16.   *PART NUMBER              A/N       9       X(9)        ORDERS
17.    PART DESCRIPTION         A/N      20       X(20)       ORDERS
18.    QUANTITY ORDERED          N      3.0       ZZ9         ORDERS
19.    QUANTITY BACKORDERED      N      3.0       ZZ9         ORDERS
20.    UNIT OF MEASURE          A/N       2       X(2)        ORDERS
21.   *PRICE                     N      3.2      ZZZ.99       ORDERS
22.   *EXTENDED PRICE            N      4.2    Z,ZZZ.99    Calculated:
                                                           EXTENDED  PRICE  =
                                                  QUANTITY ORDERED X PRICE
23.   *TOTAL EXTENDED PRICE      N      5.2   ZZ,ZZZ.99    Calculated:
                                                      TOTAL EXTENDED PRICE =
                                                      Sum of EXTENDED PRICEs
24.   *TOTAL ORDER COST          N      6.2  $$$$,$$$.99   Calculated:
                                                           TOTAL ORDER COST =
                                              TOTAL EXTENDED PRICE + SALES TAX
25.   *SALES TAX                 N      3.2      ZZZ.99    Calculated:
                                                                 SALES TAX =
                                          TOTAL EXTENDED PRICE X SALESTAX RATE

 (A)  (F)

*  The repeating  data elements 16-22 are to be  printed in ascending order by
   PART NUMBER.
*  The decimal point is not to be printed for data elements 21 through 25.
```

(D) You may recognize the entries under **EDIT MASK** as being standard COBOL picture entries. This communicates the editing requirements to the computer programmer. Because COBOL is one of the most commonly used programming languages, we used its editing syntax to *mask* the data element to be output. Look for a moment at Figure 11.9 which reviews these editing symbols and shows how they can be used to specify a wide variety of editing requirements.

Ⓔ The source column (Figure 11.7) tells the computer programmer where the data element to be printed comes from. The possible sources for output data include:

- The operating system (for example, DATE and TIME).
- An input (to the program producing the report).
- A file (read by the program producing the report).
- A calculation (performed by the program producing the report). In this instance, you will need to specify what data elements are involved in the calculation, the source of each data element, and the appropriate formula to be used.

Ⓕ Notice (on Figure 11.7) that an asterisk was used to reference special design requirements listed at the bottom of the form.

Figure 11.8 presents the layout of the ZONE ORDER. If different copies of the ZONE ORDER were to be different, we would have used multiple spacing charts. Let's examine the ZONE ORDER printer spacing chart in Figure 11.8. The following external report guidelines were applied to the printer spacing chart:

Ⓐ The size of the form, in terms of number of lines and columns, was drawn on the spacing chart with bold lines. Perforations can be drawn with dashed lines.

Ⓑ We drew and printed the constant information to be preprinted by the forms manufacturer. This includes title, company name, address, phone numbers, logos, form name and form number, unique identification number (if that is to be preprinted), lines and blocks that divide the document into sections, and column and field headings. Because these items are preprinted, you are not constrained to the print positions on the spacing chart. Different sizes and styles of type may be used.

Ⓒ We used our edit masks from the data element dictionary to record fields to be printed by the computer. The number in parentheses refers back to the corresponding field in the data element dictionary ("REF."). Don't record edit masks in fields to be completed by hand—that would confuse the programmer.

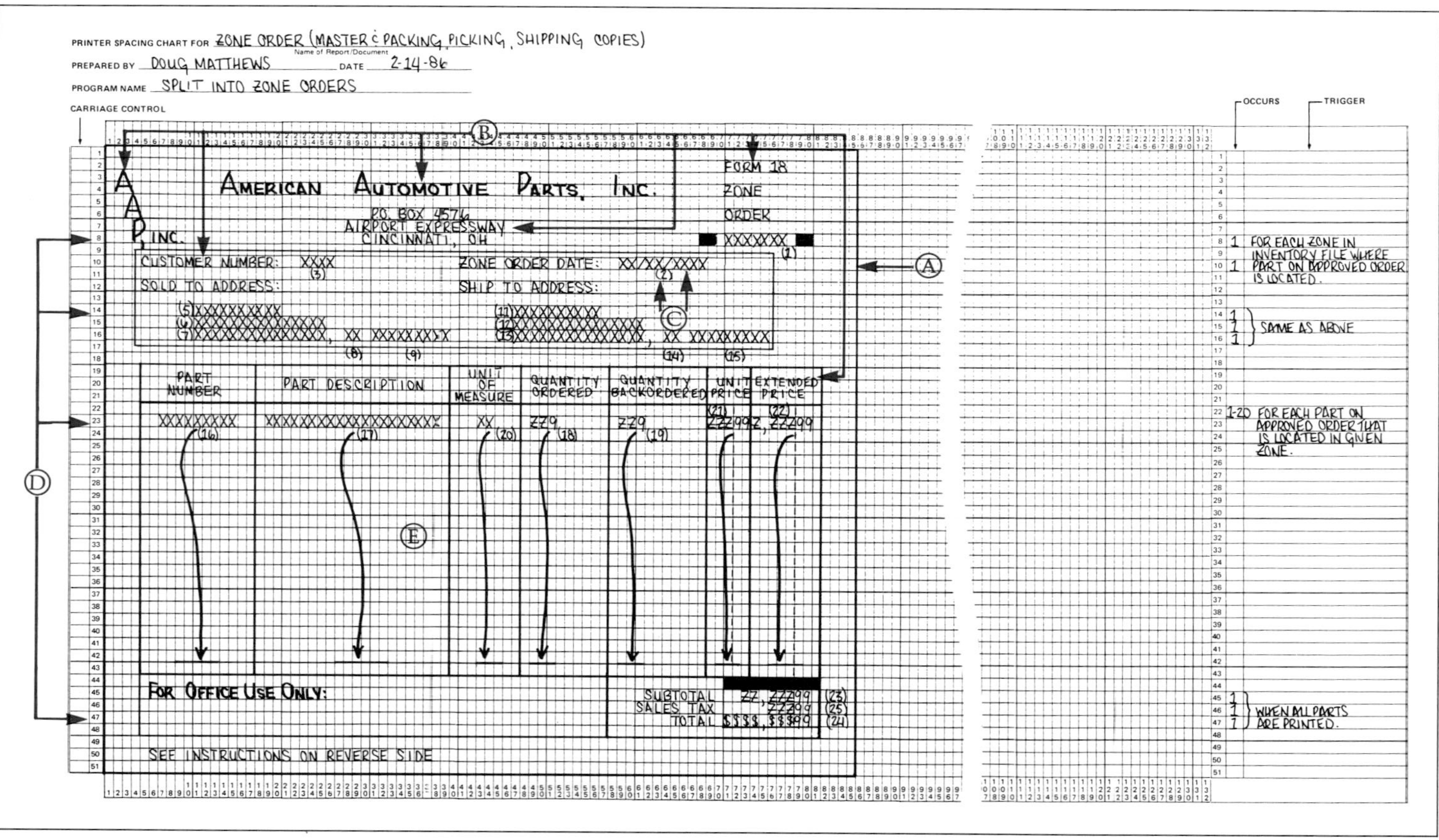

Figure 11.8

Format for the ZONE ORDER. A printer spacing chart for an external document not only specifies computer output but also serves as a model for preprinted form design.

SYMBOL	EDITING REQUIREMENT	EDIT MASK	SAMPLE DATA	HOW DATA WILL APPEAR TO USER
9	Print any numeric digit (0-9) in this position. Used for numeric fields.	999	000 005 346	000 005 346
X	Print any character in this position. Used for alpha-numeric fields.	XXXXX -or- X(15)	HORSE NO. 3	HORSE NO. 3
A	Print any letter of the alphabet (or blank space) in this location. Used for alphabetic fields.	AAAAA -or- A(5)	CAT CAT	CAT CAT
Z	Suppress leading zeroes. Use only for numeric fields.	Z9 ZZ	07 00 10 00	7 0 10
B	Print a blank character at this position.	99B99 XXBXX AABAA	1234 FRT6 SSNO	12 34 FR T6 SS NO
$	Print a dollar sign at this position. Used only for numeric fields.	$999 $ZZZ $$$$	015 015 015	$015 $ 15 $15
.	Print a decimal point at this location. Use only for numeric fields.	99.99 ZZ.ZZ $$.99	05.75 05.75 05.75	05.75 5.75 $5.75
/	Print a slash at this position in the field.	XX/XX 99/99 AA/AA	AB61 5533 SSSN	AB/61 55/33 SS/SN
-	Print a hyphen at this location in the field.	XX-XX 99-99 AA-AA	FRT6 1266 SSNO	FR-T6 12-66 SS-NO
,	Print a comma at this position if the digit to the left is 1-9. Use for numeric fields only.	9,999 Z,ZZ9	1356 2241 0225	1,356 2,241 225

Figure 11.9

COBOL syntax for defining editing requirements.

(D) Carriage controls were established because this is a nonstandard form size. The printer needs to have its top-of-page and bottom-of-page redefined when printing this form.

(E) There may be from one to twenty parts on any one order. Notice how we used vertical lines with arrowheads to indicate

Figure 11.10 ►

Output design sketch intended for user. Instead of showing users printer spacing charts for the new zone order, we would sketch or type a sample of the output that includes sample data in the fields. This sketch would actually be prepared before the printer spacing chart because we want user feedback before we commit the design to the spacing chart. A forms manufacturer is usually commissioned to design the final form and print them for AAP's use.

that the line describing a single part, may be printed repeatedly. The line spacing is assumed to be single (more about this later).

The boundary of the form was drawn in by the analyst. The printer spacing chart is *not* a scale drawing.

We again remind you that the documentation prepared in this example is primarily intended for the analysts and programmers. The edit masks recorded on our printer spacing chart, even the printer spacing chart itself, will likely be considered too difficult for users to interpret and evaluate. For the user, we recommend one or more samples of the output be generated, such as the sample illustrated in Figure 11.10.

Design of a Typical Internal Report

Internal reports include historical reports, detail reports, summary reports, and exception reports. Their design specifications are similar; therefore, we need demonstrate only one. The PART SALES SUMMARY REPORT for AAP is an internal summary report. Figures 11.11 through 11.13 present the design specifications for the PART SALES SUMMARY REPORT. The expanded data dictionary entry in Figure 11.11 is self-explanatory. Look at the data structure in OUTPUT COMPOSITION. This is a classic structure using multiple control breaks (from your programming courses). The data element design specifications for the summary report are provided in Figure 11.12.

The design layout for the PART SALES SUMMARY REPORT is depicted in Figure 11.13. Notice how the layout of the report presents the information very clearly. The following guidelines were followed when using printer spacing charts to design internal reports:

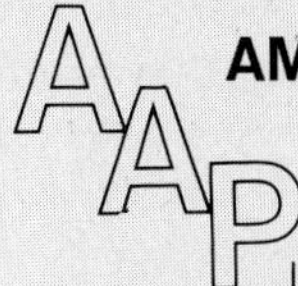

AMERICAN AUTOMOTIVE PARTS, INC.

P.O. BOX 4576
AIRPORT EXPRESSWAY
CINCINNATI, OH 45208

FORM 18
ZONE
ORDER
0525861

CUSTOMER NUMBER: 0344 ZONE ORDER DATE: 05/25/86

SOLD TO ADDRESS:
Wheeler Automotive Supply
124 State Street
Findlay, OH 45840

SHIP TO ADDRESS:
Wheeler Automotive Supply
124 State Street
Findlay, OH 45840

PART NUMBER	PART DESCRIPTION	UNIT OF MEASURE	QUANTITY ORDERED	QUANTITY BACKORDERED	UNIT PRICE	EXTENDED PRICE
BK 789	Fanbelt	Ea	10	0	1.25	12.50
BK 790	Fanbelt	Ea	5	0	1.25	6.25
BK 794	Fanbelt	Ea	5	4	1.50	7.50
MS Q 348	Paint--Supra White	Qt	1	0	4.25	4.25
MS P 348	Paint--Supra White	Pt	1	0	2.00	2.00
MS P 456	Paint--Majestic Blue	Pt	1	0	2.35	2.35

FOR OFFICE USE ONLY

SUBTOTAL	34.85
SALES TAX	1.75
TOTAL	36.60

```
DATA DICTIONARY: OUTPUT (Page 1)

DEFINITION

   NAME OF OUTPUT:  PART SALES SUMMARY
   PREPARED BY:  Doug Matthews (Feb. 20, 1986)
   DESCRIPTION:  Identifies zone, product line, and part sales over a daily,
                 weekly, and monthly basis.
   MEDIUM:  Paper
   OUTPUT TYPE:  Internal/Summary
   OUTPUT CHARACTERISTICS:  Tabular format on Standard Stock 11" X 14"
   FREQUENCY PREPARED:      7:45 A.M.  on last  working day  of week or when
                            requested.
   VOLUME:  40 pages
   NUMBER OF COPIES:  3
   COPYING METHOD:  Duplicate Printing
   OUTPUT RECIPIENT(S):  Will be  delivered  via  internal mail to  Customer
                         Services Manager and Marketing Department.

OUTPUT COMPOSITION

     A PART SALES SUMMARY consists of the following data elements:
          DATE  *of the report
          1 to 5 occurrences of the following:
               ZONE
                    1 to 35 occurrences of the following:
                         PRODUCT LINE
                              1 to 200 occurrences of the following:
                                   PART NUMBER
                                   PART DESCRIPTION
                                   UNIT SALES PAST DAY
                                   UNIT SALES PAST WEEK
                                   UNIT SALES PAST MONTH
                         PAST DAY UNIT SALES LINE
                         PAST WEEK UNIT SALES LINE
                         PAST MONTH UNIT SALES LINE
               PAST DAY UNIT SALES ZONE
               PAST WEEK UNIT SALES ZONE
               PAST MONTH UNIT SALES ZONE
          PAGE NUMBER
```

Figure 11.11

The expanded data dictionary for PART SALES SUMMARY (Page 1).

Ⓐ The report was given a heading that includes the title of the report, the company name, page number, and the current date. Items to be repeated at the top of every page are so indicated in the TRIGGER column. The TRIGGER column would also be used to explain if and when column headings will be printed (at a control break, for example, or at the top of every page).

Ⓑ Once again, the edit masks are used to indicate where and how the computer should print fields. The parentheses next to an edit mask correspond to the "REF." number in the data element dictionary.

Ⓒ Spacing between detail lines was done according to the guidelines illustrated in Figure 11.14. Simply show two detail lines

D A T A   D I C T I O N A R Y :   O U T P U T (Page 2)

NAME OF OUTPUT: PART SALES SUMMARY
PREPARED BY: Doug Matthews (Feb. 20, 1986)

REF.	DATA ELEMENT NAME	TYPE	SIZE	EDIT MASK	SOURCE
1.	DATE	A/N	8	XX-XX-XX	O/S
2.	*ZONE	A/N	1	X	PARTS
3.	*PRODUCT LINE	A/N	2	XX	PARTS
4.	*PART NUMBER	A/N	9	X(9)	ORDERS
5.	PART DESCRIPTION	A/N	20	X(20)	PARTS
6.	UNIT SALES PAST DAY	N	6.0	ZZZ,ZZ9	*ORDERS
7.	UNIT SALES PAST WEEK	N	7.0	Z,ZZZ,ZZ9	*ORDERS
8.	UNIT SALES PAST MONTH	N	8.0	ZZ,ZZZ,ZZ9	*ORDERS
9.	PAST DAY UNIT SALES LINE	N	6.0	ZZZ,ZZ9	*ORDERS
10.	PAST WEEK UNIT SALES LINE	N	7.0	Z,ZZZ,ZZ9	*ORDERS
11.	PAST MONTH UNIT SALES LINE	N	8.0	ZZ,ZZZ,ZZ9	*ORDERS
12.	PAST DAY UNIT SALES ZONE	N	6.0	ZZZ,ZZ9	*ORDERS
13.	PAST WEEK UNIT SALES ZONE	N	7.0	Z,ZZZ,ZZ9	*ORDERS
14.	PAST MONTH UNIT SALES ZONE	N	8.0	ZZ,ZZZ,ZZ9	*ORDERS
15.	PAGE NUMBER	N	2.0	Z9	Calculated by program

* The report is to be sequenced by warehouse ZONE. For each zone, the PRODUCT LINEs for that ZONE are to appear sequentially. And for each PRODUCT LINE, the PART NUMBER in that product line is to appear sequentially.

* Data elements 6 through 14 are calculated by summing the QUANTITY SOLD for a given PART NUMBER. QUANTITY SOLD may be derived from the ORDERS file.

Figure 11.12

The expanded data dictionary for PART SALES SUMMARY (Page 2).

and the appropriate spacing, if any. Figure 11.14(a) demonstrates single spacing. Figure 11.14(b) demonstrates double spacing. When printing several detail lines on a report, you may want to indicate that no detail line should be printed below a specific line number. Figure 11.14(c) shows how to specify such a requirement. Or perhaps you want the detail lines to continue until some control break, after which you print a control total. Figure 11.14(d) demonstrates this requirement.

Ⓓ Note how we used the OCCURS and TRIGGER columns. OCCURS indicates the number of times the line should be printed on a single page of the report. TRIGGER provides the

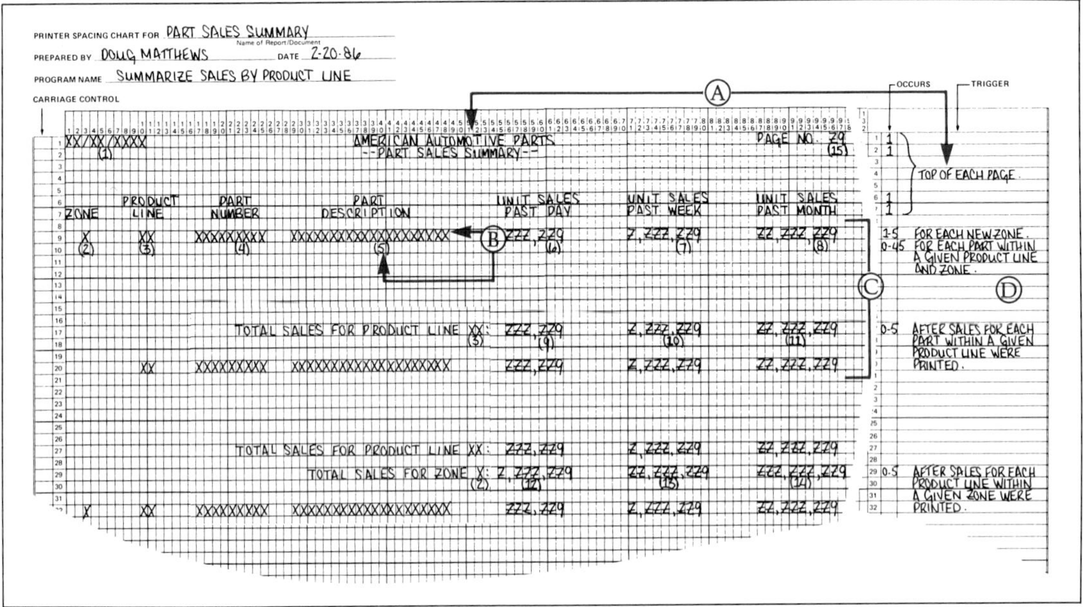

Figure 11.13

Format for the PART SALES SUMMARY output.

programmer with additional instructions on printing the corresponding line on the report.

Once again, for the users, we recommend that a sample of the report be generated. The sample should contain sample data that can be used to verify the format and content of the report with the users.

We would be remiss if we didn't point out that summary reports are the best candidates for the graphical format. Can you define a graphical version for the PARTS SALES SUMMARY REPORT?

Design of a Video Display Output

We've examined how a number of printed outputs of AAP were designed when the medium selected was paper. But the AAP customer services information system presented visual output opportunities also. Let's study the design of PART QUERY RESPONSE. Here we are interested only in the net output; in Chapter 14, you'll learn how to design the terminal dialogue that leads to the output.

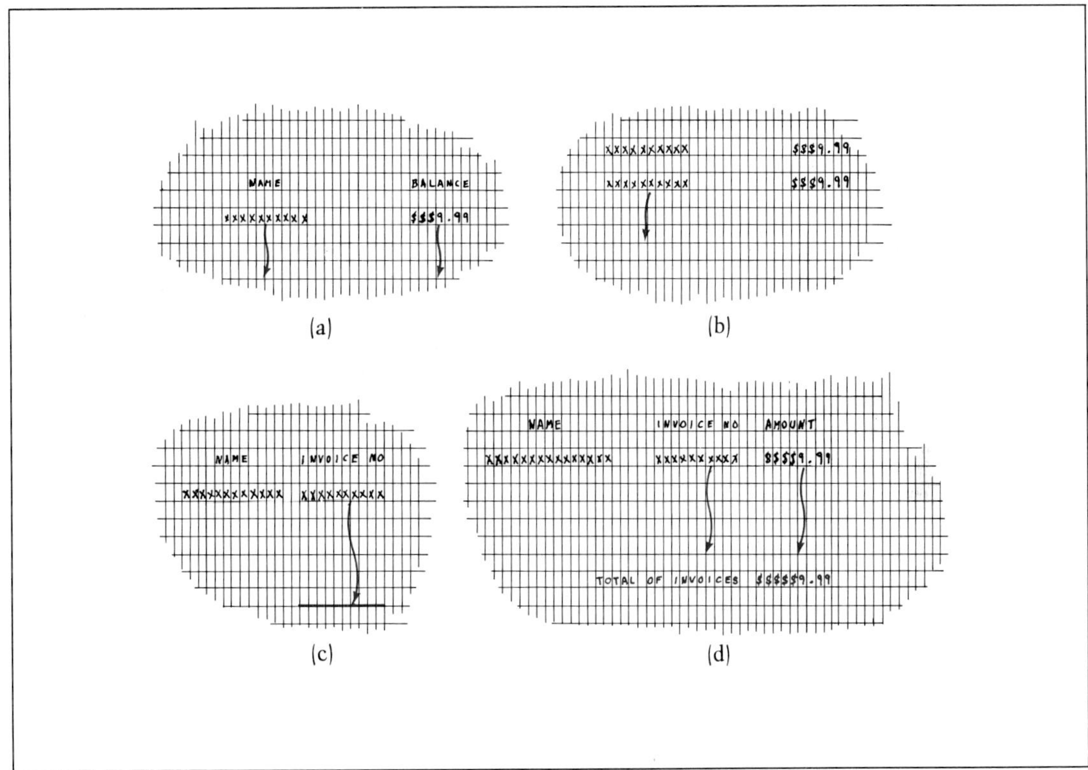

Figure 11.14

Spacing requirements for detail lines.

The design specifications for the PART QUERY RESPONSE output are presented in Figures 11.15 through 11.19. A close look at the design specifications is in order. We call your attention to the following special notes on Figure 11.15, the first part of the data dictionary:

Ⓐ We divided the display area into zones, called windows. This way, the user always knows where to look for certain things. One window is set aside to display the title, date, and page number. Another window is used to display the body of the report. The report will page or scroll through this window. A third window offers instructions to the reader for paging forward and backward, returning to the beginning of the document, and terminating the report program.

```
DATA DICTIONARY: OUTPUT (Page 1)

DEFINITION

   NAME OF OUTPUT:  PART QUERY RESPONSE
   PREPARED BY:  Cheryl Mason (March 3, 1986)
   DESCRIPTION:  Describes general part data, part-to-vehicle matchups, or
        analysis of backordered parts.
   MEDIUM:  Video          OUTPUT TYPE:  Internal
   OUTPUT CHARACTERISTICS:  Displayed on 24 (line) X 80 (column) CRT screen.
   FREQUENCY PREPARED:  On demand during the hours 8:00 A.M. to 5:00 P.M.
   OUTPUT RECIPIENT(S):  Access should be limited to order entry personnel.
   SPECIAL INSTRUCTIONS:  Each output query response is to be printed on a
        separate screen.  Line 1 must contain an appropriate title.  Lines
   (A)  2-5 should contain descriptive headings (lines 1-5 do not scroll).
        Lines 7-20 are to be used for displaying requested information.
        Lines 23-24 are used for user paging and scrolling instructions.

OUTPUT COMPOSITION

     A PART QUERY RESPONSE consists of the following data elements:
          PART NUMBER
          PART DESCRIPTION
          and one and only one of the following data groups:
               PART ORDER RESPONSE (see below)
   (B)         PART-VEHICLE MATCH RESPONSE (see below)
               PART BACKORDER RESPONSE (see below)

     PART ORDER RESPONSE consists of the following elements:
          WHOLESALE PRICE
          RETAIL PRICE
          FRANCHISE DISCOUNT RATE
          QUANTITY REQUIRED FOR VOLUME DISCOUNT
          VOLUME DISCOUNT RATE
          QUANTITY ON HAND
          QUANTITY BACKORDERED
          QUANTITY ON ORDER

     PART-VEHICLE MATCH RESPONSE consists of the following data elements:
          VEHICLE MAKE
          VEHICLE MODEL
          MODEL YEAR
          and one or more occurrences of the following element:
               PART RESTRICTIONS

     PART BACKORDER RESPONSE consists of the following elements:
          QUANTITY ON HAND
          QUANTITY ON ORDER
          TOTAL QUANTITY BACKORDERED
          and one or more occurrences of the following elements:
               SALES ORDER NUMBER
               SALES ORDER DATE
               CUSTOMER NUMBER
               QUANTITY BACKORDERED
```

Figure 11.15

The expanded data dictionary for the output PART QUERY RESPONSE (Page 1).

(B) The data structure for PART QUERY RESPONSE indicates that the output is composed of one of three possible data element groups.

D A T A D I C T I O N A R Y : O U T P U T (Page 2)

NAME OF OUTPUT: PART QUERY RESPONSE
PREPARED BY: Cheryl Mason (March 3, 1986)

REF.	DATA ELEMENT NAME	TYPE	SIZE	EDIT MASK	SOURCE
1.	PART NUMBER	A/N	9	9(9)	PARTS
2.	PART DESCRIPTION	A/N	15	X(15)	PARTS
3.	PART ORDER RESPONSE				PARTS
4.	WHOLESALE PRICE	N	3.2	ZZZ.99	
5.	RETAIL BASE PRICE	N	3.2	ZZZ.99	
6.	FRANCHISE DISCOUNT RATE	N	2	Z9	
7.	QUANTITY REQUIRED FOR VOLUME DISCOUNT	N	3	ZZ9	
8.	VOLUME DISCOUNT RATE	N	2	Z9	
9.	QUANTITY ON HAND	N	6	ZZZ,ZZ9	
10.	QUANTITY BACKORDERED	N	6	ZZZ,ZZ9	
11.	QUANTITY ON ORDER	N	6	ZZZ,ZZ9	
12.	PART-VEHICLE MATCH RESPONSE				PARTS
13.	VEHICLE NAME	A/N	10	X(10)	
14.	VEHICLE MODEL	A/N	10	X(10)	
15.	MODEL YEAR	A/N	4	X(4)	
16.	PART RESTRICTIONS	A/N	20	X(20)	
17.	PART BACKORDER RESPONSE				
18.	QUANTITY ON HAND	N	6	ZZZ,ZZ9	PARTS
19.	QUANTITY ON ORDER	N	6	ZZZ,ZZ9	PARTS
20.	TOTAL QUANTITY BACKORDERED	N	6	ZZZ,ZZ9	PARTS
21.	*SALES ORDER NUMBER	A/N	6	X(6)	ORDER
22.	SALES ORDER DATE	A/N	4	XX/XX or MM/DD	ORDER
23.	CUSTOMER NUMBER	A/N	4	X(4)	ORDER
24.	QUANTITY BACKORDERED	N	6	ZZZ,ZZ9	ORDER

* The repeating fields 21 through 24 should be displayed in ascending order by SALES ORDER NUMBER.

Figure 11.16

The expanded data dictionary for the output PART QUERY RESPONSE (Page 2).

Data element design issues for video display outputs are the same as for printed outputs. Therefore, the data element design specifications in Figure 11.16 contain information equivalent to

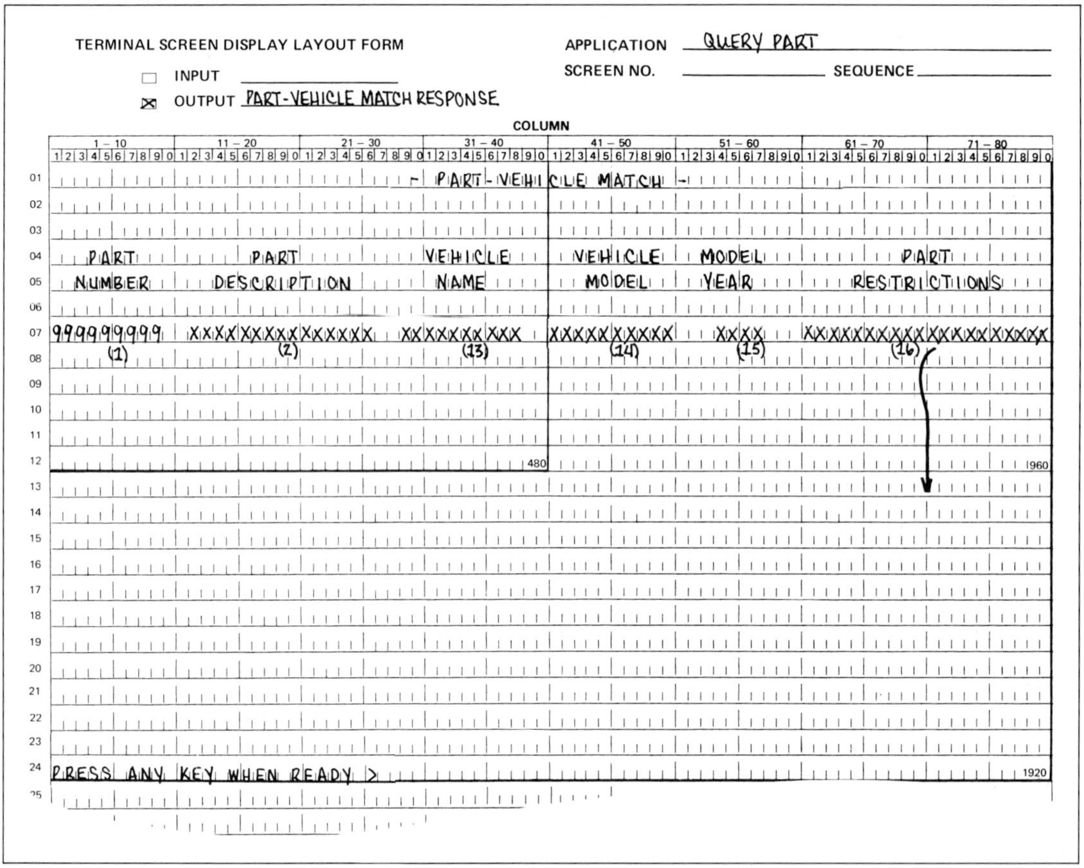

TERMINAL SCREEN DISPLAY LAYOUT FORM

APPLICATION QUERY PART

SCREEN NO. ______ SEQUENCE ______

☐ INPUT ______

☒ OUTPUT PART-VEHICLE MATCH RESPONSE

COLUMN

01 - PART-VEHICLE MATCH -

04 PART PART VEHICLE VEHICLE MODEL PART

05 NUMBER DESCRIPTION NAME MODEL YEAR RESTRICTIONS

07 999999999 XXXXXXXXXXXXXXX XXXXXXXXXXX XXXXXXXXXXX XXXX XXXXXXXXXXXXXXXXXXXXXXXXX

08 (1) (2) (13) (14) (15) (16)

480 1960

24 PRESS ANY KEY WHEN READY >

1920

Figure 11.17

Format for the PART-VEHICLE MATCH RESPONSE option of the output PART QUERY RESPONSE.

the data element specifications for our printed output design examples.

Figures 11.17 through 11.19 present the screen layouts for the PART QUERY RESPONSE. All three output screens were designed with an effort to locate the data according to the windows defined in Figure 11.15. The layout of the PART VEHICLE MATCH RESPONSE (Figure 11.17) clearly reflects the usage of the window requirements.

On the other hand, the layout for the PART ORDER RESPONSE (Figure 11.18) and the PART BACKORDER RESPONSE (Figure

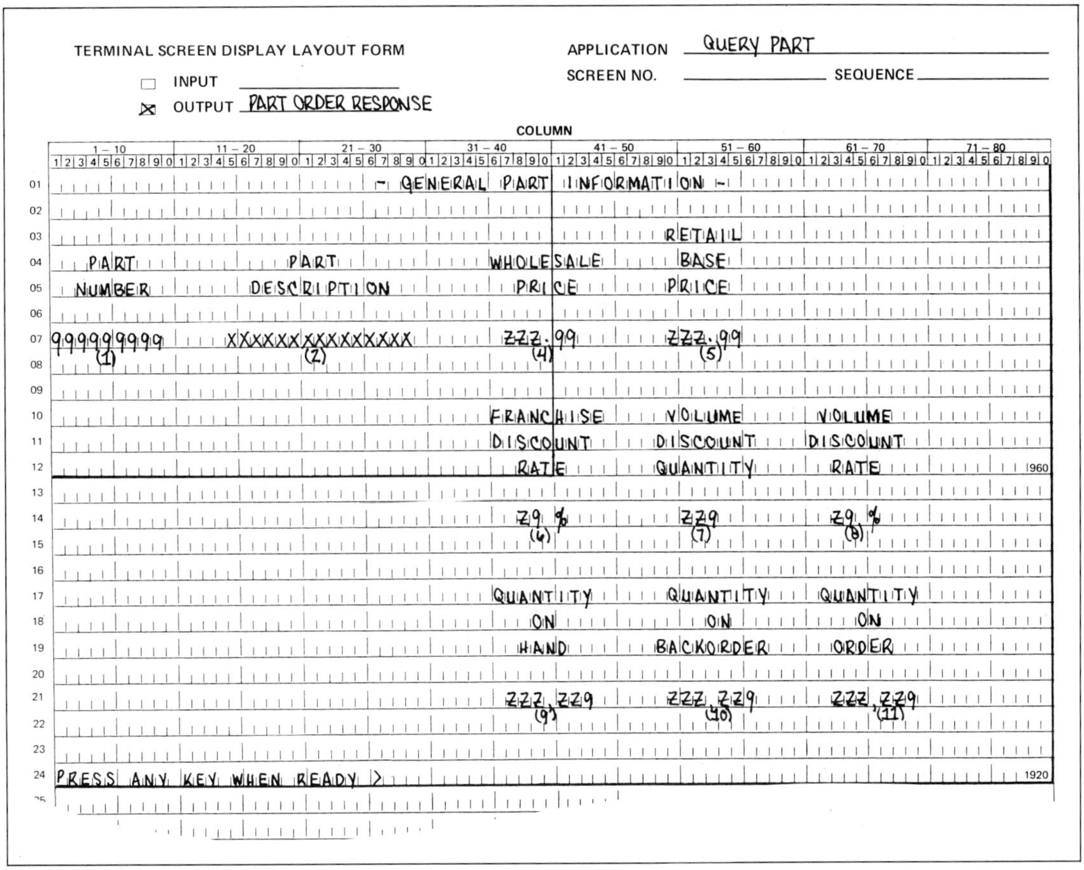

TERMINAL SCREEN DISPLAY LAYOUT FORM

APPLICATION QUERY PART

SCREEN NO. ______ SEQUENCE ______

☐ INPUT ______

☒ OUTPUT PART ORDER RESPONSE

COLUMN

01 - GENERAL PART INFORMATION -

03 RETAIL

04 PART PART WHOLESALE BASE

05 NUMBER DESCRIPTION PRICE PRICE

07 999999999 XXXXXXXXXXXXXXXXX ZZZ.99 ZZZ.99

08 (1) (2) (4) (5)

10 FRANCHISE VOLUME VOLUME

11 DISCOUNT DISCOUNT DISCOUNT

12 RATE QUANTITY RATE

14 Z9 % ZZ9 Z9 %

15 (6) (7) (8)

17 QUANTITY QUANTITY QUANTITY

18 ON ON ON

19 HAND BACKORDER ORDER

21 ZZZ,ZZ9 ZZZ,ZZ9 ZZZ,ZZ9

22 (9) (10) (11)

24 PRESS ANY KEY WHEN READY >

Figure 11.18

Format for the PART ORDER RESPONSE option of the output PART QUERY RESPONSE.

11.19) required a slight deviation. In both instances, the amount of data to be displayed across the screen restricted the ability to use the windows exactly as specified. The important point here is that there should always be an attempt to be as consistent as possible when designing terminal screens. You should also notice how we used function keys and the return key to help the user page through the output.

That completes our study of designing computer-generated outputs. In Chapter 12 we'll learn how to design computer files that will serve as a source of data for outputs.

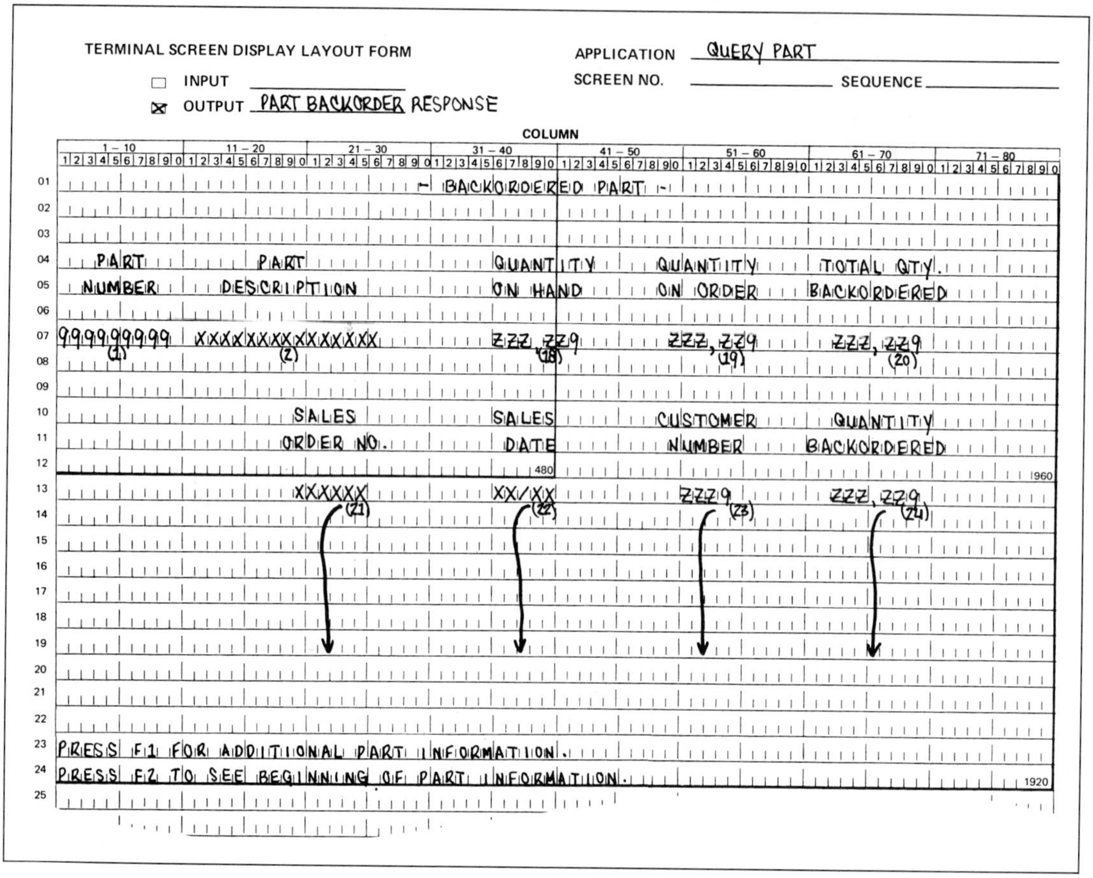

TERMINAL SCREEN DISPLAY LAYOUT FORM

APPLICATION QUERY PART

☐ INPUT

SCREEN NO. ______ SEQUENCE ______

☒ OUTPUT PART BACKORDER RESPONSE

COLUMN

- BACKORDERED PART -

PART NUMBER | PART DESCRIPTION | QUANTITY ON HAND | QUANTITY ON ORDER | TOTAL QTY. BACKORDERED

99999999 (1) | XXXXXXXXXXXXXXXX (2) | ZZZ,ZZ9 (18) | ZZZ,ZZ9 (19) | ZZZ,ZZ9 (20)

SALES ORDER NO. | SALES DATE | CUSTOMER NUMBER | QUANTITY BACKORDERED

XXXXXX (21) | XX/XX (22) | ZZZ9 (23) | ZZZ,ZZ9 (24)

480

1960

PRESS F1 FOR ADDITIONAL PART INFORMATION.

PRESS F2 TO SEE BEGINNING OF PART INFORMATION.

1920

Figure 11.19

Format for the PART BACKORDER RESPONSE option of the output PART QUERY RESPONSE.

SUMMARY

When designing outputs, the systems analyst must consider a variety of human factors. Chief among these are selection of medium and format. Media include paper, film, and video display. Format includes tabular information, graphical information, and words. Together, medium and format combinations are used to generate two basic types of outputs—external and internal. External outputs, usually transactions, exit the system to trigger or confirm actions. Internal outputs are management reports and decision support for management planning, control, and decision making.

Output design requires three basic steps. First, identify outputs as data flows on a data flow diagram for the target information system. Review the contents specified during systems analysis. Second, specify important design criteria—medium and format, to name just a couple. This requires that you understand the purpose and use of the output. Third, lay out the report, form, or display screens.

There are a number of useful tools for output design. First, an expanded data dictionary can be used to catalog important design requirements and decisions. Second, printer spacing charts are used to lay out the format of printed documents. Finally, display layout charts are used to lay out the format of terminal screens.

PROBLEMS AND EXERCISES

1. Differentiate between internal and external outputs. Why is it important that a systems analyst recognize an output as either internal or external?
2. To what extent should knowledge workers be involved in output design? How would you get your knowledge workers involved? What would you ask them to do for themselves?
3. Prepare an expanded data dictionary to describe the following outputs:
   (a) Your driver's license
   (b) Your course schedule
   (c) Your bank statement
   (d) Your phone bill
   (e) Your W-2 statement (for taxes)
   (f) A bank or credit card account statement and invoice
   (g) An external document printed on a computer

   You may invent numbers for timing and volume. Don't forget internal controls.
4. Using the sample outputs from problem three, document the layout of the output using a printer spacing chart. Be sure to make appropriate entries in the carriage control, occurs, and trigger columns for all computer printed lines. List any im-

provements that could be made to improve the readability, interpretation, and acceptability of the output.

5. How would the expanded data dictionary in problem four differ if the external output were designed as an internal visual output? Use a display layout chart to describe the format of a visual version of the sample output.

6. Prepare an expanded data dictionary for one or more internal outputs from any computer programming assignment. If a printer spacing chart was not supplied by your instructor, prepare one. If you had to change your output to make it more readable and usable, how would you do it?

7. Prepare an expanded data dictionary for the following internal output:

   The sales manager for Soundstage Record Company has requested a daily report. This report should describe the nearly 1,000 customer order responses received for a given day. A response is a member decision on whether to accept the record-of-the-month selection, request an alternate selection, request both, or request no selection be sent that month. The report is to be sequenced by MEMBERSHIP NUMBER and CATALOG NUMBER. The data dictionary for the report follows:

   The ORDER RESPONSE REPORT consists of the following elements:

   DATE * of the report

   PAGE NUMBER

   1 to 1,000 of the following:

      MEMBERSHIP NUMBER * 5 digits

      MEMBER NAME * which consists of the following:

         MEMBER LAST NAME * 15 characters

         MEMBER FIRST NAME * 15 characters

         MEMBER MIDDLE INITIAL * 1 character

      MUSICAL PREFERENCE * possible values are

         "EASY LISTENING" "TEEN HITS"

         "CLASSICAL" "COUNTRY" "JAZZ"

SELECTION OF MONTH DECISION * possible values are

"YES" "NO" "NONE"

1 to 15 of the following:

CATALOG NUMBER * 5 digits

MEDIA * possible values are

"RECORD" "CASSETTE"
"AUDIOPHILE" "8 TRACK" "REEL"

NUMBER OF PURCHASE CREDITS NEEDED * 2 digits

PERIOD AGREEMENT EXPIRES * date membership expires

Using a printer spacing chart, lay out the format for the printed report. Be sure to include appropriate report headings, edit masks with reference numbers to the expanded data dictionary, occurs, and trigger entries.

8. The sales manager has also requested that the sales staff be able to obtain information concerning a *particular* customer's order response at any time during normal working hours. Prepare an expanded data dictionary and display layout chart for the visual output CUSTOMER ORDER RESPONSE.
9. What data flows crossing the person/machine boundary on a bounded data flow diagram should be designed as computer outputs?
10. What are some of the effects that may be caused by the lack of well-defined internal controls during output design?

ANNOTATED SUGGESTED READING

Fitzgerald, Jerry. *Internal Controls for Computerized Information Systems.* Redwood City, Calif.: Jerry Fitzgerald & Associates, 1978. This is our reference standard on the subject of designing internal controls into systems. Fitzgerald advocates a unique and powerful matrix tool for designing controls. This book goes far beyond any introductory systems textbook — This is *must* reading.

12 Designing Computer Files

Minicase: Westcoast Hardware

Barney Stone, a programmer/analyst for Westcoast Hardware, was sitting at his desk reviewing design specifications for the new computer-based purchasing information system. Barney had been responsible for this project from the very beginning. Most of the programs for the system had been implemented, but the final two programs had been returned by the programmer with a note explaining that they were impossible to write according to the specifications. Because Barney had been in a hurry to implement this new system, design specifications had been passed along to the programmer as soon as they were completed. Now, Barney was frustrated. Barney's boss, George Jesson, entered the office.

George What's the matter, Barney? You look like you've just lost your best friend.

Barney Oh, I've worked so hard implementing that darn purchasing system. But I've encountered a problem with the last two programs.

George What type of problem? What do the programs involve?

Barney One of them produces a scheduled report and the other an on-line output.

George Why can't you just generate the programs to produce the reports? I don't understand, we do that all the time. You know that.

Barney It's not all that simple. The on-line program requires quick response. The file to be accessed is organized as a sequential file. The other report requires data to be retrieved and printed by product number. That presents a problem because the file is organized as an indexed file with purchase order number as the primary key. I didn't set this file up with any secondary keys because none of the previous programs needed to access the file by anything other than the purchase order number.

George You mean you have already designed and implemented the files?

Barney Yes, we were behind schedule. I figured that the highest volume of transactions against the files would be executed by the programs that maintained the files. I organized the files to make those programs run efficiently. Then I passed the specifications for the files and those particular programs on to the programmers so we could begin writing those programs.

George And now you find that the file organization is not best for the way the new programs need to access the file.

Barney That's right.

George What are you going to do?

Barney I guess I'm going to have to choose between the lesser of two evils. First, we could write programs to extract data from the existing files and place it in a temporary file whose organization suits the new programs. I can tell by the look on your face that you're not crazy about the idea of creating a redundant file every time we want to produce this report. Second, I could redesign the original files. But that means rewriting the programs. Either way, the project is behind schedule.

George I hate to add to your problems, but what are you going to do if your users think up another report that causes this same problem?

Discussion

1. What should Barney do?
2. Barney made a big mistake. Where did he go wrong?
3. Can you describe how the two files should have been implemented?

WHAT WILL YOU LEARN IN THIS CHAPTER?

You will know that you have mastered the tools and techniques of file design when you can:

1. Define fixed- and variable-length logical records for master and transaction file records in a computer-based information system.
2. Determine the optimal storage format for fields in the logical record (given the constraints imposed by common computer systems).
3. Explain why logical records are blocked into physical records, and determine the blocking factor for a given file.
4. Differentiate between file access methods and file organization techniques. Also, determine the best file organization for a given file by studying that file's required access methods.
5. Design internal controls into computer files.
6. Define file design requirements, and record those requirements in an expanded data dictionary format.
7. Use record layout charts to format logical record designs.

Computer files are the heart and lifeblood of any computer-based information system. They are also one of the fundamental components in your information system model (see margin). Almost every computer program will require access to data that has been previously captured and stored in files. Computer files store data for later use. By storing data in files, we eliminate the need to re-input those data. The design of computer files can be difficult because the storage and organization of data on a computer media requires the analyst to consider complex and often conflicting issues, such as storage capacity and performance. In this chapter, you will learn how to design and document computer files.

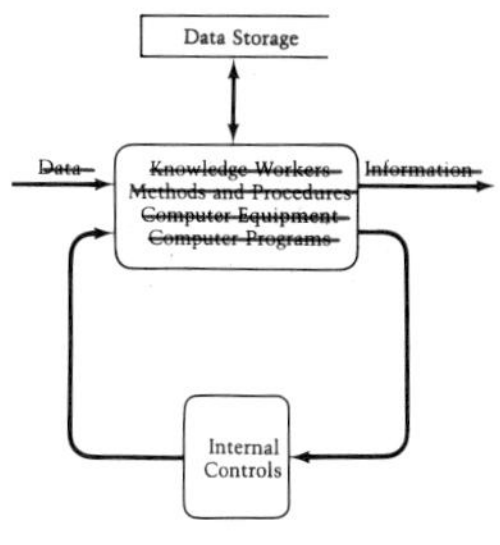

IPO Components

We continue to assume you've had an introductory data processing course and at least one course in computer programming. Therefore, we assume you are familiar with the different file storage devices, such as tape and disk. But it has become apparent to us that many of the technical issues important to file design are taught in different courses — which you may or may not have taken. Because of this, some of the technical concepts discussed here may be old hat to some of you. Please bear with us. We will try to focus on the technical issues that are pertinent to the systems analyst's responsibilities.

TECHNICAL CONCEPTS FOR FILE DESIGN

We are going to cover several technical concepts in this section. The framework that appears in the margin should be useful as an overall outline of the discussion. It depicts a model we'll call the data storage hierarchy. We'll start at the bottom of the model and work our way to the top. We'll not discuss specific storage devices because they are covered in virtually every introductory data processing course.

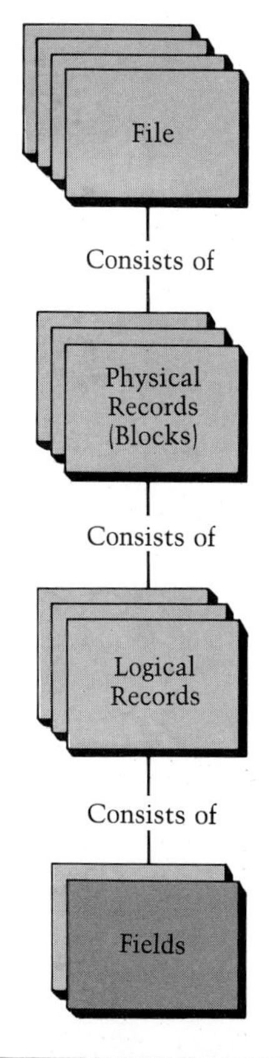

Data Storage Hierarchy

Fields and Data Formats

Field is another name for a data element. **Fields** are the smallest unit of data to be stored. As an analyst, you will define fields to be stored in files. As you do so, you will need to consider *field types* and how data will be stored in fields. There are three types of fields that can be stored: primary keys, secondary keys, and descriptors.

Primary keys uniquely identify an entity in the business. For instance, CUSTOMER NUMBER uniquely identifies a customer, and ORDER NUMBER uniquely identifies an order. The important concept is *uniqueness.* No two occurrences of CUSTOMER will have the same value for CUSTOMER NUMBER. It is your responsibility, through discussions with your users, to define primary keys for files.

Secondary keys identify a subset of all occurrences of an entity. For example, SEX defines two subsets of the entity EMPLOYEE, male employees and female employees. An entity may be defined by several secondary keys. For instance, EMPLOYEE may be subset on the secondary keys GENDER and RACE. You will also need to define the secondary keys for appropriate files.

Finally, most fields, including keys, are descriptors of such business entities as customers, employees, accounts, orders, invoices, and parts. For example, given the business entity EMPLOYEE, some descriptor fields include EMPLOYEE NAME, DATE HIRED, PAY RATE, and YEAR-TO-DATE WAGES. As an analyst, you will define all descriptive fields for computer files. These descriptive fields can be identified by studying existing forms and files (including noncomputerized files). More importantly, these fields can be defined by studying the existing output data dictionaries you generated in Chapter 11 — many of those elements are retrieved from files or calculated using elements that are retrieved from files.

Because space can be a limited resource in any computer system, the analyst is responsible for economizing space when storing any field. This requires a knowledge of the way in which data is stored.

Data Storage Formats There are three basic field-storage formats: binary codes, fixed-point numbers, and floating-point numbers. In most business-oriented systems, all fields are usually stored as binary codes. A **binary code** is a unique combination of ones and zeros that represents a number, character, or symbol. There are three common binary codes: EBCDIC (also called zoned decimal), ASCII, and packed decimal. During file design, your choice of storage formats for fields will determine how much disk or tape capacity will be needed for your files.

EBCDIC (Extended Binary Coded Decimal Interchange Code) is a popular code used on IBM mainframe computers and compatibles. Each letter, number, and special symbol is represented by an eight-bit code. Each code consists of a four-bit zone and a four-bit digit. Thus, a field value "Bill" would be stored as "11100010" (B), "10001001" (i), "10010011" (l), and "10010011" (l). This field required four bytes of storage (a byte is eight bits long on most business-oriented machines).

ASCII (American Standard Code for Information Exchange) is another popular code used by many computer manufacturers (among them are Digital Equipment Corporation and the IBM Personal Computer). ASCII represents each letter, number, or symbol with a unique seven-bit code. Actually, ASCII uses an eight-bit code, but the last bit is called a *parity bit* and is used only to check a stream of ASCII characters for correct transmission from one place to another (such as computer to printer). Standard tables for EBCDIC and ASCII codes are widely available.

Although EBCDIC and ASCII codes can be used for numeric fields, most computers do not use such codes in arithmetic operations. Some computers perform arithmetic only on fixed- and floating-point binary numbers. These pure binary formats significantly economize on space. On the other hand, IBM mainframe computers (and others) do arithmetic on packed-decimal numbers. **Packed decimal** is equivalent to EBCDIC, except that the zone bits are not used. By storing numeric fields in packed-decimal format, we realize two advantages:

1. The field does not have to be converted before an arithmetic operation is performed. This improves the performance of the computer programs.

2. The field requires only half as much storage space. Using the full EBCDIC code, the number 36 is stored as "11110011" (3) and "11110110" (6). That's two bytes of storage. Using the packed-decimal format, 36 is stored as "0011" (3) and "0110" (6). That's only one byte of storage!

Actually, packed decimal uses the codes "1100," "1101," and "1111" for the *plus sign*, *minus sign*, and *unsigned* numbers respectively. Therefore, the number "36" would actually be stored as "1100" (+), "0011" (3), and "0110" (6). That's a total of twelve bits. Unfortunately, most computers can only address a **byte,** which is usually an increment of eight bits. Thus, 36 requires two full bytes of storage, although only one and a half bytes are actually used. The rule for calculating the storage space required in packed decimal is to add 1 to the number of decimal digits (for the sign), divide by 2, and round up to the next integer.

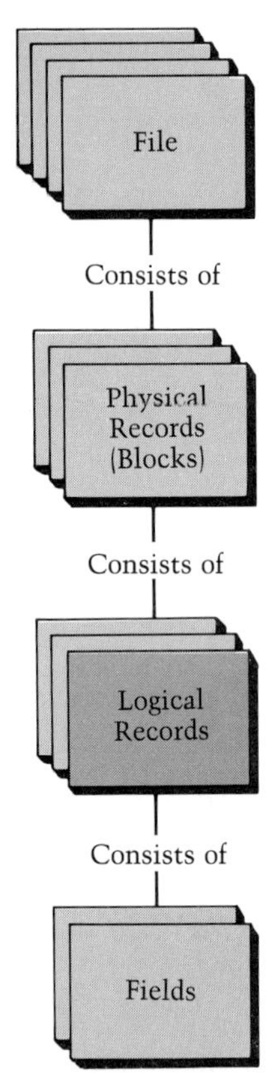

Data Storage Hierarchy

CUSTOMER NUMBER
CUSTOMER NAME
CUSTOMER ADDRESS
DATE INITIATED
CUSTOMER CREDIT LIMIT
CUSTOMER BALANCE
BALANCE PAST DUE

Implications of Data Formats for the Systems Analyst How you store fields will determine the size of files. Therefore, it is important for you to understand the storage formats available on your computer system. Files are managed through file management or database management software (possibly part of the operating system). This software may limit (or even predetermine) the data storage formats.

To economize on storage requirements, you will often make use of elaborate coding schemes. Codes allow you to store large amounts of nonarithmetic data in a relatively small amount of space. Coding schemes were discussed in Chapter 8. A review may be in order.

Logical Records

The next level in our data storage hierarchy is the logical record (see margin). A **logical record** is a collection of fields arranged in a predefined format to describe a single entity. It is also the unit of data storage that is operated upon by a computer program. For example, a logical record for CUSTOMER PAYMENT may be described by the fields listed in the margin. The primary key is underlined.

Logical records and their descriptive fields are designed by the systems analyst during systems analysis and design. During systems design, logical records will be classified as either fixed-length or variable-length records. The distinction will become important during design.

Occurrences of **fixed-length records** will be equal in length. Normally, every record occurrence will also be defined by the same fields. Fixed-length logical records are easy to identify. The data structure, as specified by using your data dictionary notation, contains no repeating groups of elements. (*Note:* Small-sized fields may be allowed to repeat within a fixed-length record; for example, DOLLAR SALES for each of the past three months).

On the other hand, if the data dictionary entry for a record (or data store) contains a repeating group of elements, the logical record is designed as a **variable-length record.** For example, the following data structure defines a variable-length record:

The record ORDER consists of the following data elements (fields):

ORDER NUMBER

ORDER DATE

CUSTOMER NUMBER

One or more occurrences of the following elements (fields):

PRODUCT NUMBER

PRODUCT DESCRIPTION

QUANTITY ORDERED

UNIT OF MEASURE

Occurrences of variable-length records normally contain a fixed-length unit (fields that will occur only once) and a repeating-group unit (fields that occur one or more times). The fixed-length unit (called the *root*) of ORDER record contains the fields ORDER NUMBER, ORDER DATE, and CUSTOMER NUMBER. And the repeating group unit contains the fields PRODUCT NUMBER, PRODUCT DESCRIPTION, QUANTITY ORDERED, and UNIT OF MEASURE. The length of any given occurrence of the record will depend on how many products are on the order. Transaction record files are typically variable-length records. Figure 12.1 demonstrates the difference between occurrences of fixed- and variable-length logical records.

For the analyst, the specification of fixed- or variable-length records will effect file size and performance in ways we'll study later in this chapter.

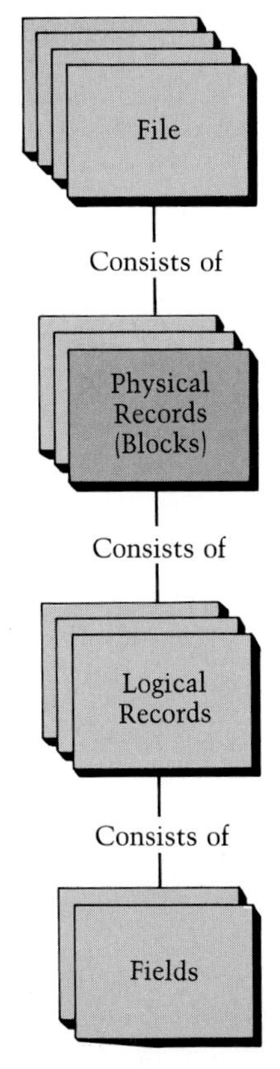

Data Storage Hierarchy

Physical Records and Blocking

As we move up our data storage hierarchy, the next level is physical records (see margin). Consider the following question: When you execute a read or write instruction to a file from your computer program, what are you reading or writing? A logical record? Think about that for a second! It would be inefficient if you read or wrote a single logical record at a time. To improve efficiency in computer systems, the operating system usually reads and writes blocks of logical records to and from your programs. How does it work? When writing a record, you are not writing the record directly to the file. Instead, you are writing the record to a buffer in the computer. When the buffer is full, the entire block of records you have written into the buffer is written to the file. The computer system handles

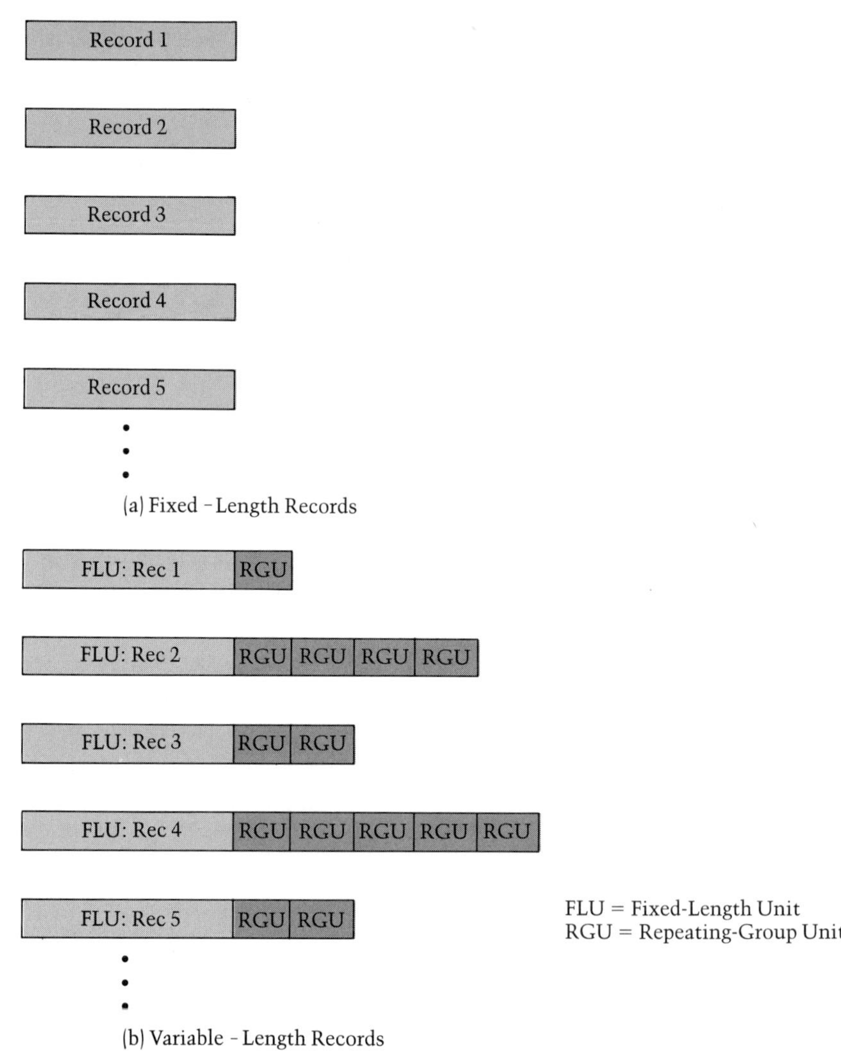

Figure 12.1

Fixed-length versus variable-length record. All occurrences of a fixed-length record will be the same size and contain the same fields. Variable-length records are usually composed of a fixed size root segment followed by some number of occurrences of the other fields.

this feature for you. The buffer is also used for reading from the file device. A block of records is read from the device into the buffer. Your subsequent read commands actually read the logical records from the buffer.

A block of logical records is also called a **physical record.** The number of logical records in a physical record is called the **blocking factor** for the file. As a systems analyst, you may have to specify the blocking factor during file design. What do we mean by *may?* On some computer systems, the blocking factor is determined by the computer's operating system — that is the blocking factors are out of your control. In other environments, operations specialists may decide on blocking factors. And in still other environments, blocking factors may be calculated by the analyst — which is why it is important for you to understand the concept of physical records and blocking.

If the blocking factor is one (meaning one physical record contains one logical record), then the physical record and the logical record are identical. Why can't you just make the blocking factor equal to the number of records in the file and thus read or write the whole file with one read or write command? The following limitations prevent such a solution:

1. The main computer memory is not nearly large enough to hold the entire file. The main memory of the computer must store the operating system, *all* active computer programs, and the read or write buffers for all those programs. This main memory is a fraction of the size of most files.
2. If the read/write buffer is too large, there won't be enough room for the computer program.
3. The storage device may impose limitations on the maximum size for the physical record. For instance, most systems cannot read or write more than one disk track at a time. This would obviously limit the blocking factor to the number of logical records that can be placed on a single track of the disk.

The typical blocking factor is normally a compromise between these three factors. The physical block size may also be restricted by the computer to be some fixed portion of a track (such as $\frac{1}{4}$ track or $\frac{1}{3}$ track). The blocking factor should try to utilize as much of the fixed portion as possible because any leftover space is wasted.

We should note that blocking is also used to maximize the number of logical records that can be recorded on magnetic tape. If you are familiar with magnetic tape, you know that an *interrecord gap* is left between physical records to permit the tape drive to start and stop. Blocked records reduce the number of interrecord gaps and

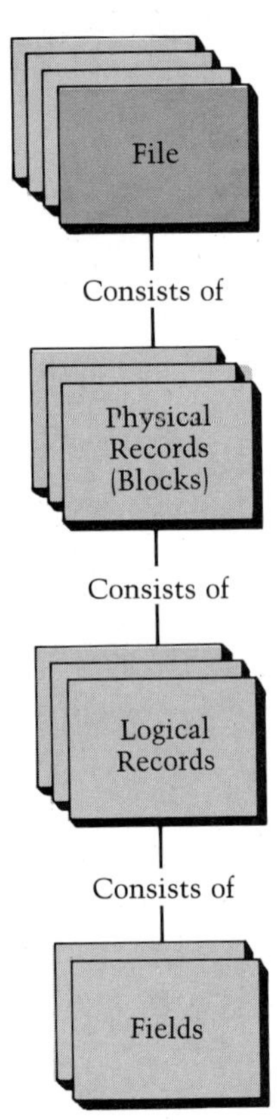

Data Storage Hierarchy

therefore increase the number of logical records that can be placed on the tape.

You'll learn how to calculate the blocking factor for a file later in this chapter.

Types of Files

The next level in our data storage hierarchy is the file itself (see margin). A **file** is the data set of all occurrences of a logical record (or physical record, which is a superset of the logical record). Typically, several types of files are encountered in information systems.

1. A **master file** contains records that are relatively permanent. Once a new master file record has been added to the file, it remains in the system indefinitely. The values of fields for the record will change over its lifetime, but the record occurrence normally remains active for a long period of time. Master file records normally contain the basic data that describe the business. Examples of master file records include CUSTOMER ACCOUNT, EMPLOYEE, and INVENTORY. Most master file records are fixed length.
2. **Transaction files** contain records that describe business events. The data describing these events normally has a limited useful lifetime. For instance, an INVOICE record is useful until the invoice has been paid off. In data processing systems, transaction records are frequently retained on-line (for example, on disk) for some period of time, after which they are migrated to off-line storage (such as tape). The inactive, off-line records are retained as an archive file. Examples of transaction files include ORDER, INVOICE, and MATERIAL REQUISITION. Many, if not most, transaction files contain variable-length records.
3. **Scratch files** (also called *work files* or *temporary files*) are special files that contain temporary duplicates or subsets of a master or transaction file. A scratch file is created, used by the appropriate computer program, and then disposed of. In other words, it is created for a single task and must be recreated each time that task is performed. A simple and common scratch file is a re-sorted CUSTOMER file in which the only difference is the sequence of the records in the file.
4. **Table files** are used to store tabular data that changes relatively infrequently. Examples include payroll system tax tables and

insurance actuary tables. Table files are typically loaded, as is, into the programs that use them. Those programs don't usually update such tables.

File Access and Organization

Files are a shared data resource. Because several programs will likely use and maintain the same file, the records should be organized so each program can easily access them. One of the major responsibilities for the systems analyst is to determine file access and organization. File organization is a function of file access. Therefore, we will begin with access.

File access is the method by which a computer program will read records from a file. Every computer program will access a file in one of two ways: sequentially or directly. The **sequential access method** starts reading or writing with a record in the file (normally the first) and proceeds — one record after another — until the entire file has been processed. Sequential access is used when a program needs to look at a relatively high percentage of all records in a file. For instance, a monthly invoice program may need to access virtually every record in the ACCOUNT file. Sequential access is normally required for batch transaction processing as well as for management reporting.

Direct access (also called *random access*) permits access of any record in a file without reading all previous records in that file. Direct access is appropriate for programs that need to access only one or a few records in a file (queries, for example). Such a program shouldn't have to read all the records sequentially until it finds the desired record. Instead, this program requires direct access to specific records in the file. Direct access is normally needed for on-line transaction processing and decision support.

File organization defines how logical records in a file are related to one another. There are three common file organizations:

1. Sequential file record occurrences are arranged according to the value of a primary key field or a descriptor field. For instance, customer records could be organized sequentially according to CUSTOMER NUMBER or CUSTOMER NAME. Sequential records can be stored one after the other, physically adjacent to one another (see Figure 12.2[a]).Or they can be arranged sequentially with a linked list (see Figure 12.2[b]).

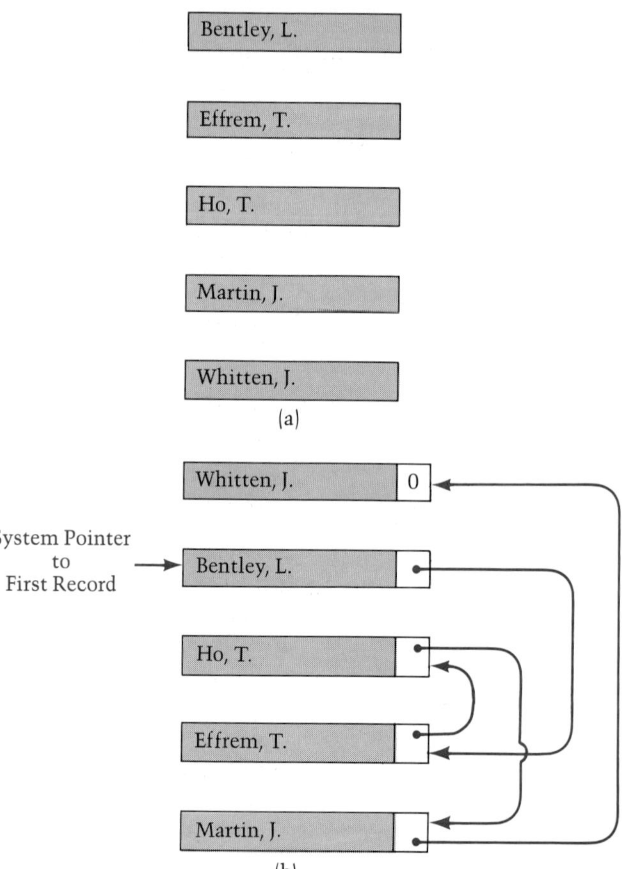

Figure 12.2

Alternative sequential file organization of records. There are two ways to store records in a sequential file. First, you can store the sequential records one after the other (Figure 12.2[a]). Second, you can implement the sequence using a linked list (called a *logically sequential file*) of records (Figure 12.2[b]).

2. Direct file record occurrences are physically located at an address that is calculated from its primary key field. The calculation of the address from the key field is called **hashing.** Thus record occurrences are scattered on the storage device instead of being arranged next to one another or linked via pointer fields. Records can be retrieved rapidly by applying the hashing formula to the primary key field of the desired record. You should

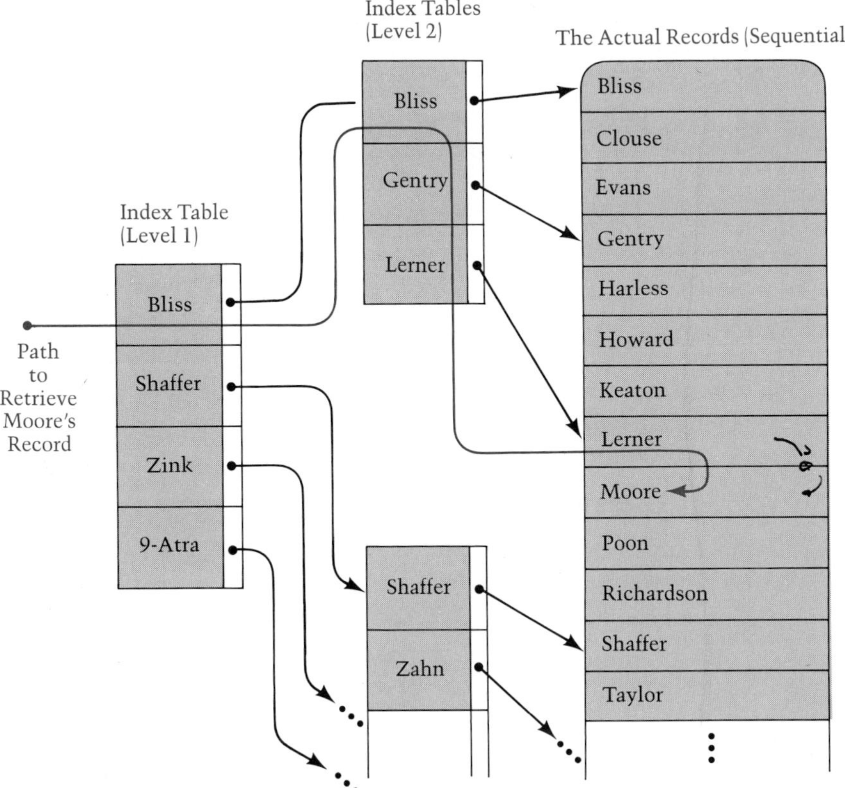

Figure 12.3

Indexed file organization. This employee file is organized as an indexed file. In indexed files, the actual records (shown on the right-hand side of the figure) are usually stored sequentially (although some approaches, such as VSAM, offer other options). As records are entered into the sequential file, index tables are built that allow the sequential files to be retrieved without sequentially reading through the whole file. The path for retrieving Moore's record is indicated.

become familiar with various hashing techniques. Some of the more common hashing techniques include the division remainder, digit analysis, mid-square, folding, and alphabetic keys methods.

3. Indexed file organization is illustrated in Figure 12.3. Records are arranged sequentially (in contiguous locations or using a linked list or both). However, the file also contains an index of

record keys and their physical addresses that can be used to semidirectly access records within the sequential file. Each program determines how it wants to access the records, sequentially or directly (via the index).

Indexed file organization is supported by software so that, when records are added to or deleted from the sequential file, the index is also maintained automatically. Two of the more common indexed file access methods are VSAM (Virtual Storage Access Method) and ISAM (Indexed Sequential Access Method). VSAM and ISAM differ primarily in the manner in which the physical files are organized. This has a greater impact on the programmer than on the analyst. Although some periodic maintenance is usually required for indexed files, a discussion of this topic is beyond the scope of this book.

The selection of the best type of organization for a file is a function of the file access methods required by programs that will use that file. If all programs need sequential access, the file should be organized sequentially. Similarly, if all programs require direct access, the file should be organized randomly. Finally, if a combination of access methods is needed, an indexed organization is recommended. Some data processing standards dictate that all master and transaction files must be organized as indexed files. Why? Because future requirements may dictate a combination of sequential and direct access even if that combination is not needed today.

HOW TO DESIGN AND DOCUMENT MASTER AND TRANSACTION FILES

In this section, we discuss how files are designed. We'll introduce some important issues and guidelines. And we'll design a couple of files to demonstrate this important systems design task.

File Design Considerations

We'd like to impress upon you two important and related issues that will affect file design: redundancy and integrity. These issues impact the value and usefulness of the files you will design.

The minimization of redundant data in files has long been a suggested philosophy of file design. Ideally, no single field would be included in more than one logical record. Take a moment and ask yourself why. Yes, redundantly stored fields will use considerably more storage space. But the problem is even more significant. If the same field is stored in more than one logical record, the data must be updated in more than one place when they change. Otherwise the *same* field could take on different values in different records. This is a data integrity problem and can be improved by reducing redundant data.

So why do systems frequently store redundant data? The reasoning is not unsound. First, there are natural relationships between files. If we need to use the data in one file (for example, CUSTOMER) to cross reference the data in another file (say, INVOICE), we redundantly store some customer fields in both files. Second, to improve performance of some programs, we can reduce the number of files needed by a program (thus reducing the number of files opened, read from, and written to) by redundantly storing some common data in more than one file.

Redundancy, as a term, has an undeserved reputation. Redundancy is not necessarily wrong. Uncontrolled redundancy is the problem! We suggest you restrict duplication of fields in different records to primary key fields (needed to cross-reference files) and relatively stable descriptor fields (those that don't change values often). For instance, CUSTOMER ADDRESS is relatively stable, but CUSTOMER BALANCE is not. The more volatile the field, the greater the danger that lies in storing that field redundantly.

The problems of data integrity and redundancy can be addressed in another way — through the use of database technology. Database technology is special purpose software that allows files to be integrated into a single data set. Actually, the notion of files, as we have defined them, disappears in a database environment. Logical record occurrences of one type (say, CUSTOMER) can be directly linked to occurrences of another type (say, ORDER). Thus by following these links (or pointers), we can retrieve all of the order records for a customer or we can retrieve the customer record for an order. There is no need to store redundant customer fields in the ORDER record or order fields in the CUSTOMER record. Hence, data integrity is improved.

Database is a complex subject. Not all introductory systems analysis and design courses consider it appropriate. For that reason, we defer any further discussion to Module E in Part IV of this book. This module can be studied at your instructor's discretion (or your

The Next Generation — Looking Beyond Files and Databases: Can We Store Expertise?

First there were files and then databases. Today we are seeing data banks, large databases owned by a company that sells access to the data banks (sort of a computerized library — a good example is *The Source,* which can be accessed via long-distance telephone calls from most popular microcomputers). Both databases and data banks store data and information. But consider the possibility of storing knowledge and expertise. That's the next generation.

Knowledge is the ability to apply information. When you generate a report for a manager, that report is information. Putting that report to use requires knowledge and expertise. Wouldn't it be nice to be able to capture and store that expertise? For example, wouldn't it be nice if the computer could periodically scan the business environment the way that a manager does, examine various databases, recognize the need for a decision or immediate attention, and make the decision (or at least inform a manager of the need for the decision and provide options and analyses of those options)? Sounds too scary?

Well, that is exactly what researchers and vendors are looking at right now! The current buzzword for this concept is *expert systems.* In an **expert system,** the expertise and knowledge associated with decision making is stored in a knowledge base. Programs are written to access the knowledge bases and databases to identify and make decisions (computerized chess programs have always been based on this idea). These programs attempt to define solutions to problems, evaluate the impact of those solutions, possibly predict how the environment may react to those solutions, and select a course of action. The expert system applications are based on the development of artificial intelligence technology, both hardware and software. These systems will require extremely rapid data and knowledge access methods ▶

own). In any event, you should be aware that most companies using database technology employ database specialists who can help the systems analyst design the database for any system.

Internal Controls for Files

We return now to the continuing topic of internal controls. Internal controls are designed into files to ensure the integrity and security of the data in those files. Internal control issues for files include the following:

- Access controls should be specified for all files. Access controls determine who will be able to read and write the file. Some users will have read and write access. Other users will have only read

The Next Generation (continued)

and processing speeds.

Knowledge bases must be combined with databases to make expert systems. Some such systems have already been built. Medical expert systems allow doctors and nurses to input symptoms and conditions. The expert system simulates the expertise of many more doctors than a hospital or clinic can afford to keep on staff. It gives the medical staff access to diagnoses and alternative treatments that may be unfamiliar to some doctors. And in all cases, the system provides a second opinion. Similar expert systems are being used to provide advanced expertise to pharmacists (for example, which drugs don't mix with other medications) and geologists (perhaps indicating where to drill for oil).

On the business front, future expert systems may try to simulate the expertise of managers and staff specialists. For instance, production schedules, quality control, accounting, marketing, and other business fields may benefit from expert systems. This is especially true if the systems could be designed not only to respond to data stored in databases but also to sense business conditions via cameras and analog sensing devices (this has already been done in applications such as environmental control, manufacturing process controls and robotics).

As systems analysts, we may become increasingly involved in applying artificial intelligence technology to develop expert systems. We may be called on to interface these systems into current information systems. And we will have some tough decisions to make. For instance, expert systems could potentially put a lot of managers and knowledge workers out of work. In other words, there are some social implications to this trend. And lest you take this too lightly, don't forget — systems analysts (and all data processing professionals) are themselves knowledge workers! ■

access. If corrections must be made to file data, *who* will authorize those changes? Authorization should not come from a data processing professional. The data belongs to the user, and changes should be authorized by members of the user community.

- Length of retention of files is another control issue. Master files are retained indefinitely. However, how long should transaction records be retained in the file? If retained indefinitely, valuable storage capacity will be wasted on records that have little probability for use. When should such records be archived? How long should the records be maintained off-line? In some cases, government regulations may dictate a long retention cycle.
- Backup methods and procedures should be defined for all data

files. Backups are used to recover data when files have been lost or destroyed. All master and transaction files should be periodically copied to tape.

- Recovery procedures complement the backup methods and procedures by defining how files will be restored if they are lost, damaged, or stolen. For any lost file, the previous update is reloaded, but this step only restores the files to the point in time when the last backup was performed. What about updates that have occurred since that backup? The easiest way to recover those updates is to design the system so that, as transactions that result in changes to any file stored on disk are processed, a continuous record of each change be kept and stored off-line on a medium such as tape. That tape can easily be reprocessed without duplicate data entry. Of course, if tape backup is undesirable or infeasible, the updates can be re-input from the history reports you designed to confirm transaction processing.

An Overview of File Design

Computer files that need to be designed are easily identified by studying either the data flow diagrams prepared during systems analysis or the outputs designed as the first task of system design. On the data flow diagram, files appear as *data stores*. Given a file to be designed, the following general procedure can be followed:

1. *Determine the contents of the file.* Actually, the contents of the file (data stores on the DFD) may have been specified during systems analysis. A data dictionary entry may have been created to define the fields (data elements) that need to be stored. If the file contents haven't been specified, they can be determined by studying the outputs and the data needed to generate those outputs. The contents of the logical record are usually recorded on a **record layout chart** (to be discussed later in this chapter).
2. *Determine file size.* To calculate the storage requirements for a new file, you need to determine how fields will be stored (EBCDIC, ASCII, packed decimal, or some other appropriate method). You will also need to know how many records will be stored in the file and how fast the file will grow. And you'll need to know how long a record should be retained before it is archived. These are questions that can only be answered by your

users. Therefore, users will have to be intimately involved in file design.

3. *Determine the best organization for the file.* You do this by studying the access methods needed by each program that will use the file. Some organizations provide guidelines for determining file organization. Others organizations standardize on VSAM or ISAM so that all files can be accessed sequentially and randomly. We'll soon offer some general hints concerning what to do in the absence of standards or guidelines.
4. *Design internal controls.* These were just discussed in the preceding section of this chapter.
5. *Determine optimal blocking factors if needed.* As mentioned earlier, some computer systems determine their own blocking factors. And in some data processing shops, the analyst is not responsible for calculating blocking factors.

So much for our overview of the file design task. Let's study a few examples of file design to see how this procedure is applied.

Design of a Master File

In Figures 12.4 through 12.6, we see the design specifications for the CUSTOMER file. This is one of the many files that appeared on the DFDs for the AAP Order Entry Information System. The CUSTOMER file is an example of a master file because customer records are relatively permanent once they have been added to the file. Figures 12.4 and 12.5 are an expanded data dictionary for the file design (similar to the data dictionaries used for outputs in Chapter 11). Skim through the entries on these forms. Then direct your attention to the following:

Ⓐ There are no repeating groups of data elements in the data structure (Figure 12.4). Therefore, the record is fixed length.

Ⓑ The record size (from Figure 12.4) is the sum of the field sizes, in bytes, from Figure 12.5 (see p. 460), a data element dictionary. Editing symbols, such as commas, dashes, and dollar signs, aren't stored and are not included in field size. For fields, we've used the code "Z" for EBCDIC storage (also called *zoned decimal*) and "P" for packed-decimal storage (again, see Figure 12.5).

```
D A T A  D I C T I O N A R Y :  F I L E (Page 1)

DEFINITION

   NAME OF FILE:  CUSTOMER
   PREPARED BY:  Doug Matthews (March 13, 1986)
   DESCRIPTION:  Contains record on each AAP customer's account
          balances, credit details, and billing information.
   MEDIUM:  Disk                        PRIMARY KEY(S):  CUSTOMER NUMBER
(A) FIXED/VARIABLE LENGTH?  Fixed       RECORD SIZE (bytes):  107 <---(B)
   BLOCKING FACTOR:  24 <---(C)         BLOCK SIZE (bytes):  2,603
   AVERAGE VOLUME (in records):  600
   ANTICIPATED GROWTH (percent and time period):  5% per year
   FILE SIZE (bytes):  75,487
(D) FILE SIZE (tracks or inches):  10 tracks
   FILE SIZE (cylinders):  2
   LIFETIME UNTIL ARCHIVE:  Indefinite
   BACKUP TIMING:  Daily 12 P.M. & 4 P.M.     BACKUP RETENTION:  7 years
   SPECIAL INSTRUCTIONS:  Only A/R Dept. is permitted to update CREDIT RATING,(E)
         CREDIT CEILING, CURRENT BALANCE DUE, and BALANCE PAST DUE.

ACCESS AND ORGANIZATION
```

PROGRAM/PROCESS NAME		ACTIVITY RATIO	UPDATE?	ACCESS METHOD
CHECK CUSTOMER CREDIT	(F)	41%	YES	SEQUENTIAL
BILL CUSTOMER		100%	YES	SEQUENTIAL
RECORD CUSTOMER PAYMENT		16%	YES	DIRECT
CREDIT CUSTOMER ACCOUNT		2%	YES	DIRECT
PRODUCE A/R SUMMARY REPORT		100%	NO	SEQUENTIAL
QUERY CUSTOMER A/R ACCOUNT		< 1%	NO	DIRECT
CHECK CUSTOMER DETAILS		45%	YES	SEQUENTIAL

```
   FILE ORGANIZATION METHOD:  Indexed (ISAM)

FILE COMPOSITION

     A CUSTOMER consists of the following data elements:
          CUSTOMER NAME
          BILLING ADDRESS which consists of:
               One or both of the following elements:
                    STREET ADDRESS
                    POST OFFICE BOX NUMBER
               CITY
               STATE
               ZIP CODE
          BILLING PHONE
          CUSTOMER TYPE
          CREDIT RATING
          CREDIT CEILING
          CURRENT BALANCE DUE
          BALANCE PAST DUE
          CUSTOMER ACTIVE FLAG
```

Figure 12.4

An expanded data dictionary for CUSTOMER master file (Page 1). An expanded data dictionary can be used to record the detailed design requirements for a file. We prepared our dictionary using a simple word processor to read in blank forms. Blank forms could, of course, be printed for use. Blank form masters can be found in your student workbook.

Ⓒ If they are required, blocking factors (Figure 12.4) are not difficult to calculate. There is usually a limit to the size of a block (for example, half of a track on the disk). And some DP shops establish a standard for block size. For any given disk drive, there are tables that provide blocking reference data for that disk drive. Different tables are used for files to be stored with and without keys. The blocking factor table tells you how big the block can be. For example, for files that require keys, the following block sizes might be found:

Track Size	*Minimum Block Size (bytes)*	*Maximum Block Size (bytes)*
1	4,026	8,293
$\frac{1}{2}$	2,604	4,025
$\frac{1}{3}$	1,892	2,603
$\frac{1}{4}$	1,466	1,891

Note that these numbers apply to one particular disk drive and the use of primary keys (see REMARK column for CUSTOMER NUMBER). This disk drive was assumed for our example. Blocking factor (BF) is calculated as follows:

BF = Maximum block size/Logical record size

We have assumed that AAP's Data Processing Shop has adopted a $\frac{1}{3}$ track blocking standard. Therefore a block size consists of 2,603 bytes. The blocking factor was then calculated as:

$$\text{Blocking Factor} = 2{,}603\,\frac{\text{bytes}}{\text{block}} \bigg/ 107\,\frac{\text{bytes}}{\text{record}}$$

$$= 24.33\,\frac{\text{records}}{\text{block}}$$

This is read "24.33" records *per* block. Blocking factors are always rounded down because a portion of a logical record cannot be stored in a physical record.

Ⓓ File size is an important calculation because we can't store data for which we don't have capacity. To calculate file size, we first determined, by consulting the users, that there are currently 600 customers and that the customer base is growing 5 percent

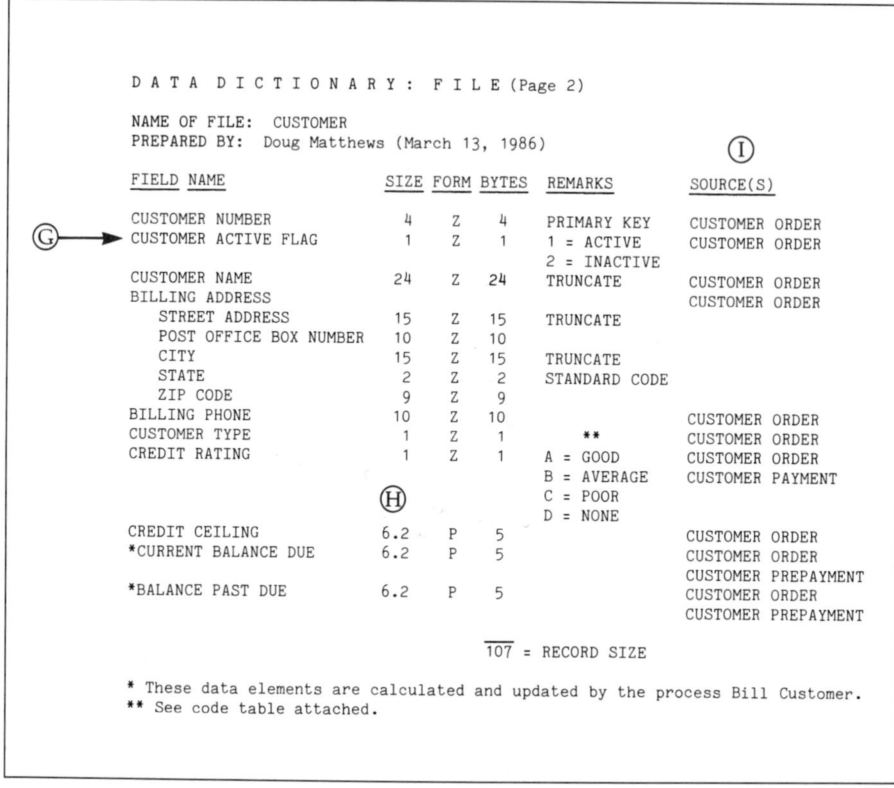

D A T A   D I C T I O N A R Y :   F I L E (Page 2)

NAME OF FILE: CUSTOMER
PREPARED BY: Doug Matthews (March 13, 1986)

FIELD NAME	SIZE	FORM	BYTES	REMARKS	SOURCE(S) (I)
CUSTOMER NUMBER	4	Z	4	PRIMARY KEY	CUSTOMER ORDER
(G) → CUSTOMER ACTIVE FLAG	1	Z	1	1 = ACTIVE 2 = INACTIVE	CUSTOMER ORDER
CUSTOMER NAME	24	Z	24	TRUNCATE	CUSTOMER ORDER
BILLING ADDRESS					CUSTOMER ORDER
STREET ADDRESS	15	Z	15	TRUNCATE	
POST OFFICE BOX NUMBER	10	Z	10		
CITY	15	Z	15	TRUNCATE	
STATE	2	Z	2	STANDARD CODE	
ZIP CODE	9	Z	9		
BILLING PHONE	10	Z	10		CUSTOMER ORDER
CUSTOMER TYPE	1	Z	1	**	CUSTOMER ORDER
CREDIT RATING	1	Z	1	A = GOOD B = AVERAGE C = POOR D = NONE	CUSTOMER ORDER CUSTOMER PAYMENT
	(H)				
CREDIT CEILING	6.2	P	5		CUSTOMER ORDER
*CURRENT BALANCE DUE	6.2	P	5		CUSTOMER ORDER CUSTOMER PREPAYMENT
*BALANCE PAST DUE	6.2	P	5		CUSTOMER ORDER CUSTOMER PREPAYMENT
			107	= RECORD SIZE	

* These data elements are calculated and updated by the process Bill Customer.
** See code table attached.

Figure 12.5

The expanded data dictionary for CUSTOMER master file (Page 2). This second page of our design data dictionary is used to record facts about fields.

per year. To calculate the file size in bytes, tracks, and cylinders, the following calculations were used:

$$\text{Bytes} = 600 \text{ records} \times 1.158 \Big/ 24 \frac{\text{records}}{\text{block}} \times 2{,}603 \frac{\text{bytes}}{\text{block}}$$

$$= 75{,}487 \text{ bytes of storage}$$

Notice that the blocking factor had to be considered because the wasted storage in any block cannot be reclaimed (because block size is fixed at 2,603 bytes per physical record). Also note that we included anticipated growth $(5\% = 1.05)$ over three years $(1.05^3 = 1.158)$ in our formula. Finally, after dividing by the blocking factor, that result was rounded up. Why? If you divided a result from the first operation of this formula by the number of records per block, the result may include a remainder. A file and a block must both contain entire records.

It is also useful to express file size in terms of tracks and cylinders because those tracks and cylinders might have to be dedicated to the file.

$$\text{Tracks} = 600 \text{ records} \times 1.158 \Big/ 24 \frac{\text{records}}{\text{blocks}} \Big/ 3 \frac{\text{blocks}}{\text{track}}$$

$$= 10 \text{ tracks (We rounded up)}$$

To determine the number of cylinders required to store the file, you need to understand another characteristic of the disk packs used by AAP. The disk packs currently in use have 9 tracks per cylinder (this may vary for other disk packs).

$$\text{Cylinders} = 10 \frac{\text{tracks}}{\text{file}} \Big/ 9 \frac{\text{tracks}}{\text{cylinder}}$$

$$= 2 \text{ cylinders/file}$$

The number of cylinders should be rounded up if necessary.

Ⓔ Notice that we recorded internal control and security comments into our expanded data dictionary.

Ⓕ Assuming there are no internal standards or guidelines for selecting the file organization, then the following technique might prove useful. To determine the access and organization of the file, we first identified each program requiring access to that file. These programs can be identified on your DFDs. For each program, we recorded whether the program should be permitted to update the file and what percentage of the records a single execution of the program will read or update (this is called an *activity ratio*). Then we applied the following rules of thumb:

> If the activity ratio is greater than or equal to 40 percent, we select the sequential access method for the program. Otherwise we select the direct access method.

In our example, both sequential and direct access against the file are required. Indexed was the logical choice for file organization because it's the only method that provides both access methods. (Please note that opinions may vary concerning the 40 percent guideline we used for our rule of thumb.)

Referring specifically to Figure 12.5, we note the following:

Ⓖ We added an element, CUSTOMER ACTIVE FLAG. Although not an element defined by our users, this flag can be set to indicate that we want to delete this customer but cannot do so at this time. For instance, the customer might still owe on invoices. This flag, if set to 'inactive' could be used to prevent that customer from submitting additional orders while retaining our ability to access the record.

Ⓗ Look at the field size column. The entry "6.2" means that the field size is 8, with 6 digits to the left of the decimal point and two to the right. You can adopt any similar convention with which you're comfortable. Notice that the 8-digit field requires 5 bytes to store. Each digit requires $\frac{1}{2}$ byte using the indicated packed-decimal format. But we need an extra $\frac{1}{2}$ byte for a sign digit. Thus, the field size in bytes is $\frac{9}{2}$, rounded up — 5 bytes.

Ⓘ The SOURCE column indicates the source of any update to that field. This may include an input name or calculation. Some fields may have several sources of update. For example, CUSTOMER BALANCE may be updated by a new order, credit, or payment.

Now that we've addressed the file design issues, we can prepare the layout for the file. The record layout chart is a tool we'll use to prepare an easy-to-read, graphical layout of the fields in a record. Figure 12.6 is the record layout chart for the CUSTOMER file. Notice that the primary key, CUSTOMER NUMBER, was located in the first field position. To be consistent, the field names used corresponded with the field names used in the data dictionary. Notice how we used the *Characteristics* portion of the form to record field storage formats. The applicable codes include:

FX = fixed point binary
FL = floating point binary
P = packed decimal (or EBCDIC)
A = ASCII
Z = zoned decimal

RECORD LAYOUT CHART FOR CUSTOMER (name of file) FILE

PREPARED BY: DOUG MATTHEWS

DATE PREPARED: MARCH 13, 1986

Field Name	CUSTOMER NUMBER	CUSTOMER ACTING FLAG	CUSTOMER NAME	STREET ADDRESS	POST OFFICE BOX NUMBER	CITY	STATE	ZIPCODE	BILLING PHONE	CUSTOMER TYPE	CREDIT RATING	CREDIT CEILING	CURRENT BALANCE DUE	BALANCE PAST DUE	
Characteristics*	Z	Z	Z	Z	Z	Z	Z	Z	Z	Z	Z	P	P	P	
Position**	0-3	4	5-28	29-43	44-53	54-68	69-70	71-79	80-89	90	91	92-96	97-101	102-106	

Figure 12.6

Record layout for CUSTOMER master record. Record layout charts are used to communicate logical record design to the programmer.

In Figure 12.6, we used Z and P. Remember, the storage formats may be constrained by your computer system.

Design of a Transaction File

The ORDER file is a transaction file used by a number of the programs in the system. This file contains data describing each customer order received by AAP. Figures 12.7 through 12.9 represent the design specifications for this transaction file. Most of these entries are similar to those in the last example. We call your attention to the following exceptions:

Ⓐ The data structure for the ORDER (Figure 12.7) contains a repeating group. Therefore, the record is set up as variable length.

Ⓑ Consequently, there is a minimum and maximum record size (Figure 12.8). Maximum record size is based on the maximum number of times that the repeating group can occur (in our case, 40). Minimum record size is easy to calculate. Because every order must have at least one ordered part, we simply sum the sizes of the individual fields (shown in Figure 12.8).

Maximum field size is a little more difficult to determine than minimum. Notice, on Figure 12.8 that, when we specified the number of bytes necessary for storing each of the repeating fields, we entered both the number of times the field may be stored *and* the size of the field in bytes. The maximum record size equals the sum of the field sizes in the fixed-length portion of the record plus the sum of 40 times the sum of the repeating elements. This enabled us to calculate maximum file size as follows:

$$27\,\frac{\text{bytes}}{\text{record}} + \left(16\,\frac{\text{bytes}}{\text{record}} \times 40 \text{ groups}\right) = 667\,\frac{\text{bytes}}{\text{record}}$$

Returning to Figure 12.7, the data dictionary, we note that

Ⓒ The range we just calculated was entered on Figure 12.7.

Ⓓ We then used the maximum record size, 667 bytes, to determine the blocking factor, just as we did in the last example. Try it for yourself. The other file size requirements can be calculated by using the formulas used in the previous example. Give

```
D A T A   D I C T I O N A R Y :   F I L E (Page 1)

DEFINITION

    NAME OF FILE:  ORDERS
    PREPARED BY:  Cheryl Mason (March 12, 1986)
    DESCRIPTION:  Contains a record of all AAP orders and their status.
    MEDIUM:  Disk                       PRIMARY KEY(S):  SALES ORDER NUMBER
    SECONDARY KEY(S):  CUSTOMER NUMBER, PART NUMBER
(A) FIXED/VARIABLE LENGTH?  Variable    RECORD SIZE (bytes):  43-667 <---(C)
    BLOCKING FACTOR:  3 <----------(D)  BLOCK SIZE (bytes):  2603
    AVERAGE VOLUME (in records):  1000 PEAK VOLUME (in records):  1300
    ANTICIPATED GROWTH (percent and time period):  8% per year
    FILE SIZE (bytes):  1,421,238 (based on peak volume)
    FILE SIZE (tracks or inches):  182 tracks
    FILE SIZE (cylinders):  21"
    LIFETIME UNTIL ARCHIVE:  Daily       BACKUP TIMING:  8:35 P.M.
    BACKUP RETENTION:  1 Year

ACCESS AND ORGANIZATION
```

PROGRAM/PROCESS NAME	ACTIVITY RATIO	UPDATE?	ACCESS METHOD
RECORD CUSTOMER ORDER	25%	YES	DIRECT
RELEASE ORDER HELD FOR PREPAYMENT	4%	YES	DIRECT
RELEASE ORDER HELD FOR CLARIFICATION	3%	YES	DIRECT
RELEASE STANDING ORDER FOR MONTHLY DELIVERY	4%	YES	DIRECT
PRODUCE SALES ORDER LOG	100%	NO	SEQUENTIAL
SUMMARIZE SALES BY PRODUCT LINE	100%	NO	SEQUENTIAL
QUERY CUSTOMER ORDER	< 1%	NO	DIRECT
QUERY PART	< 9%	NO	DIRECT

```
    FILE ORGANIZATION METHOD:  Indexed (ISAM)

FILE COMPOSITION

      A ORDER consists of the following data elements:
           SALES ORDER NUMBER
           CUSTOMER NUMBER
           PREPAYMENT AMOUNT
           ORDER DATE
           ORDER TYPE
           ORDER STATUS
           1 to 40 occurrences of the following:
                PART NUMBER
                QUANTITY ORDERED
                QUANTITY BACKORDERED
                UNIT PRICE
      (E)  NUMBER OF ORDERED PARTS
```

Figure 12.7

The expanded data dictionary for ORDERS transaction file (Page 1).

them a try and see if you come up with the same numbers for the file size entries.

(E) Notice that we added the field NUMBER OF ORDERED PARTS to the record. Variable-length records require this type of a field to indicate to the computer how much storage space is

DATA DICTIONARY: FILE (Page 2)

NAME OF FILE: ORDERS
PREPARED BY: Cheryl Mason (March 12, 1986)

FIELD NAME	SIZE	FORM	BYTES	REMARKS	SOURCE(S)
SALESORDER NUMBER	7	Z	7	PRIMARY KEY	CUSTOMER ORDER
CUSTOMER NUMBER	4	Z	4	SECONDARY KEY	CUSTOMER ORDER
PREPAYMENT AMOUNT	5.2	P	4		CUSTOMER ORDER
ORDER DATE	8	Z	8	MMDDYYYY	CUSTOMER ORDER
ORDER TYPE	1	Z	1	R = REGULAR W = RUSH E = EMPLOYEE S = STANDING	CUSTOMER ORDER
ORDER STATUS	1	Z	1	S = STANDING F = FILLING B = BACKORDERED	CUSTOMER ORDER
PART NUMBER	9	Z	40X9		CUSTOMER ORDER
QUANTITY ORDERED	3	P	40X2		CUSTOMER ORDER
QUANTITY BACKORDERED	3	P	40X2		CUSTOMER ORDER
UNIT PRICE	3.2	P	40X3		CUSTOMER ORDER
NUMBER OF ORDERED PARTS	2	P	2 (B)	Contains the number of parts on the CUSTOMER ORDER.	CUSTOMER ORDER

RECORD SIZE = 43-667

Figure 12.8

The expanded data dictionary for ORDERS transaction file (Page 2).

allocated for a particular occurrence in the ORDER. These special fields are called *repeating factors.* Notice that we didn't forget to add the repeating-factor field NUMBER OF ORDERED PARTS to the data structure for ORDER.

The rest of the entries in Figures 12.7 and 12.8 are either self-explanatory or similar to those in the master file example.

And what about the layout of this variable-length record? The layout is documented in Figure 12.9. Yes, it looks somewhat different from the layout for our sample master record in Figure 12.6. But, it's actually not that much different.

(A) We prefer to separate the root and repeating portions of the record. By referring back to the expanded data dictionary, we were able to identify those fields that were to occur only one time per logical record. The layout of the repeating fields was then depicted on the line below the line that shows the fixed portion of the record (see Figure 12.9). Notice that we did not

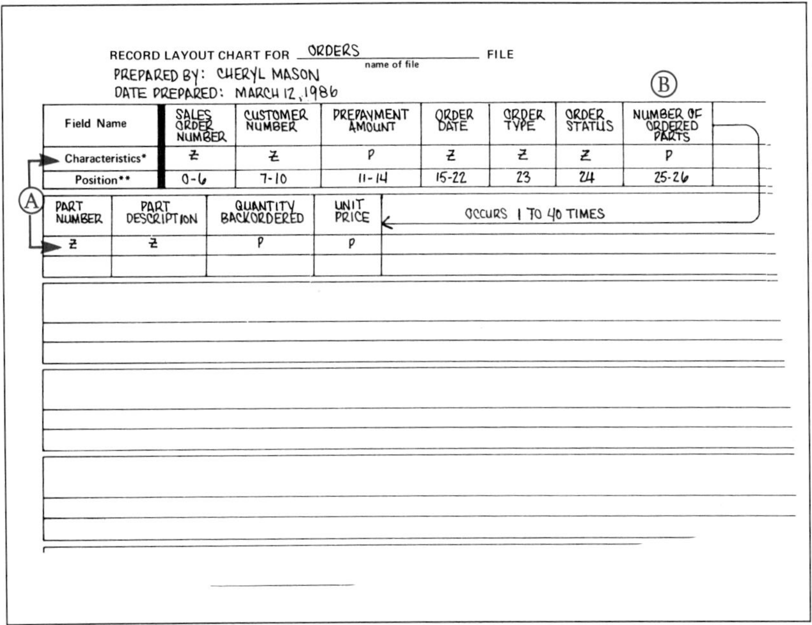

RECORD LAYOUT CHART FOR ORDERS (name of file) FILE

PREPARED BY: CHERYL MASON

DATE PREPARED: MARCH 12, 1986

Ⓑ

Field Name	SALES ORDER NUMBER	CUSTOMER NUMBER	PREPAYMENT AMOUNT	ORDER DATE	ORDER TYPE	ORDER STATUS	NUMBER OF ORDERED PARTS
Characteristics*	Z	Z	P	Z	Z	Z	P
Position**	0-6	7-10	11-14	15-22	23	24	25-26

Ⓐ

PART NUMBER	PART DESCRIPTION	QUANTITY BACKORDERED	UNIT PRICE
Z	Z	P	P

OCCURS 1 TO 40 TIMES

Figure 12.9

Format for ORDER transaction record.

enter the position of each of these fields. Why? Because the different occurrences of the repeating group will place the fields in different positions in the record.

Ⓑ The repeating factor field for any variable-length record should be located as the last field in the fixed portion of a record. Therefore, the field NUMBER OF ORDERED PARTS was appended to the fixed portion of the ORDER record. Notice that we drew an arrow from the repeating-factor field to the variable portion of the ORDER record. This was done to clarify to the programmer that NUMBER OF ORDERED PARTS serves as a repeating factor and that occurrences of the fields that follow are dependent upon its value. The line was labeled to clearly indicate the possible number of occurrences.

So you've now seen how our tools can be used to document the design of a master and transaction file. Unfortunately, the design of some files is not nearly as simple.

DATA DICTIONARY: FILE

NAME OF FILE: VENDOR
PREPARED BY: Chuck Balmer (March 19, 1986)

FIELD NAME	SIZE	FORM	BYTES	REMARKS	SOURCE(S)
VENDOR NUMBER	6	Z	6	PRIMARY KEY	VENDOR UPDATES
VENDOR NAME	20	Z	20	SECONDARY KEY TRUNCATE	VENDOR UPDATES
VENDOR ADDRESS					VENDOR UPDATES
STREET	15	Z	15	TRUNCATE	
P.O. BOX NUMBER	10	Z	10	TRUNCATE	
CITY	15	Z	15	TRUNCATE	
STATE	2	Z	2	STANDARD CODE	
ZIP CODE	9	P	5		
ITEM NUMBER	5	Z	100X5		VENDOR UPDATES
ITEM DESCRIPTION	20	Z	100X20	TRUNCATE	VENDOR UPDATES
UNIT PRICE	2.2	P	100X3		VENDOR UPDATES
DISCOUNT RATE	2.1	P	100X2		VENDOR UPDATES
NUMBER OF LATE SHIPMENTS	2.0	P	2		SHIPMENT RECEIPTS
NUMBER OF ITEMS	3.0	P	2	Contains the number of items on the VENDOR UPDATES.	VENDOR UPDATES

Figure 12.10

Partial data dictionary for a VENDOR master file. This file may have to be split into two files because the logical-record size exceeds the maximum standard physical record size.

Design of Complex Data Stores

Let's discuss a couple of difficult yet common file design problems you are likely to encounter and see how these problems might be solved. Examine the expanded data dictionary for a VENDOR file that contains variable-length records (Figure 12.10). What problem(s) might you encounter in designing this file? If we calculate the record size, we will find the minimum length to be 107 bytes and the maximum length to be 3,077 bytes. The maximum length of the record is unacceptable because AAP uses $\frac{1}{3}$-track blocking, with a block size of 2,603 bytes. One logical record will not fit within this block size.

What can we do? One alternative would be to use $\frac{1}{2}$-track blocking or some other blocking criterion that would allow for a larger block size. But you will pay a penalty if you opt for this solution. You'll need a bigger input buffer for the program (to handle the larger block).

DATA DICTIONARY: FILE

NAME OF FILE: VENDOR PRODUCTS
PREPARED BY: Chuck Balmer (March 19, 1986)

FIELD NAME	SIZE	FORM	BYTES	REMARKS	SOURCE(S)
VENDOR NUMBER	6	Z	6	PRIMARY KEY	VENDOR UPDATES
ITEM NUMBER	5	Z	5		VENDOR UPDATES
ITEM DESCRIPTION	20	Z	20	TRUNCATE	VENDOR UPDATES
UNIT PRICE	2.2	P	3		VENDOR UPDATES
DISCOUNT RATE	2.1	P	2		VENDOR UPDATES

(a)

DATA DICTIONARY: FILE

NAME OF FILE: VENDOR
PREPARED BY: Chuck Balmer (March 19, 1986)

FIELD NAME	SIZE	FORM	BYTES	REMARKS	SOURCE(S)
VENDOR NUMBER	6	Z	6	PRIMARY KEY	VENDOR UPDATES
VENDOR NAME	20	Z	20	SECONDARY KEY TRUNCATE	VENDOR UPDATES
VENDOR ADDRESS					VENDOR UPDATES
STREET	15	Z	15	TRUNCATE	
P.O. BOX NUMBER	10	Z	10	TRUNCATE	
CITY	15	Z	15	TRUNCATE	
STATE	2	Z	2	STANDARD CODE	
ZIP CODE	9	P	5		
NUMBER OF LATE SHIPMENTS	2.0	P	2		SHIPMENT RECEIPTS

(b)

Figure 12.11

Partial data dictionaries resulting from split of VENDOR master file. The VENDOR file in Figure 12.10 was split into two separate files. The VENDOR PRODUCTS file (Figure 12.11[a]) was created to contain the repeating fields. The VENDOR file (Figure 12.11 [b]) was created to store the fixed or nonrepeating fields. Note that it is common for one of the new files to retain the same name as the original file.

A second alternative would be to split the VENDOR file into two files. Some of the fields would be placed in one file and some in the other. Figure 12.11(a) and (b) contain the expanded data dictionaries for the resulting files. We chose to place the repeating elements in a separate file called VENDOR PRODUCTS. Notice that we duplicated the VENDOR NUMBER in both files. This will permit us to move back and forth between the two files by using the common keys.

Size is not the only reason we might replace a single file with two files. For example, if you study the contents of the BILL OF MATERIALS FILE (Figure 12.12), you should see that it is a variable-length record. In fact, the data structure contains *nested* (one within another) repeating groups. A PRODUCT consists of COMPONENTS that, in turn, consist of RAW MATERIALS. You may be tempted to design the layout of the BILL OF MATERIALS record as illustrated in Figure 12.13. Although logically correct, most file processing systems (such as COBOL) can handle repeating groups but do not support repeating groups *within* repeating groups. So what do we do? Once again, the record can be split into two records and files: the first file indicates all components for a product and the second file indicates all materials for a component (see Figures 12.14[a] and [b]).

SUMMARY

Computer files consist of physical records, logical records, and fields. A field or data element is the smallest unit of data to be stored. There are three types of fields: primary keys, secondary keys, and descriptors. Most business-oriented systems store fields as binary codes. There are three common binary codes: EBCDIC, ASCII, and packed decimal. An understanding of storage formats is important during file design because storage format affects file size.

A logical record is a collection of fields arranged in a predefined format to describe a single entity. A logical record is also the unit of data storage that is operated on by a computer program. Logical records for a system are specified by the systems analyst. Depending on the data structure to be stored, the logical record will have fixed or variable length. The logical record for a file is normally documented by using a record layout chart.

Occurrences of logical records are blocked into physical records, the smallest number of occurrences of logical records that can be read or written at one time. The analyst often determines the number of logical records in the block because this can affect performance.

DATA DICTIONARY: FILE

NAME OF FILE: BILL OF MATERIALS
PREPARED BY: Paula Thompson (May 2, 1986)

FIELD NAME	SIZE	FORM	BYTES	REMARKS	SOURCE(S)
PRODUCT NUMBER	5	Z	5		BOM UPDATES
PRODUCT DESCRIPTION	15	Z	15	TRUNCATE	BOM UPDATES
UNIT OF MEASURE	2	Z	2		BOM UPDATES
COMPONENT NUMBER	6	Z	20X6		BOM UPDATES
COMPONENT DESCRIPTION	15	Z	20X15	TRUNCATE	BOM UPDATES
COMPONENT UNIT OF MEASURE	2	Z	20X2		BOM UPDATES
QUANTITY REQUIRED PER PRODUCT UNIT	3	P	20X2		BOM UPDATES
RAW MATERIAL NUMBER	8	Z	20X25X8		BOM UPDATES
RAW MATERIAL DESCRIPTION	15	Z	20X25X15	TRUNCATE	BOM UPDATES
MATERIAL UNIT OF MEASURE	2	Z	20X25X2		BOM UPDATES
QUANTITY REQUIRED PER COMPONENT UNIT	3	P	20X25X2		BOM UPDATES

Figure 12.12

Partial data dictionary for BILL OF MATERIALS master file.

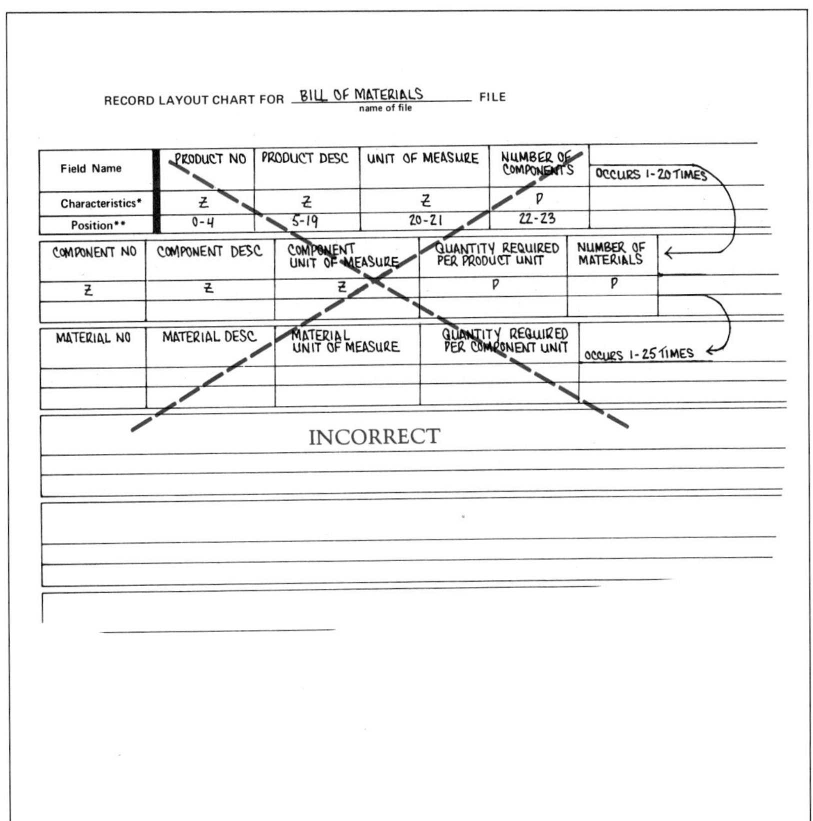

RECORD LAYOUT CHART FOR BILL OF MATERIALS FILE
name of file
Field Name
Characteristics*
Position**
PRODUCT NO
PRODUCT DESC
UNIT OF MEASURE
NUMBER OF COMPONENTS
Z
Z
Z
P
0-4
5-19
20-21
22-23
OCCURS 1-20 TIMES
COMPONENT NO
COMPONENT DESC
COMPONENT UNIT OF MEASURE
QUANTITY REQUIRED PER PRODUCT UNIT
NUMBER OF MATERIALS
Z
Z
Z
P
P
MATERIAL NO
MATERIAL DESC
MATERIAL UNIT OF MEASURE
QUANTITY REQUIRED PER COMPONENT UNIT
OCCURS 1-25 TIMES
INCORRECT

Figure 12.13

Sample incorrect record design layout. Although the layout for the BILL OF MATERIALS record is mechanically correct, records with nested repeating groups are not permitted.

DATA DICTIONARY: FILE

NAME OF FILE: BILL OF MATERIALS PRODUCT
PREPARED BY: Paula Thompson (May 2, 1986)

FIELD NAME	SIZE	FORM	BYTES	REMARKS	SOURCE(S)
PRODUCT NUMBER	5	Z	5		BOM UPDATES
PRODUCT DESCRIPTION	15	Z	15	TRUNCATE	BOM UPDATES
UNIT OF MEASURE	2	Z	2		BOM UPDATES
COMPONENT NUMBER	6	Z	20X6		BOM UPDATES
COMPONENT DESCRIPTION	15	Z	20X15	TRUNCATE	BOM UPDATES
COMPONENT UNIT OF MEASURE	2	Z	20X2		BOM UPDATES
QUANTITY REQUIRED PER PRODUCT UNIT	3	P	20X2		BOM UPDATES

(a)

DATA DICTIONARY: FILE

NAME OF FILE: BILL OF MATERIALS COMPONENT
PREPARED BY: Paula Thompson (May 2, 1986)

FIELD NAME	SIZE	FORM	BYTES	REMARKS	SOURCE(S)
COMPONENT NUMBER	6	Z	6		BOM UPDATES
RAW MATERIAL NUMBER	8	Z	25X8		BOM UPDATES
RAW MATERIAL DESCRIPTION	15	Z	25X15	TRUNCATE	BOM UPDATES
MATERIAL UNIT OF MEASURE	2	Z	25X2		BOM UPDATES
QUANTITY REQUIRED PER COMPONENT UNIT	3	P	25X2		BOM UPDATES

(b)

Figure 12.14

Partial data dictionaries resulting from split of BILL OF MATERIALS transaction file. The BILL OF MATERIALS transaction file in Figure 12.12 was split into two separate files, each file containing a single repeating group of fields.

Finally, occurrences of records, both logical and physical, make up files. There are several types of files, but the two most important classes are master files, whose records (usually fixed length) describe basic business entities (such as parts, customers, and employees), and transaction files, whose records (frequently variable length) describe business events (such as orders and invoices).

One of the most important performance decisions made by the systems analyst is file organization. File organization defines how logical records in a file are related to one another. Three common file organizations are sequential, direct, and indexed. The best way to determine an optimal file organization is by studying the file access methods required by the programs that will use and update the file.

To ensure the integrity and security of the data, internal controls should be designed for files. Internal controls for files include access, retention, backup, and recovery controls.

PROBLEMS AND EXERCISES

1. Given the numeric field UNIT SALES THIS QUARTER, calculate the field size using the following storage formats:
   (a) Binary
   (b) Zoned decimal
   (c) Packed decimal

   Assume that the value range for UNIT SALES THIS QUARTER is 0 – 500,000. Critique the three formats. When, if ever, would you use each format to store this field?

2. Given the field LIBRARY BOOK CODE, a six-digit number that uniquely identifies the books in a company library, how would you store this field? (*Hint:* Is the field numeric or alphanumeric?)

3. Differentiate between a physical and logical record. Which one is defined in the data dictionary? Which one is read or written to or from a disk? Which one is operated on by the read or write instructions in a computer program?

4. Calculate the blocking factor for a fixed-length record file, given the following factors:

   $\frac{1}{4}$ track blocking ($\frac{1}{4}$ track = 1,891 bytes)
   Logical record size = 210 bytes

   How much storage space is wasted in each physical record? How much storage space is required to store 1,000 logical records? Specify your answer in bytes.

5. Calculate the blocking factor for a variable-length file record, given the following factors:

$\frac{1}{3}$ blocking ($\frac{1}{3}$ track = 2,603 bytes)
minimum logical record size = 115 bytes
maximum logical record size = 315 bytes

How much storage space is wasted in each physical record? Specify minimum and maximum.

6. Describe the relationship between file access and file organization.
7. Determine the best organization for a file given the following data:
   (a) The file contains 2,000 logical records.
   (b) The following programs access the file:

Program	*Number of Records Accessed*
1	1
2	25
3	10
4	200
5	500
6	1

   To defend you answer, show the activity ratio and access method for each program. Why might you want to choose an indexed organization regardless of activity ratios and program access requirements?

8. Design a file for the following data store structure. State all assumptions, and prepare complete documentation including an expanded data dictionary and record layout chart.

	FIELD SIZE
EMPLOYEE consists of the following elements	
<u>EMPLOYEE NUMBER</u>	5
<u>SOCIAL SECURITY NUMBER</u>	9
EMPLOYEE NAME	20
EMPLOYEE HOME ADDRESS which consists of:	
STREET ADDRESS	20
CITY	10

STATE	2
ZIP CODE	5
EMPLOYEE HOME PHONE	10
EMPLOYEE BUSINESS PHONE	10
DEPARTMENT CODE	2
DATE EMPLOYED	6
DATE OF BIRTH	6
MARITAL STATUS	1
SEX CODE	1
RACE CODE	1
One of the following:	
MONTHLY SALARY	5
HOURLY RATE	2.2
VACATION DAYS DUE	2
SICK DAYS DUE	2
TAX EXEMPTIONS	2
GROSS PAY YEAR TO DATE	6.2
FEDERAL TAX YEAR TO DATE	6.2
STATE TAX YEAR TO DATE	5.2
FICA TAX YEAR TO DATE	6.2

10. Design a file for the following data store structure. State all assumptions, and prepare complete documentation including an expanded data dictionary and record layout chart.

	FIELD SIZE
VENDOR PART consists of the following elements:	
<u>VENDOR NUMBER</u>	6
VENDOR NAME	15
VENDOR ADDRESS which consists of:	
P.O. BOX NUMBER (optional)	2
STREET ADDRESS	20
CITY	10

STATE	2
ZIP CODE	9
VENDOR PHONE	10
VENDOR TERMS which consists of:	
DISCOUNT RATE FOR EARLY PAYMENT	1.1
EARLY PAYMENT PERIOD	2
NET PAYMENT PERIOD	2
1 to 15 occurrences of the following:	
MATERIAL NUMBER	5
MATERIAL DESCRIPTION	10
UNIT OF MEASURE	2
UNIT PRICE	4.2
QUANTITY REQUIRED FOR DISCOUNT	4
QUANTITY DISCOUNT RATE	2.1
LEAD TIME	2

ANNOTATED REFERENCES AND SUGGESTED READINGS

Fitzgerald, Jerry. *Internal Controls for Computerized Information Systems.* Redwood City, Calif.: Jerry Fitzgerald & Associates, 1978. This is our reference standard on the subject of designing internal controls into systems. Fitzgerald advocates a unique and powerful matrix tool for designing controls. This book goes far beyond any introductory systems textbook — Must reading.

Johnson, Leroy F., and Rodney H. Cooper. *File Techniques for Data Base Organization in COBOL.* Englewood Cliffs, N.J.: Prentice-Hall, 1981. We haven't found too many books that exclusively cover file structures and processing (there are several books that cover the underlying data structures). This book is both readable and comprehensive, even if you've never had a COBOL course or experience with COBOL. It explains the various file (and database) structures in relatively simple terms.

Analysts in Action

Input and Terminal Dialogue Design for the New System

When we left Cheryl and Doug, they had completed the design of outputs and files for the new order-entry system. Now they must design the inputs and terminal dialogue for the new system.

Episode 6

We begin this episode in the conference room where Cheryl has scheduled a Saturday morning meeting to review input design specifications with the entire order-entry staff. Joey suggested the Saturday morning overtime because he wanted everyone to become familiar with the input and online methods that would be used with the new system.

Input Specifications for the New System

Cheryl called the meeting to order. "Thank you all for coming. Before I begin, Doug and I want to thank all of you for your cooperation during the early phases of this project. We realize that the early phases seemed preoccupied with the existing system and too concerned with *what* you wanted. We purposefully avoided a premature concern with the computer because we didn't want to build you a system you would curse and regret. Thanks to your cooperation, *your* system is looking very good. We cannot overemphasize that this is *your* system, not ours. So interrupt at any time."

"What we want to do today is to review system inputs. Let's begin with the customer order." Cheryl placed a transparency (Figure 1) on the overhead projector and continued. "This is the proposed Customer Order Form 17. It looks similar to your current Form 17. You will no longer have to assign the sales order number. That will be done by the system. Notice . . ."

Pamela Lentl interrupted, "Wait a minute, Cheryl. If the sales order number isn't assigned until the order is processed, how will we uniquely identify an order before that time?"

Cheryl replied, "I'm not sure why you need to."

Pamela continued, "I do it frequently! Let's say a customer mails in an order and realizes a mistake has been made. Often, that customer will call us and say 'If you haven't processed my order, I'd like to make some changes.' I need to be able to identify that order somehow."

Doug interrupted. "I'm embarrassed. We talked about that point, and I forgot. There will be a preprinted sequence number at the bottom of every form. That number is imprinted on the form by the forms manufacturer. I forgot to include it on the sketch. Sorry!"

"I've got a question, Cheryl." The speaker was Karen Link, a senior order-entry clerk. "How much of this form has to be filled out to initiate computer processing?"

"All you would have to complete is the ORDER DATE, ►

Figure 1

Sketch of a source document.

AAP, INC

AMERICAN AUTOMOTIVE PARTS, INC
P.O. BOX 4576
AIRPORT EXPRESSWAY
CINCINNATI, OH 45208

FORM 17

SALES ORDER

ORDER DATE:	CUSTOMER NO:	CUSTOMER ORDER NO.
SOLD TO:		SHIP TO:

#	PART NUMBER	DESCRIPTION	QUANTITY	UNIT MEASURE	DISCOUNT RATE	DISCOUNT	UNIT PRICE	EXT. PRICE
1								
2								
3								
4								
5								
6								
7								
8								
9								
10								

FOR OFFICE USE ONLY
DATE RECEIVED
CLERK
PREPAYMENT AMOUNT $____

ALL SALES SUBJECT TO THE TERMS AND CONDITIONS ON REVERSE SIDE

SIGNATURE OF CUSTOMER OR REPRESENTATIVE

SUB TOTAL	
SALES TAX	
TOTAL	
PAID	
BALANCE	

ORIGINAL COPY TO SALES DEPARTMENT

CUSTOMER NUMBER, CUSTOMER ORDER NUMBER (when it's appropriate), SOLD TO and SHIP TO ADDRESSes, PREPAYMENT AMOUNT, PART NUMBERs, and QUANTITIES. The rest will be done by the computer," Cheryl replied.

Karen looked concerned. "Sometimes we approve special discounts and preinflation unit prices. How can your system make such subjective decisions?"

Cheryl looked over to Joey. "Joey, is this correct?"

"Yeah," replied Joey. "Can we say that if UNIT PRICE and DISCOUNT RATE are filled out those values override the values in the files?"

Karen rejoined the discussion. "That won't work, Joey. Our sales representatives routinely complete most of those columns. How will you be able to tell if the column was filled out by a salesperson or by our clerks? For that matter, what keeps customers from entering their own prices?"

"Karen's right," said Doug. "We need a better mechanism. But I think we'd better take this one back to the sales reps and see what they have to offer. We probably should have invited a few of them to this meeting."

Cheryl answered, "Okay. We'll resolve that problem. This is exactly the kind of thing we're trying to uncover in this meeting. Where was I? Oh yes, notice that we've included a place to record prepayment ▶

Figure 2

Typical specifications for input fields.

Data Element Dictionary: Input

Name of Input CUSTOMER ORDER

Ref.	Field Name	Type	Size	Memo	Edit Mask	Editing/Validation
1	SALES ORDER NUMBER	A/N	7		999999X	MUST BE UNIQUE MODULUS II
2	ORDER DATE	A/N	8		MMDDYYYY 99999999	MUST CONTAIN VALUES & VALID MONTH DAY & WEEK
3	CUSTOMER NUMBER	A/N	4		9999	OPTIONAL
4	CUSTOMER ORDER NUMBER	A/N	6		999999	OPTIONAL
5	BILLING ADDRESS					MUST CONTAIN VALUES
6	BILL TO STREET ADDRESS	A/N	15		X (15)	
7	BILL TO POST OFFICE BOX NUMBER	A/N	10		X (10)	
8	BILL TO CITY	A/N	15		X (15)	
9	BILL TO STATE	A/N	2		AA	STANDARD CODE
10	BILL TO ZIPCODE	A/N	9		999999999	MUST BE NUMENC
11	SHIPPING ADDRESS					OPTIONAL IF SAME AS REFERENCE 5
12	SHIP TO STREET ADDRESS	A/N	15		X (15)	X (15)
13	SHIP TO POST OFFICE BOX NUMBER	A/N	10		X (10)	

— CONTINUED

* Chemical carbon is preferred!

amounts. You won't have to write them in the margins anymore!

"What we need from you now is some verification on the sizes of each field and some feel for the range of values that each field can assume. This will help us write edit programs that guarantee the accuracy of the data before it's processed. We've recorded the fields you'll enter on this transparency (see Figure 2). I'm going to go through these one ▶

by one and verify the size and editing columns. Don't be put off by this form. Most of the information on the form is intended for our computer programmers. During this session, all we need to do is to verify size and value ranges. Let's get started. As you know, you each will have a computer terminal at your workstation to enter customer orders directly into the computer."

"Oh my God!" The unidentified voice was accompanied by some genuine fear, if facial expressions can be trusted.

"Don't worry!" said Cheryl. "I remember my first experience with the terminal. I thought I'd blow up Cleveland if I pressed the wrong key. It won't happen! First off, we are going to develop a very pleasant conversational dialogue between you and the computer. To as great an extent possible, you will forget that you're communicating with a machine. Beginning next week, we'll start walking you through that dialogue. Right now, I'd like to discuss the final input that'll result from that dialogue: the CUSTOMER ORDER. Can I continue?"

Noting that there were no questions, Cheryl went on, "We thought that, to make your job easier, we'd try to make the input similar to the customer order form we just discussed. With the understanding that we have some changes to make to that form, the only difference here is that the form will be painted on your terminal screen and you'll fill in the blanks."

Jeannine Black, another senior clerk, replied, "That sounds nifty. But I find it hard to believe we're going to immediately understand exactly what to do. I worked on this kind of system at another company, and I wish I had a dollar for every time I couldn't figure out what to do. The computer jocks would tell us just press this key or press that key. But we'd get confused, especially if we didn't have our reference guide with us!"

Cheryl responded to Jeannine's concerns. "Believe me, I know how you feel. I've seen some of those poorly designed systems. Would you feel better if you didn't need a reference guide? What if everything you need to know is right on the screen?"

"That would be terrific," replied Jeannine. "But you'd need a screen the size of a large television set."

"Not really," countered Cheryl. "All we have to do is make sure simple key explanations and instructions always appear on the screen. Look at this transparency (Figure 3). Notice that the instructions appear in lines 3 through 5. They will always appear there. As you enter each field, you press the return key. The cursor will automatically go to the next field. If you press the backspace key, the cursor will automatically go to the previous field. When you press the return key after the last field, the data will be input to the computer for processing."

"What if I accidentally press the return key after the last field and I made a mistake?" Karen asked.

Doug answered, "I'll tell you what we can do. How about if we have the computer ask you a simple 'Are you sure?' question before the computer processes the input? That would give you time to check the form for errors."

Karen smiled, "Now that's a good idea!"

Cheryl continued, "But that's not the only safeguard. After you enter any field and press the return key, the system will automatically check the data against the value ranges we discussed earlier in this meeting. If the value is incorrect, the system will give you an appropriate error message and ask you to reenter the same field instead of moving on to the next field."

Karen and Jeannine almost simultaneously countered, "But what if you forget what to put in the field? You may never get to the next field."

Cheryl answered again, ▶

Figure 3

Typical input screen.

TERMINAL SCREEN DISPLAY LAYOUT FORM

☒ INPUT CUSTOMER ORDER

☐ OUTPUT

APPLICATION

SCREEN NO. SEQUENCE

COLUMN

```
01                       ON-LINE ORDER ENTRY SUBSYSTEM
02
03    TYPE IN THE FIELD AT THE CURSOR'S CURRENT POSITION AND PRESS RETURN KEY.
04    RETURN KEY WILL TAKE YOU TO NEXT FIELD. BACKSPACE KEY WILL TAKE YOU TO
05    PREVIOUS FIELD. RETURN KEY AFTER LAST FIELD WILL INPUT AND PROCESS ORDER.
06    PRESS F9 KEY FOR HELP AT ANY TIME.
07
08    A                    AMERICAN AUTOMOTIVE PARTS, INC.             FORM 17
09     A                            P.O. BOX 4576                       ON-LINE
10      P INC.                    AIRPORT EXPRESSWAY
11                                  CINCINNATI, OH       SALES ORDER 050184-083
12
13    ORDER DATE 5-1-84 CUSTOMER NUMBER 85     CUSTOMER ORDER NO 73562851
14
15    SOLD TO:                             SHIP TO:
16      LEMON LIME AUTO PARTS               LEMON LIME AUTO PARTS
17      33 MAIN STREET                      33 MAIN STREET
18      LAUGHALOT, IN 47906                 LAUGHALOT, IN 47906
19
20
21    #  PART NUMBER   DESCRIPTION  QUANT U/M  DISC  DISC    UNIT    EXTENDED
22                                                  RATE    PRICE     PRICE
23    1  BK-858-0001   BELT           5     EA   0   0.00   0.75      3.75

                                                    SUBTOTAL    25.80
                                                    SALES TAX    1.29
                                                    TOTAL       27.09
                                                    PAID        00.00
23    PRESS F10 KEY TO EXIT SYSTEM                  BALANCE     27.09
24    PRESS F7 KEY TO START THIS ORDER OVER
35
```

Figure 4a

Typical terminal dialogue screens.

TERMINAL SCREEN DISPLAY LAYOUT FORM

☐ INPUT

☐ OUTPUT

APPLICATION

SCREEN NO. SEQUENCE

COLUMN

Line	Content
01	CUSTOMER SERVICES SYSTEM
02	MAIN MENU
03	
04	TYPE THE NUMBER OF THE DESIRED OPTION AND PRESS RETURN.
05	
06	
07	SELECT ONE OF THE FOLLOWING OPTIONS:
08	
09	1 = PROCESS AN ORDER
10	
11	2 = QUERY PART FILE
12	
	3 = QUERY CUSTOMER FILE

"That's highly unlikely. Because the form on the screen is identical to the paper form you'll be using, it's unlikely you won't know what to enter. But in the event that you do forget, look at line 5. This line will always remind you that you can press the F9 key to get detailed instructions. When you press F9, the system remembers where you are and then displays detailed help screens. These screens provide greater assistance and examples. When you press F9 again, it takes you right back to where you were in the order screen."

Jeannine replied, "If this system works the way you're describing it, we can't get lost. That'll be a monumental improvement over some of the systems I've worked with."

Cheryl concluded her discussion of the on-line sales order input. "Like I said, we're planning to walk through an entire terminal session with selected clerks. I think we'll include both you and Karen on the list; especially you, Jeannine, since you've had some experience with unfriendly on-line systems.

Terminal Dialogue Specifications for the New System

It's one week later. Doug and Cheryl have prepared some sample screens of real terminal situations. Various users have been walked through a typical terminal session. Doug conducts the session while Cheryl makes appropriate modifications to the design specifications. We haven't much time, but let's eavesdrop on a small part of the walkthrough.

Doug begins, "Jeannine, this is the screen (see Figure 4[a]) ►

Figure 4b

Typical terminal dialogue screens.

TERMINAL SCREEN DISPLAY LAYOUT FORM

☐ INPUT ________

☐ OUTPUT ________

APPLICATION ________

SCREEN NO. ________ SEQUENCE ________

COLUMN

1 – 10 | 11 – 20 | 21 – 30 | 31 – 40 | 41 – 50 | 51 – 60 | 61 – 70 | 71 – 80

Row	Screen content
01	CUSTOMER SERVICES SYSTEM
02	MAIN MENU
03	
04	TRY AGAIN.
05	TYPE THE NUMBER OF THE DESIRED OPTION AND PRESS RETURN.
06	
07	→ SELECT ONE OF THE FOLLOWING OPTIONS ○
08	
09	1 = PROCESS AN ORDER
10	
11	2 = QUERY PART FILE
12	480 … 1960
13	3 = QUERY CUSTOMER FILE
14	
15	
16	
17	
18	
19	INVALID OPTION
20	YOU MUST SELECT 1, 2, OR 3

that will appear on your terminal when you correctly enter your password. Tell me what you're going to do."

"Well," replied Jeannine, "I'm going to see if you guys know what you're doing. The screen says select option 1, 2, or 3. I choose 4."

Doug responded by showing Jeannine a new terminal screen (Figure 4[b]). "As you can see," he said, "the system has identified your response as invalid. Notice the new instruction. What are you going to do now?"

"Okay, so you got me on this one." Jeannine seemed surprised that Cheryl and Doug had anticipated her invalid response. "I'll select option 1."

Once again, Doug shuffled through his stack of forms. He came up with Figure 4(c). "What are you going to do now?" he asked.

"I'll bet you have another error message if I choose anything other than option 1, 2, or 3," suggested Jeannine. Noting Doug's smile, she assumed she was correct. "I'll take option 1."

And once again, Doug shuf- ▶

Figure 4c

Typical terminal dialogue screens.

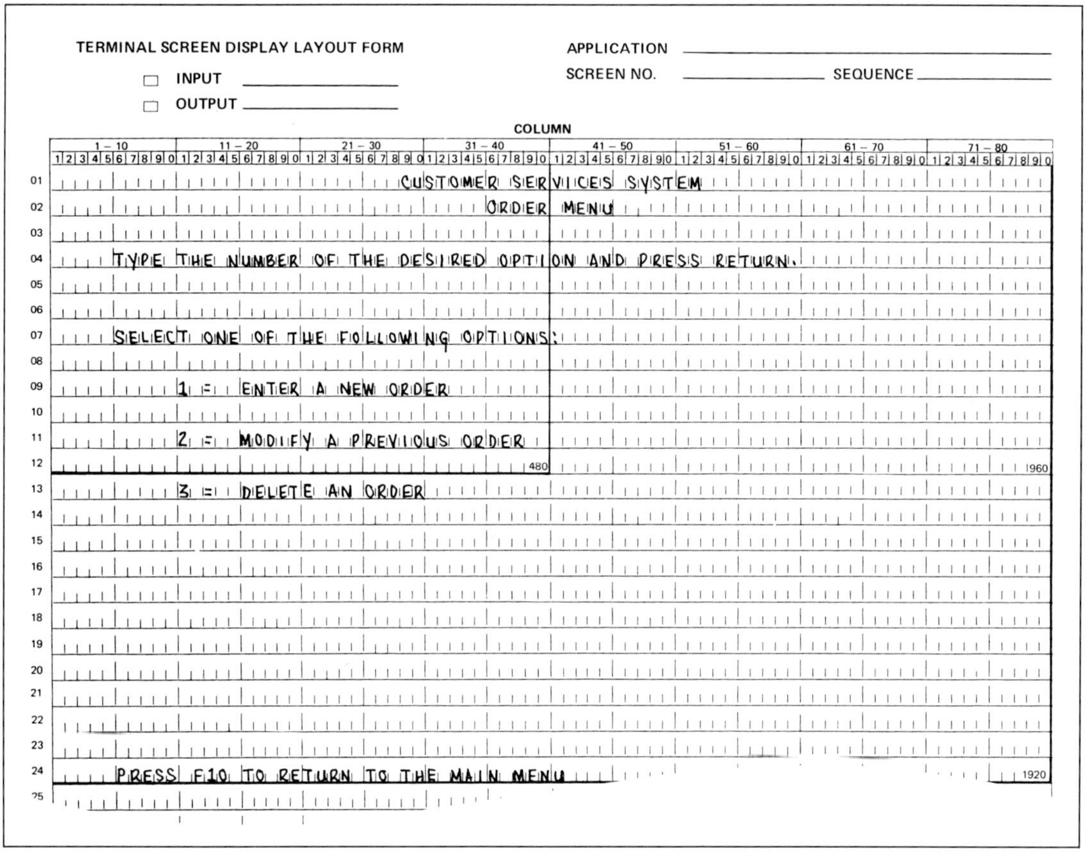

TERMINAL SCREEN DISPLAY LAYOUT FORM

☐ INPUT ______

☐ OUTPUT ______

APPLICATION ______

SCREEN NO. ______ SEQUENCE ______

COLUMN

```
01                                   CUSTOMER SERVICES SYSTEM
02                                         ORDER MENU
03
04     TYPE THE NUMBER OF THE DESIRED OPTION AND PRESS RETURN.
05
06
07     SELECT ONE OF THE FOLLOWING OPTIONS:
08
09          1 = ENTER A NEW ORDER
10
11          2 = MODIFY A PREVIOUS ORDER
12
13          3 = DELETE AN ORDER
14
15
16
17
18
19
20
21
22
23
24     PRESS F10 TO RETURN TO THE MAIN MENU
25
```

fled through his papers. This time he came up with Figure 5. "Does this look familiar? It's the blank sales order screen we discussed at the meeting last Saturday. We've made the changes suggested during that meeting. You all know how to deal with that screen. Let's move on to another sample terminal session."

The walkthrough continued along in the same manner.

Where Do We Go from Here?
This chapter introduced you to two important tasks of systems design: the design of computer inputs and terminal dialogue design. There are several important issues that must be addressed when designing inputs and terminal dialogue. You have been exposed to several of ▶

Figure 5

Typical input screen.

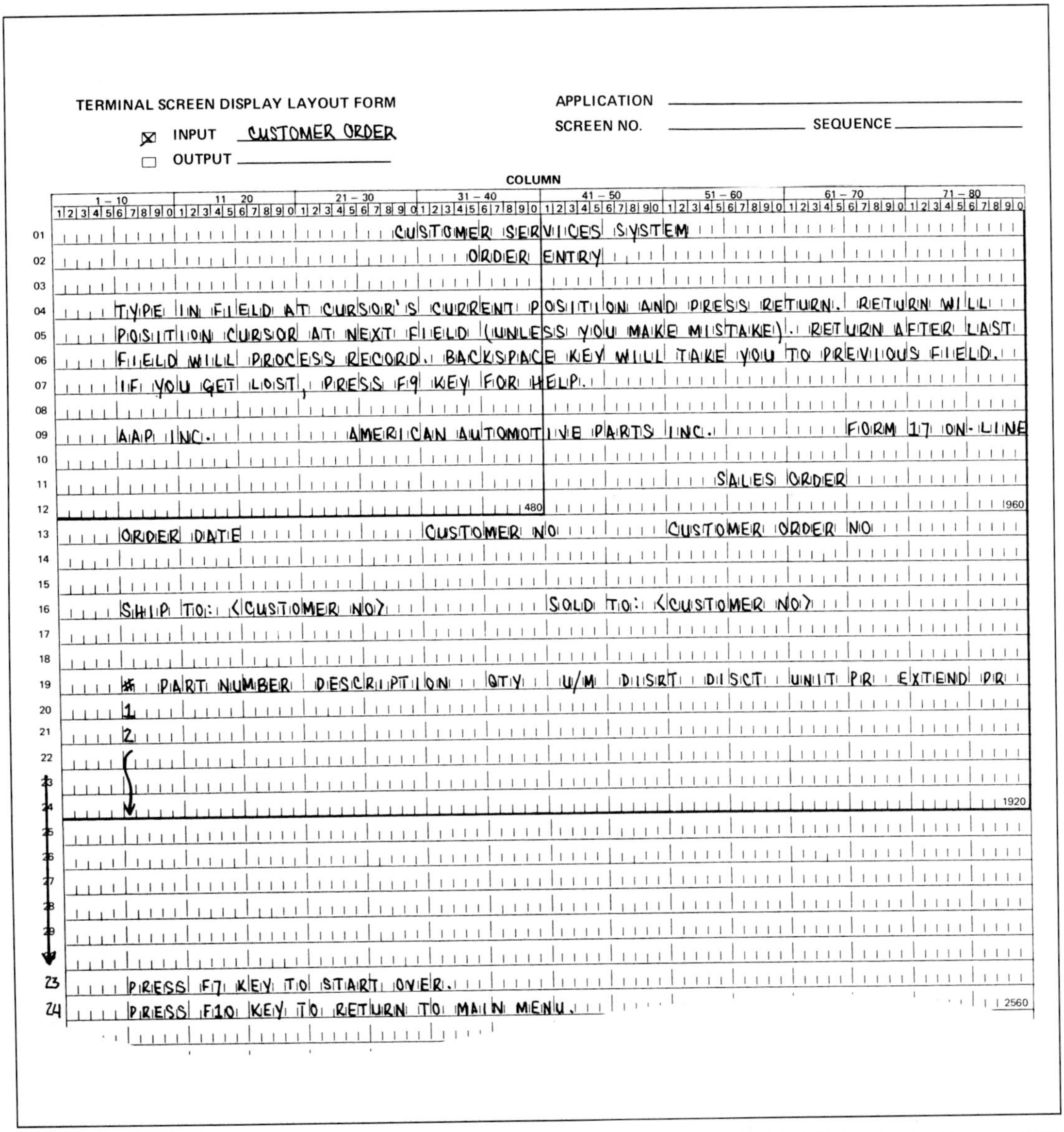

TERMINAL SCREEN DISPLAY LAYOUT FORM

☒ INPUT CUSTOMER ORDER

☐ OUTPUT

APPLICATION

SCREEN NO. SEQUENCE

COLUMN

Row	Content
01	CUSTOMER SERVICES SYSTEM
02	ORDER ENTRY
03	
04	TYPE IN FIELD AT CURSOR'S CURRENT POSITION AND PRESS RETURN. RETURN WILL
05	POSITION CURSOR AT NEXT FIELD (UNLESS YOU MAKE MISTAKE). RETURN AFTER LAST
06	FIELD WILL PROCESS RECORD. BACKSPACE KEY WILL TAKE YOU TO PREVIOUS FIELD.
07	IF YOU GET LOST, PRESS F9 KEY FOR HELP.
08	
09	AAP INC. AMERICAN AUTOMOTIVE PARTS INC. FORM 17 ON-LINE
10	
11	SALES ORDER
12	
13	ORDER DATE CUSTOMER NO CUSTOMER ORDER NO
14	
15	
16	SHIP TO: <CUSTOMER NO> SOLD TO: <CUSTOMER NO>
17	
18	
19	# PART NUMBER DESCRIPTION QTY U/M DISRT DISCT UNIT PR EXTEND PR
20	1
21	2
22	
23	
24	
23	PRESS F7 KEY TO START OVER.
24	PRESS F10 KEY TO RETURN TO MAIN MENU.

the tools systems analysts have at their disposal for documenting the input and terminal dialogue specifications.

In Chapter 13, you will learn about issues and tools for designing computer inputs. You will learn about important terminal dialogue design issues and tools in Chapter 14.

Communication skills are very important in designing computer inputs and terminal dialogue. In addition to obtaining an understanding of the issues and tools for input and terminal dialogue design, we strongly encourage you to read Part IV, Module C, "Communication Skills for the Systems Analyst." ■

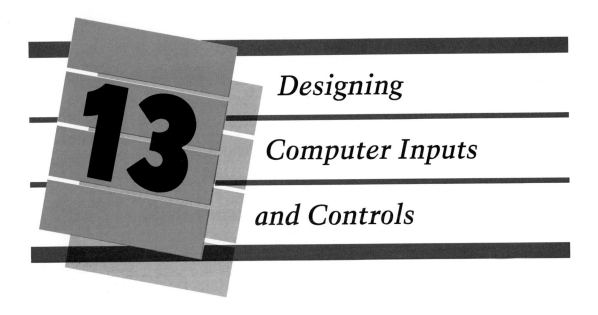

13 Designing Computer Inputs and Controls

Minicase: Soft Shoe, Inc. (Part I)

Carey Carmichael, manager of the Information Systems Department at Soft Shoe, had just returned to his office after an hour-long meeting with the Order-Entry Department. Order Entry was irate about the new order-entry system, and Carey had taken a lot of heat. Now he was faced with the problem of smoothing things out. Unfortunately, Carey didn't know much about the recently installed system. He had turned the project over to Judy Lucas, who had been a programmer at Soft Shoe for five years before her recent promotion to systems analyst. This was her first systems project. Judy entered Mr. Carmichael's office. Let's listen in:

Judy Good afternoon, Mr. Carmichael. What did you want to see me about?

Carey Judy, I'm going to get straight to the point. The Order-Entry Department is unhappy with the new order-entry system you installed. Before they officially cut over to the new system, they want some changes.

Judy What are they unhappy about? That may be the first interactive system that I've implemented, but it's a darn good one.

Carey They claim it's not easy to use, that it takes them longer than it should to enter a sales order because the dialogue is confusing. They also claim that they're experiencing an increase in customer complaints.

Judy I don't see how that can be. The program is very easy to use. You should see it. I used a lot of fancy terminal functions—blinking screens, reverse video, and things like that—to make their job of entering sales orders more interesting. And besides, what do their customer complaints have to do with my system?

Carey They claim the new system isn't recording the customer sales orders accurately.

Judy I don't see how that can be either. The program asks the data-entry clerk to enter all the information that's on the sales order form. If they filled the form out right, there wouldn't be any problems.

Carey Sit down. I think there are a few things we need to talk about.

Discussion

1. Is it possible Judy has made some mistakes?
2. What do you think Judy should have done differently?

WHAT WILL YOU LEARN IN THIS CHAPTER?

In this chapter, you will learn how to use input record layout charts and display layout charts to design inputs. You will know that you have mastered input design tools and techniques when you can:

1. Explain the difference between *data capture, data entry,* and *data input.*

2. Define the appropriate input method and medium alternative for a computer input.
3. Apply human factors to the design of computer inputs.
4. Design internal controls into computer inputs.
5. Identify data flows on the BDFD (bounded data flow diagram) that must be designed as computer inputs.
6. Define input design requirements, and use an expanded data dictionary format to record them.
7. Design a source document for data capture.
8. Use input record layout charts and display layout charts to format batch and on-line computer inputs.

"Garbage in! Garbage out!" This overworked expression is no less true today than it was when we first studied computer programming. You have studied the design of computer outputs and computer files. Outputs are produced from data that is either input or retrieved from files. And data in files must have been input to those files. In this chapter, you are going to learn how to design computer inputs. Input design serves an important goal: Capture and get the data into a format suitable for the computer. And data, as you recall, constitute one of the fundamental components of your information system model (see margin).

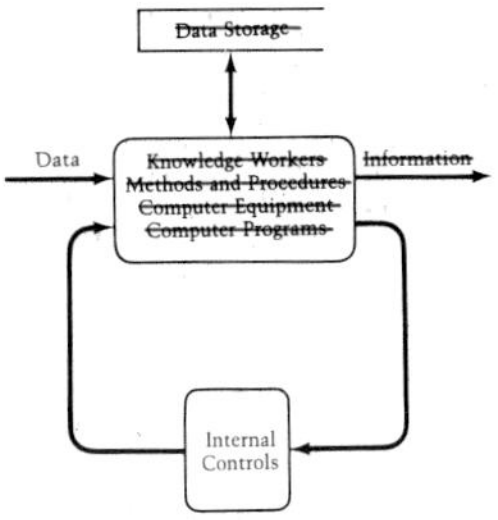

IPO Components

One of the first things you must learn is the difference between data capture and data input. Alternative input media and methods must also be understood prior to designing the inputs. And because accurate data input is so critical to successful processing, file maintenance, and output, you should also learn about human factors and internal controls for input design. After learning these fundamental concepts, we will study the tools and techniques of input design.

METHODS AND ISSUES FOR DATA CAPTURE AND INPUT

Information = f(Data, Processing)! Do you remember that formula from Chapter 3? Well, this topic is about data. Where does data originate? How is data captured? How is data input to the computer? And how do we know the input is valid? We will answer these and other important issues as we study input concepts and principles.

Data Capture Versus Data Entry Versus Data Input

When you think of input, you usually think of input devices, such as card readers and terminals. But input begins long before the data arrives at the device. Therefore, let's begin with an overview of the data input cycle.

Where does data originate? Let's examine one typical situation. A computer operator has just mounted the DAILY SALES ORDER tape on the tape drive to input today's sales orders to the computer for processing. Where did the tape come from? The tape was created in the Data-Entry Department. The Data-Entry Department is responsible for getting business data into a format suitable for input to a computer system. Our computer tape input file was created on a key-to-disk system. Data-Entry clerks key(punch) the data that was directly recorded on magnetic disks. Special key-to-disk workstations were used. The disk files were then copied to the computer tape, which we introduced at the beginning of our story. But how did the data-entry clerks get the data in the first place?

The data is presented to the data-entry clerks on SALES ORDER forms. And where do the forms come from? They are periodically delivered to the Data-Entry Department in batches. Where do the batches originate? In our case, the SALES ORDER form is initiated in one of two ways. Either a salesperson completed the form or the customer telephoned an order to a sales clerk who completed the form. The data originated in the business! The sales orders were collected into a batch and delivered to the Data-Entry Department.

To get the sales order data into the computer, the analyst had to design the form, design the input record, and design methods for getting the data into the computer (from *customer* to *form* to *data-entry clerk* to *disk* to *tape* to *computer*).

This brings us to our fundamental question. What is the difference between data capture, data entry, and data input? *Data happens!* The sales order in our example will occur as long as the business exists. What we must do is determine *when* and *how* to capture the data. **Data capture** is the identification of new data to be input. *When* is easy! It's always best to capture the data as soon as it's originated. *How* is another story! Creating a **source document** (a term commonly associated with forms used to record data that will eventually be input to a computer) is not easy. Source documents (or their equivalent) should be easy for the knowledge worker to fill out and should facilitate rapid data entry into a machine-readable format.

Data entry is not the same as data capture. As you may have gathered from our early example, **data entry** is the process of translating the source document into the machine-readable format. That format may be a punched card, an optical mark form, a magnetic tape, or a floppy diskette, to name a few. Only after the data has been entered to one of the machine-readable formats do we have **data input** for the computer. Let's examine some of the data capture and data entry alternatives you should consider during systems design.

Input Methods and Media

The system analyst usually selects the method and medium for all inputs. Let's compare and contrast the different input methods and the medium alternatives available for modern information systems. Input methods can be broadly classified as either batch or on-line.

Batch Methods and Media Batch input is the oldest and most traditional input method. Source documents are collected and then periodically forwarded to Data Entry. Data-entry operators key the data using a data-entry device that translates the data into the machine-readable format. The DAILY SALES ORDER example we presented earlier in this chapter conforms to this description. There are numerous medium alternatives for batch inputs. Figure 13.1 illustrates the input procedures required for these different media.

For many years, punched cards were the most common medium for batch input data. In Figure 13.1(a) you see that data-entry clerks transcribe (or keypunch) the data from the source document to the punched card (at keypunch workstations). In many shops, the punched cards are rekeyed at verifier workstations to determine if keying errors have been made. The verifier workstation does not repunch the card. Instead, it compares the original punched card with the keystrokes being re-entered and reports any discrepancies. After cards have been punched and verified, they can be input to the computer.

For the most part, the punched card medium has been replaced by *magnetic* media. Key-to-disk (KTD) and key-to-tape (KTT)

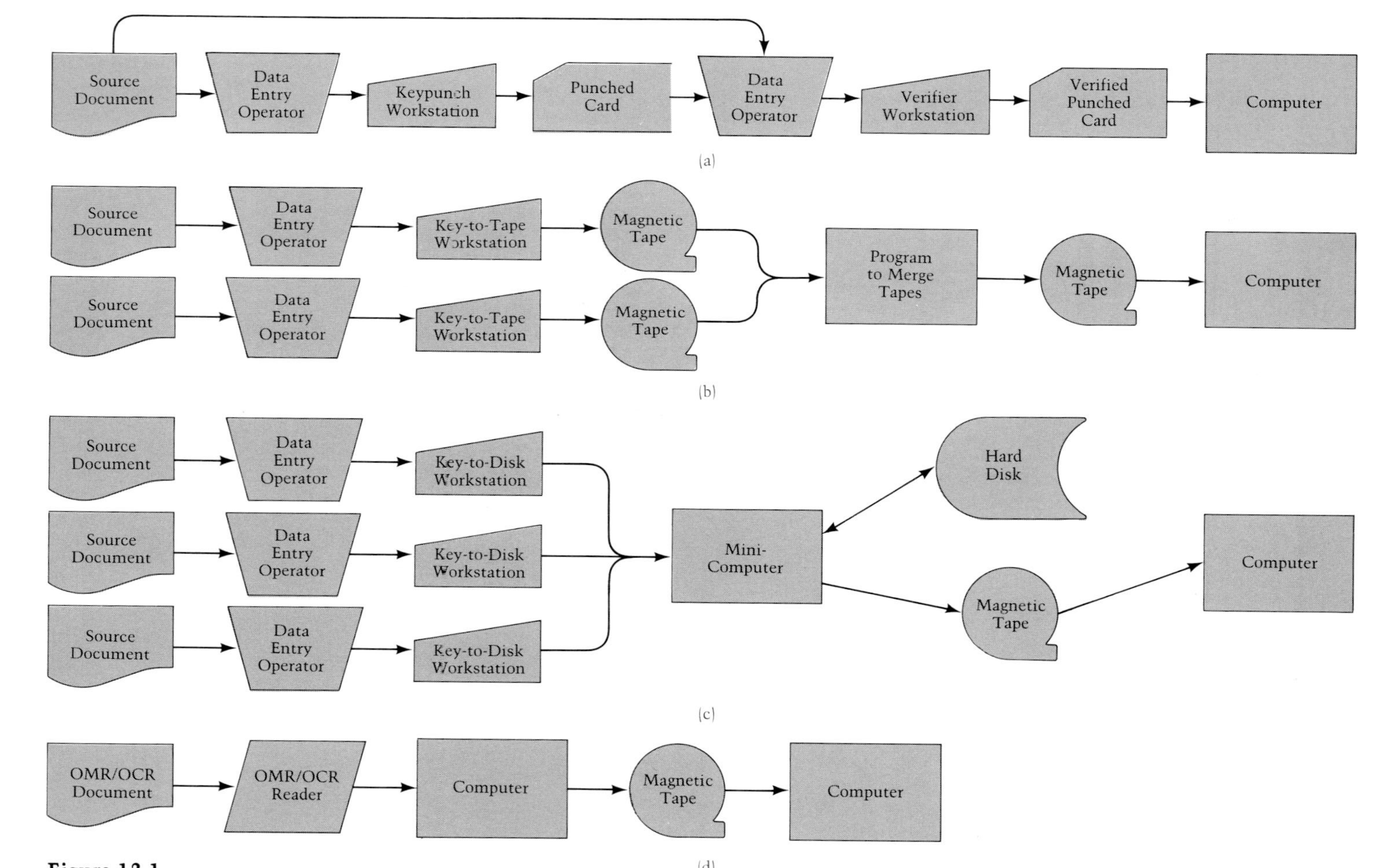

Figure 13.1

Alternative input procedures for batch input media. These illustrations show the similarities and differences between the most typical batch input methods.

workstations transcribe data to magnetic disks and magnetic tape. Several advantages are gained from KTD and KTT technology. The workstations are much quieter, which makes life as a data-entry clerk more bearable. As each input record is keyed, it is displayed. The data can be corrected because it is initially placed into a buffer. The data is released to the magnetic media after the data-entry clerk has verified it. The resulting input file, possibly merged from several KTD or KTT workstations, permits much faster data input rates to the computer than those achieved with punched cards.

Figures 13.1(b) and 13.1(c) illustrate the key-to-tape and key-to-disk input procedures. Key-to-tape workstations (13.1[b]) are normally standalone or clustered. Data is initially recorded on individual reel or cassette tapes. The tapes normally have to be merged or copied to a single tape that is input to the computer. Key-to-disk workstations (13.1[c]) are normally connected to a special-purpose minicomputer. Data is initially transcribed to the minicomputer's disk. The data is then either copied from disk to tape for input to the main computer or directly transferred to the main computer.

Figure 13.1(d) illustrates another batch input medium, the optical mark form. You are likely familiar with this medium because most machine-scored tests, including the Scholastic Aptitude Tests, are machine-scored from this medium. Optical mark forms eliminate most or all of the need for data entry. Essentially, the source document becomes the input medium, or so it seems. As Figure 13.1(d) illustrates, the source document is directly read by an optical mark reader (OMR) or optical character reader (OCR). The computer records the data to magnetic tape, which is then input to the computer. OCR and OMR input are generally suitable only for high-volume input activities. By having data directly recorded on a machine-readable document, the cost of data entry is eliminated.

One characteristic of all of these batch media is the significant possibility of error when moving from the source document to the input medium. Before data can be processed, it must be edited. Have you written edit programs in your programming courses? If so, you know that edit programs require significant effort. We'll discuss this issue further when we present internal controls for inputs.

On-Line Methods and Media The current trend in data input revolves around on-line methods. This trend makes sense — capture data at its point of origin, in the business, and directly input that data to the computer. At one time, the cost of on-line applications was prohibitive. Today, inexpensive, improved on-line technology has made on-line applications more common. Many batch input applications have been redesigned for on-line input.

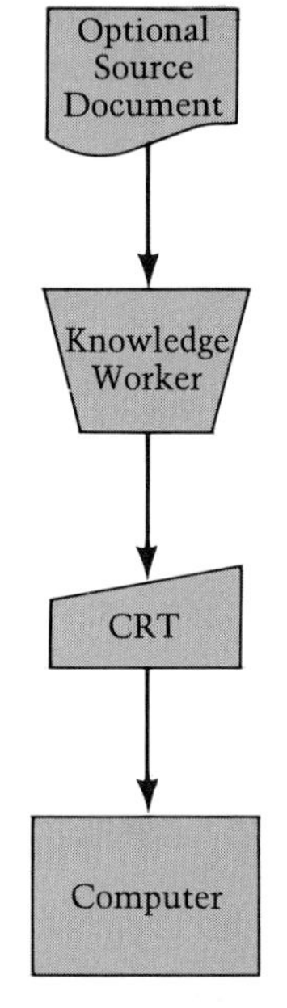

On-Line Input Method

The most common on-line medium cannot really be classified as a medium; it is the cathode ray tube (CRT) terminal, also referred to as video display terminal (VDT) or video display unit (VDU). The CRT or *tube* consists of a monitor screen and keyboard that are directly connected to the computer system. The CRT operator, a knowledge worker, directly enters the data when that data originates (see the figure in the margin). No data entry by a separate data entry staff! No need to record data onto a medium that is later input to the computer! This is direct input! If data is entered incorrectly, the computer's edit program detects the error and immediately requests the CRT operator to make a correction.

But on-line data input can become even more sophisticated than this. With today's technology, we can *completely* eliminate human intervention. Point-of-sale terminals in retail and grocery stores frequently include bar-code and optical-character readers. You've all seen the bar codes recorded on today's food store products (see the example printed in the margin). These bar codes eliminate the need for traditional keyed data entry. Instead, sophisticated laser readers interpret the bar code and send the data represented by that code directly to the computer for processing.

Batch Versus On-Line To hear some people talk, *all* systems should be designed for on-line input. The technology is certainly cheaper than it used to be. So why bother with batch input? No matter how cheap and fast on-line processing gets, an on-line program simply cannot be nearly as fast as its batch equivalent. Why? Because most on-line programs require human interaction, and people are slow relative to computers. Also, for large-volume transactions, too many CRT terminals and operators may be needed to meet demand. As the number of on-line CRTs grows, the overall performance of the computer declines. Furthermore, many inputs naturally occur in batches. For instance, our mail may include a large batch of customer payments on any given day. Postal delivery is, at least today, a batch operation. Additionally, some transaction input data may *not* require immediate attention. Finally, batch processing may be preferable because internal controls (discussed shortly) are

Universal Product Code

simpler. In an era of scarce computing resources, on-line input should perhaps be reserved for inputs that benefit most from immediate processing.

Human Factor Considerations for Input Design

Because inputs originate with knowledge workers, human factors play a significant role in input design. Furthermore, if batch methods are used, data-entry clerks' needs must also be considered. With this in mind, several human factors should be evaluated.

The volume of data to be input should be minimized. The more data that is input, the greater the potential number of input errors and the longer it takes to record and input the data. The following general principles should be followed:

1. *Enter only variable data.* Do not enter constant data. For instance, when deciding what elements to include in the SALES ORDER input, we need PART NUMBERs for all parts ordered. But do we need to input PART DESCRIPTIONs for those parts? Think about it! PART DESCRIPTION is probably stored in a computer file. If we input PART NUMBER, we can look up PART DESCRIPTION. Permanent (or semipermanent) data should be stored in files. Of course, inputs must be designed for maintaining those files.
2. *Do not input data that can be calculated or stored in computer programs.* For example, if you input QUANTITY ORDERED and PRICE, you don't need to input EXTENDED PRICE (= QUANTITY ORDERED × PRICE). Another example is incorporating FEDERAL TAX WITHHOLDING data in tables (arrays) instead of keying in that data every time.
3. *Use codes for appropriate data elements.* Codes were introduced in Chapter 8. Codes can be translated in computer programs by using tables as described in item 2 of this list.

Source documents should be easy for users to complete. The following suggestions may help:

- *Include instructions for completing the form.* By the way, did you know that people don't like to have to read instructions printed on the back side of the form?
- *Minimize the amount of handwriting.* Most people suffer from

notorious penmanship. The data-entry clerk or CRT operator may misread the data and input incorrect data. Use check boxes wherever possible so the user needs only to check the appropriate value.

Design documents so they can be easily and quickly entered into the system. We suggest the following:

- Data to be entered (keyed) should be sequenced so it can be read like this book, top to bottom and left to right (see Figure 13.2[a]). The data-entry clerk should not have to move from right to left on a line or jump around on the form (see Figure 13.2[b]) to find data items to be entered.
- Input data should not be mixed with data not to be entered. Preferably, similar types of input data should be grouped together. For instance, groups of numeric and non-numeric fields should not be mixed.
- Ideally, portions of the form that are not to be input are placed in the lower right portion of the source document (the last portion encountered when reading top to bottom and left to right).

Please note that these are only guidelines. Your users have the final say on source document design. (Customers are always right—even when they're wrong!)

Internal Controls for Inputs

Once again, we expand our coverage on the continuing topic of internal controls. Input controls ensure the accuracy of data input to the computer. The following internal control guidelines are offered:

1. *The number of inputs should be monitored.* This is especially true with the batch method because source documents may be misplaced, lost, or skipped.

    - In batch systems, each batch should be recorded on a batch control slip. Data includes BATCH NUMBER, NUMBER OF DOCUMENTS, and CONTROL TOTALS (for example, total number of line items on the documents). These totals can be compared with the output totals on the history report after processing has been completed. If the totals are not equal, the cause of the discrepancy must be determined.

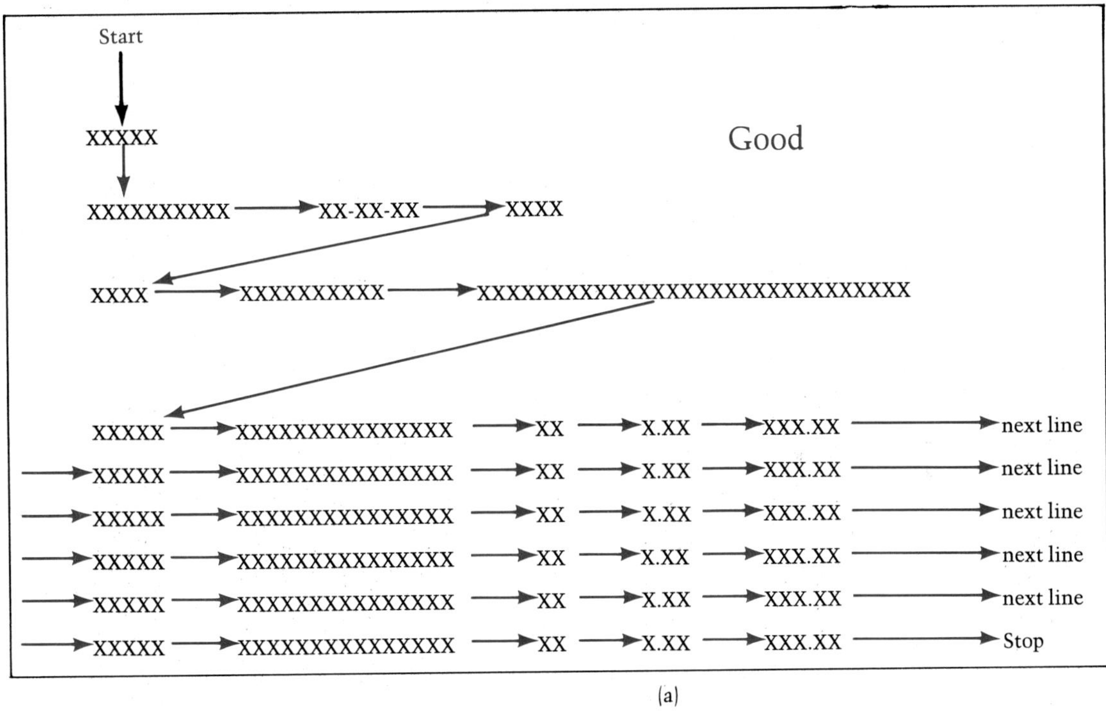

(a)

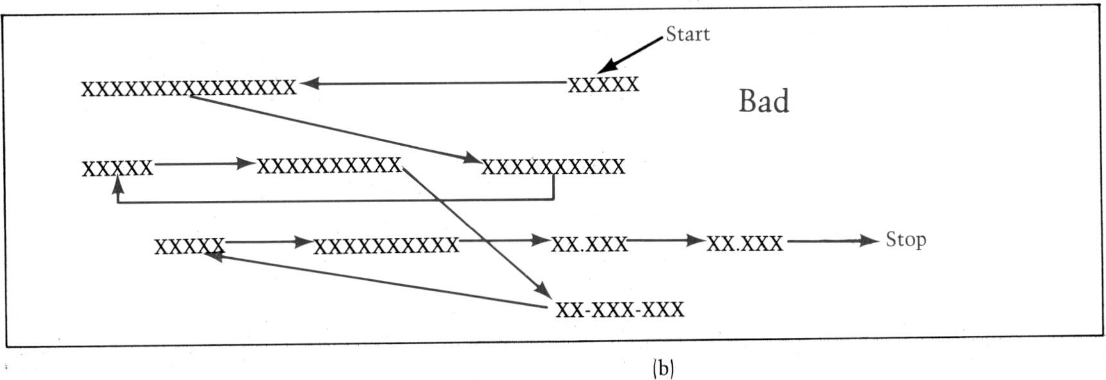

(b)

Figure 13.2

Keying from source documents. Source documents should be designed to aid in rapid data entry. The source document in part (a) was designed to allow the data entry clerk to locate and key data in a natural top-to-bottom, left-to-right sequence. The source document in part (b) will be likely to negatively affect the data entry clerk's ability to quickly locate and enter data.

- In batch systems, an alternative control would be *one-for-one* checks. Each source document would be matched against the corresponding historical report detail line that confirms that the document has been processed. This control check may only be necessary when the batch control totals don't match.
- In on-line systems, each input transaction should be logged to a computer file so it can be recovered in the event of a processing error or if data is lost.

2. *Care must also be taken to ensure that the data is valid.* Two types of errors can infiltrate the data: invalid data recorded by users and data-entry errors. Data-entry errors include copying errors, transpositions (typing 132 as 123), and slides (keying 345.36 as 3453.6). The following techniques are widely used to validate data:

   - **Completeness checks** determine whether all *required* fields on the input have actually been entered.
   - **Limit and range checks** determine whether the input data for each field fall within the legitimate set or range of values defined for that field. For instance, an upper-limit range may be put on PAY RATE to ensure that no employee is paid at a higher rate.
   - **Combination checks** determine whether a known relationship between two fields is valid. For instance, if the VEHICLE MAKE is Pontiac then the VEHICLE MODEL must be one of a limited set of values that comprise cars manufactured by Pontiac (Firebird, Grand Prix, Bonneville, to name a few).
   - **Self-checking digits** are a technique for determining data-entry errors on primary keys. A *check digit* is a number or character that is appended to a primary key field. The check digit is calculated by applying a formula, such as Modulus 11, to the actual key (see Figure 13.3). How does the check digit verify correct data entry? There are two methods. Some data-entry devices can automatically validate data by applying the same formula to the data as it is entered by the data-entry clerk. If the check digit entered doesn't match the check digit calculated, an error is displayed. Computer programs can also validate check digits by using readily available subroutines.
   - **Picture checks** compare data entered against the known edit mask or picture defined for that program. For instance, the

MODULUS 11

The following procedure is used to assign a check digit to a key field:

STEP 1: Determine the size of the key field in digits.

2 4 1 3 5 = 5 digits

STEP 2: Number each digit location from *right to left* beginning with the number "2".

2 4 1 3 5
6 5 4 3 2

STEP 3: Multiply each digit in the key field by its assigned location number.

$2 \times 6 = 12$
$4 \times 5 = 20$
$1 \times 4 = 4$
$3 \times 3 = 9$
$5 \times 2 = 10$

STEP 4: Sum the products from Step 3.

$12 + 20 + 4 + 9 + 10 = 55$

STEP 5: Divide the sum from Step 4 by 11.

55 / 11 = 5   Remainder 0

STEP 6: If the remainder is less than 10, append the remainder digit to the key field. If the remainder is equal to 10, append the character "X" to the key field.

2 4 1 3 5 0

Figure 13.3

Modulus 11 self-checking digit technique. Modulus 11 is a common self-checking digit technique used to verify that the original data has been correctly transcribed into machine-processable form. For example, if a user read the key field value 241350 (the number derived in the Modulus 11 example) and mistakenly keyed in the value 243150, the incorrect data could have been detected by applying the Modulus 11 formula to the key values.

input field may have an edit mask XX999AA (where X can be a letter or number, 9 must be a number, and A must be a letter. The field "A4898DH" would pass the picture check but the field "A489ID8" would not.

Data validation requires that special input edit programs be written to perform input checks. However, the input validation requirements should be designed when the inputs themselves are designed.

HOW TO DESIGN BATCH AND ON-LINE INPUTS

How do you design on-line and batch inputs? In this section, we'll give an overview of the process, tools, and techniques. Then we'll look at some sample input designs. We'll also be applying the concepts and controls you learned in the last section.

Identify the Input Requirements of the New System

The bounded data flow diagram (BDFD) identifies those inputs to be designed. In Figure 13.4, you see an input data flow called COURSE REQUEST for a student course registration system. Any data flow that enters the machine side of the boundary is an input to be designed.

Given the inputs to be designed, there are two ways to identify the data elements to be input. First, we can learn more about these inputs by reviewing their data dictionary entries. The basic content of these inputs may have been defined during the definition phase of systems analysis using the data dictionary syntax covered in Chapter 8. Alternatively, we can define input requirements by studying the output and file designs. An output data element that can't be retrieved from files or calculated from elements that are retrieved from files, *must be input!* Additionally, inputs must be designed to maintain the files in the system.

Determine the Design Parameters

As we did with outputs and files, we can now expand our data dictionary to include input design factors. These factors address many issues introduced earlier in this chapter. Furthermore, many of the design factors introduced in the file design chapter are equally appropriate here. Why? Especially in the case of batch inputs, the input is a file and that input file contains input records. Important considerations for designing inputs include:

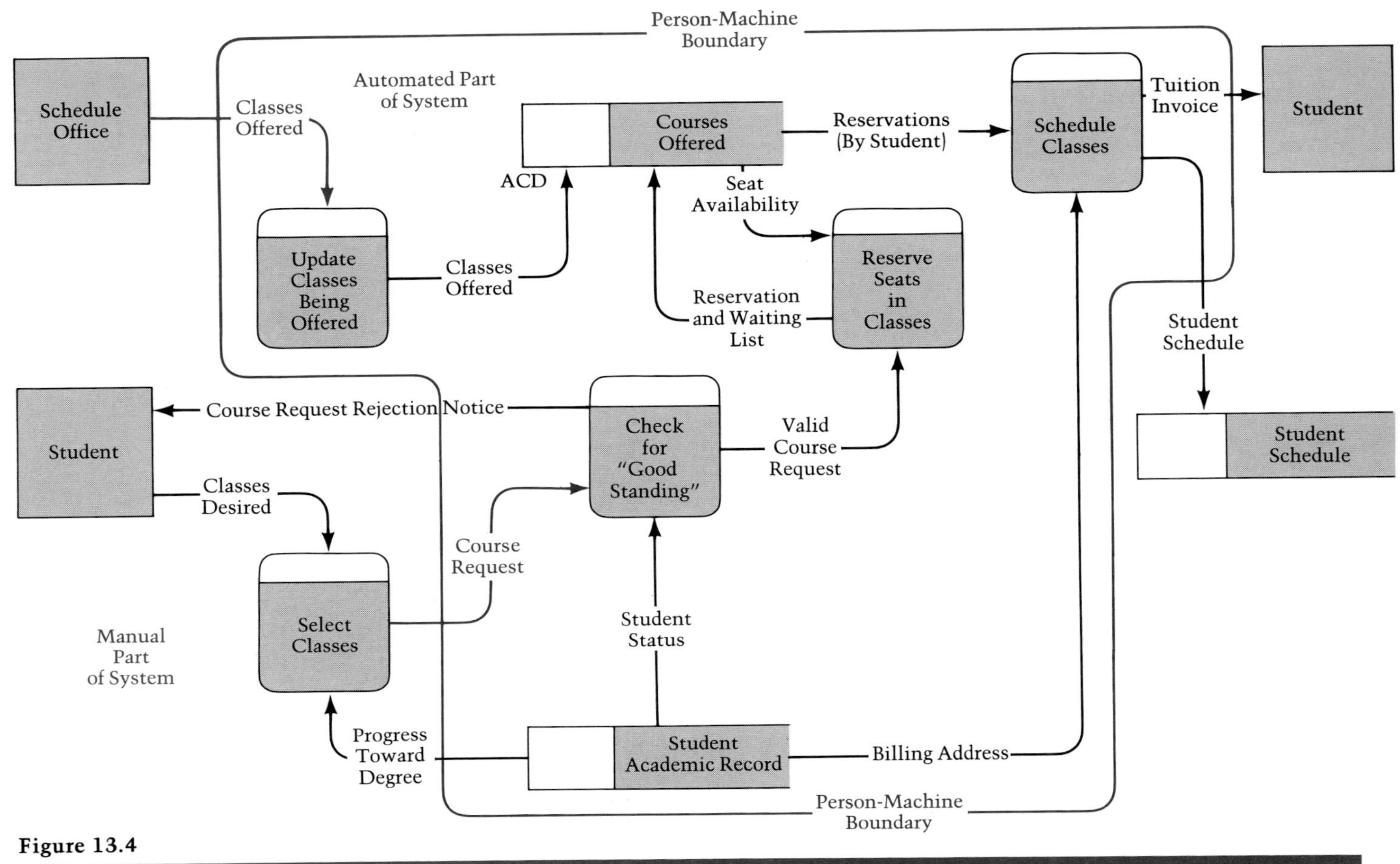

Figure 13.4

A sample bounded data flow diagram. Those data flows entering the person/machine boundary of a data flow diagram represent inputs that must be designed. The data flows CLASSES OFFERED and COURSE REQUEST would need to be designed as computer inputs. The analyst must focus on the data capture, data entry, and data input for these data flows.

1. *Identify source documents that need to be designed or modified.*
2. *Determine the input method to be used.* Batch? On-line? What specific media? KTT? KTD? OCR? Remember, input may be restricted to media available in the current environment, especially if funds are not available for new media or services.
3. *Determine the timing and volume of input.* **Timing** is how often the input will be done (for instance, "Once Daily," "Hourly," "On demand, 24 hours," "On demand, 8A.M.—5P.M., Weekdays"). **Volume** is the number of inputs in a batch or time period. This data is needed to predetermine data-entry personnel requirements and schedules or determine how many terminals will be needed.
4. *Specify internal controls and special instructions to be followed for the input* (create an audit trail file for an on-line input, create batch control slips for a batch input, and so forth).
5. *Study the input data elements to determine which data really need to be input.* Remember the guidelines for data reduction presented earlier in this chapter, and don't forget the value of a good code for reducing data volume.

Lay out the Source Document

We prefer to design the source document first. The source document is for the user. If at all possible, we'll try to get some user sketches of the document *before* we make our suggestions. A well-designed source document will be divided into zones.

Some zones are used for identification; these include company name, form name, official form number, date of last revision (an important element that is often omitted), and logos. Other zones contain data that identify a specific occurrence of the form, such as form sequence number (possibly preprinted) and date. The largest portion of the document is used to record transaction data. Data that occur once and data that repeat should be logically separated. Totals should be relegated to the lower portion of the form because they are usually calculated and, therefore, not input. Many forms include an authorization zone for signatures. Instructions should be placed in a convenient location, preferably not on the back of the form. A template for a hypothethical source document is provided in Figure 13.5.

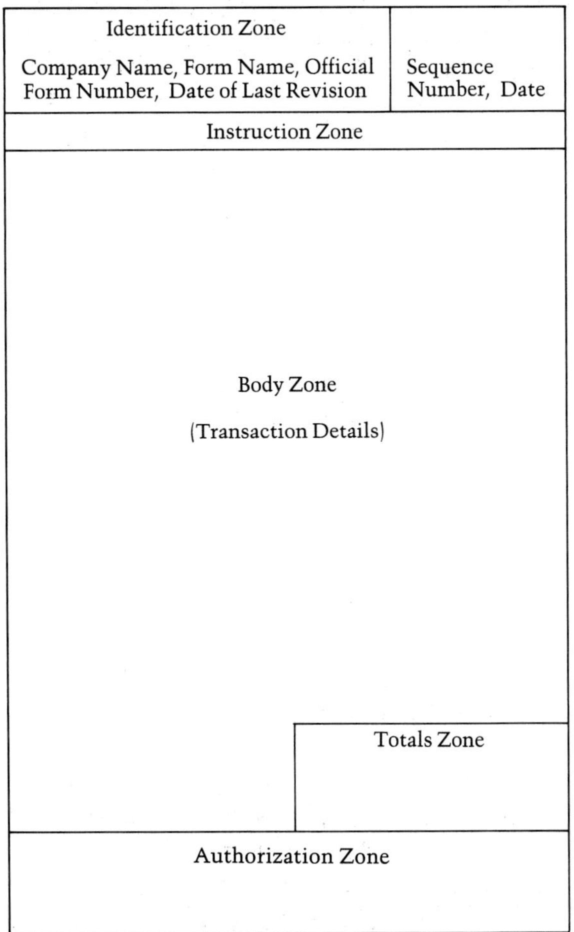

Figure 13.5

Source document design zones. A source document for input can be designed in zones such as those indicated on this template. The locations are fairly typical with the exception of the instructions zone, which may be located almost anywhere on the form (or separate from the form).

Design the Input Records or Screens

Finally, we can design the layout of the input record (batch) or input screens (on-line). The format or layout of an input is a very important design requirement and must be communicated clearly to computer programmers. Two tools available for describing the for-

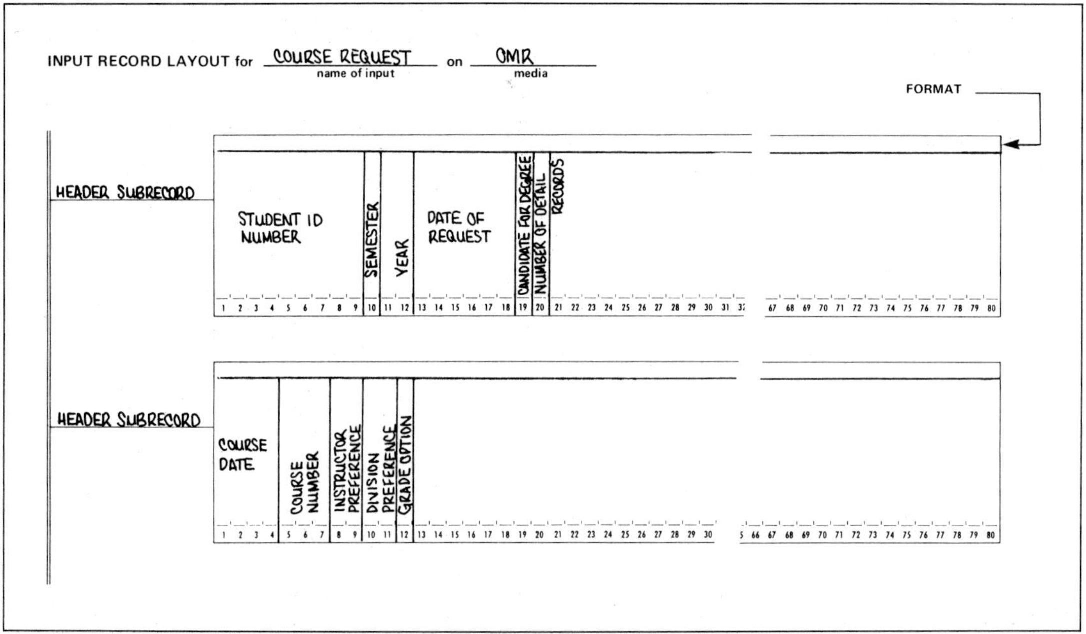

Figure 13.6

Sample input record layout chart for batch COURSE REQUEST input. Input record layout charts are used to format batch inputs. This chart varies from the record layout chart used to define the format of a file in that it does not contain a portion in which to indicate the storage characteristics (for example, character or packed decimal) and the storage position(s) are already noted on the form.

mat of inputs include the input record layout chart and the display layout chart.

The **input record layout chart** is used to lay out the format of batch inputs. Figure 13.6 is a sample input record layout chart for the batch input COURSE REQUEST appearing on the BDFD in Figure 13.4. The form is not hardware dependent and can be used to document virtually any type of medium including punched card images and key-to-tape (or disk) images. Four 80-column punched card images (a common punched card size) or one 320-character record (for magnetic media) can be accommodated. The form is read and prepared in the same manner as a record layout chart. One final note—the input record layout chart is primarily intended for the computer programmer, not the user.

The display layout chart for on-line outputs was introduced in Chapter 11. Figure 13.7 provides the layout for the on-line input of COURSE REQUEST. This form should be familiar to you. As was the case with input record layout charts, display layout charts are intended for the programmer, not the user.

Now let's use our tools to design some inputs.

Design of an On-Line Input

Because the trend is toward on-line systems, let's begin by examining an on-line input design for AAP. There are two generally accepted ways of designing on-line inputs, question and answer dialogues and form filling. In the **question/answer** mode, the system asks several questions and the operator responds with the appropriate answer. Default answers are often provided in brackets (as in <default>). Care must be taken to design input dialogues to include responses that must occur when improper data is entered. The windows concept introduced in Chapter 11 is especially useful for this requirement.

Form filling is another on-line input technique. A blank form is *painted* on the screen. The screen cursor moves to the first field to be entered on the form. When the operator enters that field, the return key sends the cursor to the next field to be entered. The automatic movement of the cursor from field to field is often assisted by dialogue software (such as IBM's CICS, a teleprocessing monitor). Fields are edited as they are entered, and appropriate error messages are displayed. After all fields have been entered, the operator presses a function key to release the data to the computer program. Most of the screen must be used for the form; however, small windows should be set aside for *MESSAGES* and *ESCAPE.* Instructions and expanded messages can be placed in a separate file that can be displayed when a function key assigned to HELP is pressed.

Specifically, we will present here the design of the input transaction, CUSTOMER ORDER. The detailed design specifications for the CUSTOMER ORDER are presented in Figures 13.8 through 13.13. Let's walk through some of the design entries. In Figure 13.8, we draw your attention to the following.

Ⓐ We initially defined the data structure for the CUSTOMER ORDER from the original data dictionary description. Notice

TERMINAL SCREEN DISPLAY LAYOUT FORM

☒ INPUT COURSE REQUEST

☐ OUTPUT

APPLICATION STUDENT REGISTRATION

SCREEN NO. SEQUENCE

COLUMN

```
01                                     COURSE REQUEST
02
03      ANSWER QUESTIONS AS THEY ARE ASKED.  TYPE HELP FOR ASSISTANCE.
04
05
06      1.    STUDENT-ID-NUMBER?          XXX-XX-XXXX (1)
07            XXXXXXXXXXXXXXXXXXXXXXXXX   XXX-XX-XXXX (a)
08
09      2.    SEMESTER? X (2)      YEAR? XX   (3)
10            XXXXXXXXXXXXXXXXXXXXXXXXXXXXX   (b)
11
12      3.    DATE OF REQUEST? <TODAY>        XX-XX-XX (4)
13            XXXXXXXXXXXXXXXXXXXXXXXXXXX     XX-XX-XX (c)
14
15      4.    CANDIDATE FOR DEGREE? <NO>      X   (5)
16            XXXXXXXXXXXXXXXXXXXXXXXXX       X   (d)
17
18      5.    ENTER COURSES? <YES>            X
19
20            COURSE  COURSE   INSTR  DIV     GRADE          SYSTEM RESPONSE
21             DEPT   NUMBER   PREFC  PRF     OPTION
22
23            XXXX    XXX      XX     XX      X              XXXXXXXXXXXXXXXXXXXXXXXXXXXXXX
24                                                           XXXXXXXXXXXXXXXXXXXXXXXXXXXXXX
25            XXXX    XX       XX     XX      X
 ↓              ↓      ↓        ↓      ↓      ↓                       ↓
23
24      PRESS F1 TO STOP ENTERING COURSES FOR THIS STUDENT.
```

FUNCTION KEY ASSIGNMENTS

PF1	RETURN TO MAIN MENU	PF9		PF17	
PF2		PF10		PF18	
PF3		PF11		PF19	
PF4		PF12		PF20	
PF5		PF13		PF21	
PF6		PF14		PF22	
PF7		PF15		PF23	
PF8		PF16		PF24	

◄ **Figure 13.7**

Sample display layout chart for on-line COURSE REQUEST input. Display layout charts are used to format on-line inputs.

D A T A D I C T I O N A R Y : I N P U T (Page 1)

DEFINITION

NAME OF INPUT RECORD: CUSTOMER ORDER
NAME OF SOURCE DOCUMENT: SALES ORDER (FORM 17)
PREPARED BY: Doug Matthews (April 4, 1986)
DESCRIPTION: A customer order for products.
INPUT METHOD: On-line
INPUT MEDIUM: Terminal Display Unit
FREQUENCY PREPARED: On demand during the hours 8 A.M. to 5 P.M.
AVERAGE VOLUME (in records): 300
PEAK VOLUME (in records & time period): 400 (May - August)
SPECIAL INSTRUCTIONS: Line 1 of the terminal screen should be used to display a descriptive title to the operator. Lines 2 through 4 should be used to display instructions to the operator. Lines 5 through 22 should be used for scrolling questions and answers. Line 23 should be used to display error messages to the user. Finally, line 25 should be used to tell the operator how to get out of the question/answer input screens.

INPUT COMPOSITION:

A CUSTOMER ORDER consists of the following data elements:

- SALES ORDER NUMBER
- BILLING ADDRESS
- optionally, the following:
  - SHIPPING ADDRESS
  - CUSTOMER NUMBER
  - CUSTOMER ORDER NUMBER
- ORDER DATE
- PAYMENT AMOUNT
- 1 to 20 of the following elements:
  - PART NUMBER
  - ~~PART DESCRIPTION~~
  - QUANTITY ORDERED
  - UNIT OF MEASURE
  - (A) DISCOUNT RATE
  - ~~DISCOUNT~~
  - ~~UNIT PRICE~~
  - ~~EXTENDED PRICE~~
- ~~SUB TOTAL~~
- ~~SALES TAX~~
- ~~TOTAL ORDER AMOUNT~~
- ~~AMOUNT OWED FOR ORDER~~

Figure 13.8

The expanded data dictionary for on-line CUSTOMER ORDER input (Page 1). A form should be developed to record the many input design requirements. Notice that the authors' form allows space for entries concerning all the input design issues discussed earlier in the chapter.

that we crossed out a number of the elements. Why? Recall that we stated earlier that not all data on a source document should be entered by the data entry operator. We eliminated on the source document those elements that could be read from files or calculated within the computer programs.

It is also important to note that some of the data elements are optional, meaning that they may or may not be entered from all forms. Finally, notice that the data structure includes a repeating group of fields.

The data-element design requirements for the CUSTOMER ORDER input are provided in Figure 13.9.

Ⓐ We identified each field as alphabetic, numeric, or alphanumeric. It is important to know the type of field because each field should be edited to conform to the proper type.

Ⓑ We also specified field size. Unlike outputs and files, input field sizes may include decimal points — and they have to be entered! However, do not include editing symbols, such as dollar signs, dashes, and slashes in the input field size. Remember, we are trying to reduce the volume of input. Numeric input fields are *not* normally *packed*, as was the case in storage files. All fields — numeric, alphabetic, and alphanumeric — are input as character strings (ASCII or EBCDIC).

Ⓒ The concept of an edit mask was first introduced in Chapter 11. An input edit mask should not include such special editing symbols as dollar signs and dashes because, as we have already noted, they are not included in the field. However, the edit mask should indicate which positions of a field can be numeric, alphabetic, and alphanumeric. The mask also indicates the decimal point position in some numeric fields. The edit mask defines the picture check for the field. For example, SALES ORDER NUMBER must be entered with six digits followed by either a digit or a letter.

Ⓓ Input-validation controls are crucial to the information system. You should define any data-element validation checks to be performed. For instance, key fields may require check digits. Other fields may require limit checks (record the value ranges).

After reviewing AAP's existing customer order form, we decided that the design layout could be improved. The existing form

D A T A   D I C T I O N A R Y :   I N P U T (Page 2)

NAME OF INPUT RECORD: CUSTOMER ORDER
PREPARED BY: Doug Matthews (April 4, 1986)

	FIELD NAME	TYPE	SIZE	EDIT MASK	EDITING/VALIDATION
1.	SALES ORDER NUMBER	A/N	7	999999X	Must be unique and pass Modulus 11.
2.	ORDER DATE	A/N (A)	8 (B)	99/99/9999 mm/dd/yyyy	Must contain values and valid month, day, and year.
3.	CUSTOMER NUMBER	A/N	4	9999	Optional
4.	CUSTOMER ORDER NUMBER	A/N	6	999999	Optional
5.	BILLING ADDRESS				Must contain values
6.	STREET ADDRESS	A/N	15	X(15)	
7.	POST OFFICE BOX NUMBER	A/N	10	X(10)	
8.	CITY	A/N	15	X(15)	
9.	STATE	A/N	2	AA	Standard code.
10.	ZIP CODE	A/N	9	9(9)	
11.	SHIPPING ADDRESS			(C)	Optional if same as BILLING ADDRESS
12.	STREET ADDRESS	A/N	15	X(15)	
13.	POST OFFICE BOX NUMBER	A/N	10	X(10)	(D)
14.	CITY	A/N	15	X(15)	
15.	STATE	A/N	2	AA	Standard code.
16.	ZIP CODE	A/N	9	9(9)	Must be numeric.
17.	PAYMENT AMOUNT	N	6.2	999,999.99	Optional If present must be less than or equal to TOTAL ORDER COST.
18.	PART NUMBER	A/N	9	9(9)	Must be valid AAP part number.
19.	QUANTITY ORDERED	N	3	9(3)	Must be > 0.
20.	DISCOUNT RATE	N	2.1	99.9	Optional. If present must be < 20%.
21.	UNIT OF MEASURE	A/N	10	X(10)	Optional

Figure 13.9

The expanded data dictionary for on-line CUSTOMER ORDER input (Page 2). The expanded data dictionary also includes entries to describe data elements.

would require the user to skip around to find specific data to be keyed in by the user is read in the left-to-right, top-to-bottom improved form. Notice that we did not use a special chart of any kind. Instead, the form was simply sketched on an eight-and-a-half by eleven-inch sheet of paper. Notice how the design layout of the new form facilitates the user's keying efforts. Data that will be keyed in by the user is read in the left-to-right, top-to-bottom sequence. The sketch can be reviewed with a professional forms manufacturer who will compose and print the form.

Now we're ready to present the terminal screens that will be used to input the appropriate data from the new customer order form. We chose the form-filling method for input. Figure 13.11 represents what the user will initially see on the CRT screen. The screen cursor will initially be positioned in column 20, row 6. As the instructions indicate, the user will be permitted to move around the screen from one item to the next or back to the previous item. In the escape area, we show the user how to discontinue the input of customer orders.

AAP, INC

AMERICAN AUTOMOTIVE PARTS, INC
P.O. BOX 4576
AIRPORT EXPRESSWAY
CINCINNATI, OH 45208

FORM 17

SALES ORDER

ORDER DATE: | CUSTOMER NO: | CUSTOMER ORDER NO.

SOLD TO: SHIP TO:

#	PART NUMBER	DESCRIPTION	QUANTITY	UNIT MEASURE	DISCOUNT RATE	DISCOUNT	UNIT PRICE	EXT. PRICE
1								
2								
3								
4								
5								
6								
7								
8								
9								
10								

FOR OFFICE USE ONLY
DATE RECEIVED
CLERK
PREPAYMENT AMOUNT $____

ALL SALES SUBJECT TO THE TERMS AND CONDITIONS ON REVERSE SIDE

SIGNATURE OF CUSTOMER OR REPRESENTATIVE

SUB TOTAL	
SALES TAX	
TOTAL	
PAID	
BALANCE	

ORIGINAL COPY TO SALES DEPARTMENT

Figure 13.10 ▲

The source document for CUSTOMER ORDER. Compare the source document with the display layout chart for CUSTOMER ORDER. Notice that the form can be easily completed and that its top-to-bottom, left-to-right flow aids in rapid data entry.

Figure 13.11 ►

Display layout chart for on-line CUSTOMER ORDER input form. The initial screen seen by the user is a blank order form to be filled in.

TERMINAL SCREEN DISPLAY LAYOUT FORM

☒ INPUT CUSTOMER ORDER

☐ OUTPUT ______________

APPLICATION ______________

SCREEN NO. ______________ SEQUENCE ______________

COLUMN

1 – 10 | 11 – 20 | 21 – 30 | 31 – 40 | 41 – 50 | 51 – 60 | 61 – 70 | 71 – 80

CUSTOMER ORDER

ENTER THE FOLLOWING ITEMS FROM SALES ORDER (FORM 17). USE "LEFT ARROW" KEY
TO BACKSPACE TO PREVIOUS ITEM. USE "RIGHT ARROW" KEY TO ADVANCE TO NEXT
ITEM. PRESS "RETURN" KEY WHEN ALL ITEMS HAVE BEEN ENTERED.

SALES ORDER # ORDER DATE

CUSTOMER # CUSTOMER ORDER #

BILLING ADDRESS SHIPPING ADDRESS
STREET STREET
P. O. BOX P. O. BOX
CITY CITY
STATE STATE
ZIPCODE ZIPCODE

PART NUMBER QUANTITY UNIT MEASURE DISCOUNT AMOUNT PAID

PRESS "PF1" TO RETURN TO MENU OFFERING OTHER ORDER ENTRY PROGRAM OPTIONS

480 1960 1920 2560 3440

FUNCTION KEY ASSIGNMENTS

PF1	RETURN TO O/E MENU	PF9		PF17	
PF2		PF10		PF18	
PF3		PF11		PF19	
PF4		PF12		PF20	
PF5		PF13		PF21	
PF6		PF14		PF22	
PF7		PF15		PF23	
PF8		PF16		PF24	

But what about the actual entry of data elements? A programmer would need more specific input requirements than those depicted in Figure 13.11. A more appropriate display layout chart is provided in Figure 13.12. This chart shows the programmer how data is actually input.

Ⓐ We have indicated the exact location and edit mask for each data element. In addition to the edit mask, a reference number has been provided (usually just below the edit mask). This reference number corresponds to the data element in the expanded data dictionary. But what about the letters within the parentheses? These letters are used to reference a memo that discusses system messages and display attributes.

Ⓑ The portion of the screen will scroll upward, thus allowing the user to enter data for a large number of parts. Downward arrows were drawn after elements numbered 18 through 21 to indicate that the user may enter several values for these elements.

Ⓒ If at any time, the user enters incorrect data values for an element, a descriptive error message will appear. We explained these error messages with a reference letter and appropriate memos. The memos are shown in Figure 13.13. Notice that we've used Structured English to document when specific error messages may occur. No, we don't consider this documentation as "doing the programmer's job." By conveying these editing requirements in Structured English, we are reducing the time we have to spend conveying the requirements to the programmer.

Well, that's about it for this input. What would we do differently if the CUSTOMER ORDER were designed as a batch input? We'll show you right now.

Design of a Batch Input

Our design of the CUSTOMER ORDER as a batch input isn't much different from that for the on-line input. The primary difference is the use of an input record layout chart in place of the display layout chart. Because data from a batch of customer orders must be keyed by a data entry clerk and stored in a temporary file, we had to design that input file. The expanded data dictionary for the batch input

TERMINAL SCREEN DISPLAY LAYOUT FORM

APPLICATION ______ SCREEN NO. ______ SEQUENCE ______

☒ INPUT CUSTOMER ORDER

☐ OUTPUT ______

COLUMN

01	*CUSTOMER ORDER*
02	ENTER THE FOLLOWING ITEMS FROM SALES ORDER (FORM 17). USE "LEFT ARROW" KEY
03	TO BACKSPACE TO PREVIOUS ITEM. USE "RIGHT ARROW" KEY TO ADVANCE TO NEXT
04	ITEM. PRESS "RETURN" KEY WHEN ALL ITEMS HAVE BEEN ENTERED.
05	
06	SALES ORDER # 999999X ← (A) ORDER DATE 99/99/9999
07	(1)(a) (2)(a)
08	CUSTOMER # 9999 CUSTOMER ORDER # 999999
09	(3)(a) (4)(a)
10	BILLING ADDRESS SHIPPING ADDRESS
11	STREET XXXXXXXXXXXXXXX (6)(a) STREET XXXXXXXXXXXXXXX (12)(a)
12	P. O. BOX XXXXXXXXXX (7)(a) 480 P. O. BOX XXXXXXXXXX (13)(a) 1960
13	CITY XXXXXXXXXXXXXXX (8)(a) CITY XXXXXXXXXXXXXXX (14)(a)
14	STATE AA (9)(a) STATE AA (15)(a)
15	ZIPCODE 999999999 (10)(a) ZIPCODE 999999999 (16)(a)
16	
17	PART NUMBER QUANTITY UNIT MEASURE DISCOUNT AMOUNT PAID
18	999999999 999 XXXXXXXXXX 99.9 999,999.99
19	(18)(a) (19)(a) (21)(a) (20)(a) (17)(a)
20	(B)
21	
22	(C)
23	XXXXXXXXXXXXXXXXXXXXXXXXXXXXXXXXXXXXXXXXXXXXXXXXXXXXXXXXXXXXXXXXX (b)
24	PRESS "PF1" TO RETURN TO MENU OFFERING OTHER ORDER ENTRY PROGRAM OPTIONS 1920
42	
43	3440

FUNCTION KEY ASSIGNMENTS

PF1	RETURN TO O/E MENU	PF9		PF17	
PF2		PF10		PF18	
PF3		PF11		PF19	
PF4		PF12		PF20	
PF5		PF13		PF21	
PF6		PF14		PF22	
PF7		PF15		PF23	
PF8		PF16		PF24	

Figure 13.12

Display layout chart for on-line CUSTOMER ORDER input fields to be input. This screen shows the proper edit masks for the fields to be entered by the user.

Memo For CUSTOMER ORDER Input Record

Ref. No. Memo

a These fields are to be displayed as a "red" background.

b This field is used to provide the user with a descriptive error message when invalid commands or data have been entered. Otherwise the field is not printed. When the message is displayed, it should "blink" to grab the user's attention. As a reminder, the editing criteria were explained in the expanded data dictionary. The following specifies the conditions and types of messages to be displayed to the user:

```
Select the appropriate case:

     Case 1:  SALES ORDER NUMBER is invalid

          If the SALES ORDER NUMBER is equivalent to the SALES
          ORDER NUMBER of any previously entered DAILY SALES
          ORDER then:

               error message = "Sales order number was assigned
               to previously entered sales order, please re-
               enter."

          If the SALES ORDER NUMBER fails the Modulus 11 check
          then:

               error message = "Sales order number was illegal,
               possible keying error, please re-enter."

     Case 2:  ORDER DATE is invalid

          Select appropriate case:

               Case 2.1  ORDER DATE contains no values, then:

                    error message = "The order date must be
                    provided on all orders, please enter."

               Case 2.2  ORDER DATE contains invalid values for
                    MONTH, DAY, or YEAR then:

                    error message = "The order date is not
                    valid, please re-enter."

     Case 3:  Select appropriate case for BILLING ADDRESS:

               Case 3.1  BILL TO STREET ADDRESS, BILL TO POST
                    OFFICE BOX NUMBER, BILL TO CITY, BILL TO
                    STATE, or BILL TO ZIPCODE contains no
                    values, then:

                    error message = "A complete billing address
                    is required on all sales orders, please re-
                    enter."

               Case 3.2  BILL TO STATE contains invalid state
                    code, then:

                    error message = "Standard state codes must
                    be entered, please re-enter."

               Case 3.3  BILL TO ZIPCODE contains non-numeric
                    value:

                    error message = "Zipcodes must be numeric,
                    please re-enter."
```

(continues)

```
Memo for CUSTOMER ORDER Input Record
(continued)

Case 4:  Select appropriate case for entered SHIPPING
     ADDRESS:

          Case 4.1  SHIP TO STREET ADDRESS, SHIP TO POST OFFICE
               BOX NUMBER, SHIP TO CITY, SHIP TO STATE, or SHIP
               TO ZIPCODE contains no values, then:

               error message = "Shipping addresses must be
               complete for all sales orders, please enter."

Case 5:  PAYMENT AMOUNT entered invalid, then:

          If PAYMENT AMOUNT is not numeric, then:

               error message = "Payment amount must be a numeric
               dollar amount, please re-enter."

          If PAYMENT AMOUNT is greater than the TOTAL ORDER COST
          (sum of EXTENDED PRICE, plus SALES TAX), then:

               error message = "Payment amount exceeds the total
               cost of the sales order, please re-enter."

Case 6:  PART NUMBER is not a valid AAP part number, then:

     error message = "Entered an incorrect AAP part number,
     please re-enter."

Case 7:  QUANTITY ORDERED is not greater than 0, then:

     error message = "Quantity ordered must be greater than
     0, please re-enter."

Case 8:  DISCOUNT RATE provided is not less than 20 percent, then:

     error message = "AAP allowed discount rates may not
     exceed 20 percent, please re-enter."
```

Figure 13.13

Memo attachment for the design of on-line CUSTOMER ORDER input. Memos are used to describe display attributes (such as blinking fields) and error messages.

CUSTOMER ORDER differs only slightly from the on-line version. The primary differences are noted on the partial expanded data dictionary displayed in Figure 13.14.

Ⓐ Batch input files frequently contain variable-length records. We were able to determine the record size only after addressing the data-element design considerations (for example, field sizes).

Ⓑ The data structure for the CUSTOMER ORDER is very similar to the data structure we defined when we designed the on-line

The Next Generation Have You Written Your Last Edit Program?

Input design has always carried with it the burden of data validation. People—both data-entry operators and end users—make mistakes. Therefore, the systems analyst is responsible for specifying type, size, picture, and value checks on all fields to be input to a computer information system. And programmers often spend as much time writing the associated edit programs to check input data as they spend writing the functional parts of the programs. Clearly, there's room for productivity improvement.

Today, software packages are emerging that promise to eliminate the need for writing new edit programs. Some of these packages may be offered as add-on functions intended to work with such traditional languages as COBOL. Others are sold as part of database management systems or fourth-generation programming languages. In either case, the principle is both simple and common to all editing requirements.

How do these editors work? First, inputs are defined in a computerized dictionary. The dictionary specifies the type of field (for instance, *numeric*), size of field, edit mask (like a PICTURE in the COBOL language), and legal values. Values may be specified as a range or as a table of codes. The dictionary may also specify combination criteria, such as restricting the codes that may be used for one field according to the value of another field.

After the dictionary has been defined, your conventional programs may be written. However, instead of using standard INPUT or READ instructions, you use commands that automatically perform input. When the data is read, the data dictionary's programs compare the data against editing requirements defined in the dictionary. Discrepancies are reported either on the terminal screen (for an on-line system) or via a printed report (for a batch system). Consequently, the programmer can skip straight to the functional programs that need to be written.

As always, we are interested in how this technology may change the systems analyst's job. The change is subtle but significant. In most environments, the analyst has always been responsible for specifying input editing requirements for the programmer. But it seems silly to record these in a standard data dictionary (of the type you've been learning and using in this book) only to have the programmer input them to the input editing dictionary described here. The programmer (who is often not as familiar with the business problem as the analyst) may make a transcription mistake. It makes more sense for the analyst to learn about these input editing technologies and directly record the editing requirements for the programmer. ■

version. The only difference is that the data element NUMBER OF ITEMS ORDERED has been added. Why? Because, as you should recall from the previous chapter, variable-length records require a repeating factor field.

```
D A T A   D I C T I O N A R Y :   I N P U T

DEFINITION

   NAME OF INPUT RECORD:  CUSTOMER ORDER
   NAME OF SOURCE DOCUMENT:  SALES ORDER (FORM 17)
   PREPARED BY:  Doug Matthews (April 4, 1986)
   DESCRIPTION:  A customer order for products.
   INPUT METHOD:  Batch
   INPUT MEDIUM:  Key-to-disk
   FREQUENCY PREPARED:  Daily - 7:30 A.M. and 12:00 N.
   RETENTION:  2 days
   AVERAGE VOLUME (in records):  300
   PEAK VOLUME (in records & time period):  400 (May - August)
(A) FIXED OR VARIABLE LENGTH?:  Variable
   RECORD SIZE (characters):  162 - 637
   SORTING REQUIREMENTS:  SALES ORDER NUMBER and PART NUMBER

INPUT COMPOSITION:

     A CUSTOMER ORDER consists of the following data elements:
          SALES ORDER NUMBER
          BILLING ADDRESS
          optionally, the following:
               SHIPPING ADDRESS
               CUSTOMER NUMBER
               CUSTOMER ORDER NUMBER
          ORDER DATE
          PAYMENT AMOUNT
          1 to 20 of the following elements:
               PART NUMBER
               QUANTITY ORDERED
               UNIT OF MEASURE
               DISCOUNT RATE
      (B) NUMBER OF ITEMS ORDERED
```

Figure 13.14

Expanded data dictionary for batch CUSTOMER ORDER input.

The input record layout chart is presented in Figure 13.15. Looks pretty simple, right? It should! It's not much different from the record layout charts introduced in the previous chapter. What do we see that is different on this chart? The storage format (for example, character or packed decimal) for each field is not specified. Why? Normally, all fields on an input record are stored as character strings. Therefore, there is no need for specifying alternative formats.

In Chapter 11, you learned how to design computer-generated outputs. Recall that the data flow diagram helped you identify the outputs that must be designed. Be careful though. Because DFDs show only net data flows (input or output), not all outputs that must be designed will show up on the DFD! For instance, not until we

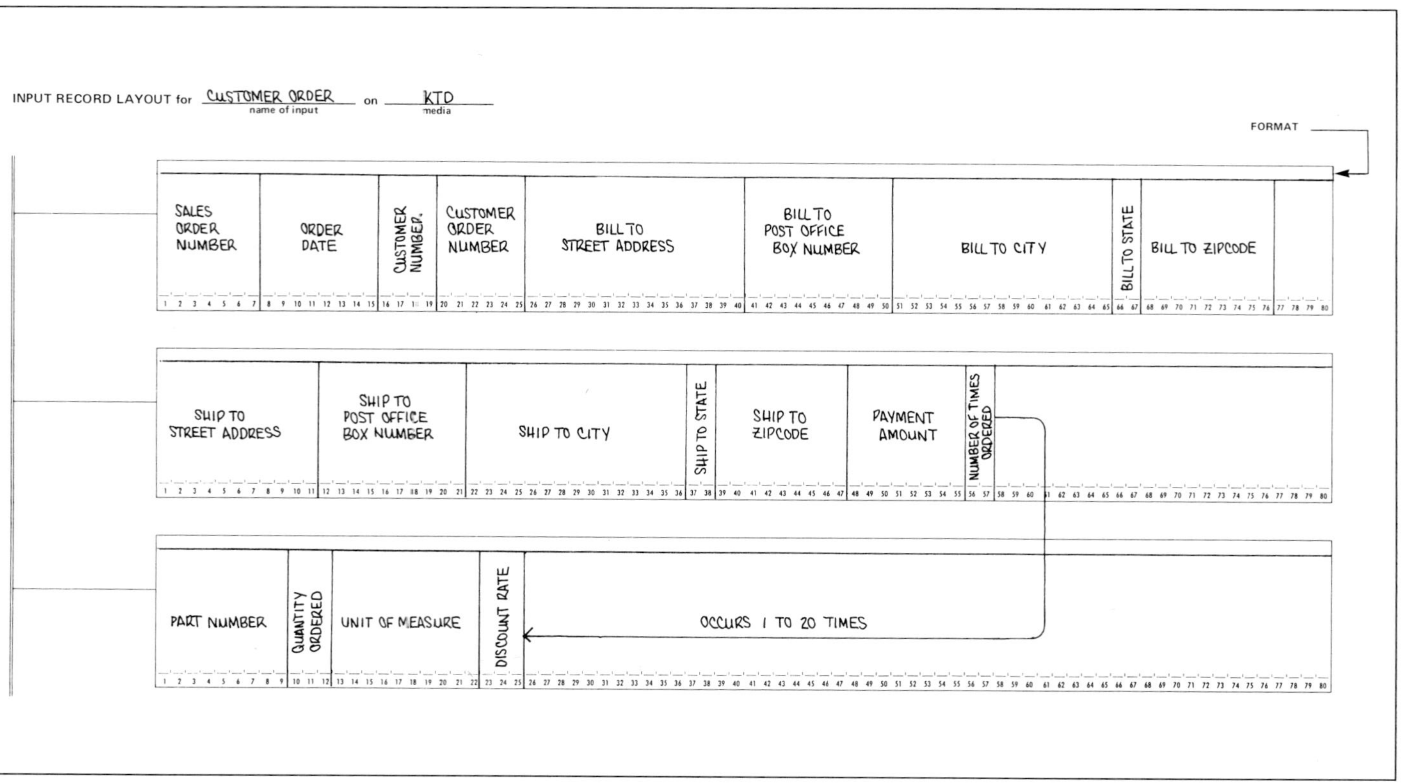

Figure 13.15

Input record layout chart for batch CUSTOMER ORDER input format.

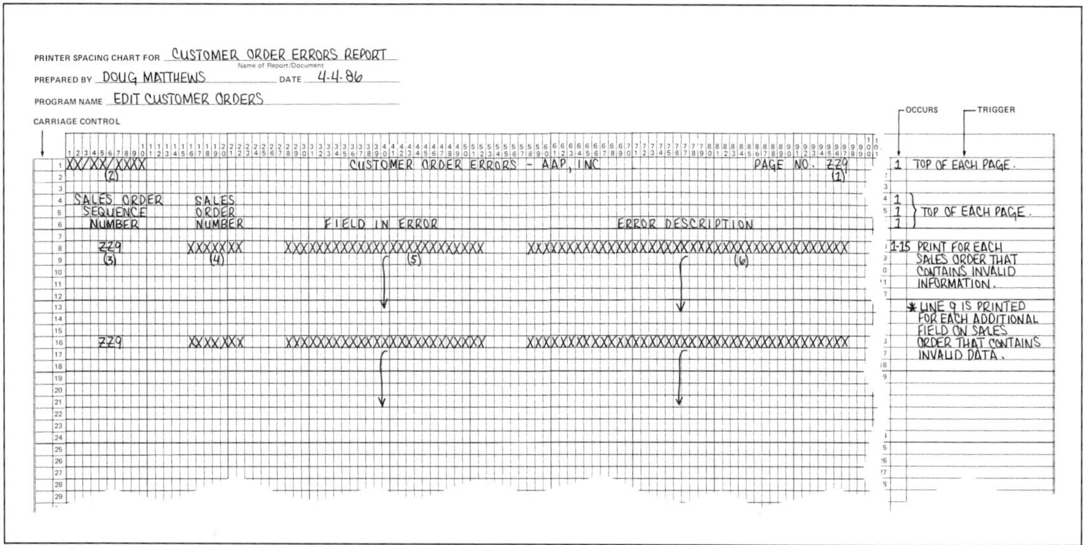

Figure 13.16

Sample printer spacing chart for DAILY CUSTOMER ORDER ERRORS REPORT format. Input design will likely send you back to output design because you should always design edit reports and transaction-processing historical reports for all inputs.

selected the batch input method for entering customer orders, did we recognize the need for a new report: the DAILY CUSTOMER ORDER ERRORS REPORT. This edit report will identify all CUSTOMER ORDERS that contain incorrect data. The order-entry clerk will be able to use this report to follow up on the customer order documents to ensure their accuracy. Because you already know how to design computer outputs, we won't spend time discussing the design of this report. However, we've included the printer spacing chart for DAILY CUSTOMER ORDER ERRORS REPORT in Figure 13.16. Notice that the report clearly indicates the customer orders, specific fields, and errors that were encountered.

Designing Batch Inputs Involving Multiple Record Types

It's quite common for a systems analyst to design a batch input file that contains more than one type of input record. For instance, a system may include a program that allows the marketing department to update a product file. The program might (1) place new

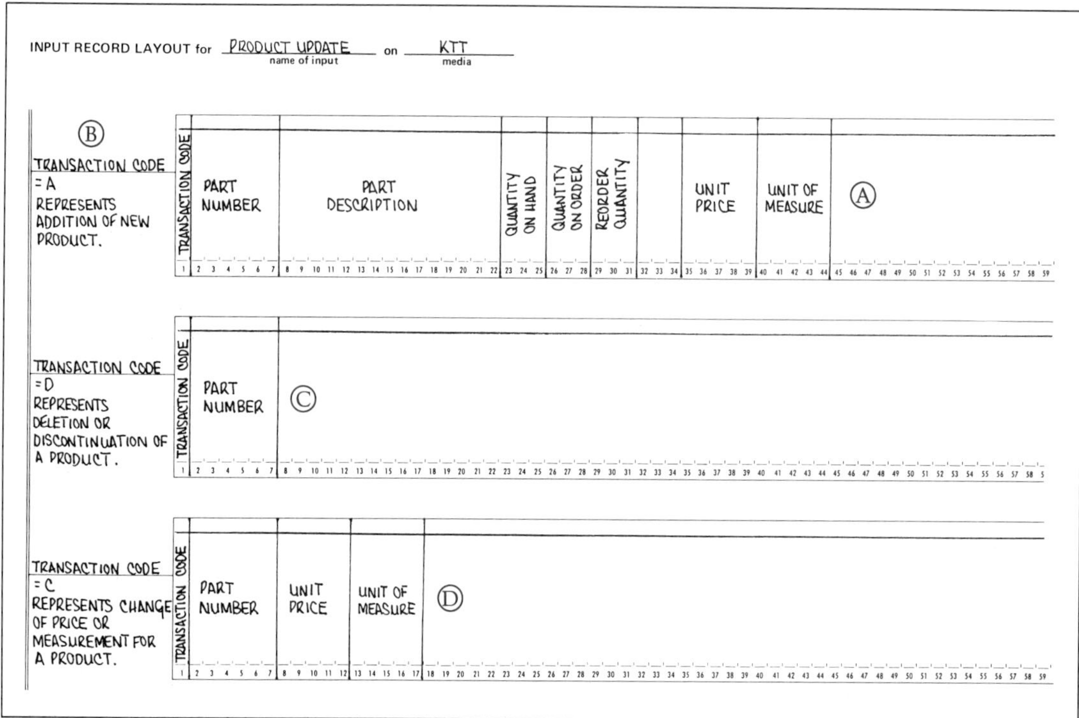

Figure 13.17

Sample input record layout chart for multiple input records.

products into the file, (2) delete from the file products that are to be discontinued, (3) change the contents of a product record to reflect a new price or unit of measurement. It's obvious that the input data necessary for performing these three tasks varies significantly. To add a product, all the data elements describing the product are needed. To delete a product, only the product number is necessary. Finally, to change the contents of a product record, the product number and only those data elements to be changed are required.

The batch input file that would contain the input transaction data necessary for the program to update the product file can be designed easily, using the same tools as those we used for the batch input file. However, we have to make one small adjustment. How do we complete the input record layout chart when the content and format of the input record is dependent on the particular type of update to the product file?

In Figure 13.17, you can see how the design of the input layout record could be defined. Because the content and format of the input record is dependent on the particular type of update, we simply showed the three possible design layouts. Let's examine the record layout closely.

Ⓐ The portion represents the contents and layout of the input record that is required when a new product is to be added to the product file. Notice that we included in the record a special field called TRANSACTION CODE. This field will be included in each of the three input record types. The value of this field will identify the particular type of input task to be performed.

Ⓑ The label is provided to let the programmer know which record layout corresponds to which input record type.

Ⓒ The portion of the input record layout chart specifies the data elements and layout for an input record that represents the deletion of an existing product record in the product file.

Ⓓ The portion of the input record layout chart specifies the data elements and layout for an input record that represents updates to the contents of an existing product record in the product file.

SUMMARY

The goal of input design is to capture data and get that data into a format suitable for the computer. Input methods can be broadly classified as either batch or on-line. The systems analyst must be familiar with the advantages and disadvantages of each method as well as with the various media used to implement both methods. Because input is highly visible to the end user, analysts should consider a number of *human factors* when designing computer inputs. The volume of data to be input by the user should be minimized because every data element input carries with it the risk of error. Source documents for capturing data should be designed for easy completion by users and for rapid data entry by data-entry clerks and CRT operators.

Internal controls are also essential for inputs. Internal controls should be established for monitoring the number of inputs and for ensuring that the data are valid. Internal control techniques for ensuring the validity of data include completeness checks, limit and range checks, combination checks, self-checking digits, and picture clauses.

To design computer inputs, the systems analyst should begin by identifying the input requirements of the new system. Bounded data flow diagrams (BDFDs) identify data to be captured and input to the system. The data dictionary defines the basic content of the inputs to be designed. Next, the analyst must specify the design parameters — issues concerning data capture, data entry, and data input — for the input. Then the analyst designs the source document. Finally, the analyst must lay out the format of the batch or on-line input. An input record layout chart is used to format batch inputs. A display layout chart is used to format on-line inputs. Both tools allow the analyst to define the format of fixed- and variable-length inputs.

PROBLEMS AND EXERCISES

1. Explain the difference between *data capture*, *data entry*, and *data input*. Relate the three concepts to the processing of your school's course request or course registration.
2. To what extent should the knowledge worker be involved during input design? What would you ask the knowledge worker to do? When? What would you do for the knowledge worker? When?
3. Define an appropriate input method and medium for each of the following inputs:
   (a) Customer magazine subscriptions
   (b) Hotel reservations
   (c) Bank account transactions
   (d) Customer order cancellations
   (e) Customer order modifications
   (f) Employee weekly time cards
4. What data flows crossing the person/machine boundary of a bounded data flow diagram should be designed as computer inputs?
5. What effects can be caused by lack of internal controls for inputs?

6. Obtain a copy of an application form (such as loan, housing, or school) or any other document used to capture data (such as a course scheduling form, credit card purchase slip, or time card). Do not be concerned whether the application is currently input to a computer system. How do the people who initiate or process the form feel about it? Comment on the human engineering. How well is it divided into zones? Comment on the suitability of the application for data entry. Are elements that wouldn't be keyed properly located? What changes would you make to the form?

7. The order-filling operation for a local pharmacy is to be automated. The pharmacy processes 50 to 200 prescriptions per day. Customer prescriptions are to be entered on-line by the pharmacist. Prepare an expanded data dictionary and display layout chart for documenting the design of the on-line input PRESCRIPTION. A working data dictionary for PRESCRIPTION follows:

   A PRESCRIPTION contains the following elements:

   CUSTOMER NAME

   DOCTOR NAME

   1 to 10 occurrences of the following:

   DRUG NAME

   QUANTITY PRESCRIBED

   MEDICAL INSTRUCTIONS

   RX NUMBER * a federal licensing number — 6 digits

   1 to 10 occurrences of the following * added by pharmacist

   DRUG NUMBER * a number that uniquely identifies a prescription drug — 6 characters

   LOT NUMBER * a number that uniquely identifies the lot from which a chemical was produced — 6 characters

   DOSAGE FORM * the form of the medication issued, such as "pill". P= PILL C = CAPSULE L = LIQUID I = INJECTION R = LOTION

   UNIT OF MEASURE * G = GRAMS

O = OUNCES M = MILLILITERS

QUANTITY DISPENSED

NUMBER OF REFILLS

and optionally:

EXPIRATION DATE

8. A moving company maintains data concerning fuel tax liability for its fleet of trucks. When truck drivers return from a trip, they submit a journal describing mileage, fuel purchases, and fuel consumption for each state traveled through. This data is to be batch input daily to maintain records on trucks and fuel stations. The TRIP JOURNAL data dictionary follows:

   A TRIP JOURNAL consists of the following elements:

   TRUCK NUMBER

   DRIVER

   CODRIVER NUMBER

   TRIP NUMBER

   DATE DEPARTED

   DATE RETURNED

   1 to 20 of the following:

   STATE CODE

   MILES DRIVEN

   FUEL RECEIPT NUMBER

   GALLONS PURCHASED

   TAXES PAID

   STATION NAME

   STATION LOCATION

   Design the batch input TRIP JOURNAL. Be sure to design an appropriate source document. Fuel receipts are to be stapled to the source document.

ANNOTATED REFERENCES AND SUGGESTED READINGS

Fitzgerald, Jerry. *Internal Controls for Computerized Information Systems.* Redwood City, Calif.: Jerry Fitzgerald & Associates, 1978. This is our reference standard on the subject of designing internal controls into systems. Jerry advocates a unique and powerful matrix tool for designing controls. The discussion of input controls is especially thorough. This book goes far beyond any introductory systems textbook — Must reading.

Designing On-Line Terminal Dialogues

Minicase: Soft Shoe, Inc. (Part II)

In Chapter 13, we listened in on a conversation between Carey Carmichael, manager of the Information Systems Department, and Judy Lucas, a systems analyst. Carey was telling Judy about complaints the Order-Entry Department had voiced about the new order-entry system Judy had implemented. At the tail end of their conversation, Carey was preparing to tell Judy, in detail, of the many mistakes she had made. Judy spent the following two weeks improving the on-line portion of the order-entry system. The majority of her efforts were spent adding data editing features to screens used to input customer sales orders.

Customer complaints decreased in the weeks that followed. Judy had done a fine job of ensuring the accuracy of the data input by the order-entry clerks. But Judy was constantly receiving phone calls concerning problems the order-entry clerks were encountering. The clerks called Judy with the following questions and problems.

"What does it mean when the terminal says *HIT FUNCTION KEY 5?*"

"Judy, I really goofed! I pressed the wrong key and a new screen appeared on the CRT. How do I get back to the previous screen?"

"I keep typing in a date and that dumb computer won't accept it. Can you come fix it?"

"Judy, I'm using the terminal to do something I've never done before. I have a screen that appeared, and I don't know how to go about typing in the information. Can you give me directions?"

"I keep trying to see one of our customer orders, but the screen runs it by me so fast I don't have a chance to see all the information I need to see."

"Judy, isn't it about time you make the terminal screen stop displaying that joke of yours? I get tired of seeing that thing appear across the screen."

These types of phone calls come at all hours of the day. Needless to say, Judy still has improvements to make to the terminal dialogue of the order-entry system.

Discussion

1. Can you tell from the phone calls what mistakes Judy has made in designing the terminal dialogue?
2. What are some other mistakes a systems analyst might make when designing terminal dialogue?

WHAT WILL YOU LEARN IN THIS CHAPTER?

In this chapter you will learn how to design the terminal dialogue that results in the on-line outputs and inputs that were designed in Chapters 11 and 13, respectively. You will know that you've mastered terminal dialogue design when you can:

1. Determine which features on the available display terminal(s) can be used for effective terminal dialogue design.
2. Identify the type(s) of users who will use an on-line system.

3. Design or evaluate the human engineering in a terminal dialogue for a typical information system.
4. Apply appropriate terminal dialogue strategies to an on-line information system.
5. Use a dialogue chart to plan and coordinate a terminal dialogue for an on-line information system.
6. Use display layout charts (for net inputs and outputs from Chapters 11 and 13 as well as for dialogue from this chapter) to format the screens in an on-line system.

The current trend is toward on-line information systems that permit the knowledge worker to directly converse with the computer to input data and output information. The design of conversational terminal dialogue has taken on greater importance because of this trend. You have already learned how to design, on-line, *net* inputs and outputs. In this chapter, you will learn how to bring these net inputs and outputs together into a dialogue that is controlled by the user of a display terminal. How will the system first present itself to the user? How will the user get to various input and output functions? And how will the system deal with user errors? These are all important questions to be addressed in this chapter.

WHEN PEOPLE TALK TO COMPUTERS

Terminal dialogue design is the specification of a conversation between the knowledge worker and the computer. This conversation results in input of new data to the information system, output of information to the knowledge worker, or both. The information system components pertinent to this chapter are indicated in the margin. What makes a terminal dialogue good? Does the available technology limit or enhance dialogue possibilities? How can a terminal dialogue be organized?

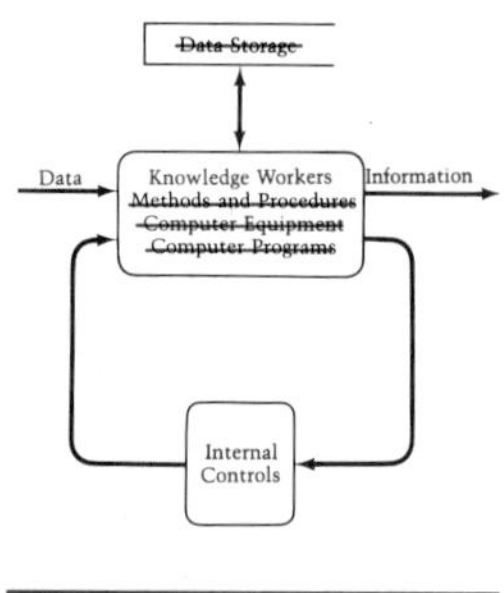

IPO Model

We assume you know what a display terminal is, but we suspect that many of you are not familiar with the various features offered by many terminals. Your exposure may be somewhat limited by the technology your school or business can afford. Because display terminal features affect terminal dialogue design, we'll begin with an overview of features. Then we can examine some of the fundamental human factors and design strategies that underlie terminal dialogue design.

Display Terminals and Features That Affect Dialogue Design

The design of terminal dialogue can be enhanced or restricted by the available features of the display terminal itself. Before we discuss these features, you should become aware of an important technical trend in our industry. Display terminals are gradually being supplemented or replaced by microcomputers that can be used to emulate display terminals. By *emulate,* we mean that software is used to make the microcomputer *think* and *behave* as a display terminal. The advantage is significant. The microcomputer becomes a more flexible resource. When not being used as a CRT terminal, it can be used as a computer, and vice versa. Furthermore, technology that is rapidly evolving allows the microcomputer to move data to and from a larger computer. Thus the microcomputer can (1) be used as a terminal to get data from a host computer (this is called *downloading*), (2) become a microcomputer to process that data, and then (3) become a terminal again to send processed data back to the host computer (called *uploading*). We want to emphasize that, when we talk about display terminal features in this chapter, we are implicitly including microcomputers that can behave as display terminals. Let's outline some display terminal features that can affect terminal dialogue design.

Display Area The size of the display area is critical to terminal dialogue design. The two most common display areas are 25 (lines) by 80 (columns) and 25 by 132. Some terminals, such as Digital Equipment Corporation's VT-102, can be easily shifted between these two display sizes. Some newer terminals are designed to display more lines, so that an entire page of a standard letterhead can be displayed. Other specialized terminals, such as those used at some teller stations in banks, restrict the display area to 12 or fewer lines.

Character Set Every display terminal uses a predefined character set. Most terminals use the character set available through the ASCII character codes that were introduced in Chapter 12. Many intelligent terminals and microcomputers allow the programmer to supplement or replace the predefined character set. Additionally, many terminals offer graphics character codes that allow pictures and charts to be mapped to the display screen. Graphics capabilities must be supported by graphics software that allows the programmer to take advantage of the graphics display capabilities.

Paging and Scrolling The manner in which the display area is shown to the user is controlled by both the technical capabilities of the terminal and the software capabilities of the computer system. Paging and scrolling are the two most common approaches to showing the display area to the user. **Paging** displays a complete screen of characters at a time. The complete display area is known as a page, screen, or frame. The page is replaced on demand by the next or previous page; this is much like turning the pages of a book. **Scrolling** moves the display up or down, *one line at a time.* This is similar to the way movie and television credits scroll up the screen at the end of a movie. We'll discuss the choice of paging or scrolling for a dialogue when we discuss human factors.

Color Displays and Display Attributes Greater numbers of display terminals are using color display capabilities. Color can be used to highlight specific messages, data, or areas of the screen.

Many display terminals permit a variety of display and audio attributes. Some of these attributes include:

- Double brightness on selected fields or messages.
- Blinking for selected fields or messages.
- Nondisplay for selected fields (for example, passwords).
- Reverse video for selected fields, messages, or display areas. Reverse video permits the color of the background (such as black) and the color of selected fields and messages (such as green) to be reversed.
- Audible alarm such as a bell or whistle.

Each of these features, when available, is activated by predefined codes that the programmer must learn or apply.

Split-Screen or Window Capability Windows were introduced in Chapter 13. Split-screen capability is a simpler variation on the windows concept. In either case, the screen, *under software control,* can be divided into areas (called *windows*). Each area can act independently from the other windows, using features such as paging, scrolling, display attributes, and color. Each window can be defined to serve a specific purpose for the user.

Function Keys Most modern terminals have special keys called function keys (usually labeled *F1*, *F2*, and so on). These keys can be used to implement certain common, repetitive operations in a terminal dialogue (for example, START, HELP, PAGE UP, PAGE DOWN, EXIT). Normally, these keys are defined to perform the desired operations under software control. That is to say, you program the keys. We'll discuss some of the more common uses of function keys when we discuss human factors later in this chapter. In any event, the analyst often defines the functions of these keys and the programmer implements those functions.

Input Options We are no longer restricted to the keyboard as the input technology for terminals. Today, we are encountering other options, such as *touch-sensitive screens, voice recognition,* and *mice.* The last of these may not be familiar to you. A mouse is a small hand-sized device that sits on a flat surface near the terminal. It has a small roller ball on the underside. As you move the mouse on the flat surface, it causes the cursor to move on the screen. Under software control, the mouse can be used to select menu options and to reposition the cursor with ease.

The Importance of Human Factors in Good Terminal Dialogue Design

Nowhere are human factors as important as they are in terminal dialogue design. Just ask the typical systems analyst who spends half the day answering phone calls like these:

> "Mary, what the heck does the message *Error 56 in GETRECV.CBL* mean?"
>
> "Lonnie, my keyboard just locked up! I can't get the system to accept anything I type. Help!"
>
> "Jenny, how do I get back to the last screen in the order system? I think I made a terrible mistake. Can I change data that was previously entered?"
>
> "John, what does it mean when the tube says *DATA FILE LOST?*"

Don't laugh! We've talked to analysts who field these type questions at all hours of the day. That's why we want to discuss the subject of human engineering.

Terminal users can be broadly classified as either dedicated or casual. A **dedicated user** is one who will spend considerable time using the display terminal. This user is likely to become comfortable and familiar with the terminal's operation. The **casual user,** on the other hand, will only use the terminal on an occasional basis. This user may never become truly comfortable with the terminal. The casual user is becoming less common in this computer-literate age. It is difficult to imagine today's youth as being ill at ease with the computer or display terminal. Still, most of today's systems are being designed for the casual user, with an emphasis on user friendliness.

General Human Engineering Guidelines Given the type of user for an on-line system, there are a number of important human engineering factors that should be incorporated into the design:

- *The user should always be aware of what to do next.* The system should always provide instructions on how to proceed, back up, exit, and the like.
- *The screen is always formatted so that the various types of information, instructions, and messages always appear in the same general display area.* This way, the user always knows approximately where to look for specific information. To achieve this goal, we suggest that *windows* or areas be defined as indicated in Figure 14.1. A sample screen, divided into windows, is illustrated in Figure 14.2. The windows concept can easily be implemented with screen formatting software that is generally available for most computers. Even without such software, windows can be defined and followed by using conventional programming techniques.
- *Within the body window, the dialogue should be limited to one idea per frame,* whether paging or scrolling through the window. For instance, the window should display one menu, one input, one report, or one query response.

  The choice between *paging* and *scrolling* for the body window depends on the information content to be displayed in that window. If the information to be displayed is continuous in nature, such as most reports, scrolling can be used. The cursor

SUGGESTED WINDOW DEFINITIONS

Title window	The title window identifies the screen from the user's point of view.
Instruction window	The instruction window is normally required only for input screens. The window displays input instructions to the user.
Flag window	The flag window is used to *point to* some specific line in one of the other windows to highlight the location of an error or problem. For example, if the user has made a mistake, the symbol "↲" might appear in the flag window on the line in which the mistake occurred. To discover the specific nature of the problem, the user should look at the message window, (the window described next). Display attributes such as blinking fields and reverse video can accomplish the same purpose and eliminate the need for a flag area.
Message window	The message window is used to display system messages to the user. For instance, error messages and/or suggestions may be recorded in this window. Most of the time, this window would be blank.
Escape window	The escape window is used to suggest how the user can exit the current system or subsystem. For example, the escape window may display a message on how to get back to the main system menu or to the previous menu of options.
Body window	The body window is the largest display area. It is in the body that the user inputs new data or views output information. The body is also used to display *help* messages that are too long to display in the message or instruction windows. This window is also used to display menu options or direct question and answer type dialogues (more about these options later).

Figure 14.1

Window areas on the terminal screen. Terminal screens are much easier to read if the screen is partitioned into areas, called windows, into which similar data and specific types of messages are always recorded. Adapted from Mehlmann, 1981.

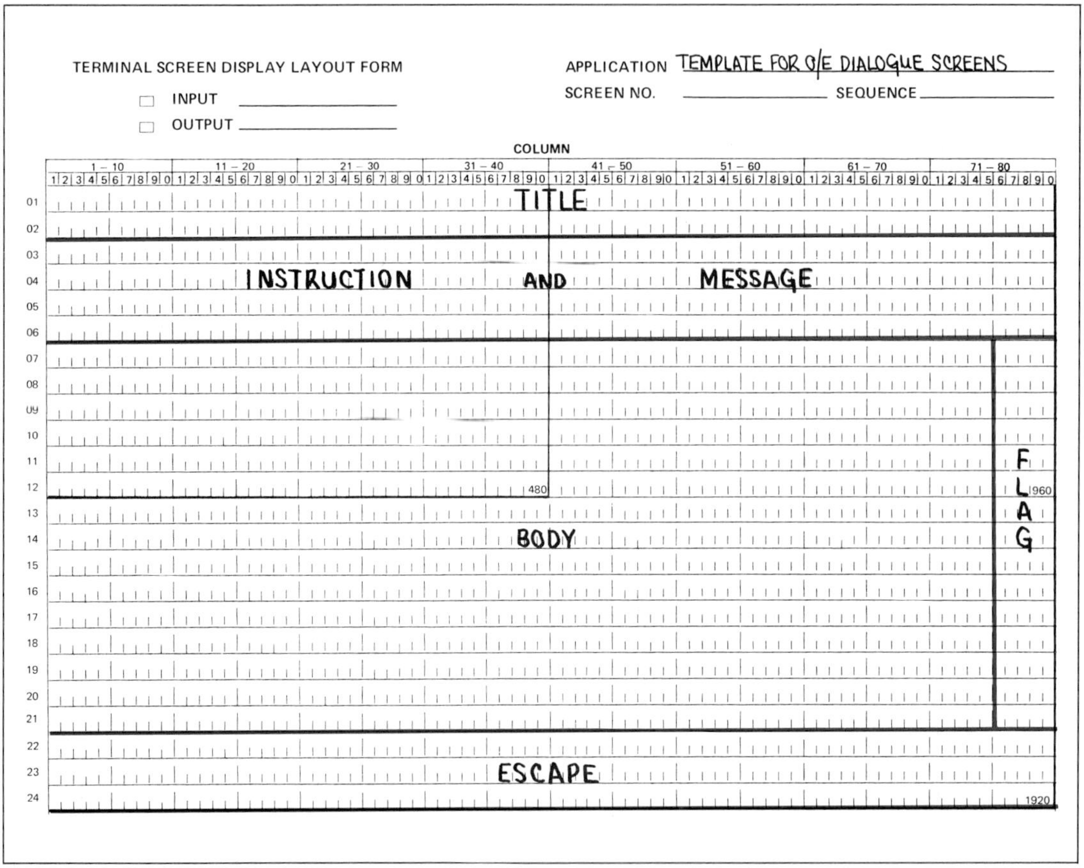

TERMINAL SCREEN DISPLAY LAYOUT FORM

☐ INPUT ______

☐ OUTPUT ______

APPLICATION TEMPLATE FOR O/E DIALOGUE SCREENS

SCREEN NO. ______ SEQUENCE ______

COLUMN

1 – 10 | 11 – 20 | 21 – 30 | 31 – 40 | 41 – 50 | 51 – 60 | 61 – 70 | 71 – 80

01 TITLE

04 INSTRUCTION AND MESSAGE

12 480 1960

11–14 FLAG

14 BODY

23 ESCAPE

24 1920

Figure 14.2

Sample windows for a terminal screen. This is one alternative for window design on a terminal screen. Different partitions are possible; however, once a partition has been created, it should be used consistently.

can be moved up and down such a listing line by line. If the information to be displayed is to be viewed one record at a time or depicted as a form, paging is preferred.

- *Messages, instructions, or information should remain in the window long enough to allow the user to read them.* For instance, data should not be allowed to scroll out of a window before it can be read. One way to accomplish this is to print only as much information as the window can display at one time and then freeze the screen. A message to press either any key or some

TYPICAL FUNCTION KEY ASSIGNMENTS

- *START a program or function.*
- *HELP: display help text.*
- *Cursor Movement.* Many systems have predefined keys for moving the cursor forward and backward one character, word, or field at a time as well as for moving the cursor up and down one line or page at a time. If these functions don't exist, they can be developed and used by all systems.
- EXIT *or* TERMINATE *the session.* If data can be lost, appropriate messages and instructions should be used to make sure the user hasn't made a mistake.
- ESCAPE from an operation (input or output) that is currently being done. This might be used to "start over" if the operator feels a serious mistake has been made.
- *Keystroke combinations.* Microcomputers and some intelligent terminals can take advantage of special software called keyboard enhancers (such as RoseSoft's *Prokey*). Keyboard enhancers allow single keys (not restricted to function keys) to automatically execute long sequences of common and predefined keystrokes.

Figure 14.3

Common function key uses.

specific key to continue can be displayed in the instruction window. The system can then page or scroll through the next set of information.

- *Use display attributes sparingly.* Display attributes, such as blinking, highlighting, and reverse video, can be distracting if overused. Judicious use allows you to call attention to something important (for example, the next field to be entered, a message, or an instruction).
- *Simplify complex functions and reduce typing by providing the user with function keys.* Some of the functions most commonly defined on function keys are described in Figure 14.3.
- *Default values for fields and answers to be entered by the user should be specified.* A common practice is to place the default

value in brackets (for example, ORDER DATE? <Today's Date>). The user can press the enter key to get the default date.

- *Anticipate the errors users might make.* Users will make errors, even when given the most obvious instructions. If the user can potentially execute a dangerous action, let it be known (a message ARE YOU SURE? is nice). An ounce of prevention goes a long way!

  With respect to errors, a symbol in the flag window should point to the error. Also, an appropriate error message should appear in the message window. The user should not be allowed to proceed without correcting the error. Instructions to correct the error can be displayed in the instruction window. A HELP key can be defined to display additional instructions or clarification in the body window. In any event, the user should never get an operating system message or fatal error. If the user does something that could be catastrophic, the keyboard should be locked to prevent any further input. An appropriate instruction to call the analyst or computer operator should be displayed in this situation.

Dialogue Tone and Terminology The overall tone and terminology of a terminal dialogue is another important human engineering consideration. The session should be user-friendly (an overused, frequently unachieved goal) and noncomputerese (an underemphasized factor). With respect to the tone of the dialogue, the following guidelines are offered:

- *Use simple, grammatically correct sentences.* It is best to use conversational English rather than written English. Written English is often *stuffy.* However, slang and profanity are taboo!
- *Don't be funny or cute!* When someone has to use the system fifty times a day, intended humor is about as funny as any joke you've just heard for the fiftieth time.
- *Don't be condescending;* that is, don't insult the intelligence of the user. For instance, don't offer rewards or punishment (*That's correct* or *You should know better*). Although these techniques are fine for computer-assisted instruction for children, adults can be insulted by such tactics!

With respect to terminology used during the dialogue, the following suggestions may prove helpful:

1. *Don't use computer jargon.*
2. *Avoid most abbreviations.* Abbreviations assume the user understands how to translate the abbreviation. Check first!
3. *Avoid symbology that may be foreign to the user* (such as mathematical notation).
4. *Use simple terms.* Use *NOT CORRECT* instead of *INCORRECT.* There is less chance of misreading or misinterpretation.
5. *Be consistent in your use of terminology.* For instance, don't use *EDIT* and *MODIFY* to mean the same instruction.
6. *Instructions should be carefully phrased, and appropriate action verbs should be used.* The following recommendations should prove helpful:
   - Try SELECT instead of PICK when referring to a list of options. Be sure to indicate whether the user can select more than one option from the list of available options.
   - Use TYPE, not ENTER, to request the user to input specific data or instructions.
   - Use PRESS, not HIT or DEPRESS, to refer to keyboard actions. Where possible, refer to keys by the symbols or identifiers that are actually printed on the keys. For instance the ↵ is used on some terminals to designate the RETURN or ENTER key.
   - When referring to the cursor, use the term POSITION THE CURSOR, not POINT THE CURSOR.

These suggestions may seem like nit-picking. But remember, most of you are much more familiar with the display terminal than the average knowledge worker.

Terminal Dialogue Strategies

So much for the human engineering factors. Are there any specific strategies you can employ to design *better* terminal dialogue? Indeed, there are a number of such strategies, and the choice of strategy depends on the nature of the function to be performed and the characteristics of the knowledge worker who will use the terminal. Let's briefly survey these strategies.

Menu Selection The most popular dialogue strategy currently being used is **menu selection.** A menu of alternatives or options is presented to the user. The user selects the desired alternative or option by keying in the number or letter that is associated with that option. More sophisticated technology allows menu selection by touching the screen, pointing to the desired item with a light pen, or using cursor keys or a mouse to move the cursor to the desired alternative. A sample menu is illustrated in Figure 14.4.

Menu-driven systems are particularly popular with the casual or semicasual user who doesn't have the time or inclination to learn about computers. Menu-driven systems also place production processing under the control of the user. It should be mentioned that by placing control in the hands of the users, production efficiency may deteriorate. Menu items should be self-explanatory and should contain neither jargon nor vague abbreviations or statements. If there are so many menu alternatives that the menu screen is too small or becomes cluttered, menus can be designed hierarchically. Small lists of related menu options can be grouped together into a single menu. These menus can then be grouped into a higher-level menu. This approach was applied in Figure 14.4. If the option DISPLAY WARRANTY REPORTS is selected, the submenu WARRANTY SYSTEM REPORT MENU will appear. And if the PART WARRANTY SUMMARY option is then selected, the bottom screens shown in Figure 14.4 will appear. Specific reports can be selected from that screen. There is no technical limit to how deeply hierarchical menus can be nested. However, the deeper the nesting, the more you should consider providing direct paths to deeply rooted menus for the experienced user who may find navigating through the multiple levels annoying.

Eventually, the menus will get you to a basic input or output operation or screen. The design of on-line inputs and outputs was covered in Chapters 11 and 13, respectively. Those screens can now be merged into the overall dialogue. For example, the display layout chart depicted in Figure 14.5 represents the design of an on-line output that could be derived from the on-line terminal dialogue shown in Figure 14.4.

Instruction Sets Instead of menus (or in addition to menus) you can design an on-line dialogue around an instruction set. Because the user must learn this syntax, this approach is suitable only for dedicated terminal users. There are three types of syntax that can be defined. Which type is used depends on the available technology.

1. A form of *Structured English* can be defined as a set of com-

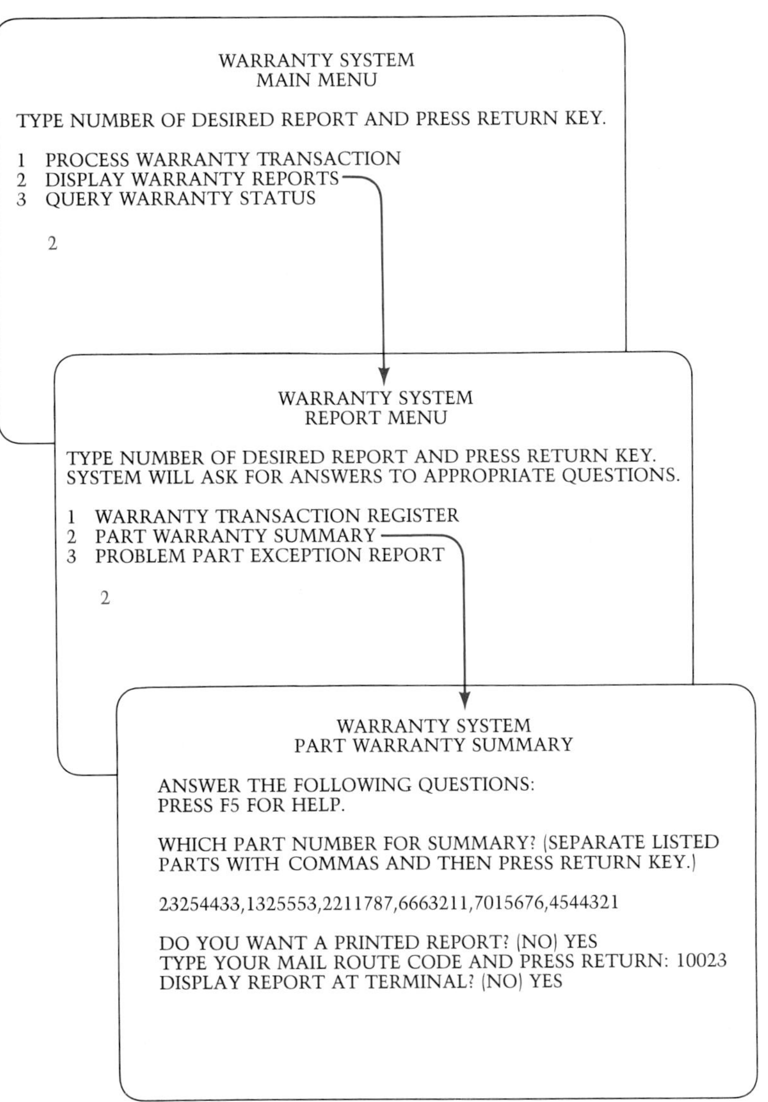

WARRANTY SYSTEM
MAIN MENU
TYPE NUMBER OF DESIRED REPORT AND PRESS RETURN KEY.
1 PROCESS WARRANTY TRANSACTION
2 DISPLAY WARRANTY REPORTS
3 QUERY WARRANTY STATUS
2
WARRANTY SYSTEM
REPORT MENU
TYPE NUMBER OF DESIRED REPORT AND PRESS RETURN KEY.
SYSTEM WILL ASK FOR ANSWERS TO APPROPRIATE QUESTIONS.
1 WARRANTY TRANSACTION REGISTER
2 PART WARRANTY SUMMARY
3 PROBLEM PART EXCEPTION REPORT
2
WARRANTY SYSTEM
PART WARRANTY SUMMARY
ANSWER THE FOLLOWING QUESTIONS:
PRESS F5 FOR HELP.
WHICH PART NUMBER FOR SUMMARY? (SEPARATE LISTED
PARTS WITH COMMAS AND THEN PRESS RETURN KEY.)
23254433,1325553,2211787,6663211,7015676,4544321
DO YOU WANT A PRINTED REPORT? (NO) YES
TYPE YOUR MAIL ROUTE CODE AND PRESS RETURN: 10023
DISPLAY REPORT AT TERMINAL? (NO) YES

Figure 14.4

Sample menu selection for terminal dialogue. Menu selection is the most popular dialogue strategy in use today. It is particularly effective when dealing with the casual user who knows little about computers. This menu demonstrates a multiple hierarchical menu structure.

mands that control the system. In this type of dialogue, an elaborate HELP system should be created so the user who forgets the syntax can get assistance quickly.

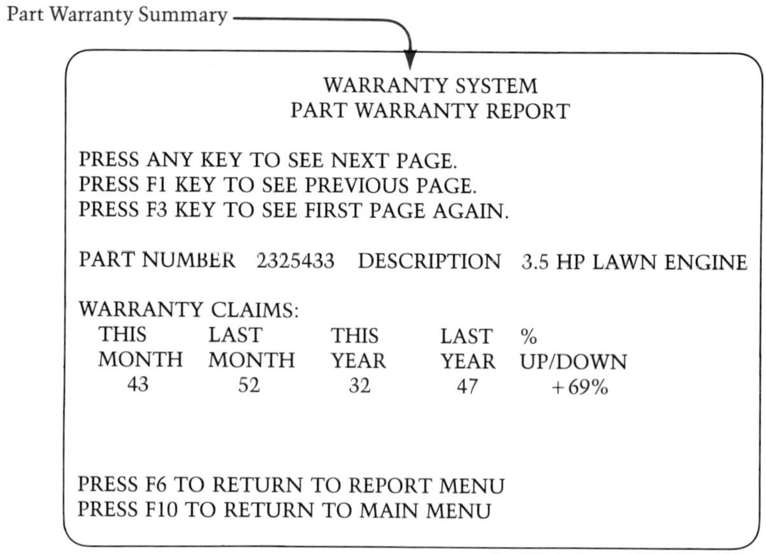

Part Warranty Summary

```
                  WARRANTY SYSTEM
               PART WARRANTY REPORT

PRESS ANY KEY TO SEE NEXT PAGE.
PRESS F1 KEY TO SEE PREVIOUS PAGE.
PRESS F3 KEY TO SEE FIRST PAGE AGAIN.

PART NUMBER  2325433  DESCRIPTION  3.5 HP LAWN ENGINE

WARRANTY CLAIMS:
  THIS     LAST     THIS    LAST   %
  MONTH    MONTH    YEAR    YEAR   UP/DOWN
   43       52       32      47       +69%


PRESS F6 TO RETURN TO REPORT MENU
PRESS F10 TO RETURN TO MAIN MENU
```

Figure 14.5

On-line output screen. Terminal dialogue design is concerned with specifying the dialogue required for the user to arrive at the input and output screens. This on-line output can be arrived at by the user through entering the appropriate options and commands for the dialogue screens depicted in Figure 14.4.

2. A *mnemonic syntax* can be defined. A **mnemonic syntax** is built around meaningful abbreviations for all commands. Once again, a HELP system is highly recommended.
3. *Natural language syntax* interpreters are now becoming available (for example, ON-LINE ENGLISH™). When using **natural language syntax,** the user enters commands using natural English (either conversational or written). The system interprets these commands against a known syntax and requests clarification if it doesn't understand what the user wants. As new interpretations become known, the system learns the user's vocabulary by saving it for future reference. As we go to press, this is an emerging technology.

Question/Answer Dialogues To supplement either menu-driven or syntax-driven dialogues, you can use **question/answer strategies** where appropriate. The simplest questions involve yes or no answers — for instance, "Do you want to see all records? <NO>." Notice how we offered a default answer! Questions can be more elaborate. For instance, the system could ask, "Which part number are you interested in <last part number queried>?" Just make sure you consider all possible *correct* answers and deal with the actions to be taken if incorrect answers are entered. Question/answer dialogue is difficult because you must try to consider everything the user might do wrong!

The three strategies we've suggested should be considered together with the human factors discussed earlier. If you evaluate your dialogue against these fundamental concepts, you may save yourself from that dreaded 2 A.M. phone call, "Betty? Did I wake you? Sorry! But we have a problem with what the system is asking us for . . ."

HOW TO DESIGN AND DOCUMENT A TERMINAL DIALOGUE

The typical approach to designing a terminal dialogue is to throw together a few display layout charts. This strategy doesn't fare too well — the final dialogue ends up being designed by the programmer, on the fly. It shouldn't surprise you that a typical terminal dialogue may involve many possible screens, perhaps hundreds! Each screen can be laid out with a display layout chart. But what about the coordination of these screens?

Screens will occur in a specific order. Perhaps you can move forward and backward through the screens. Additionally, some screens may occur only under certain conditions. And to make matters more difficult, some screens may occur repetitively until some condition is fulfilled. This almost sounds like a programming problem, doesn't it? We need a tool to coordinate the screens that can occur in terminal dialogue. Enter dialogue charts! Dialogue charts are a variation on program flowcharts and hierarchy charts.

A sample dialogue chart is illustrated in Figure 14.6. The arrows indicate that a screen can get to another screen in that sequence. Note that the arrows can be bidirectional, meaning that you can get to either screen in either direction. The treelike structure suggests that, at some point in the dialogue, the user will select an option and execute only those screens in that branch of the tree. This IF-THEN

Figure 14.6

Sample dialogue chart. Dialogue charts are used to coordinate terminal dialogue screens. This tool can depict the sequence and variations of screens viewed by the user.

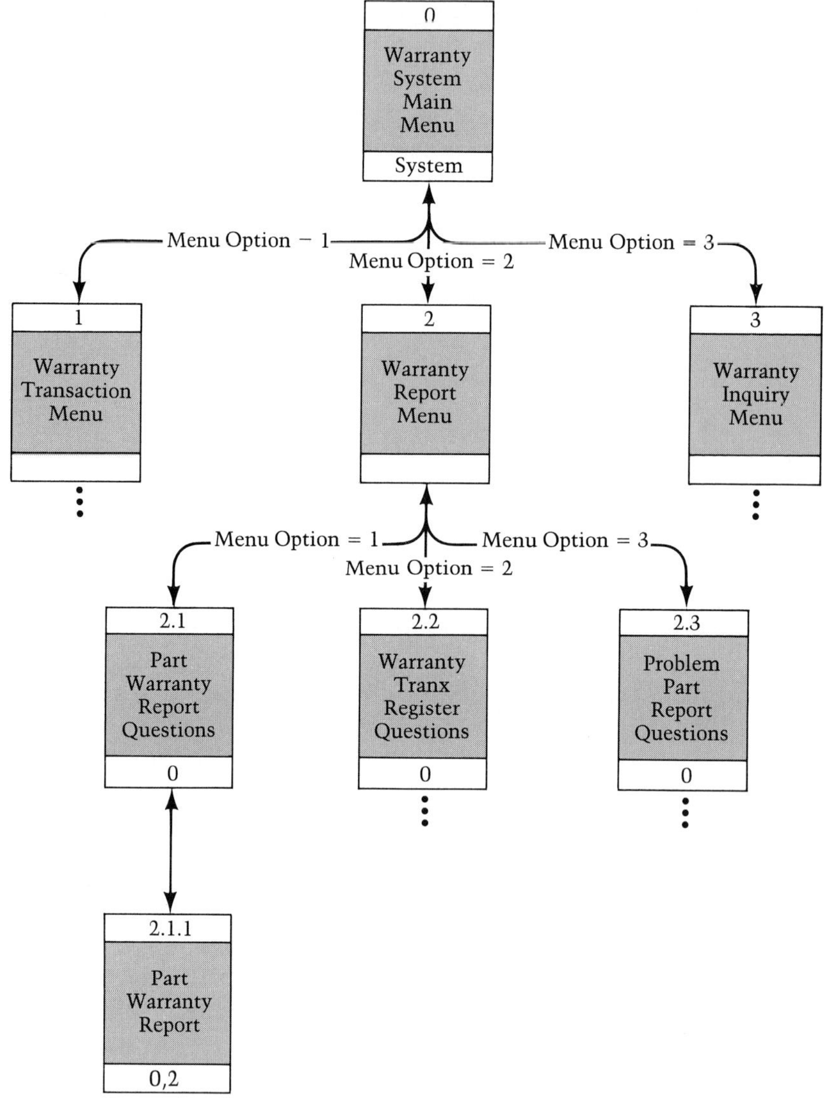

structure is perfect for menu-type dialogues. Figure 14.6 shows a simple dialogue chart. Let's study this tool in greater detail.

Dialogue Chart Conventions

The purpose of the dialogue chart is to depict the sequence and variations of screens that can occur when the user sits at the terminal. You can think of it as a roadmap. Each screen is analogous to a city. Not all roads go through all cities. Figure 14.7 depicts all of our dialogue chart conventions. The rectangles represent display screens (formatted by display layout charts). The arrows represent the flow of control through the various screens.

Ⓐ Notice that the rectangles are divided into three sections. The top section contains a reference number that corresponds to the SCREEN NUMBER that appears on the display layout chart.

Ⓑ To keep things simple, we'll follow the same numbering convention you learned in the data flow diagrams chapter. The middle section names or describes the screen. Most dialogues permit the user to get from one screen to another in either direction (hence, the arrowhead at each end of the arrow).

Ⓒ Because it is desirable in many systems to provide shortcuts back to previous screens, the bottom section of the rectangle describes the allowable shortcuts, called *escapes.*

Ⓓ A screen drawn behind another screen indicates that special HELP screens have been (or will be) designed to assist the user with the screen behind which the HELP screen has been drawn. These help functions are said to be in the *background.*

The rectangles only describe *what* screens can appear during the dialogue. The arrows describe *when* these screens occur. Earlier, we stated that the flow of screens in a terminal dialogue occurs with almost programming-like precision. Indeed, the three constructs of a well-structured computer program apply equally to the dialogue chart:

① *Sequence.* The screens occur in a natural sequence one after the other.

② ⑤ *Selection.* Based upon the user's answer to a question or selection of a menu alternative, a different path through the screens is selected (similar to programming's if-then-else construct).

④ ③ *Repetition.* Until some condition is fulfilled a sequence of screens is repeated. This is similar to programming's repeat-until or do-while constructs.

⑥ The small triangle that contains a letter indicates the return of control to that point indicated by the letter.

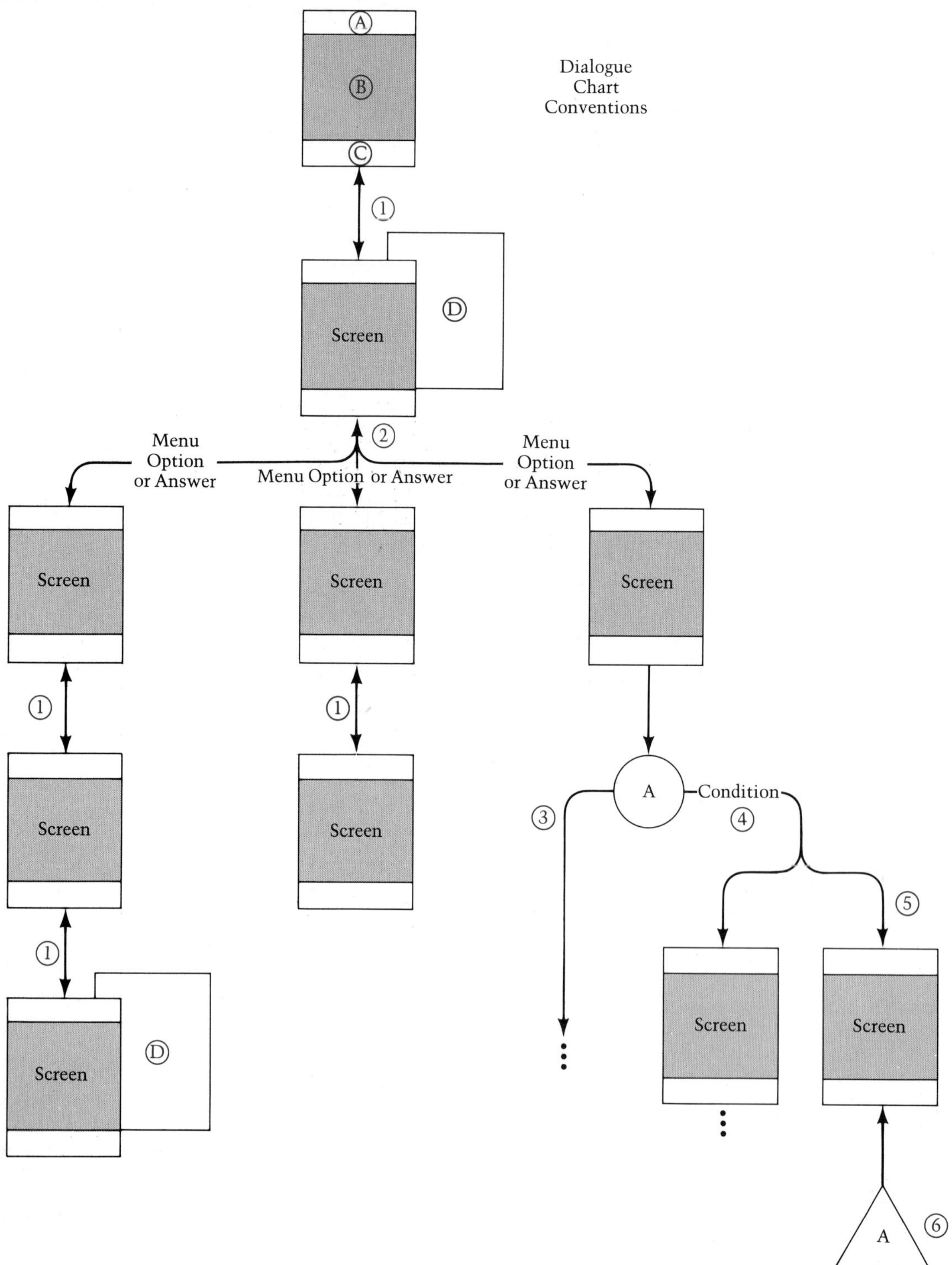

A
B
C
Dialogue
Chart
Conventions
1
Screen
D
2
Menu
Option
or Answer
Menu Option or Answer
Menu
Option
or Answer
Screen
Screen
Screen
1
1
Screen
Screen
A
Condition
3
4
1
5
Screen
D
Screen
Screen
6
A

◄ Figure 14.7

Dialogue chart conventions. A dialogue chart consists of rectangles that represent display screens and arrows that represent flow of control through various display screens.

The constructs can be nested just like programming constructs. Unlike program flowcharts, most arrows in a dialogue chart are bidirectional. This indicates that the user can also move backward through the screens. The escape numbers in the screen rectangles help us avoid sloppy *go-to* arrows on the dialogue chart. Using these simple notations, the analyst (and possibly users) can design a complete dialogue. The dialogue chart serves as a table of contents for the display layout charts for all of the screens we've just discussed.

Let's examine the terminal dialogue for some of the AAP, Inc. project. Recall that in Chapter 11, we designed the on-line output PART QUERY RESPONSE. Recall also, that in Chapter 13 we designed the on-line input CUSTOMER ORDER. Think back. Did you happen to wonder how the user was going to request the output PART QUERY RESPONSE or how the user was going to initiate the input of a CUSTOMER ORDER? By designing the terminal dialogue for AAP, we can answer these questions.

Design of a Dialogue Structure

The on-line portion of the AAP order-entry system can be partitioned into several levels of screens with each level aimed toward accomplishing a more well-defined function. For example, the on-line portion of the AAP order-entry system can initially be decomposed into three on-line support capabilities: transaction processing, management reporting, and decision support. Each of these capabilities can be assigned screens that will assist the user. In addition, these support capabilities might be decomposed into more specific support functions for which screens are also assigned.

In Figure 14.8, we present a dialogue chart that depicts the sequence and variations of screens that can occur when the user sits at the terminal. Notice that some of the screen names appear below a horizontal line rather than inside a rectangle. In order to keep this chapter down to a reasonable length, we did not design and discuss the segments of the dialogue that appear below the horizontal lines.

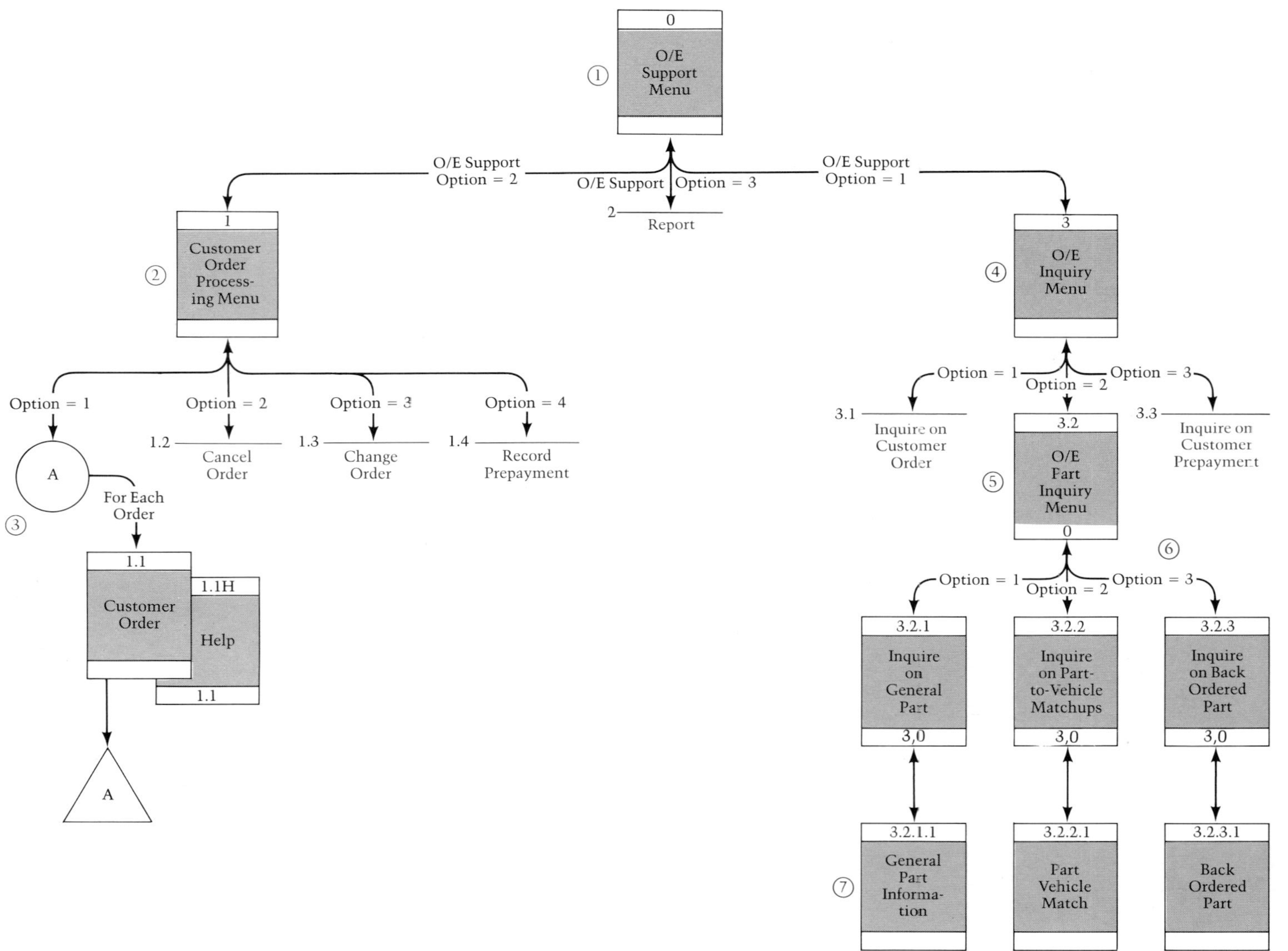

0
O/E Support Menu
①
O/E Support Option = 2
O/E Support
Option = 3
2 Report
O/E Support Option = 1
1
Customer Order Processing Menu
②
Option = 1
Option = 2
Option = 3
Option = 4
1.2 Cancel Order
1.3 Change Order
1.4 Record Prepayment
A
③
For Each Order
1.1
Customer Order
1.1H
Help
1.1
A
3
O/E Inquiry Menu
④
Option = 1
Option = 2
Option = 3
3.1 Inquire on Customer Order
3.3 Inquire on Customer Prepayment
3.2
O/E Part Inquiry Menu
0
⑤
⑥
Option = 1
Option = 2
Option = 3
3.2.1
Inquire on General Part
3,0
3.2.2
Inquire on Part-to-Vehicle Matchups
3,0
3.2.3
Inquire on Back Ordered Part
3,0
3.2.1.1
General Part Information
⑦
3.2.2.1
Part Vehicle Match
3.2.3.1
Back Ordered Part

◂ **Figure 14.8**

Dialogue chart for AAP order-entry on-line support functions. This dialogue chart shows the relationship between the many display screens needed to describe the dialogue of the AAP order-entry on-line support functions. The labeled horizontal lines represent portions of the order-entry system for which the display screens needed to support a function have not yet been defined.

We call your attention to the following points of interest in Figure 14.8:

① The O/E (order-entry) SUPPORT MENU is the first screen to be viewed by the terminal user. Because this is the first screen seen by the user, there are no escapes. The function of this screen is to provide the user with on-line support options. The AAP order-entry system contains several such options, which are conveniently grouped into submenus. The O/E SUPPORT MENU will provide the user with the option of processing a customer order, obtaining a report, and performing inquiries. Each of these options, when chosen, will result in the user seeing a new screen: the CUSTOMER ORDER PROCESSING MENU, the REPORT MENU, or the O/E INQUIRY MENU screen. The menu options selected are recorded on the branching lines.

② The CUSTOMER ORDER PROCESSING MENU screen will offer the user a number of transaction-processing options. No escapes were specified for this screen because O/E SUPPORT MENU is the only previous screen seen by the user so far, and thc arrow already handles this escape option.

③ The ORDER PROCESSING OPTION sends the user into a repeating screen, CUSTOMER ORDER, that can be filled in until there are no more orders to input (at which time the user selects one of the escapes). Notice that screen 1.1 overlaps screen 1.1.H. Screen 1.1.H will supplement the CUSTOMER ORDER screen, providing help instructions as needed. Help should always return to the screen from which it was called.

④ The O/E system will allow the user to do three types of on-line inquiries. The O/E INQUIRY MENU screen displays the inquiry options to the user.

⑤ The user will be provided with the O/E PART INQUIRY MENU screen if the user's choice was to do an inquiry on an AAP part. The user may request three different types of information concerning a part. Screen 3.2 will provide the user with the option of retrieving general information on a part, identifying part and vehicle matchups, and retrieving information concerning backordered parts.

⑥ Either screen 3.2.1, 3.2.2, or 3.2.3 will be displayed to the user, depending on the part inquiry option selected from the O/E PART INQUIRY MENU screen. The purpose of these screens is to determine which part the user wants to receive information on. Notice that the escape options shown on each of these screens allows the user to return to the O/E PART INQUIRY MENU screen, O/E INQUIRY MENU screen, or O/E SUPPORT MENU screen. As we design more levels of screens, the escape options become more beneficial to the user.

⑦ Screens 3.2.1.1, 3.2.2.1, and 3.2.3.1 represent outputs. Look familiar? These screens were designed in Chapter 11. They always appear immediately after the user has supplied appropriate information called for on the previous screen. Notice that there are no escape mechanisms other than the ability to return to the previous screen.

Given the dialogue structure, we can design the actual dialogue using display layout charts.

Design of the Actual Dialogue

Referring back to the dialogue chart shown in Figure 14.8, there are several paths that the dialogue will follow. For the sake of brevity, we will design screens only for those rectangles defined on the chart. These screens were chosen because they serve as the dialogue that would be required for the user to arrive at the input and output screens that were designed in Chapters 11 and 13.

If one hasn't already been constructed, we suggest that a template for the windows or areas be defined. We used the template shown in Figure 14.9 for our design.

The initial screen seen by the user is presented in Figure 14.10. It is the main system menu. The screen number on the display layout chart should match the screen number in the dialogue chart. Line 22 is a message field for error messages. The accompanying letter in

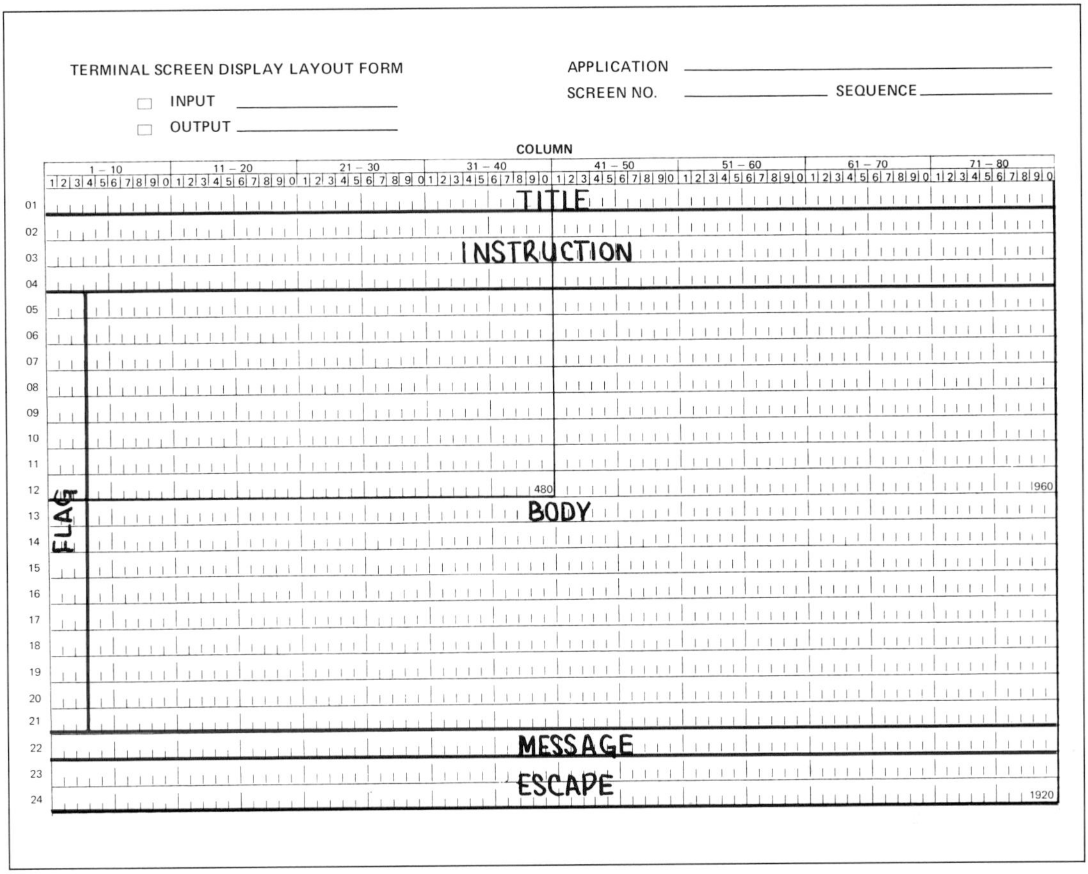

TERMINAL SCREEN DISPLAY LAYOUT FORM

☐ INPUT ______

☐ OUTPUT ______

APPLICATION ______

SCREEN NO. ______ SEQUENCE ______

COLUMN

TITLE

INSTRUCTION

FLAG

BODY

MESSAGE

ESCAPE

480 1960 1920

Figure 14.9

Template for order-entry system windows. We recommend that a template for your window areas be defined. In fact, create an overlay template using a blank transparency for an overhead projector. The overlay can be placed on each screen you design to check for consistency with the windows.

parentheses directs us to a memo (Figure 14.11) that describes the messages that can be printed. Finally, notice that we used the function key assignments of the display layout chart to define an operation, TERMINATE SESSION.

Let's move on. If our user wishes to input some customer orders, then option 2 on the O/E SUPPORT MENU would be selected. According to our dialogue chart, the user would now see screen 1, the CUSTOMER ORDER PROCESSING MENU, which is shown

TERMINAL SCREEN DISPLAY LAYOUT FORM

☐ INPUT ____________

☐ OUTPUT ____________

APPLICATION O/E ON LINE CONTROL

SCREEN NO. 0 SEQUENCE ____________

COLUMN

01	- O/E SUPPORT MENU -
02	
03	
04	
05	
06	[1] INQUIRE ON PARTS, ORDERS, & CUSTOMER PREPAYMENTS
07	[2] PROCESS CUSTOMER ORDERS
08	[3] REPORT
09	
10	
11	SELECT DESIRED O/E SUPPORT OPTION ==> X
12	480 / 1960
22	XXXXXXXXXXXXXXXXXXXXXXXXXXXXXXXXXXX (a)
23	
24	PRESS "F10" TO TERMINATE SESSION 1920
25	
43	3440

FUNCTION KEY ASSIGNMENTS

PF1		PF9		PF17	
PF2		PF10	TERMINATE TERMINAL SESSION	PF18	
PF3		PF11		PF19	
PF4		PF12		PF20	
PF5		PF13		PF21	
PF6		PF14		PF22	
PF7		PF15		PF23	
PF8		PF16		PF24	

Figure 14.10

Display layout chart of the O/E SUPPORT MENU screen format. This is the first display screen that would be viewed by the user. The editing symbols have been added for the programmer's benefit. Notice that the three options appearing on the dialogue chart are displayed within the body of the screen. Selection of either one of the options will result in the display of a new screen from the dialogue.

Figure 14.11 ▶

Memo attachment for AAP order-entry dialogue design. Memos are used to describe messages and help instructions associated with the standard edit masks recorded in the display layout chart.

Memo For On-line Dialogue of AAP Order-Entry System

Ref. No.

a The error message will appear on line 22 if the user enters an incorrect option number. The error message should read "OPTION CHOSEN NOT VALID...TRY AGAIN", and the cursor should be repositioned.

b If the user enters an invalid AAP PART NUMBER, the error message "NOT VALID AAP PART NUMBER...TRY AGAIN" should appear, and the cursor should be repositioned for re-entry. If the user enters a PART DESCRIPTION that is not associated with a particular AAP part, the error message "NO PART OF THIS DESCRIPTION EXISTS...TRY AGAIN" should appear. The cursor should be repositioned for re-entry.

c If the user enters an invalid VEHICLE NUMBER the error message "VEHICLE NUMBER NOT VALID... TRY AGAIN" should appear on line 22. If the user enters a PART DESCRIPTION that is not associated with an AAP part, the error message "NO PART OF THIS DESCRIPTION EXISTS...TRY AGAIN" should appear. In either case, the cursor should be repositioned for re-entry.

d The following explanations are to appear in the "body" of the DAILY SALES ORDER screen (1.1). Each explanation corresponds to a particular data element the user is asked to enter.

Ref. #	Explanation
1	The SALES ORDER NUMBER must be provided. This item requires 7 characters. The first 6 must be numbers (0-9); the last, or 7th character, may be a number or an alphabetic letter "X".
2	The ORDER DATE must be provided. Enter the number of the Month, Day, and Year. For example, "12/03/1985" represents "December 3, 1985". The Month, Day, and Year must be separated by a "/" symbol.
3	The CUSTOMER NUMBER should be provided if known. This item requires 4 digits (0-9).
4	The CUSTOMER ORDER NUMBER is not required. However, if known, it should be entered.
6 & 12	STREET is only required for the BILLING ADDRESS (SHIPPING ADDRESS is only required if different from BILLING ADDRESS). STREET may be up to 15 characters.
7 & 13	POST OFFICE BOX NUMBER is only required for the BILLING ADDRESS (SHIPPING ADDRESS is only required if different from BILLING ADDRESS). POST OFFICE BOX NUMBER can receive up to 10 characters.
8 & 14	CITY is only required for the BILLING ADDRESS (SHIPPING ADDRESS is only required if different from BILLING ADDRESS). CITY may recieve up to 15 characters.
9 & 15	STATE is required for the BILLING ADDRESS (SHIPPING ADDRESS is only required if different from the BILLING ADDRESS). Provide the 2-character standard abbreviation for the state.
10 & 16	ZIP CODE is only required for the BILLING ADDRESS (SHIPPING ADDRESS is required only if different from the BILLING ADDRESS). ZIP CODE must contain numbers (0-9), no more than 9.
17	PAYMENT AMOUNT must be provided if payment accompanied the order. Indicate dollar and cents with a ".". For example: Ten dollars should be entered as "10.00".
18	PART NUMBER is required for each item ordered. PART NUMBERs must contain 9 digits. The PART NUMBER must also be a valid AAP part number.
19	The QUANTITY ORDERED for each part must be provided.
20	DISCOUNT RATE is only required if terms of agreement exist. This item must contain a number with a decimal point specified. For example, 10 and 1/2 percent discount would be entered as "10.5".
21	UNIT OF MEASURE is optional and may be up to 10 characters in length.

in Figure 14.12. This screen is similar to the previous screen because both screens were designed using our template and because both screens simply offer a menu of options to the user. Notice that, in accordance with our dialogue chart, this screen offers the user an escape option to return to the previous menu. The user who wishes to input customer orders would select option 1.

Option 1 should take us to a new screen. This screen should allow our user to start keying in data for customer orders. This is the input screen we designed in Chapter 13. The display layout chart for CUSTOMER ORDER has been reproduced for you in Figure 14.13. The dialogue chart indicates that this screen should be displayed to the user repeatedly until the user has input all the customer orders. The user would then press function key F4 to escape back to screen 1.

What happens if the user has problems when entering data into the CUSTOMER ORDER screen? For example, the user might not know how the SALES ORDER DATE should be entered or why the screen will not accept the PART NUMBER that was typed in. On the dialogue chart, we see screen 1.1 overlapping screen 1.1.H. 1.1.H is a special help screen that is associated with the DAILY CUSTOMER ORDER screen. The user who encounters a problem while keying a customer order can press the function key, F5, and the HELP screen will be displayed. Figure 14.14 represents the layout of the HELP screen. The possible explanations that may appear on this screen were documented in Figure 14.11. Each explanation given to the user corresponds to a particular data element the cursor was positioned at when the user pressed the F5 (help) key.

That completes our walkthrough of the dialogue as seen by a user wishing to input customer orders. Output dialogues would be documented similarly.

Testing a Terminal Dialogue for Effectiveness

Before we leave this chapter, let's briefly discuss testing. Terminal dialogues can be somewhat lengthy and complex. It is important to test the dialogue. We've said it once, but it's worth repeating. The standard editing symbols used on display layouts, along with the memos, are intended primarily for the computer programmer who must implement the screens and dialogue. Users are not likely to be comfortable with these symbols. Therefore, the standard display layout charts should not be proofed by users. One alternative is to

TERMINAL SCREEN DISPLAY LAYOUT FORM

☐ INPUT ________

☐ OUTPUT ________

APPLICATION O/E ON LINE CONTROL

SCREEN NO. 1 SEQUENCE ________

COLUMN

01	- CUSTOMER ORDER PROCESSING MENU -
06	[1] REGULAR ORDERS
07	[2] CANCEL ORDER
08	[3] CHANGE ORDER
09	[4] RECORD PREPAYMENT
12	SELECT DESIRED ORDER PROCESSING OPTION ==> X
22	XXXXXXXXXXXXXXXXXXXXXXXXXXXXXXXXXXXXXXXXXXXXXX (a)
24	PRESS "F9" FOR O/E SUPPORT MENU

FUNCTION KEY ASSIGNMENTS

PF1		PF9	RETURN USER TO O/E SUPPORT MENU SCREEN	PF17	
PF2		PF10		PF18	
PF3		PF11		PF19	
PF4		PF12		PF20	
PF5		PF13		PF21	
PF6		PF14		PF22	
PF7		PF15		PF23	
PF8		PF16		PF24	

Figure 14.12

Display layout chart for CUSTOMER ORDER PROCESSING MENU screen. As depicted on the dialogue chart, this screen will appear if the user elects option 2 from the O/E SUPPORT MENU screen (see Figure 14.7). In accordance with the dialogue chart, the screen will provide the user with the four processing options, as well as with a fifth option whereby the user can return to the O/E SUPPORT MENU.

TERMINAL SCREEN DISPLAY LAYOUT FORM

APPLICATION PROCESS NEW ORDERS

☒ INPUT CUSTOMER ORDER

SCREEN NO. 1.1 SEQUENCE ______

☐ OUTPUT ______

COLUMN

01 *CUSTOMER ORDER*

02 ENTER THE FOLLOWING ITEMS FROM SALES ORDER (FORM 17). USE "LEFT ARROW" KEY

03 TO BACKSPACE TO PREVIOUS ITEM. USE "RIGHT ARROW" KEY TO ADVANCE TO NEXT

04 ITEM. PRESS "RETURN" KEY WHEN ALL ITEMS HAVE BEEN ENTERED.

06 SALES ORDER # 999999X (1)(a) ORDER DATE 99/99/9999 (2)(a)

08 CUSTOMER # 9999 (3)(a) CUSTOMER ORDER # 999999 (4)(a)

10 BILLING ADDRESS SHIPPING ADDRESS

11 STREET XXXXXXXXXXXXXXX (6)(a) STREET XXXXXXXXXXXXXXX (12)(a)

12 P. O. BOX XXXXXXXXXX (7)(a) 480 P. O. BOX XXXXXXXXXX (13)(a) 1960

13 CITY XXXXXXXXXXXXXXX (8)(a) CITY XXXXXXXXXXXXXXX (14)(a)

14 STATE AA (9)(a) STATE AA (15)(a)

15 ZIPCODE 999999999 (10)(a) ZIPCODE 999999999 (16)(a)

17 PART NUMBER QUANTITY UNIT MEASURE DISCOUNT AMOUNT PAID

18 999999999 999 XXXXXXXXXX 99.9 999,999.99

19 (18)(a) (19)(a) (21)(a) (20)(a) (17)(a)

23 XXXXXXXXXXXXXXXXXXXXXXXXXXXXXXXXXXXXXXXXXXXXXXXXXXXXXXXXXXXXXXXXXX (6)

24 PRESS "F4" TO RETURN TO CUSTOMER ORDER PROCESSING MENU; "F5" FOR HELP. 1920

25

42

43 3440

FUNCTION KEY ASSIGNMENTS

PF1		PF9		PF17	
PF2		PF10		PF18	
PF3		PF11		PF19	
PF4	RETURN USER TO THE CUSTOMER ORDER PROCESSING MENU SCREEN	PF12		PF20	
PF5	DISPLAY THE HELP SCREEN	PF13		PF21	
PF6		PF14		PF22	
PF7		PF15		PF23	
PF8		PF16		PF24	

Figure 14.13

Display layout chart for CUSTOMER ORDER screen. This screen represents an on-line input. The systems analyst would likely design this screen during input design (Chapter 13). The purpose of terminal dialogue design is to specify how the user is to arrive at such input or output screens.

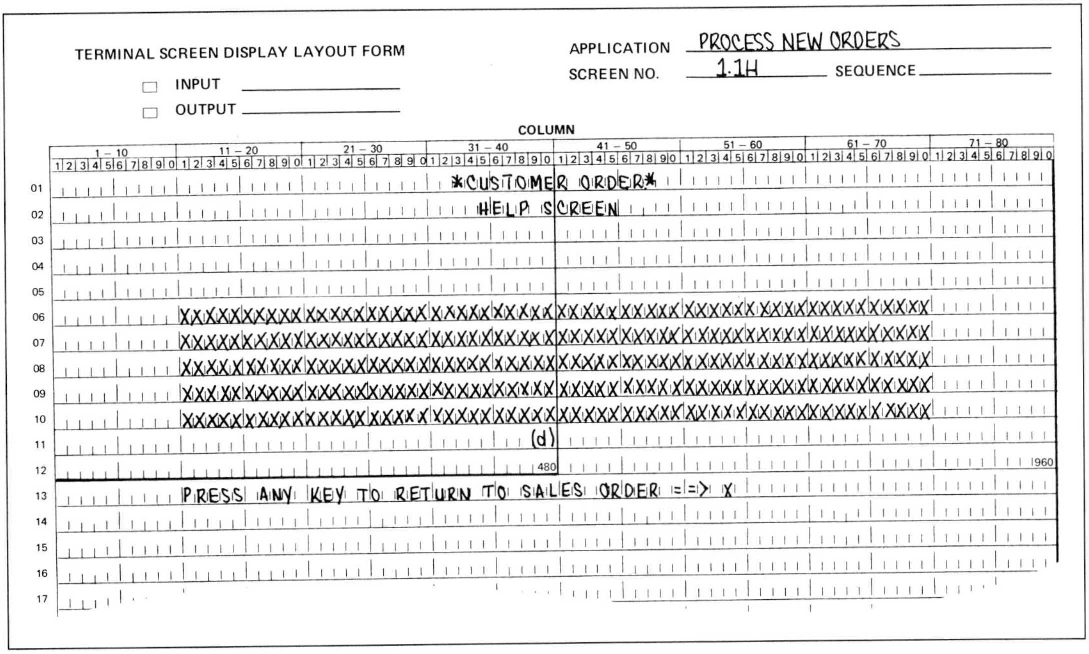

TERMINAL SCREEN DISPLAY LAYOUT FORM

☐ INPUT ____

☐ OUTPUT ____

APPLICATION PROCESS NEW ORDERS

SCREEN NO. 1.1H SEQUENCE ____

COLUMN

CUSTOMER ORDER

HELP SCREEN

(d)

480

1960

PRESS ANY KEY TO RETURN TO SALES ORDER ==> X

Figure 14.14

Display layout chart for the CUSTOMER ORDER help screen. All on-line inputs should have help screens that can be referenced by the user. Help screens should be brief, concise, and informative.

prepare sample screens using display layout charts. These screens will contain sample data and messages instead of editing symbols. Using the dialogue chart, you can then walk the user through the dialogue using these sample screens. A more modern approach to dialogue development and testing involves simulation.

Simulation is the most effective approach to testing a terminal dialogue. There are two basic approaches to simulating a dialogue for the user; these are hand coding and dialogue generators. **Hand coding** uses the dialogue chart and display layout charts to build a simple, working model of the dialogue *on the computer.* To quickly program the system, only the basic screens are implemented. Data is not edited or processed. The user can sit at a terminal and test the dialogue (with the understanding that the data are not edited or processed).

Dialogue generators are even more effective! They allow you to bypass the display layout chart altogether. The analyst and user use a *screen painting* facility (software) to develop working prototypes of the screens on the terminal. Developing and editing these screens is quick and painless. And the analyst can get immediate feedback from the user and make appropriate changes. Not only is the design being completed; the dialogue generator is creating the computer program code to create and drive the screens and dialogue. The productivity gains are substantial!

SUMMARY

The design of conversational terminal diaglogue has taken on greater importance due to the trend toward on-line information systems. Terminal dialogue design is the specification of a conversation between the knowledge worker and the computer that results in the input of new data to the information system, the output of information to the knowledge worker, or both. Display terminals and terminal features affect good dialogue design. The systems analyst should be familiar with the current technology of display terminals and their features because they can be used to improve dialogue design.

Human factors are also important considerations for good terminal dialogue design. Most of today's systems are being designed for the casual user, with an emphasis on user friendliness. Human engineering principles can guide the development of user-friendly terminal dialogues for different types of users. There are three strategies commonly used for terminal dialogue design: menu selection, instruction set, and question/answer. The choice of strategy depends on the nature of the function to be performed and on the characteristics of the knowledge workers who will use the terminal.

Typical terminal dialogues may involve many screens. The coordination of these screens is very important (for example, some screens will occur in a specific order whereas others occur under certain conditions). A dialogue chart is a tool used to depict the sequence and variations of the screens that can occur when the user

The Next Generation

Display Managers and Screen Design Facilities: Automating Terminal Dialogue Design

Designing terminal dialogue with pencil, paper, dialogue charts, and display layout charts is a long, tedious task. And even after you've documented the design, your users will likely demonstrate the uncanny ability to "bust that dialogue"—do something you hadn't anticipated. Or they won't like a particular screen—one you spent half an hour designing. Or they won't like several screens! Terminal dialogue design is a task that screams for automated tools. Display managers, screen-design managers, and dialogue managers (there are many names) promise to make the next generation of terminal dialogue design as easy as writing with word processors instead of pen and paper.

Tools that automate the dialogue process are becoming very popular. Some are available as standalone products that work in a variety of hardware and software environments (including microcomputers). Some are sold as standalone systems, used only to design and simulate the dialogue and leaving implementation to programmers. Others generate dialogue that can directly interface with application programs written in specific languages (such as COBOL). And some dialogue tools are bundled into (included in) other software packages, such as database management systems, teleprocessing monitors, compilers, and fourth-generation languages.

What can these dialogue tools do for you? They normally consist of at least two components, an *editor* and a *demonstrator.* The editor works in much the same way as a word processor (or an operating system editor). It allows you to create screens, designating specific areas for prompts, messages, input fields, and output fields. Sophisticated editors may allow you to control the color and size of any prompt, message, or the like, and to associate specific display attributes with those items (such as blinking and reverse video). Some editors can even draw boxes and special characters, allowing you to create or recreate a form that can be displayed and 'filled in' by the user.

Some editors generate working program code. For instance, an editor might allow you to redefine and program function keys. Help routines may be installed around such keys. And relative to input fields, the editor may allow you to associate complicated edit masks and data validation checks with the fields. For example, the display manager may automatically generate or use editing routines to check user inputs for proper type (such as numeric), size, format, and even value range and to print an appropriate message if the user makes an error.

The demonstrator portion of the dialogue tool is used to prototype and test the dialogue. Users can sit down at a terminal and try your design out for size. You would normally work with them, noting any action they might take that hasn't been accommodated in the dialogue. What's the net impact? Terminal dialogues take much less time to design and implement—and that's the name of the game! Few schools have been able to avail themselves of this powerful environment. But many businesses have already started moving into this specific "next generation." ■

sits at a terminal. The dialogue chart can serve as a table of contents for the numerous display layout charts for the screens.

After developing a dialogue, it should be tested on the knowledge workers who will have to use that dialogue. The users should be observed during this test period—you are trying to find flaws in the terminal dialogue. A flaw occurs when the user does something the analyst didn't consider.

PROBLEMS AND EXERCISES

1. To what extent should the knowledge worker be involved during terminal dialogue design? What would you do for the knowledge worker? What would you ask the knowledge worker to do for you? Detail a strategy that consists of specific steps you and the knowledge workers would follow.
2. Study the features on two visual display terminal(s) or microcomputers. You may need to borrow manuals to complete this assignment. How might these features be used to design effective terminal dialogue?
3. What documentation prepared during input design and output design is needed during terminal dialogue design? How does that input and output design documentation relate to terminal dialogue design?
4. Explain the difference between a dedicated and casual terminal user. How would your strategy for designing terminal dialogue for a dedicated user differ from that for designing terminal dialogue for a casual user?
5. An automated record-keeping information system is being designed for an employment agency. Some of the tasks to be automated on-line include:

   Transaction Processing

   - A. Processing clients
     - a. Recording new clients
     - b. Matching clients with job openings
     - c. Notifying clients of job openings
   - B. Processing jobs

a. Recording job openings

b. Matching jobs with clients

c. Recording job placements

Management Reporting

A. Reporting of job openings

B. Reporting weekly job placements

C. Reporting client credentials

Decision Support

A. Query clients

a. Query general client information

b. Query employee job qualifications

c. Query employee job requirements/preferences

B. Query job openings

a. Query general job opening information

b. Query job opening requirements

C. Query job placements

Assume that the terminal input and output screens have already been designed to support these on-line processes. Develop a dialogue chart to depict the sequence and variations of dialogue screens that might occur when a user sits at the terminal. Be sure to include help screens for all input screens, escape options for navigating the structure, screen reference numbers, and descriptive screen names.

6. Terminal screens should be designed for consistency. Design a template for the screens in problem 5. The template should clearly indicate windows or areas of the screen used to display common messages. Do you have windowing or similar screen design software on your computer system? If so, describe how you'd implement your windows. If not, how will you ensure that data and messages are displayed in the proper window?

7. Arrange to study an on-line or microcomputer application. It may be either a business system (such as an inventory, accounts receivable, or personnel system) or a productivity tool (such as a word processor, spreadsheet, or database system). Analyze the human engineering of the terminal dialogue. Analyze the human engineering of the display screens. If possible, discuss

the dialogue and screens with users. What do they like and dislike about the design?

8. Redesign the application in problem 7 to improve or change the terminal dialogue and screens. If possible, discuss your improved design with users. Do they like your new design better? Did they raise any concerns?

9. Using the dialogue chart from problem 5 and the screen template from problem 6, design the dialogue screens required for a user to arrive at the basic input and output screens. (Assume that the actual input and output screens have already been designed.) Be sure to include explanations of possible error messages that may appear when the user makes invalid entries.

10. Test the terminal dialogue you prepared in problem 6. Replace all display layout charts with screens that contain actual data and messages instead of editing symbols. Simulate a user terminal session by having someone walk through the dialogue using these sample screens. Challenge them to do something your dialogue wasn't designed to handle.

11. Obtain documentation or magazine reviews on an automated screen-design aid. If possible, arrange for a demonstration. How would the product improve your productivity? How would the product decrease your productivity? What features do you dislike or would you prefer to see?

ANNOTATED REFERENCES AND SUGGESTED READINGS

Fitzgerald, Jerry. *Internal Controls for Computerized Information Systems.* Redwood City, Calif.: Jerry Fitzgerald & Associates, 1978. This is our reference standard on the subject of designing internal controls into systems. Fitzgerald advocates a unique and powerful matrix tool for designing controls. This book goes far beyond any introductory systems textbook — Must reading.

Mehlmann, Marilyn. *When People Use Computers: An Approach to Developing an Interface.* Englewood Cliffs, N.J.: Prentice-Hall, 1981. We are indebted to Marilyn for the concept of zoning a screen into areas. But this book goes far beyond that. Every systems analyst can get something out of this book, which is a modern and comprehensive study of how to analyze and design intelligent terminal dialogues.

Analysts in Action

Methods, Procedures, and Program Design for the New System

When we left Cheryl and Doug, they had designed the batch and on-line inputs and the terminal dialogue for the new order-entry system. Now they must design the data processing methods and procedures required for the new system.

Episode 7

We begin this episode in Cheryl's office, two weeks later. Doug and Cheryl have just arrived and are enjoying their early morning coffee. Ed Earl Jones, Manager of the Computer Information Systems Group, has just walked into the office.

Methods and Procedures Specifications for the New System

"Well. Look who finally came back from vacation!" Cheryl smiled a welcome. "How are you, Ed Earl?"

"I'm doing fine but with all the travel I've done over the last three weeks, I had to come back to work to relax. Hey, I just wanted to check in with you on this order-entry system project. I assume things are going well?"

"Terrific!" replied Cheryl. "We're finishing up the design right now. We should start packaging the program specifications today. Better get those code cutters geared up, Ed Earl. This one's going to take some time."

Ed Earl smiled and responded, "You know, you'll get the best we have. Just let me know how many programmers you'll need. I'll even let you choose the chief programmer. Whoever it is will report to the two of you. Well, I've got to finish my check-ins with the other teams. Keep up the good work." Ed left the office.

Cheryl smiled, "I suppose we had better start earning our pay for today, eh Doug?"

Doug replied, "Let's see where we are." After shuffling through a stack of papers (sample page in Figure 1) Doug continued, "Hey, it looks like you finished the last of the basic systems flowcharts before you left yesterday."

"Yep. I haven't had a chance to tell you yet. We can start on backup and recovery procedures."

Doug hesitated for a moment and then said, "I think I'd like to start with a master file. Let's do the customer master file. Based on my conversations with Joey, this file is critical. Additionally, our own design specifications call for updates at any time during any working day."

Cheryl interrupted, "Do you have any feel for how long Joey can afford to be without the on-line order-entry and query subsystems?"

Doug replied, "Yes, we dis- ►

Figure 1

Sample systems flowchart.

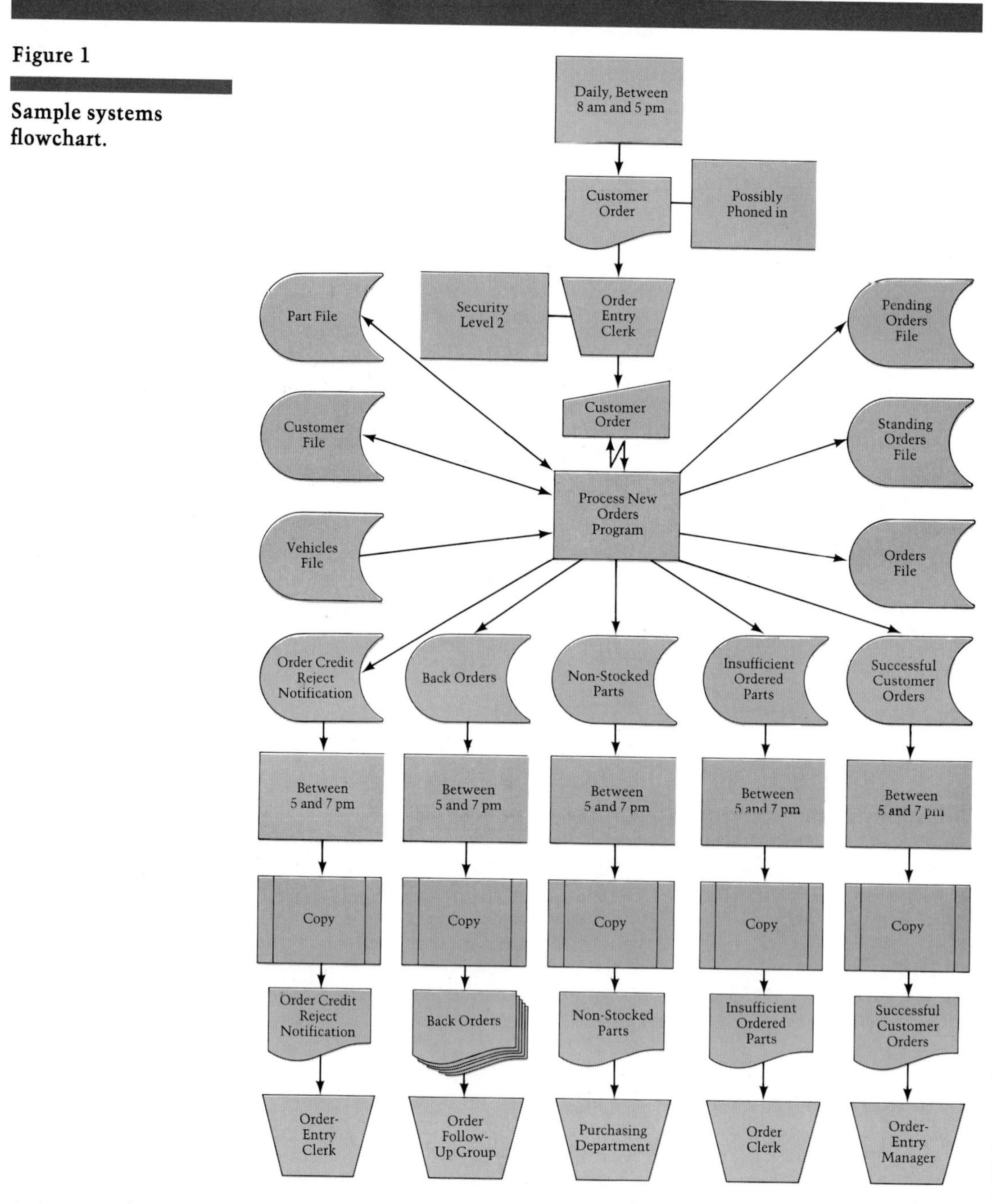

cussed that on Wednesday. Obviously, he doesn't want to lose the system ever. But he said he could afford no more than half a day; about four hours."

"Well, that's it, then," said Cheryl. "We'll backup the customer master file twice during working hours. I'll ask operations for a noon and 4 P.M. backup. Those are two slow periods for new orders anyway. And of course, if the system crashes, we'll reload the latest backup tape."

Cheryl had been drawing a picture of what she was saying. She took a few moments to finish the drawing (see Figure 2) and then gave the paper to Doug. "How's that?"

Doug answered, "Good! But to fully recover from a crash, we still have to reprocess all transactions since the last backup tape was created."

Cheryl responded, "Yeah. Did all our transaction processing procedures log successful transactions to tape files?"

"Yes," answered Doug. "And I have a list of all those transaction tapes somewhere. Here it is! I've recorded the backup transactions tape and all master and transaction files that were updated by those successful transactions."

"Great!" said Cheryl. "All we have to do is to reprocess all transaction tapes that updated the customer master file. I better make a note that only those transactions that occurred after the date and time of the last backup tape should be reprocessed." Cheryl was adding several items to her systems flowchart. "Here! How's this?" . . .

It's three hours later. Cheryl and Doug have finished defining backup and recovery procedures for the system. All system flowcharts for the new order-entry system have been delivered to operations who will review them and then schedule a meeting to discuss the new procedures. Meanwhile, Cheryl and Doug are planning their next task before they go to lunch.

Program Design Specifications for the New System

Doug pointed to the three notebooks of analysis and design specifications for the order-entry system. "Will you look at that?!" he groaned. "Now we have to get all those specifications organized so the programmers can get started."

Cheryl grinned, "I'll do implementation planning and start working on parts of the user's manual. Before you start packaging the program specifications, let's make sure we've got the format down, okay?"

Noting Doug's nod, Cheryl continued, "I want Beverly to manage the programming team. I've worked with her before. We've agreed on a specific format for program specifications. First, Bev likes to have all the file specifications included in a single packet. That includes all data dictionary forms and record layout charts. She'll assign a programmer to quickly create test files for use by all other members of the programming team. Next, we want a separate package of specifications for each program. This package will include . . ."

Doug interrupted, "Excuse me, Cheryl. Before you describe the package, do you want the programs in any specific sequence?"

Cheryl answered, "Yes, good question! Let's package the programs in the sequence in which I want Bev to implement them. Let's do the transaction processing programs first because we want to get those programs up and running first. Then we'll do decision support. We'll save the management-reporting programs until after we finish all the transaction processing and queries."

"Okay," Doug nodded. "Now, how are we going to organize each program specification?"

Cheryl responded, "Every program specification should begin with a structure chart (see Figure 3) similar to the one I was working on here and one of these IPO charts (see Figure 4). The structure chart will depict the various modules in a ▶

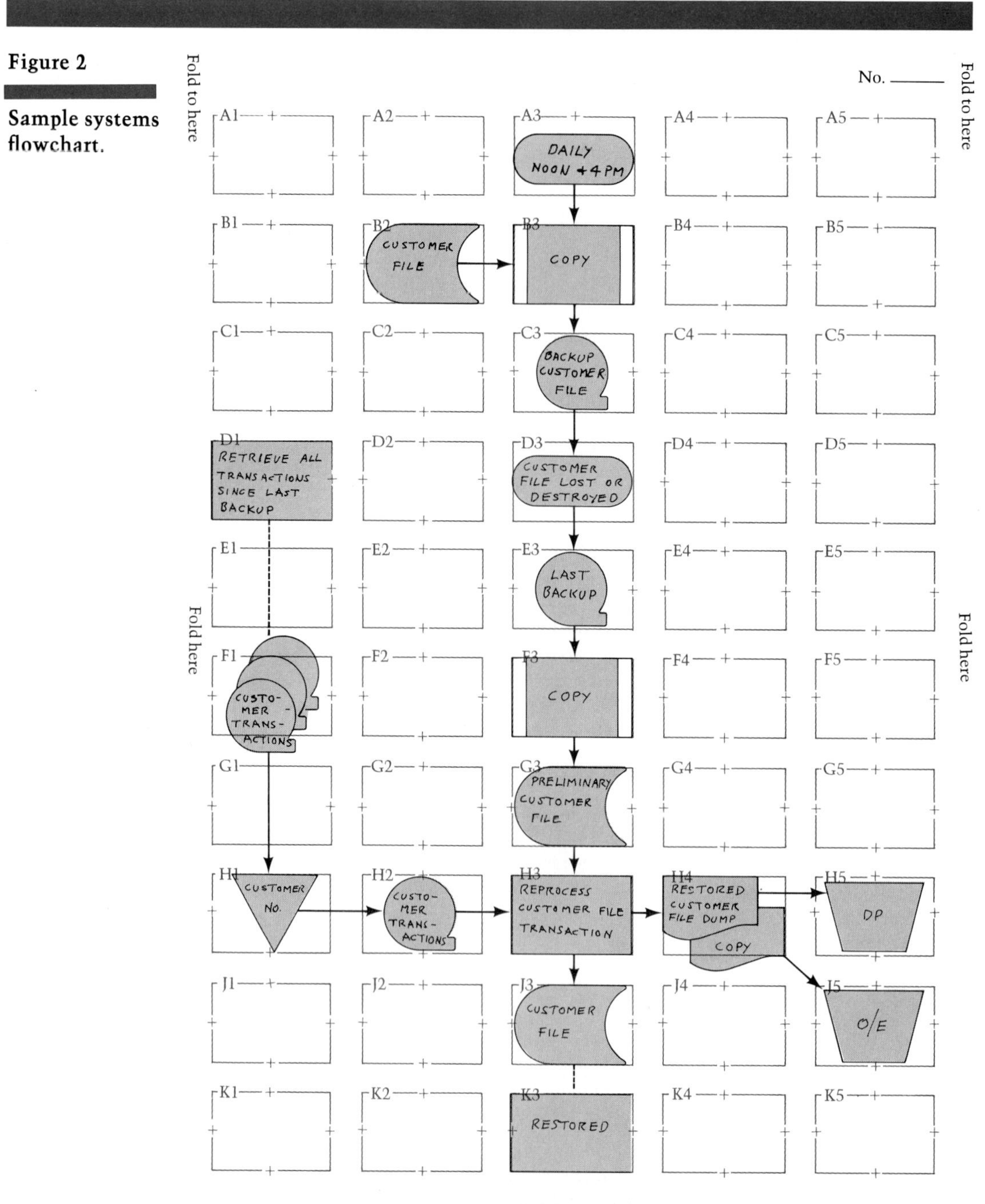

Figure 2

Sample systems flowchart.

Figure 3

Sample structure chart.

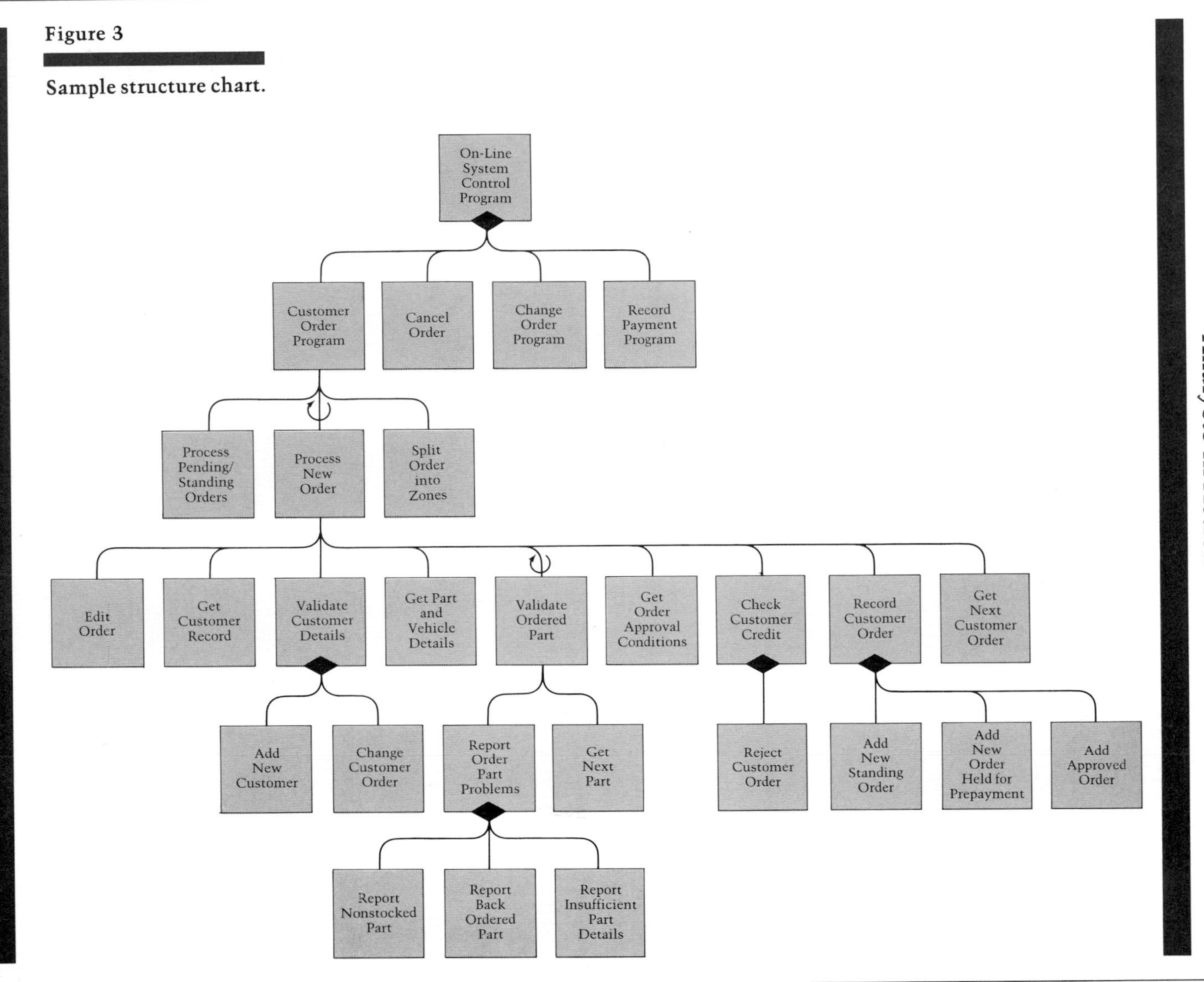

Figure 4

Sample IPO Chart.

PROGRAM ABSTRACT for ______ (name of program) Prepared by ______ Date ______ Page ___ of ___

INPUT	PROCESS	OUTPUT

program and their relationship(s). The chart will be useful in project management and in ensuring that the programs will be maintainable once they have been installed. The IPO chart will describe the program and reference the supporting detailed documentation. Have you used these charts before?"

"Yes," answered Doug. "The center column is the key. It represents the program or programs being documented. That's where I describe the program and its procedures. The input and output columns contain the systems flowchart inputs and outputs for the program."

Cheryl nodded, "Yes, but I want every systems flowchart symbol to reference the supporting detailed documentation. For inputs, outputs, and dialogue, the symbol should point to all necessary data dictionary forms, printer spacing charts, input layout charts, dialogue charts, and display layout charts. For files, we don't need the data dictionary forms, but we should reference the record layout charts. Those record layout charts will have to be duplicated because most files are shared by several programs. Any questions?"

"No," Doug answered. ►

Figure 5

Typical outline for program specifications.

PROGRAM SPECIFICATIONS FOR
AAP CUSTOMER SERVICES SYSTEM

I. System overview (with PDFDs and system flowchart)
II. Programming team organization
III. Programming schedule (with Gantt chart)
IV. Program specifications
    A. Program 1
        1. Structure chart
        2. IPO charts
        3. Terminal dialogue specifications
            a. Dialogue charts
            b. On-line input and output specifications
                1) Data dictionary
                2) Record layout charts
                3) Printer spacing and display layout charts
    B. Program 2
        .
        .
        .

"We're just reorganizing all this documentation according to programs. Is this outline (see Figure 5) what you have in mind?"

Cheryl scanned the outline and answered, "Yes."

Where Do We Go from Here?
In this episode, you observed Cheryl and Doug wrapping up the design of the new system. They used a new tool, the systems flowchart, to document data processing methods and procedures. You will learn how to draw systems flowcharts in Chapter 15. Also, Cheryl and Doug are beginning to package the final set of design specifications into programs that can be written by the computer programmers. This is when all of the documentation you've been learning comes together. You'll learn how to package those design specifications in Chapter 16.

Cheryl opted to do implementation planning for the new system. Successful implementation planning is highly dependent upon your project management skills. If you're interested in implementation planning, we suggest you read Part IV, Module A, "Project Management." ■

15 Designing Computer-Based Methods and Procedures

Minicase: Platters-by-Mail Record Club (revisited)

In the minicase for Chapter 7, we explained the operations of the Platters-by-Mail Record Club. We then challenged you to draw a picture that described the business. Since then, many of the record club's operations have been automated. Let's take a look at how the operations are performed.

At approximately 8:30 each morning, the Order-Entry Department collects all new sales order forms. These forms include orders received both in the mail and over the phone. Order Entry delivers the batch of forms to Data Entry, where the orders are keyed (typed) and stored on magnetic tape.

Data Entry then delivers the sales order tape to Data Processing, where the tape is read by a program that checks the sales orders for keying errors. The program generates an errors report that identifies incomplete and invalid sales orders. This report is delivered to order-entry clerks who correct the sales orders and send them back to Data Entry for rekeying. The same program stores all valid sales orders on a new magnetic tape. When all sales orders have been successfully processed and written to that tape, the tape is read by a program that produces another tape on which the orders are resequenced according to customer number.

This sorted tape is input to another program that checks an inventory master file to determine the availability and price of products that appear on the sales order. If the sales order cannot be filled, a back order notice is generated. The next program uses the customer accounts receivable master file to check credit on those orders that can be filled. For customers who have a poor credit rating, a payment overdue notice is printed. The program produces an order confirmation letter for orders that will be filled. A final program produces an invoice with carbons for picking, packing, and shipping the orders that have passed the credit check. That program also produces a sales order transaction file that contains all successfully processed sales orders and a sales order register. Also, all successfully processed sales orders are stored on a new magnetic tape and archived. All reports generated by this program are initially held by Data Processing. Data Processing compares the batch totals generated by the last program against a batch control slip that was generated by Data Entry when the orders were keyed. If the totals match, Data Processing will deliver the reports to Order Entry.

The new system also includes an on-line program that allows the sales manager both to query the inventory file to obtain product prices and to query the customer accounts receivable file to obtain customer credit and invoice information. This program is available to the manager from 8:00 A.M. to 5:00 P.M. each working day.

Customer order cancellations are processed immediately. When the order-entry clerk receives a cancellation request (via the mail or phone), the clerk enters the order cancellation request on the CRT. An on-line program reads the customer accounts receivable file to determine the status of the order. If the order has not yet been filled, the clerk phones the warehouse to have the order terminated. The program also generates order cancellation confirmation letters (printed as a batch at 4:30 P.M. that day).

This narrative description of the record club's operations is becoming lengthy. We haven't even talked about how the customer payments and billing operations are performed. But let's stop here — we have a challenge for you.

Challenge

Remember, we said a picture is worth a thousand words. Draw a picture to describe the data processing methods and procedures being performed in the record club, how these operations are being accomplished, and the sequence in which they are occurring.

WHAT WILL YOU LEARN IN THIS CHAPTER?

In this chapter, you will learn how to design and document computer-based methods and procedures using systems flowcharts. You will know that you have mastered the specification of methods and procedures when you can:

1. Differentiate between batch, on-line, remote batch, and distributed methods of data processing.
2. Describe the general procedures required to implement each of the data processing methods just listed.
3. Define and design methods and procedures for internal controls, including backup and recovery.
4. Explain how systems flowcharts are used for systems design and how they relate to the tools you learned in Chapters 11 through 14.
5. Read, prepare, and present systems flowcharts describing typical data processing methods and procedures. (Systems flowcharts should conform to guidelines to enhance their communication value to both technical and nontechnical audiences.)

Data processing and computer-based systems require well-defined methods and procedures to ensure that the information system functions properly. Nowhere is the absence of well-defined methods and procedures more evident than in the recent emergence of microcomputer-based information systems. When end users design their own systems, they frequently forget about methods and procedures for backup and recovery and other internal controls.

Why? Because end users aren't schooled in fundamental data processing methods and procedures. In this chapter, we will study the design of methods and procedures — they are equally applicable to mainframe and microcomputer environments.

Systems flowcharts are a graphical tool used to show the sequence of processing and activities in a computer-based information system. Why not use data flow diagrams for this purpose? Some analysts believe that data flow diagrams make systems flowcharts obsolete. This is unfortunate. True, data flow diagrams have replaced systems flowcharts as the preferred tool for many systems analysts. But systems flowcharts and data flow diagrams can and should complement one another. DFDs are useful for depicting the overall system — both manual and computer elements — with a minimum of symbols. And DFDs clearly illustrate activities that occur in parallel. Meanwhile, systems flowcharts are especially useful for describing the methods and procedures that underlie the data processing activities. And although systems flowcharts are definitely more complicated than DFDs, if they are properly drawn and presented, they can be presented to the nontechnical audience.

DATA PROCESSING METHODS AND PROCEDURES AND THEIR IMPLICATIONS

What are methods and procedures? And how do we document them? Methods and procedures (part of your information system model, reproduced in the margin) define the sequence of events that produce outputs from their requisite inputs. Specifically, a method is a way of doing something. A procedure is a step-by-step plan for implementing the method. Methods and procedures can also be described as answering the question "*who* does *what* and *when* do they do it?" Also, the question "*how* will it be done?" In this section, we will briefly discuss methods and procedures typically used to implement information systems. Most methods can be broadly classified on each of two scales:

1. Degree of centralized versus distributed processing
2. Degree of batch versus on-line processing

Systems can be partially distributed or partially on-line. Let's examine these two common methods and procedures more closely.

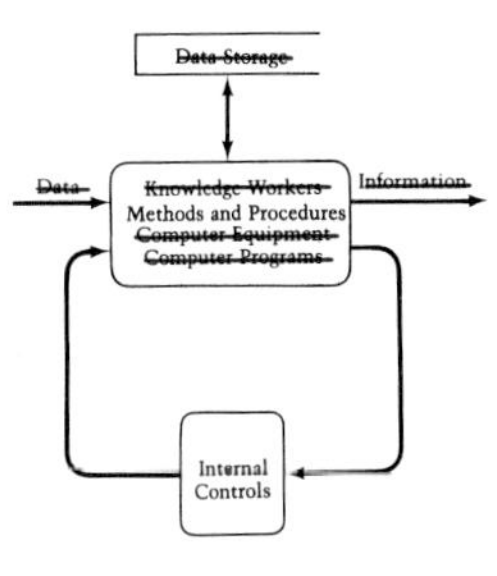

IPO Components

Centralized Versus Distributed Processing

At one time, all data processing was centralized, with data recorded, input, and processed at a central computer site. The cost of placing computers closer to the knowledge workers was prohibitive. Today, because computers have become much cheaper, many organizations have decentralized or distributed their processing workload to multiple computer sites. Distributed computing can offer several advantages including improved responsiveness, better user control over data, and reduced costs (especially with microcomputers). As an analyst, you need to be aware of the alternatives and to be able to discuss the technology with specialists and users.

There are several approaches to distributed processing. Each approach connects the computer systems through one of the network architectures listed in the margin. We'll briefly survey these options. The study of network strategies, technologies, and data communications should become an integral part of your continuing education for a career in systems analysis and design.

Network Strategies

- Point-to-Point Connection
- Bus Networks
- Star Networks
- Hierarchical Networks
- Ring Networks

Point-to-Point and Bus Networks The simplest networking strategy is to provide a direct link between any two computer systems you wish to connect. This concept is illustrated in Figure 15.1. Notice that the network can contain microcomputers, minicomputers, mainframe computers, and terminals. To completely connect all points between N computers or devices, you would need $N \times (N - 1)/2$ direct paths. Unless each data path is heavily utilized, the cost could be prohibitive. In fact, utilization of any point-to-point data path should be verified before installing that path.

What can you do if the direct paths will not be heavily utilized? You could have specific computers and devices share a single point-to-point data path (see Figure 15.2). The data path in this case is called a **bus.** Only one computer system or device can send data through the bus at any given time. Incidentally, the computer systems and devices are said to be multidropped off the bus.

Ethernet, a product developed jointly by Xerox, Intel, and Digital Equipment Corporation, is an example of a bus network strategy. *Ethernet* also happens to be an example of a special product category called *local area networks.* A **local area network** is a collection of computers, terminals, printers, and other computing devices that are connected through cable over relatively short distances (for instance, in a single building). These computers and devices can

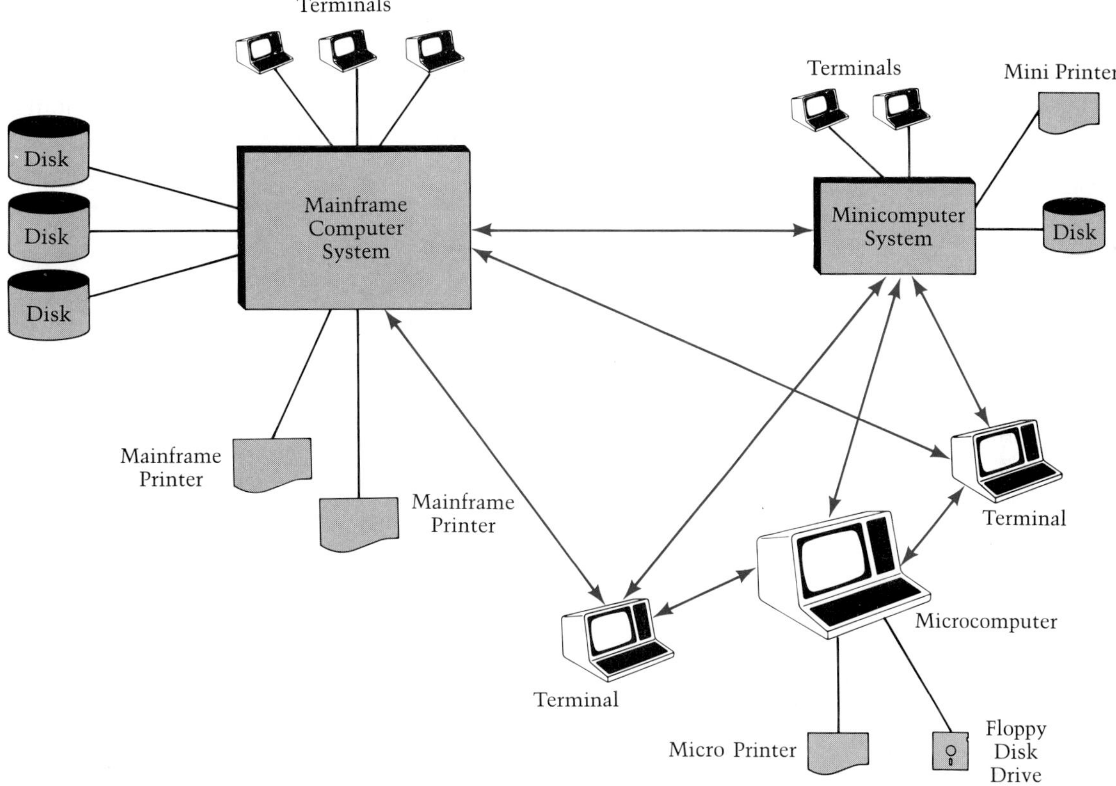

Figure 15.1

Point-to-point network. The simplest distributed processing network architecture is point to point, whereby a dedicated data path is placed between two devices. That data path only has to concern itself with understanding the devices on each end.

transmit data to one another through this network. *Ethernet's* bus architecture manages point-to-point communication to prevent collisions that can occur when multiple devices try to use the bus at the same time.

Star and Hierarchical Networks A **star network** links multiple computer systems (often called *satellite processors*) through a central computer (see Figure 15.3). Some will argue that this is a holdover from the days when centralized computing reigned supreme. However, the truth is that much data in any organization can (and

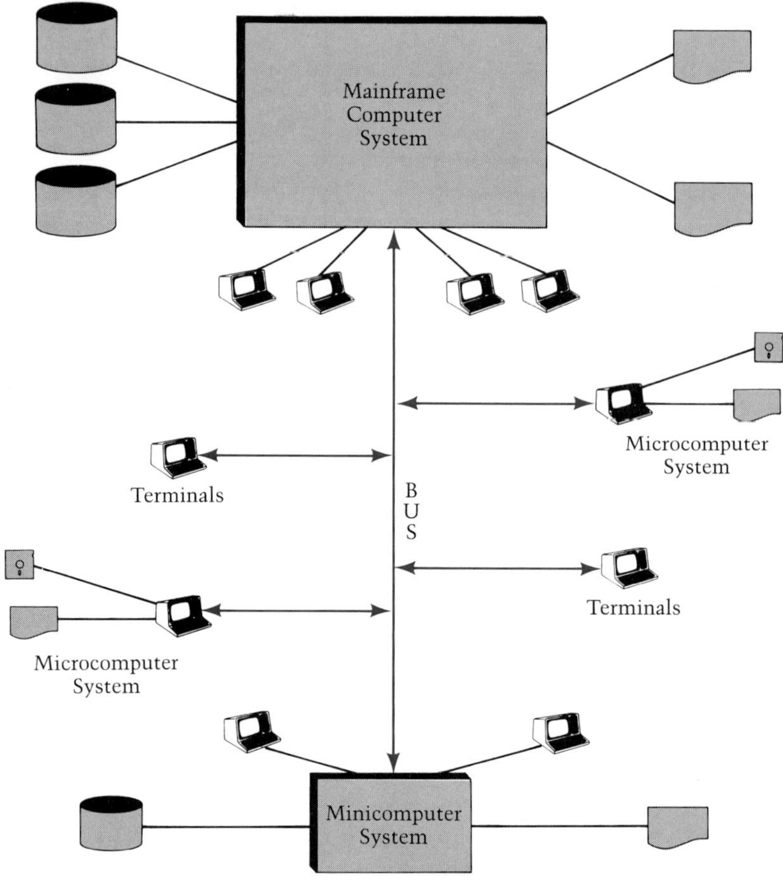

Figure 15.2

Bus network. A bus network is similar to a point-to-point network except that multiple devices share a single point-to-point pathway. Only two devices, a sender and a receiver, can use the path at any given time.

should) be maintained on and shared through the central computer. The central computer is being used as a traffic cop to control the transmission of data and information between the distributed processor sites.

A **hierarchical network** can be thought of as a multiple star network. Figure 15.4 illustrates such a network. The top computer system, usually a mainframe computer, controls the entire network. The satellite processors (in this case, minicomputers and

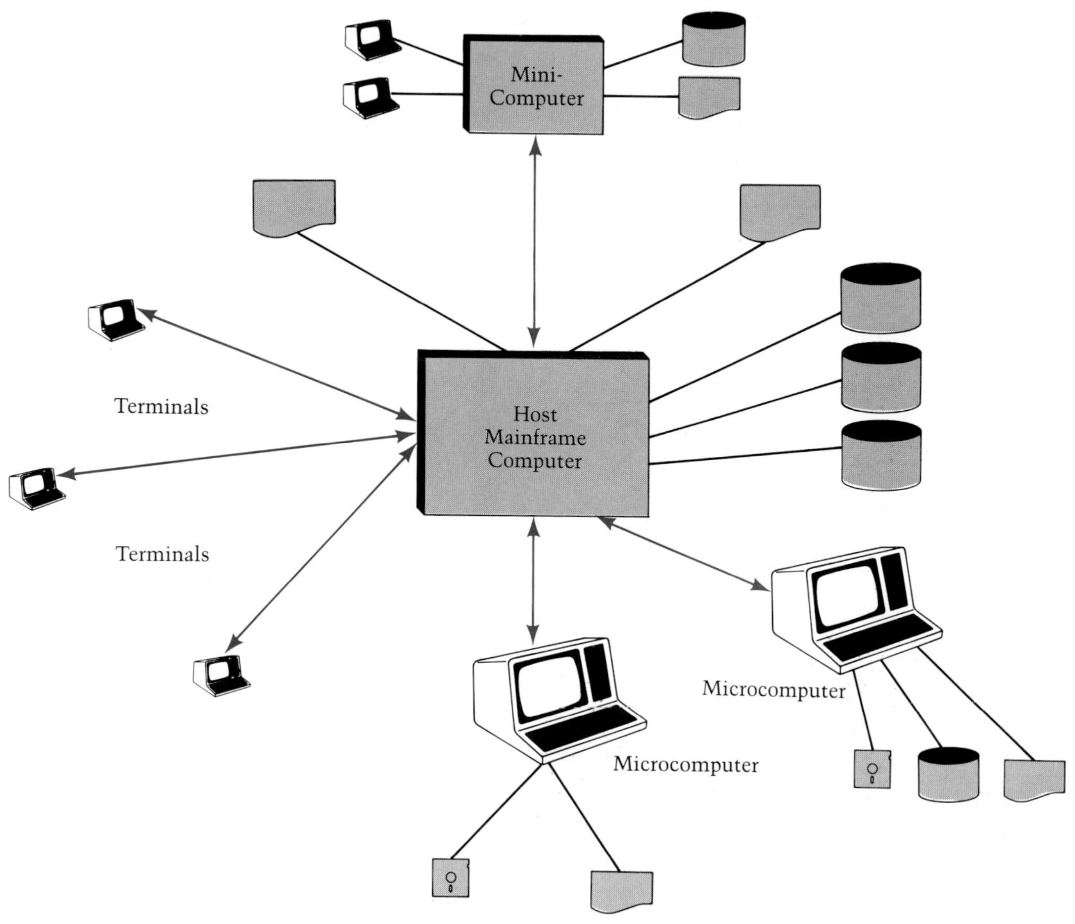

Figure 15.3

Star network. In a star network, a central computer plays traffic cop to control satellite processors and devices that are trying to communicate with each other and with the central computer.

microcomputers) have their own satellites (in this case, microcomputers and terminals). Notice that each satellite may have its own complement of *dedicated* devices (such as disk drives and terminals). IBM's *System Network Architecture* (SNA) is essentially a hierarchical network.

Ring Networks A **ring network** connects multiple computers (but not other devices) into a ringlike structure (see Figure 15.5). Each

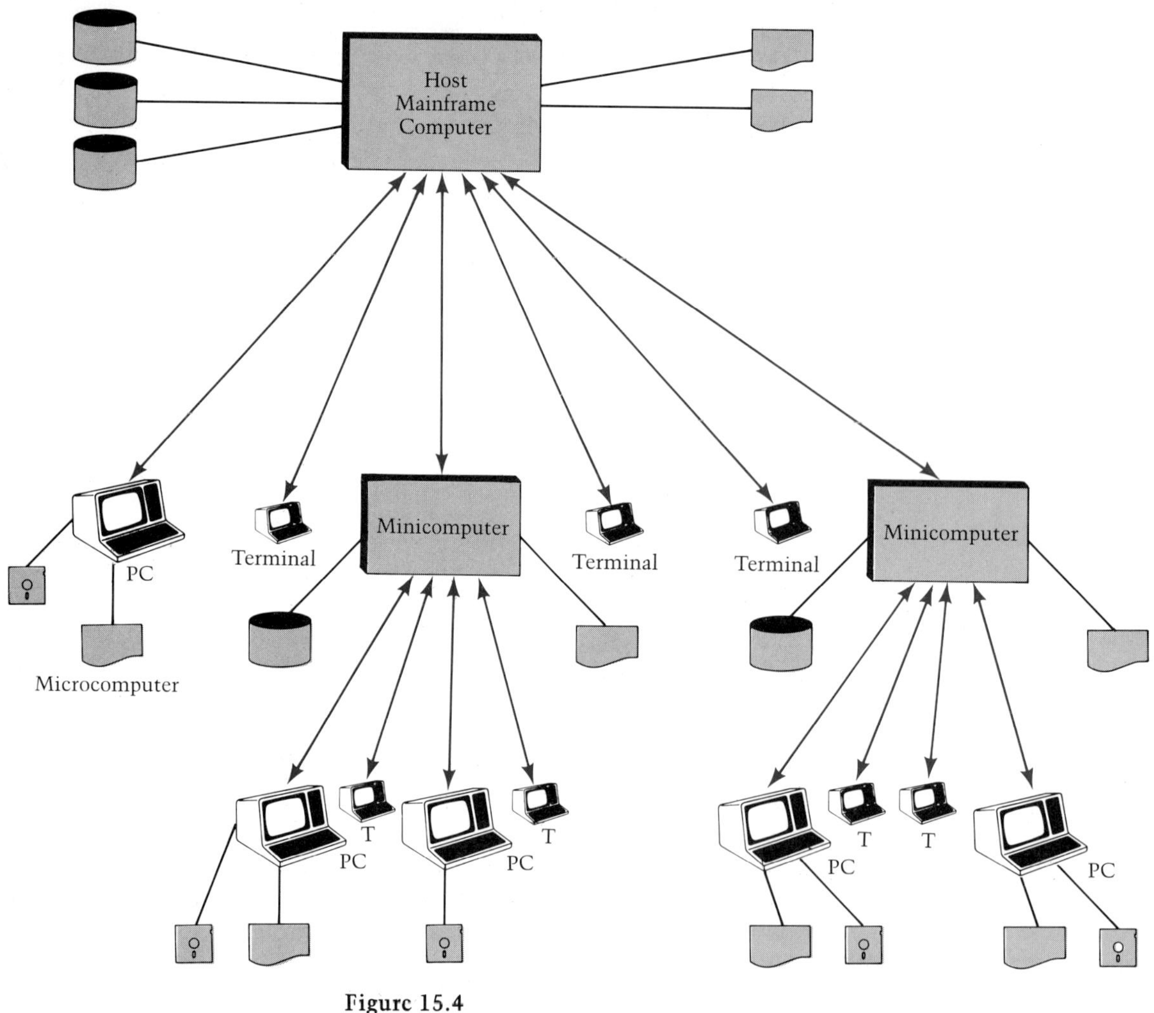

Figure 15.4

Hierarchical networks. Hierarchical networks, such as IBM's popular SNA, use a host computer to control satellite processors and devices, which in turn may control other satellite processors and devices, and so forth. The host computer supervises the entire network.

computer can transmit data to only one other computer. Every data transmission includes an address, similar to the address you write on an envelope. When a computer in the ring receives a packet, it checks the address. If the address is not for that computer, it passes it on to the next computer in the ring.

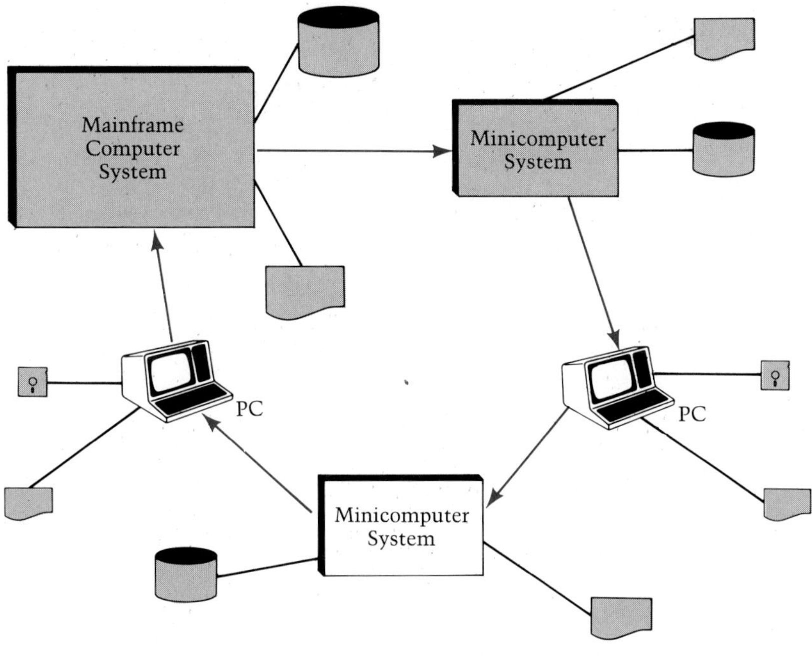

Figure 15.5

Ring networks. Ring networks link computers, one to another, but in one direction only. Data transmissions are passed around the ring until they arrive at their intended destination.

The Importance of Data Communications All of the network architectures just discussed are implemented through data communications technology. Making computers and devices *talk* with one another is one of the most exciting technologies in today's information systems world. Transmitting data through the network is not as easy as it may seem. Data can be directly transmitted through cables (as in local area networks), over telephone wires, via microwave, and even via satellite. Furthermore, data are subject to complications, such as different codes recognized by different computers and devices. Microcomputer to mainframe computer connection is a particularly *hot* issue today.

The many issues and complexities of data communications are beyond the scope of this book. As a systems analyst, you often enlist data communications and distributed processing specialists to help answer questions that arise. You'll find it easier to work with such specialists if you begin to plan your continuing education in this rapidly changing facet of technology.

Batch Versus On-Line Processing and Their Internal Control Implications

Batch and on-line processing concepts were introduced and surveyed in Chapters 11 through 14—at least with regard to inputs and outputs. Our perspective here is on batch versus on-line *processing.*

Many of the required internal controls for the system were specified when inputs, outputs, and files were designed. We must now incorporate these and other controls into the methods and procedures for the system. The purpose of internal controls for methods and procedures is to ensure the accountability, auditability, and recovery capability for the new information system.

A Review of Batch Processing Methods In the batch processing method, transactions are accumulated into batches for periodic processing. The batch inputs are processed against master files. Transaction files may also be created or updated at that time. In a batch system, management reports are generated on a scheduled basis. That is, either a report is regularly scheduled to be generated on a specific date and time or the report is scheduled *after* it has been requested.

Batch processing procedures are dependent on the organization of the computer master files. Most early files were sequential and stored on tape. Tape devices cannot retrieve records directly because all of the records prior to the desired record must be read. Therefore, standard procedures required that the input transactions be sorted into the same order as the master files. Consider the PAYROLL system shown in Figure 15.6. TIMECARDS are sorted into the same sequence as the PAYROLL MASTER FILE (keyed on EMPLOYEE NUMBER) before they can be processed. Also note that two copies of master files are used. As a result of processing, an entirely new master file is produced. The old file is normally retained as a backup. Sequential files are not as common today as they were in the past. Unless they are being used as part of systems developed long ago, sequential files have been largely replaced by more flexible direct and indexed files.

When direct and indexed files are used, the processing procedures are greatly simplified (illustrated in Figure 15.7). The input

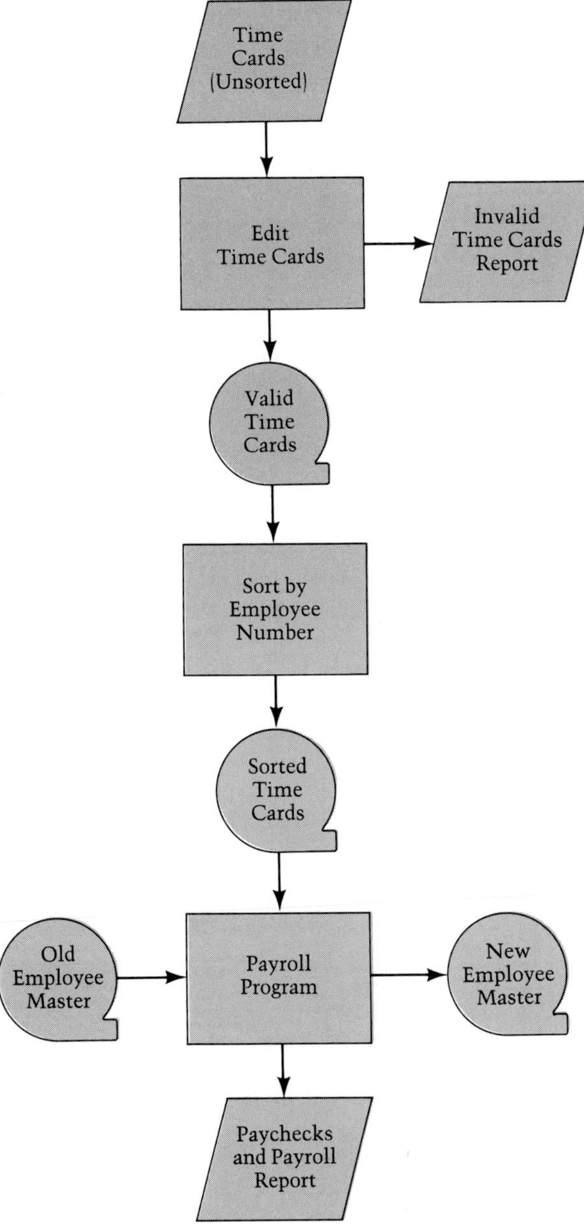

Figure 15.6

Batch processing with sequential files. This figure illustrates the batch input method using sequential tape files. Input transactions must be sorted into the same sequence as the master file. Furthermore, the old master file cannot be updated. Instead, a new master is produced when transactions are processed.

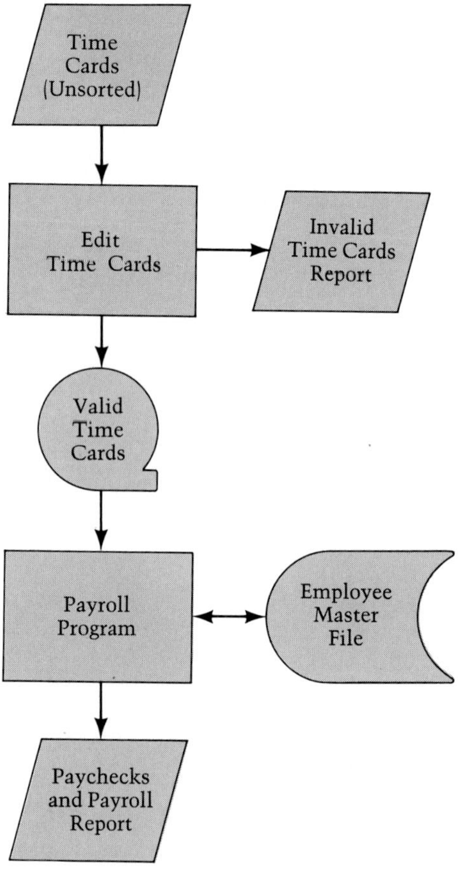

Figure 15.7

Batch processing with direct and indexed files. This picture illustrates batch input processing with direct and indexed (which may be physically sequential) files stored on disk. Disk file processing is simpler than tape file processing because master files can be directly updated and input records don't have to be sorted.

data does not need to be sorted prior to processing because specific master file data can be retrieved directly from disk without having to read the records that precede the desired record (data might still be sorted to improve efficiency). Furthermore, a record can be retrieved, changed, and then rewritten to the same file, eliminating the need for two copies of the master file.

We can also combine the concepts of batch and distributed processing. A batch of records can be created and edited at a distributed site and then transmitted to the central site for processing (see Figure 15.8). This is called a *remote batch* because the batch originates at a remote site. This processing method is appropriate for situations in which identical transactions are captured at geographically different locations. For instance, each regional sales office may capture, input, and edit their own sales orders. Those orders can be transmitted as remote batches to the central computer site where they will be merged and processed as a single batch.

Internal Controls for Batch Systems Throughout the past several chapters, you've learned to design numerous internal controls into systems. But we're not through yet. The following additional internal controls must be designed into batch systems:

1. All inputs and outputs are scheduled and logged. A runbook states when programs should be run, instructs the computer operator of any necessary setup (for instance, loading special forms on the printer), and describes which JCL (Job Control Language) file to execute (this concept should be familiar to students of programming). The runbook is also used to record the production runs and list any problems that have occurred.
2. Procedures describe how input errors (edit reports, introduced in Chapter 13) should be distributed to users and whether processing can proceed before these errors are corrected. The error correction cycle is included in the procedures.
3. Procedures require batch control totals (see Chapter 13) to be checked against the historical report generated for transaction processing. If the totals are not in agreement, output distribution should be delayed until the discrepancy has been accounted for.
4. Procedures describe how scheduled outputs are to be collated, duplicated, and distributed to users.
5. Procedures specify when and how master and transactions files are backed up. Backup copies of files are needed so they can be restored in the event of a disaster (such as equipment failure or sabotage) that destroys the main copies of those files. For most files, backup copies are written to an off-line medium, such as tape, cassette, or floppy disks.

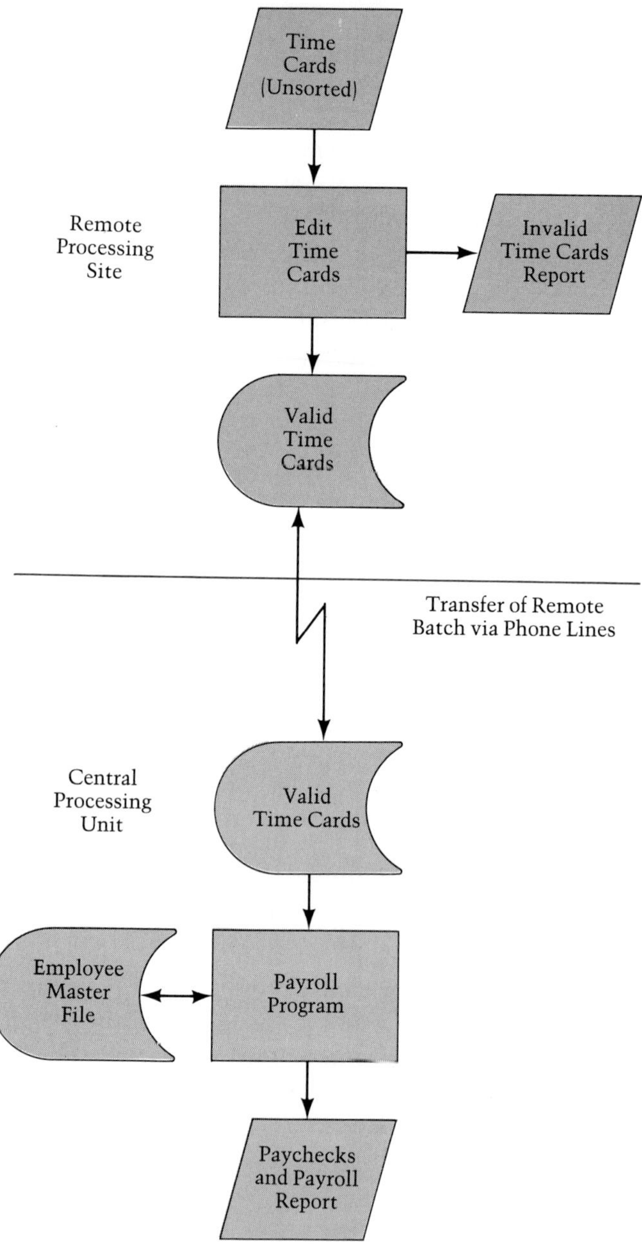

Figure 15.8

Remote batch processing. In remote batch processing, separate batches are created at remote sites (another batch system or an on-line system) and then transmitted to a central site for processing. The transmission may be made via direct cable (short distances) or telephone, microwave, or satellite (for long distances).

6. Procedures specify how files will be recovered in the event that they are lost or destroyed. The backup files (just described in #5) will only ensure the data up to the point in time when that backup was made. Transactions that occurred after that backup must be *re*processed. There are two methods for doing this. One approach is to re-input those transactions from the historical reports produced during transaction processing. This, however, means going through data entry and editing again. Another approach is to record historical data in machine-readable format (during transaction processing) and then simply to reprocess the data from this backup transaction file.

A Review of On-Line Processing Methods Modern information systems are moving away from batch methods and toward on-line methods. That is why this book has placed so much emphasis on the design of on-line inputs, outputs, and terminal dialogue. Transactions and inquiries are processed as they occur. Figure 15.9 illustrates the on-line method and procedures. Transactions are processed when they occur (no batches). Notice that on-line processing requires direct or indexed files. Sequential files simply can't provide adequate response time for on-line systems.

A completely on-line system is not common. The management reports may be *scheduled* in the same manner as they are in batch processing. Few organizations have computing resources that permit users to generate large reports as frequently as they desire. Small reports can be produced *on demand* and displayed at a terminal screen. However, printouts are usually scheduled at available printing devices when those devices become available. The exception is terminal workstations that include a printer (especially microcomputers).

Internal Controls for On-Line Systems The following additional internal controls should be designed into on-line systems:

1. Access to the on-line system is restricted to authorized users. Appropriate security measures are defined in the methods and procedures to prevent unauthorized access to data and processing. Frequently, multiple levels of security are built into the system because different users are allowed to do different things. For instance, at our local credit union, all tellers are allowed to process your basic deposits, withdrawals, transfers, and loan payments. However, modifying specific transactions, correcting

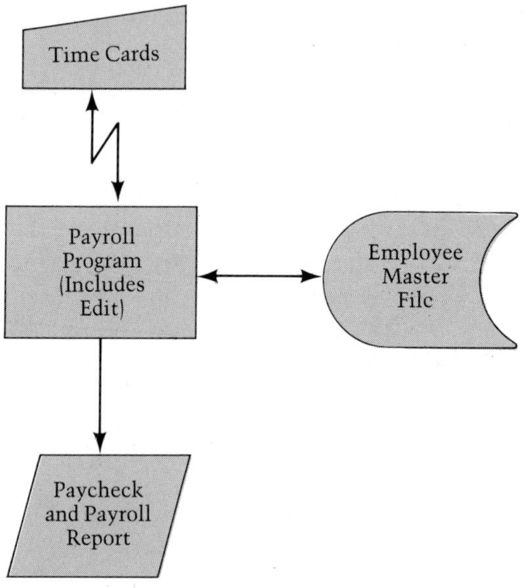

Figure 15.9

On-line processing. With on-line or interactive processing, transactions are processed as they occur. Because transactions can occur during all business hours, on-line programs must be available to users at all times. This means that the programs may also be idle (but still available) at some times.

errors, and making large withdrawals is restricted to tellers who have a *super teller* password.

2. Backup and recovery for files is more difficult for the on-line system. Master and transaction files are periodically backed up, as was the case with batch processing. However, whereas batch transactions include batch control totals that were verified after a processing run, on-line processing offers no such control. Instead, separate files are maintained for successfully processed transactions. If the main file is lost or damaged, the recovery procedure consists of two steps: (1) load the last backup of the file that was lost and (2) reprocess those transactions that occurred after the last backup of the lost file. These transactions can be processed directly from the tape journal of those transactions.

Additional Internal Controls to Be Designed As you've gone through the design chapters, you've learned that you must design internal controls for outputs, files/databases, inputs, and on-line terminal dialogue. In this chapter, we've added internal controls for batch and on-line processing. There are some other controls that must be specified for any type of system. They may include:

- *Simultaneous processing controls.* When two or more users try to update the same record in a file or database at exactly the same time, you have a problem. If user A retrieves the record, then user B retrieves the same record, then user A writes the updated record, and then user B writes its own updated record, the update for user A has been lost. The analyst should ensure that this can't happen by making sure that if simultaneous processing is possible, a record can be *locked out* to more than one user at a time.
- *Maintenance controls.* We've discussed this earlier, but as you prepare systems flowcharts, you need to ensure that all updates to master and transaction files were properly performed. Some user or manager should get a daily update report to check for any unauthorized updates that might have been recorded. This report is frequently called a *journal.*
- *Physical security.* In some cases, physical security must be established by the analyst. Who can use the computer equipment and software? This question is becoming more important as systems are installed on microcomputers that are not usually housed in a secure area. The analyst may have to investigate ways to physically restrict both the access to and the movement of computer equipment. And the analyst may also have to investigate software techniques of restricting access to software, files, and databases.
- *Physical reliability.* The analyst may have to specify controls to prevent accidental or intentional environmental problems. Some systems are susceptible to static electricity. Magnetic fields can erase data recorded on tape. Dust contamination can be a problem in some areas. Humidity and temperature can also be problems. Normally, these issues are addressed by computer operations management, not analysts. However, as microcomputer-based systems multiply, the analyst has become more responsible for such controls.

A complete survey of internal controls is a subject that can only be presented well in its own book (see the suggested reading for this chapter). What we have tried to do in the last six chapters is to briefly discuss the most important controls and to place them into the context of the design tasks (output, files, input, and so forth) during which they should be specified.

USING SYSTEMS FLOWCHARTS TO DOCUMENT METHODS, PROCEDURES, AND CONTROLS

Systems flowcharts were one of the very first tools commonly used by systems analysts and computer programmers. In fact, the American National Standards Institute (ANSI) has established certain symbols that are widely used in the data processing industry to describe the logic of both systems and computer programs. Although the symbols have been standardized, their use has not. Thus many systems flowcharts look incomprehensible to those who would use them. Is it any wonder that systems flowcharts have developed an unfavorable reputation with users?

Systems flowcharts are supposed to be the basis for communication between knowledge workers, systems analysts, computer operations personnel, and computer programmers. Now that's a tall task! But it's not impossible. You should think of systems flowcharts as a chance to prove (or disprove) that a specific technical solution to the user's requirements will work.

Systems Flowchart Symbol Categories

- Processing
- Batch Input
- Batch Output
- Files/Database
- On-Line Input and Output
- Miscellaneous

In this section, you'll learn how to draw clear systems flowcharts. Although for the most part, we will follow the ANSI standard, at some points we will go beyond that standard because it has not advanced to keep pace with advances in data processing methods, such as distributed computing, on-line computing, and newer batch input methods. Furthermore, the ANSI standard does not suggest appropriate guidelines for drawing clear systems flowcharts. We will do so. Some of the ideas are our own. Others have been suggested by fellow authors in the systems analysis and design field. We suggest that you adopt and document a standard for your organization, systems group, or individual projects.

Systems Flowchart Symbols and Conventions

Systems flowcharting symbology can be conveniently classified into the six subsets listed in the margin on the previous page. As we discuss these symbols and patterns, we'll use a cloudlike symbol to represent those symbols that haven't been introduced in the narrative. Most symbols and patterns are shown in the margin.

Processing Symbols There are only three basic symbols for processing: the computer program, the manual operation, and the auxiliary operation. The most important of these symbols, the rectangle, represents a computer program to be written or purchased for the system (top rectangle). If the program already exists (in a library of common utilities and programs), it is depicted as shown in the margin (bottom rectangle).

Sometimes, you need to indicate that a person must perform a manual operation (for example, CORRECT INPUT ERRORS) before a processing sequence can be started or continued. A trapezoid is used to depict such a process. Inside the trapezoid you should record both the operation or task to be performed *and* the person who should perform that operation as shown in the margin.

The square is a less commonly used symbol that indicates an auxiliary operation performed by auxiliary data processing equipment that is not directly connected to the computer. Examples include punched card sorters, decollators, and magnetic ink character sorters. The name of the operation or the required device should be recorded in the square.

Batch Input Symbols Batch symbology should convey how source documents originate and how they are recorded to a computer-readable medium. As you learned in Chapter 13, most data originates on business source documents or forms. Once the data is recorded, a batch of documents are sent to data-entry clerks who transcribe the data from the forms into a computer-readable format. This operation is called *keying*. The most common media to which the data is keyed are punched cards, magnetic disk (key-to-disk or KTD), and magnetic tape (key-to-tape or KTT). These batch input operations are illustrated for you in the margin on the next page.

Punched cards (labeled a in the margin) are much less common today than they were several years ago. But when the ANSI standard was adopted, most batch input was done on punched cards and

Program Name (ID # Is Optional)

Utility or Library Program Name

Computer Program Symbols

Manual Operation and Who Does It

Manual Operation Symbol

Auxiliary Operation Name or Required Equipment

Auxiliary Operation Symbol

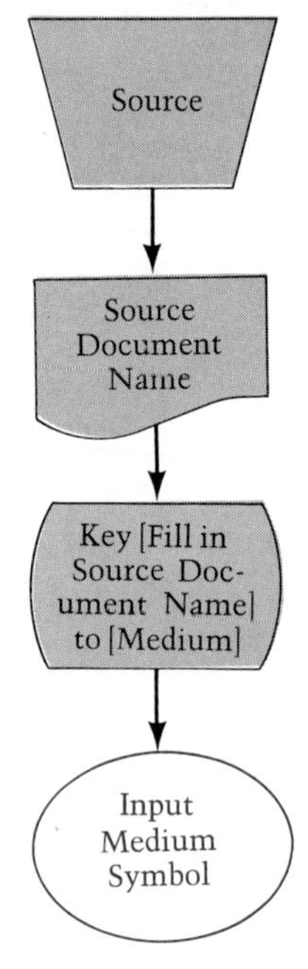

Data Capture

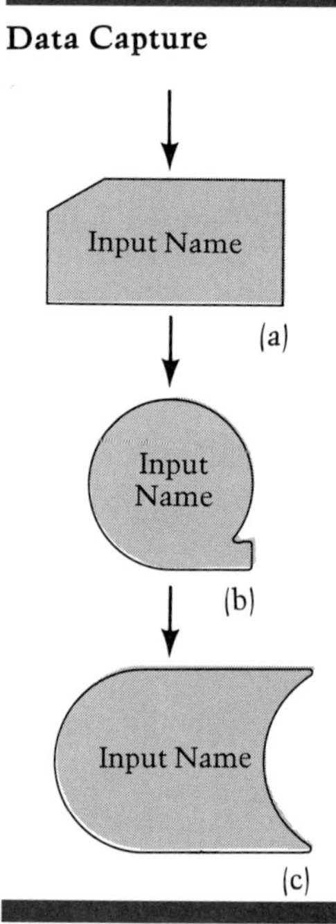

Input Medium Symbols

paper punch tape. Today, most batch input is done using key-to-tape and key-to-disk methods. We need to adopt a notation for these methods. We have tried several notations and settled on the simple notations illustrated in the margin. The keying symbol (from the preceding paragraph) represents the entire KTD or KTT system. The net output of that computer is the tape (labeled b for KTT) or disk (labeled c for KTD) file that will be read into the computer program.

There is one more input method that is not clearly defined in the ANSI standard, optical character recognition (OCR) or optical mark recognition (OMR). Because the input form is predefined, we suggest using the notation displayed in the margin on the next page. Notice that OCR and OMR forms can be directly read by the computer program (assuming you have the appropriate reader). OCR and OMR methods greatly simplify the data capture and data input procedures by eliminating the need for keying.

Batch and Scheduled Output Symbols The most common output is the printed report or form. Both were covered in Chapter 11. In all cases, the output is generated by a computer program (rectangle) and received by a person (trapezoid). Multiple copies of reports or forms are depicted as offsets of the same symbol. Each copy can have a separate destination, or all copies can go to the same destination.

If the output is to be produced on microfilm, auxiliary equipment will be necessary. Normally, the output is first written to tape. That tape is read by computer output microfilm (COM) equipment to produce the output. Once again, the ANSI standard doesn't offer a notation for this method. We suggest you use the notation depicted at the top of page 590.

File/Database Symbols Systems flowcharts show only those files and databases stored on the computer. Figure 15.10 illustrates tape file processing. Tape files may interface *only* with computer programs and auxiliary equipment; people, through manual operations (trapezoids), may not directly read or write tape files. The name of the file is recorded in the tape file symbol. Recall that tape files are automatically sequential files. The update of a sequential file requires that a new copy of that file be produced. The old copy is usually saved but eventually erased. The updated file is labeled *old* and *new* as illustrated in Figure 15.10.

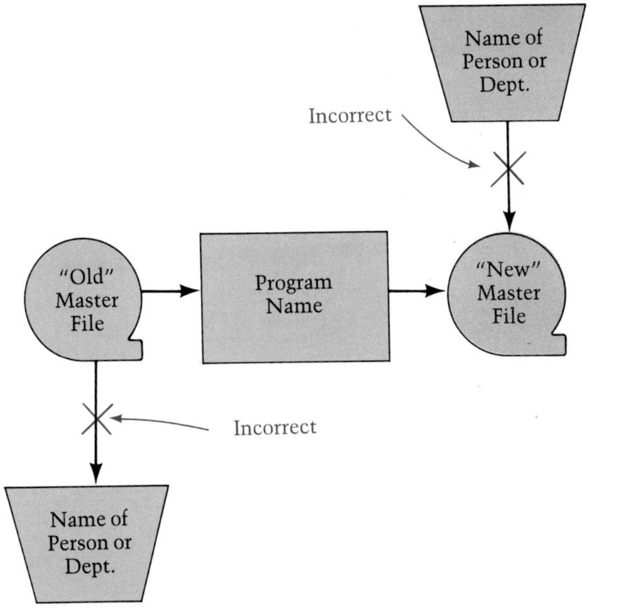

Figure 15.10

Tape file processing on systems flowcharts.

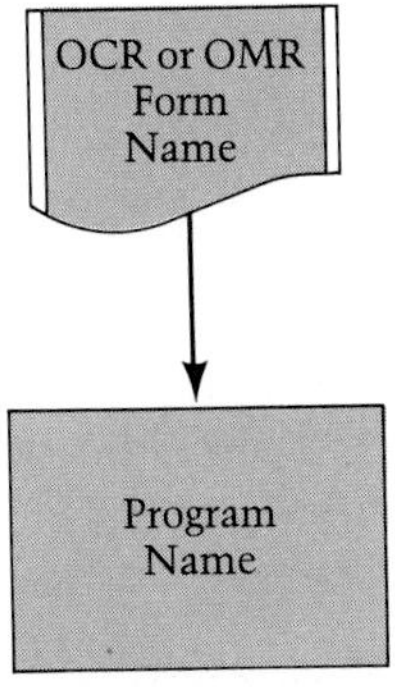

OCR and OMR Input Symbols

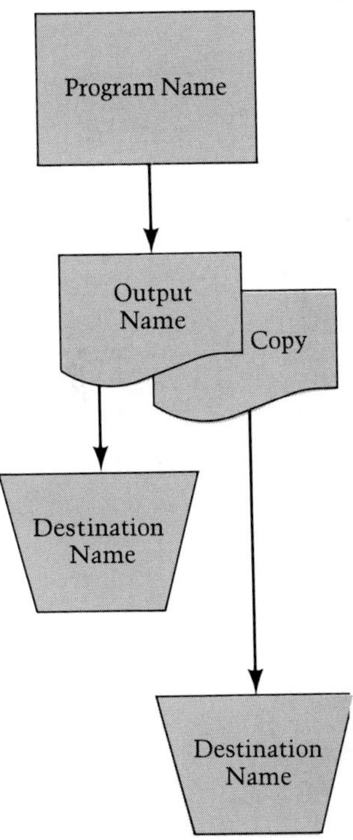

Printed Report (and Multicopy) Symbols

Disk devices can be used to store sequential, direct, and indexed files. Notice (at the top of the next page) that the arrow between the file and the program may be single-ended or double-ended. This indicates whether the program reads and uses the file or whether it reads and updates the file. As was the case with tape files, only computer programs may *read from* and *write to* disk files. Never use a manual operation (trapezoid) in place of the computer program (rectangle).

On-Line Symbology The symbology for showing on-line inputs and outputs can be somewhat tricky, so pay close attention. If we had to show every possible screen (Chapter 14) the systems flowchart would become very, very cluttered. Therefore, we adopt the DFD-like convention of showing only the *net* input and output operations for the on-line system. The ANSI standard has given us two symbols for on-line input and output. You should only use one of the two symbols with any given program. The choice depends on whether the *net* result of the given on-line program is input or output.

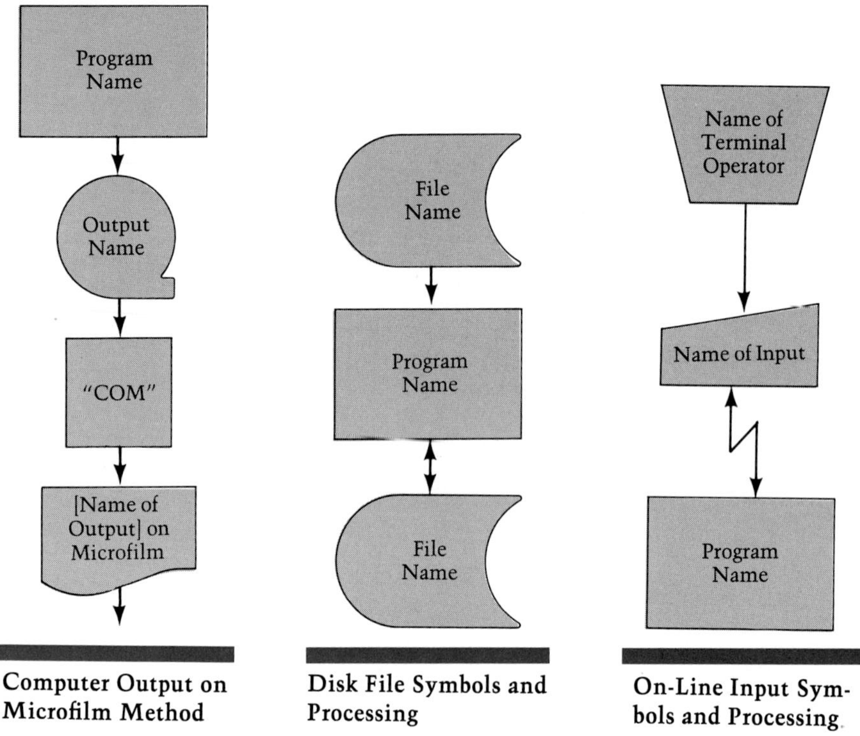

Computer Output on Microfilm Method

Disk File Symbols and Processing

On-Line Input Symbols and Processing

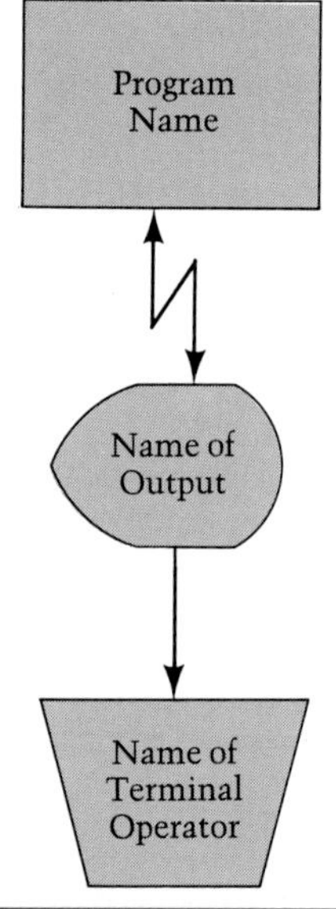

On-Line Output Symbols and Processing

A net input program is illustrated above. The authorized terminal operators are indicated by the trapezoid connected to a keyboard symbol. Notice the *ragged* communications line between the program symbol and the keyboard symbol. This double-ended arrow indicates on-line communications. It represents instructions and data from the user to the system as well as instructions and messages from the system to the user.

A net output subprogram is depicted in the left margin. Again, the authorized users are indicated by the trapezoid. And again, the double-ended-arrow communications line represents instructions, information, messages, and the like.

Now you may argue that you have programs that do both net input and net output, and so you need to show both symbols with a single program. Not typically! What you likely have are two separate on-line programs under the control of a master on-line control program, possibly driven by a menu. We recommend that you show the separate programs on systems flowcharts and use a hierarchy chart (Figure 15.11) to show that the programs are part of a single on-line system.

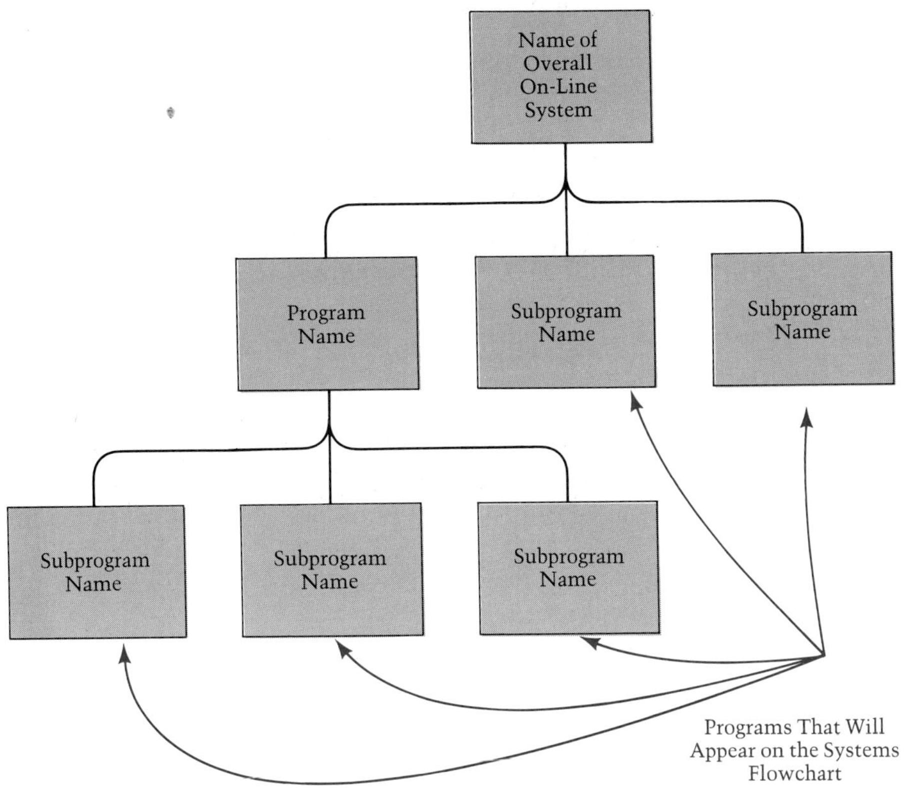

Figure 15.11

Hierarchy chart for an on-line program. Show each input and output subprogram of an on-line system in the systems flowcharts. Then use a hierarchy chart to show the relationships between these subprograms.

The trend toward distributed computing has also complicated the use of the ANSI standard. For instance, how do you show the uploading or downloading of data between files on different computers. We suggest using the notation shown in the margin. The ANSI communications arrow is used, but with only one arrow and only between file media. This is the way you would show a remote batch being transmitted to the main site. For distributed systems, a high-level systems flowchart (similar to the one shown in the margin) should be drawn to show the interface. Separate detailed systems flowcharts should be drawn for the applications performed on each computer. Modems, for telephone data communications, should be depicted using the auxiliary operation symbol (square).

Data Communications via Files

Miscellaneous Symbols There are a number of miscellaneous symbols in the ANSI standard. They can be useful for documenting aspects of methods and procedures not covered by the other symbols.

Perhaps the most important miscellaneous symbol is the *comment*, which is shown in the margin. The open-ended box is used to add any needed explanation to any other symbol on the chart. These explanations may describe security features, archiving instructions, timing, or any other important aspect of the procedure. We like to use *comments* to describe the schedule or trigger of a sequence of systems flowchart symbols (for instance, "every 4th Tuesday at 3:00 P.M." or "On demand, weekdays, 8 A.M. till 5 P.M.").

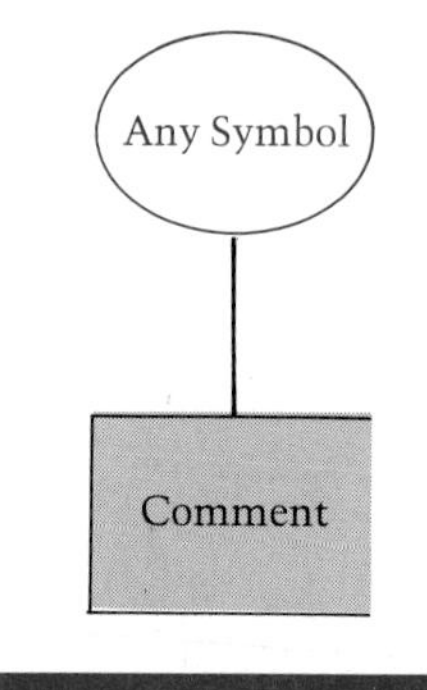

Comment Symbol

The *sort, merge,* and *extract* symbols shown in the margin are used to describe file operations. They require files as input and files as output. As a brief reminder, *sorting* is the sequencing of records in a single file. *Merging* is the sequencing of records from more than one file into a single file. These operations were much more common when tape master and transaction files were common. *Extracting,* still commonly used, is the selection of specific records from a larger file. The smaller file is usually used to produce reports and answer inquiries. Also, it is usually deleted after it has been used.

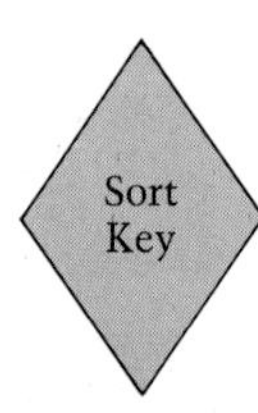

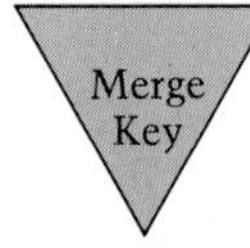

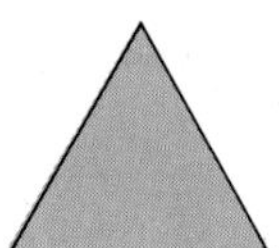

Extract Symbol (If necessary use comment symbol to describe extraction criteria.)

Sort, Merge, and Extract Symbols

Finally, the single-ended *arrow* on a systems flowchart indicates the flow of control from one step to another. Flow of control arrows, unlike data flow arrows on DFDs, *are not named!*

For your convenience, Figure 15.12 shows all of the systems flowchart symbols and their meanings.

How Systems Flowcharts Are Used

Let's take our usual look at how systems flowcharts fit into your pyramid model as a documentation tool. Unlike any other design tool we've covered, systems flowcharts document a wider spectrum of components in the IPO face of the pyramid (see margin on the next page). The principle value of systems flowcharts is to document data processing *methods and procedures* for the information system. And we've already surveyed the spectrum of possibilities for that component. But systems flowcharts, like data flow diagrams, also document *all* of the other IPO components:

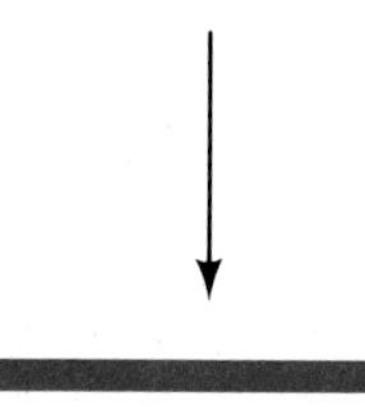

Flow of Control Symbol

Data and Information. Systems flowcharts show all of the source documents, reports, and inquiry responses that were initially documented on the data flow diagram. But whereas the DFD showed only net data flows, systems flowcharts show many other data flows that are added during the design process.

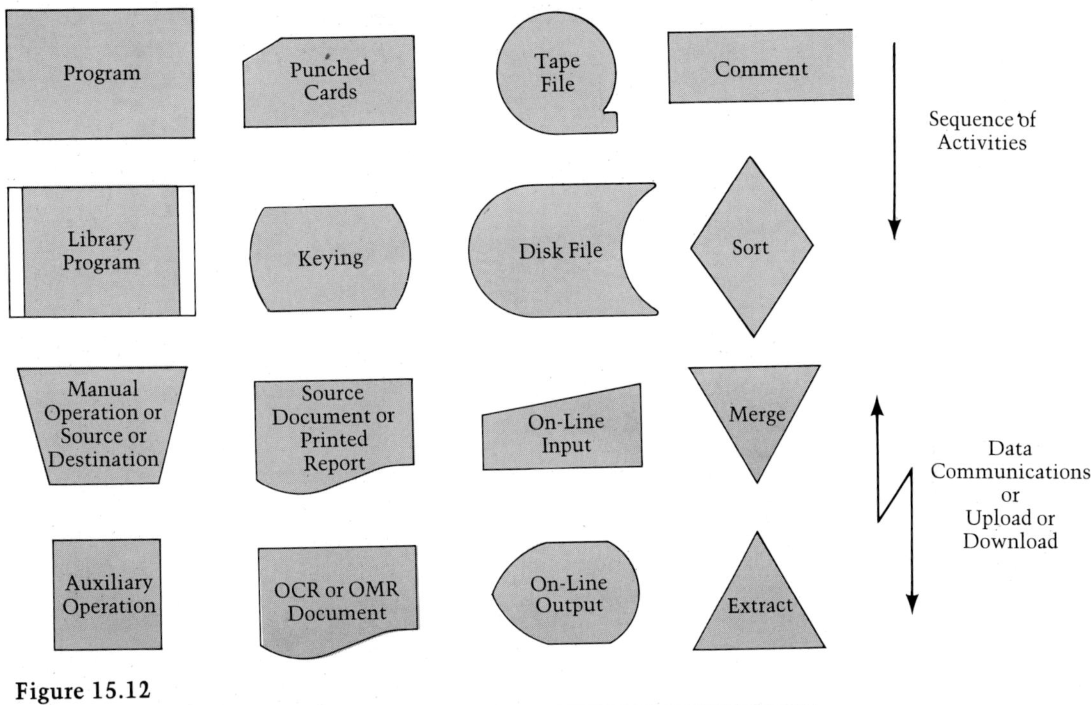

Figure 15.12

The systems flowchart symbols and their meanings.

For instance, edit reports, master file update inputs, historical reports, and batch control slips can be found on systems flowcharts but not on DFDs.

Knowledge Workers. Although systems flowcharts are not intended to show all manual activities performed by people in the system, the interfaces between specific people and the computerized components of the system are much more specific on the systems flowchart. DFDs showed only net input and output data flows—systems flowcharts show all data flows (as noted in the previous item).

Data Stores. Relative to the computerized part of an information system, DFDs show only files and databases that contain master file and transaction file data. Systems flowcharts, on the other hand, also show temporary or scratch files and audit trail files that are necessary for internal control.

Hardware and Software. Systems flowcharts use special symbols to indicate the types of hardware and software that will be

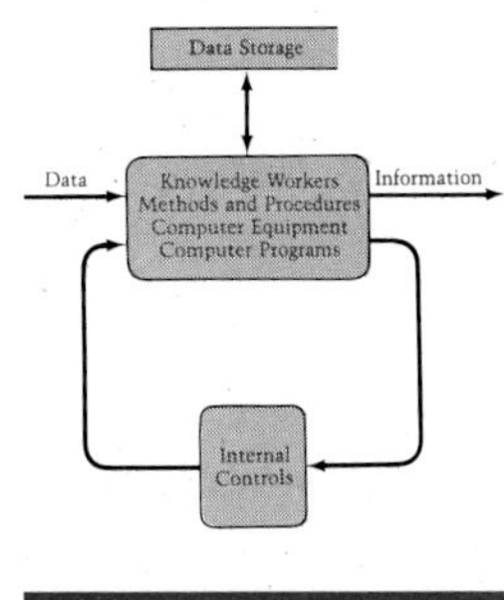

IPO Components

included in the system. Although *physical* DFDs can also do this to some degree, they are not nearly as clear!

Systems flowcharts cannot depict the level of detail we can accomplish with our data dictionaries and layout charts. But just as you used hierarchy charts as a pictorial outline for the data flow diagram, so you use systems flowcharts as pictorial outlines into your detailed input, output, file, and terminal dialogue specifications. Virtually every symbol on the systems flowchart points to a more detailed design specification of that component. If a symbol doesn't have accompanying detailed specifications, the design specifications are incomplete!

Drawing Systems Flowcharts

Systems flowcharts are not difficult to construct, especially if you follow the IPO concept. In this section, we will examine how systems flowcharts are used to document the design of batch and online methods and procedures of the AAP order-entry system. Because the inclusion of internal control features differentiates systems flowcharts from DFDs, we will pay particular attention to provisions for such controls.

Methods and Procedures for Batch Processing If you've been using data flow diagrams to define requirements, how do you shift gears to the systems flowchart? The complementary use of these tools is extremely valuable and not very difficult. Your objective is to transform a set of general requirements, expressed by the DFD, into a set of methods and procedures, expressed by systems flowcharts.

A bounded data flow diagram depicting a design solution for a subset of order processing at AAP is presented in Figure 15.13. You may recognize it as one of the logical DFDs from Chapter 7. Notice that only a portion of the subsystem is to be computerized. We will now document methods and procedures for the computerized processes in the BDFD.

Let's first document the batch transaction, CUSTOMER ORDER. How do we start flowcharting? In Figures 15.14 and 15.15

Figure 15.13 ▶

Bounded data flow diagram for AAP's order-entry subsystem. A bounded data flow diagram is a useful starting point for drawing detailed systems flowcharts. The BDFD conveys design decisions that have already been made. Of particular interest are data flows that cross the boundary (net computer inputs and outputs).

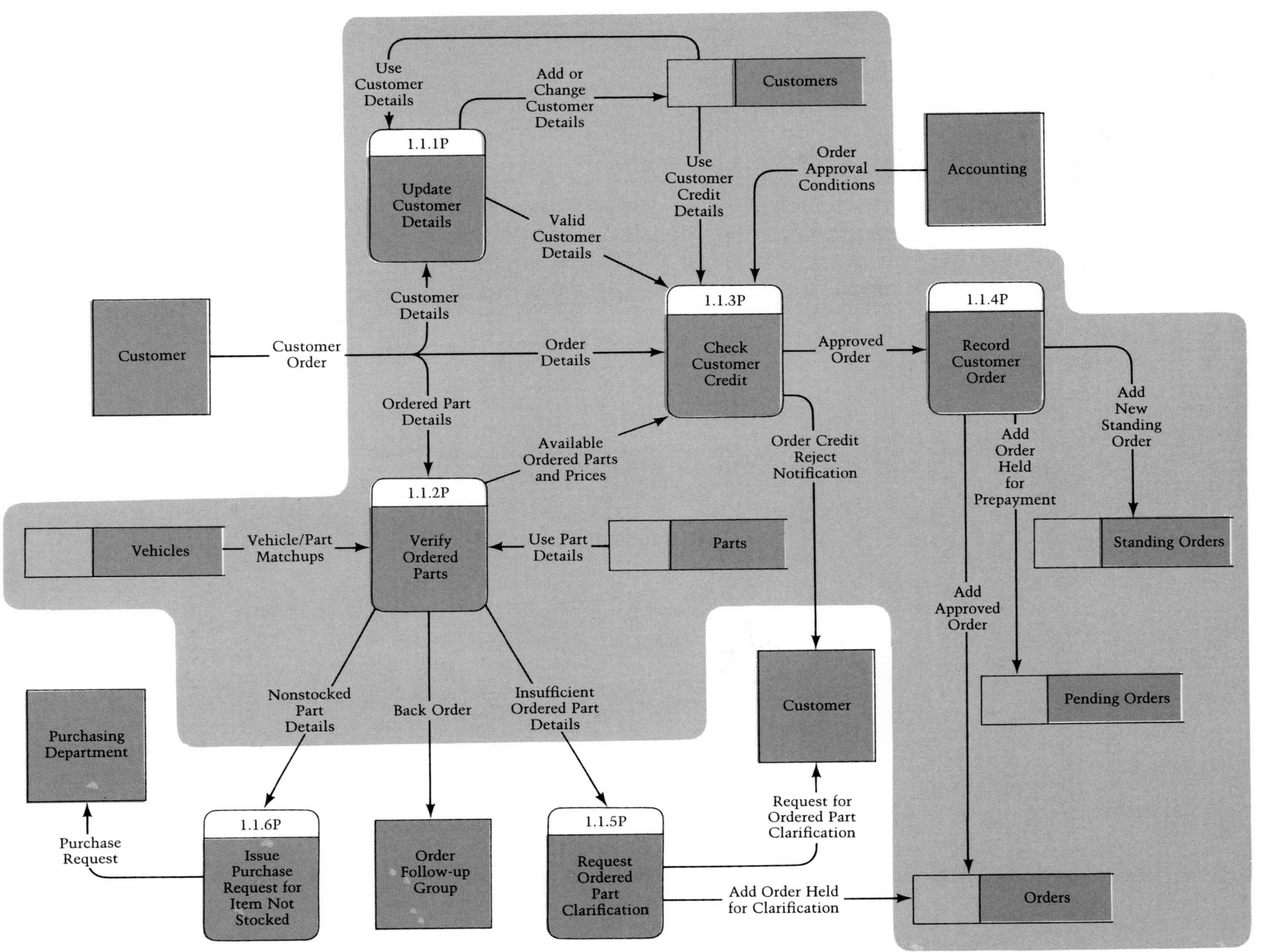

Use Customer Details
Add or Change Customer Details
Customers
1.1.1P
Update Customer Details
Use Customer Credit Details
Order Approval Conditions
Accounting
Valid Customer Details
Customer Details
Customer
Customer Order
Order Details
1.1.3P
Check Customer Credit
Approved Order
1.1.4P
Record Customer Order
Add New Standing Order
Ordered Part Details
Available Ordered Parts and Prices
Order Credit Reject Notification
Add Order Held for Prepayment
1.1.2P
Vehicles
Vehicle/Part Matchups
Verify Ordered Parts
Use Part Details
Parts
Standing Orders
Add Approved Order
Customer
Pending Orders
Nonstocked Part Details
Back Order
Insufficient Ordered Part Details
Purchasing Department
Request for Ordered Part Clarification
1.1.6P
Issue Purchase Request for Item Not Stocked
Purchase Request
Order Follow-up Group
1.1.5P
Request Ordered Part Clarification
Add Order Held for Clarification
Orders

Figure 15.14

Batch input methods and procedures for customer orders. This systems flowchart depicts the methods and procedures typically employed for batch inputs. Particularly common is the key/edit/correct loop. Not all batch systems require sorting (especially those that use disk for master and transaction files).

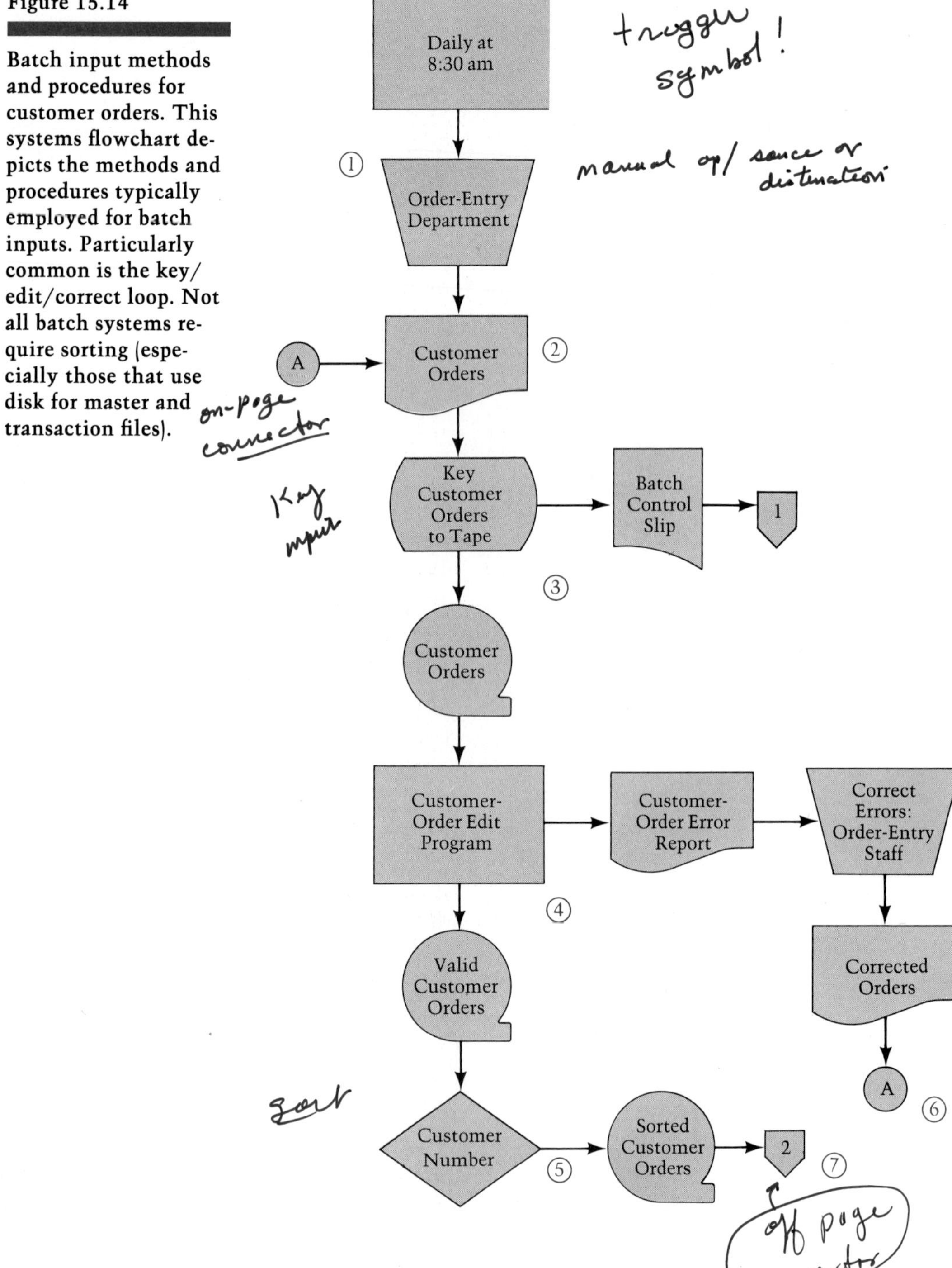

we see the systems flowchart for a batch version of PROCESS NEW ORDERS. Let's walk through the systems flowchart. Figure 15.14 illustrates the methods and procedures for batch input of customer orders (from Figure 15.13).

① A boundary (on the DFD) is the source of the net input data flow in Figure 15.13. That boundary becomes a manual operation (trapezoid) symbol on the system flowchart. Because customers can't directly deliver orders to data processing, we replaced them with their authorized representative, the ORDER-ENTRY GROUP.

② The data flow CUSTOMER ORDERS must initially be captured on a source document. For our batch system, each weekday morning the order-entry group delivers a batch of customer orders to the Data-Entry Department.

③ Because AAP's Data-Entry Department currently uses key-to-tape data entry, we have chosen that input method. Using the key-to-tape system, the Data-Entry Department will record the customer orders. Although many KTT workstations may be involved, the net result is a single tape that contains all sales orders to be processed that day. For internal control, the Data-Entry Department will also prepare a batch control slip. After customer orders have been processed, this slip will be compared with the historical report to ensure that all transactions were indeed processed.

④ The customer-orders tape from the key-to-tape system must be edited to detect keying errors made by the data-entry clerks. The CUSTOMER ORDER EDIT PROGRAM will check for these errors. Notice that this program was not depicted on the DFD. It was added here because the computerized system required internal controls to ensure valid input data. A CUSTOMER ORDER ERRORS REPORT will identify erroneous sales orders. This report will be used by the order-entry group to make corrections and resubmit corrected customer orders for rekeying. Valid orders are written to a new tape, VALID CUSTOMER ORDERS.

⑤ To improve processing efficiency, the customer orders are sorted by customer number. Notice that the field that is to serve as the sort key is recorded in the *sorting* symbol. The resulting (SORTED) CUSTOMER ORDERS can now be processed.

The Next Generation *Systems Flowcharts—Going, Going, Gone?*

In this box feature, you'll pardon us if we wax philosophical. It's hard for us to suggest the possible departure of an old friend. And systems flowcharts are an old friend. They've gotten us through a lot of information systems development projects. And they've received a lot of undeservedly bad publicity. At one time, systems flowcharts were the only popular tool the analyst had. What does the future hold for the next generation relative to methods and procedures? And what about systems flowcharts? In this chapter, we've suggested that systems flowcharts are not obsolete—that they are still useful for designing methods and procedures. And we believe that. But it saddens us to realize that systems flowcharts are finding their way into fewer and fewer books and methodologies. Some of us who have used them successfully will resist. But we may be fighting a losing battle.

You see, if we are totally honest, there is *nothing* that you can't document with systems flowcharts that couldn't be documented with *physical* data flow diagrams. The DFD is the new kid on the block. And with the current emphasis on structured tools and techniques, the trend is toward using new tools like DFDs and placing less emphasis on systems flowcharts (and, for that matter program flowcharts—pseudocode and fourth-generation techniques are the new, favored kids on that block). And we can understand the issue at hand. If we use DFDs for systems analysis, why switch tools during design, especially since it isn't really necessary. Using the PDFD conventions discussed in Chapter 7, you could draw any systems flowchart in Chapter 15. You could even use the top-to-bottom, left-to-right sequencing guidelines and the on- and off-page connectors to make them easy to read!

Advocates of a modular program design methodology called *Structured Design* have sometimes suggested that the new system's methods and procedures be specified only with data flow diagrams, not systems flowcharts. You see, Structured Design provides a formal technique for specifying the top-down modular structure of programs, working from the data flow diagrams for the system. However, Meiler Page-Jones, a leading expert on Structured Design, has clearly demonstrated the use of systems flowcharts within that methodology (Page-Jones, 1980).

Therefore, for the time being, the tools coexist. There are people out there who have never even heard of data flow diagrams. Others know what they are but are skeptical of their value. Or maybe they just haven't learned or used them. Systems flowcharts have a lot of friends in that crowd. But YOU are the next generation for systems design of methods and procedures. And most of you are being trained in the structured techniques. Consequently, you will eventually be the majority. As for our beloved systems flowcharts, we take comfort in the fact that someday a new tool will come along and probably obsolete the data flow diagram. But for the time being, you'll forgive those of us who put up a fight . . . R.I.P? ■

Time out! Let's study some of the mechanical guidelines we followed when drawing this systems flowchart. First, notice that the symbols occur in patterns of three — input-process-output. The output frequently becomes an input to the next process, thereby allowing the pattern to repeat itself. Next, notice that the flow proceeds from top to bottom and left to right. You can read the flowchart like a book. This simple guideline, suggested by many authors, could dispel the bad reputation systems flowcharts have received from users. This brings us to two new symbols that appear on our flowchart.

If we follow the last guideline, how can we indicate return to a previous step? Look again at Figure 15.14. The small circle with the letter *A* in it (labeled ⑥ on the figure) is used to indicate *return of control* to a previous step on the page. Note that we said *on the page!* The circle is called an *on-page connector.* It should only occur *in pairs* — on the same page of a systems flowchart. We used the on-page connector to illustrate the edit and corrections cycle on our systems flowchart.

What about situations in which we can't depict the entire sequence of events on one page? For example, what happens after VALID CUSTOMER ORDERS have been sorted? How is the BATCH CONTROL SLIP used later in the procedure? Just as we had an on-page connector, so we also have an *off-page connector.* Off-page connectors are demonstrated on Figures 15.14 and 15.15. The off-page connector in Figure 15.14 is labeled ⑦. The number inside the symbol on one page should match with the number in another off-page connector on another page. Make sure you don't violate the IPO pattern when you use on-page or off-page connectors. Neither connector symbol counts as an input, process, or output symbol.

All names and descriptions are written *inside* the symbols. Finally, all arrows are vertical, horizontal, or on a forty-five degree angle. Lines do not cross unless it is absolutely necessary. All of these conventions enhance the readability of the systems flowchart.

Now we can continue our example. What happens after the customer orders have been captured, keyed, edited, and sorted? For the answer, we can return to our DFD (Figure 15.13). We have to make a decision as to which processes will be consolidated into specific programs. We have two alternatives. We could treat each DFD process as a separate program. If so, we'd have to introduce temporary files (called *scratch files*) to pass data between the programs. Alternatively, we could group one or more processes into

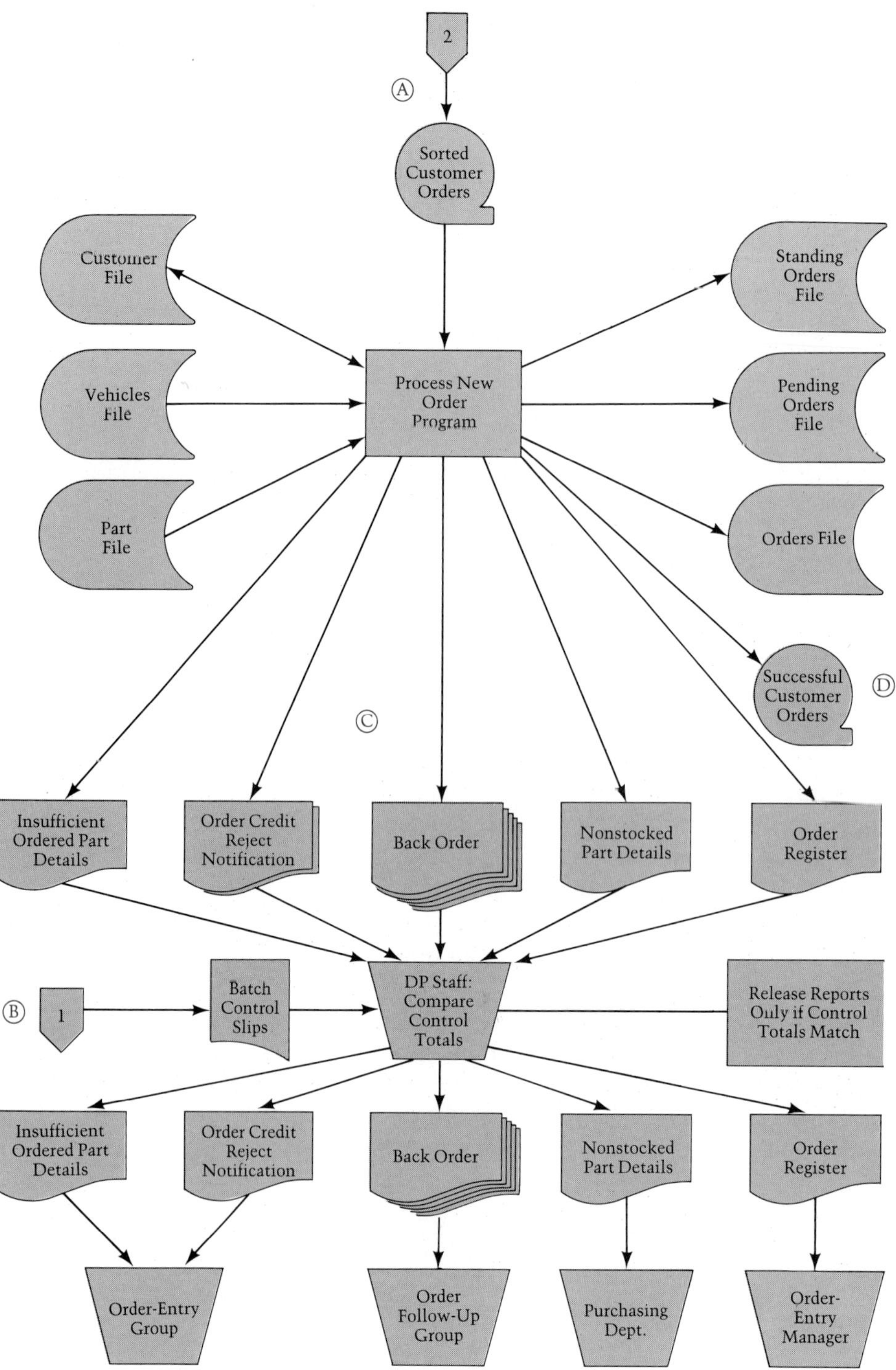
2
A
Sorted Customer Orders
Customer File
Vehicles File
Part File
Process New Order Program
Standing Orders File
Pending Orders File
Orders File
Successful Customer Orders
D
C
Insufficient Ordered Part Details
Order Credit Reject Notification
Back Order
Nonstocked Part Details
Order Register
B
1
Batch Control Slips
DP Staff: Compare Control Totals
Release Reports Only if Control Totals Match
Insufficient Ordered Part Details
Order Credit Reject Notification
Back Order
Nonstocked Part Details
Order Register
Order-Entry Group
Order Follow-Up Group
Purchasing Dept.
Order-Entry Manager

◄ **Figure 15.15**

Order processing with no limitations on number of files open to a program. This systems flowchart is a continuation of Figure 15.14. The program illustrated accomplishes all of the tasks documented inside the boundary of the DFD shown in Figure 15.13. This solution requires a computer system that allows a large number of files to be open at a single time.

separate programs. This would eliminate the need for scratch files. However, these more complex programs will have to have many more computer files open at one time.

For the sake of simplicity, let's first examine the consolidation of *all* of our DFD processes into a single program. Figure 15.15 presents this alternative. Note the following:

Ⓐ The off-page connector indicates a continuation of the input sequence depicted in the previous figure. Note that we duplicated the SORTED CUSTOMER ORDERS file for the sake of clarity. The program produces an ORDER REGISTER (a historical report) that reports transactions processed—another control feature we've added to the system.

Ⓑ Remember the BATCH CONTROL SLIP that was created for the input batch in Figure 15.14? It shows up again on this flowchart. The ORDER REGISTER is compared with the BATCH CONTROL SLIP to see if any transactions have been lost. The reports and documents that were printed are not distributed until the totals match.

Ⓒ How can so many reports be printed at one time? The answer is by spooling. The reports and documents are not printed at the same time. Output data for each report are spooled to a disk file. Reports are printed separately, when the printer becomes available and proper paper or forms is mounted.

Ⓓ All successfully processed customer orders were written to a tape file. This tape file is our *audit trail* for transactions. If, for any reason, any master file is lost or destroyed, we can reprocess lost transactions from this tape. We'll show this later in this section.

The systems flowchart in Figure 15.15 may not be technically feasible in some environments. Why? Because some computer systems restrict the number of files that can be used (open) by any one program. Suppose, for example, that our computer system allowed us to open only three files per program. We would have to change our procedures. In such a case, temporary or scratch files are intro-

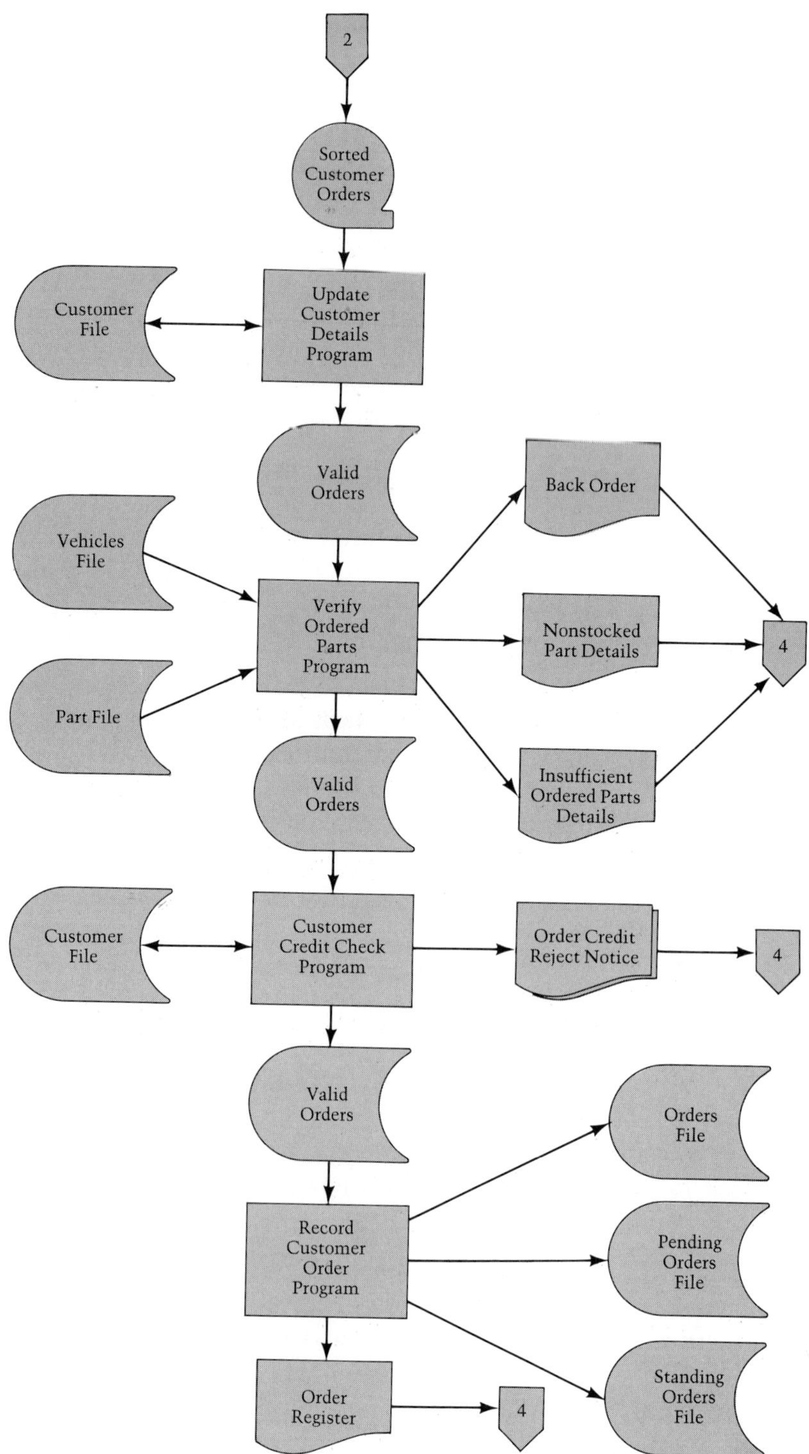
2
Sorted Customer Orders
Customer File
Update Customer Details Program
Valid Orders
Back Order
Vehicles File
Verify Ordered Parts Program
Nonstocked Part Details
4
Part File
Valid Orders
Insufficient Ordered Parts Details
Customer File
Customer Credit Check Program
Order Credit Reject Notice
4
Valid Orders
Orders File
Record Customer Order Program
Pending Orders File
Order Register
4
Standing Orders File

◄ **Figure 15.16**

Order processing using scratch files. This is a modification of Figure 15.15 to accommodate the fact that the number of files that can be open has been limited by the computer system. As a result, the single program from Figure 15.15 had to be factored into smaller programs that correspond to the original DFD tasks.

duced. A portion of the modified flowchart that would result is shown in Figure 15.16.

Methods and Procedures for On-Line Processing In Figure 15.17, we see the systems flowchart for an on-line version of processing orders. We call your attention to the following details:

Ⓐ In the on-line version, customer orders are processed immediately. The CUSTOMER ORDER form has been made optional because the Order-Entry Department will also accept orders via phone. An O/E clerk will input the sales order, via a CRT, to the PROCESS NEW ORDER PROGRAM. This program will edit the input data for errors and immediately notify the CRT operator of errors. Given a valid order, that order will be processed immediately. There is no need for the separate edit and correct cycle that we used for batch processing.

Ⓑ Note the comment indicating that the O/E Department users must have a security level of 2. The new system will have three security levels that may be assigned to users. Security level 1 will permit the user only to display reports and perform select inquiries. Users who are assigned security level 2 will be allowed to perform transaction processing and select inquiries. Finally, security level 3 permits the user to perform transaction processing, management reporting, all inquiries, and file maintenance.

Ⓒ Because the PROCESS NEW ORDER PROGRAM is available from 8:00 A.M. until 5:00 P.M., outputs will be continuously generated during that period. We can't afford to dedicate separate printers to generate each of the reports required during this period of time. Instead, reports will be dumped to a temporary file from which they will be printed, twice daily.

Ⓓ Internal controls are also very important for on-line systems. As was the case for the batch input system, we produced a historical report and backup file. But because transactions are processed on-line, over a long period of time, we couldn't dedi-

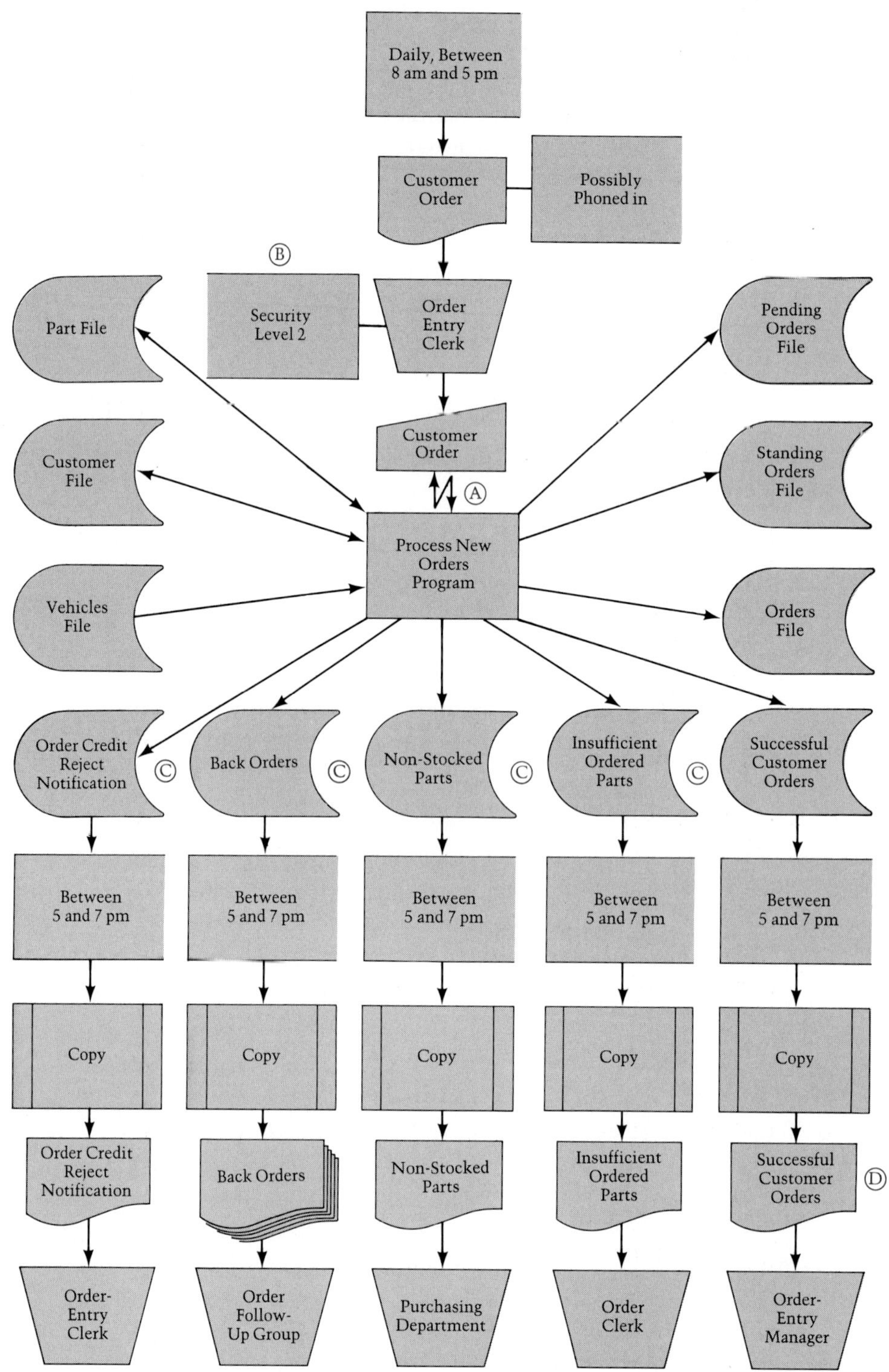

Daily, Between 8 am and 5 pm
Customer Order
Possibly Phoned in
B
Security Level 2
Order Entry Clerk
Part File
Customer File
Vehicles File
Customer Order
A
Process New Orders Program
Pending Orders File
Standing Orders File
Orders File
Order Credit Reject Notification
C
Back Orders
C
Non-Stocked Parts
C
Insufficient Ordered Parts
C
Successful Customer Orders
Between 5 and 7 pm
Between 5 and 7 pm
Between 5 and 7 pm
Between 5 and 7 pm
Between 5 and 7 pm
Copy
Copy
Copy
Copy
Copy
Order Credit Reject Notification
Back Orders
Non-Stocked Parts
Insufficient Ordered Parts
Successful Customer Orders
D
Order-Entry Clerk
Order Follow-Up Group
Purchasing Department
Order Clerk
Order-Entry Manager

◀ **Figure 15.17**

Customer-order processing in an on-line system. This is an on-line version of the customer-order processing subsystem. The program handles all the processing requirements that were depicted on the BDFD as well as the input editing requirements. As a side note, the order-processing program may be a subprogram in a hierarchy chart that depicts the structure of a complex on-line system.

cate a printer or tape drive to record the successful transactions. Instead, we record all successful transactions to an on-line file, SUCCESSFUL CUSTOMER ORDERS. Once each day, we copy the SUCCESSFUL CUSTOMER ORDERS file to an off-line medium (tape), and from that we produce our historical report, ORDER REGISTER.

What about on-line outputs? The AAP order-entry system allows users to inquire against files. One of the inquiries was about AAP parts. The systems flowchart in Figure 15.18 shows that the Order-Entry and Marketing Departments are allowed access to the QUERY PART PROGRAM. The program prompts the user for a PART NUMBER (a search key), retrieves part information from one of three files, and displays the information on the CRT. If the user wants to get a printout, the dialogue permits the user to request a printed copy. The output is generated as shown. However, the comment specifies that the printed copy of the output PART QUERY RESPONSE will not be available until the next morning (overnight printing).

Methods and Procedures for Scheduled Outputs Recall that management reports are typically scheduled in both batch and on-line systems. The systems flowchart for a typical scheduled report is shown in Figure 15.19. The data are retrieved from the files, and the report is produced and distributed. Remember, some systems may limit the number of files that can be open to a program. If so, the program may be split into separate programs. The first program would extract data from one file, creating a scratch file. The second program uses the scratch file plus other files to create the report.

Methods and Procedures for Maintenance, Backup, and Recovery of Files Transaction files are maintained by transaction-processing programs. Similar programs must be designed to maintain the master files in the system (for instance, CUSTOMER ACCOUNT and INVENTORY). These programs are similar to other transaction-processing programs except they only create, delete, and modify

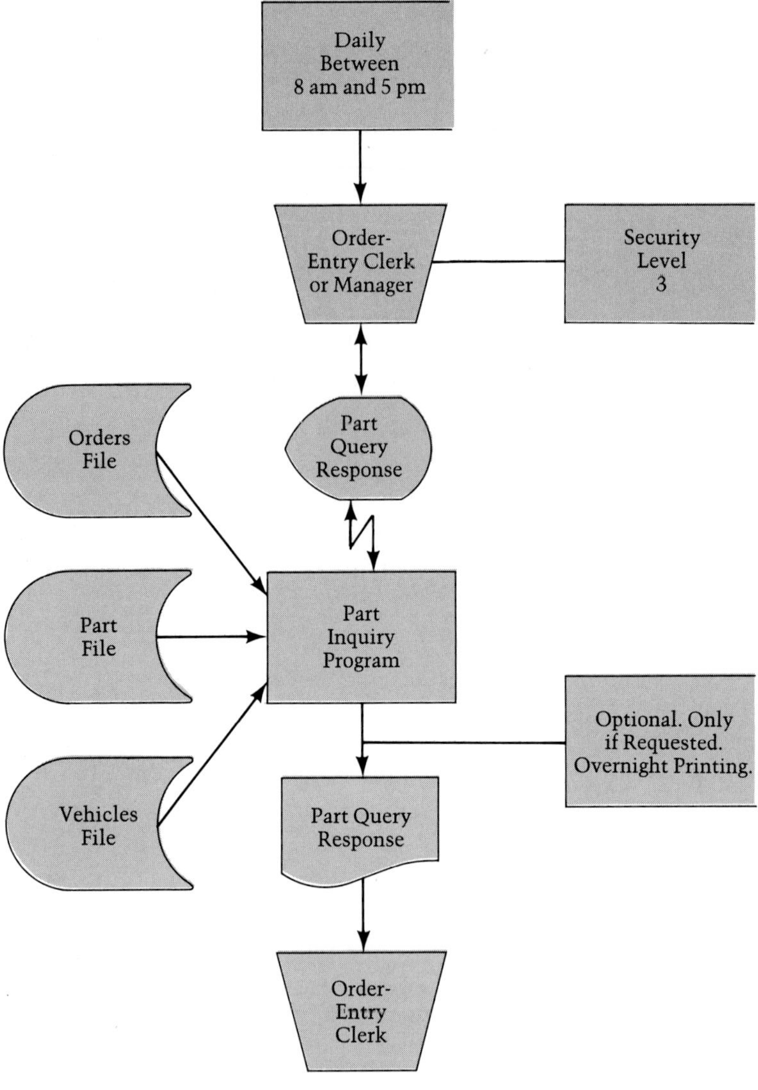

Figure 15.18

Systems flowchart for an on-line inquiry. The systems flowchart for an inquiry is relatively simple, as you can see.

records in the master file. These requirements are normally excluded from DFDs (which tend to document the net input and output activities). However, they cannot be excluded from systems flowcharts. If the file isn't created and maintained, it can't be used and updated.

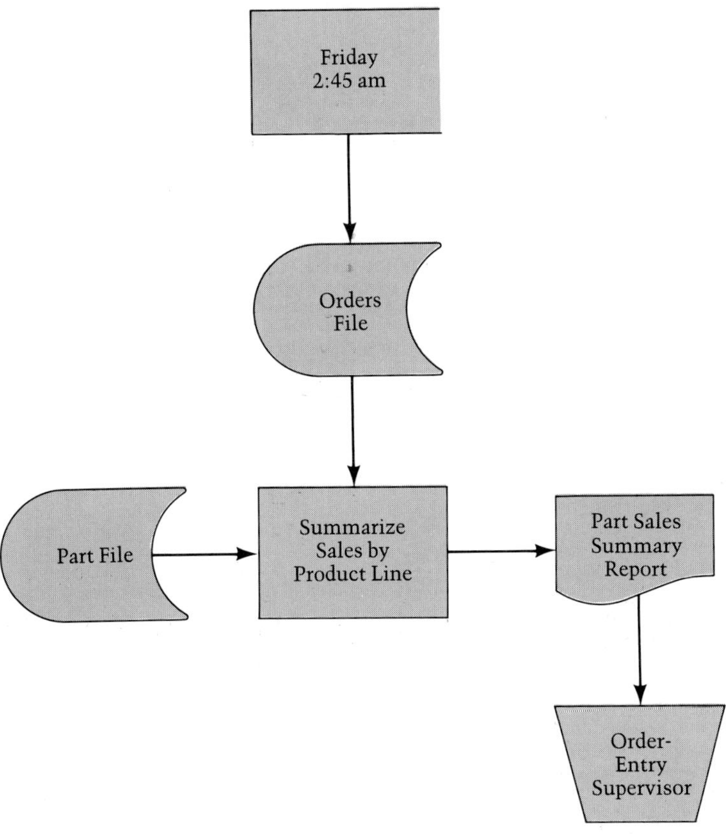

Figure 15.19

Scheduled report procedures. Management reports are usually generated on a scheduled basis in *both* batch and on-line systems. The flowcharts are straightforward.

Earlier in this chapter, you learned that one of the most important tasks in documenting the methods and procedures for a system is the inclusion of backup and recovery procedures. Let's think back. In documenting the batch and on-line versions of PROCESS NEW ORDER we made sure to generate audit files for archiving the successfully processed customer orders. Suppose we lose a master or transaction file. What will we do?

A systems flowchart to back up and, if necessary, recover the CUSTOMER master file is shown in Figure 15.20. To recover the lost file, we recreate the CUSTOMER FILE from the last backup

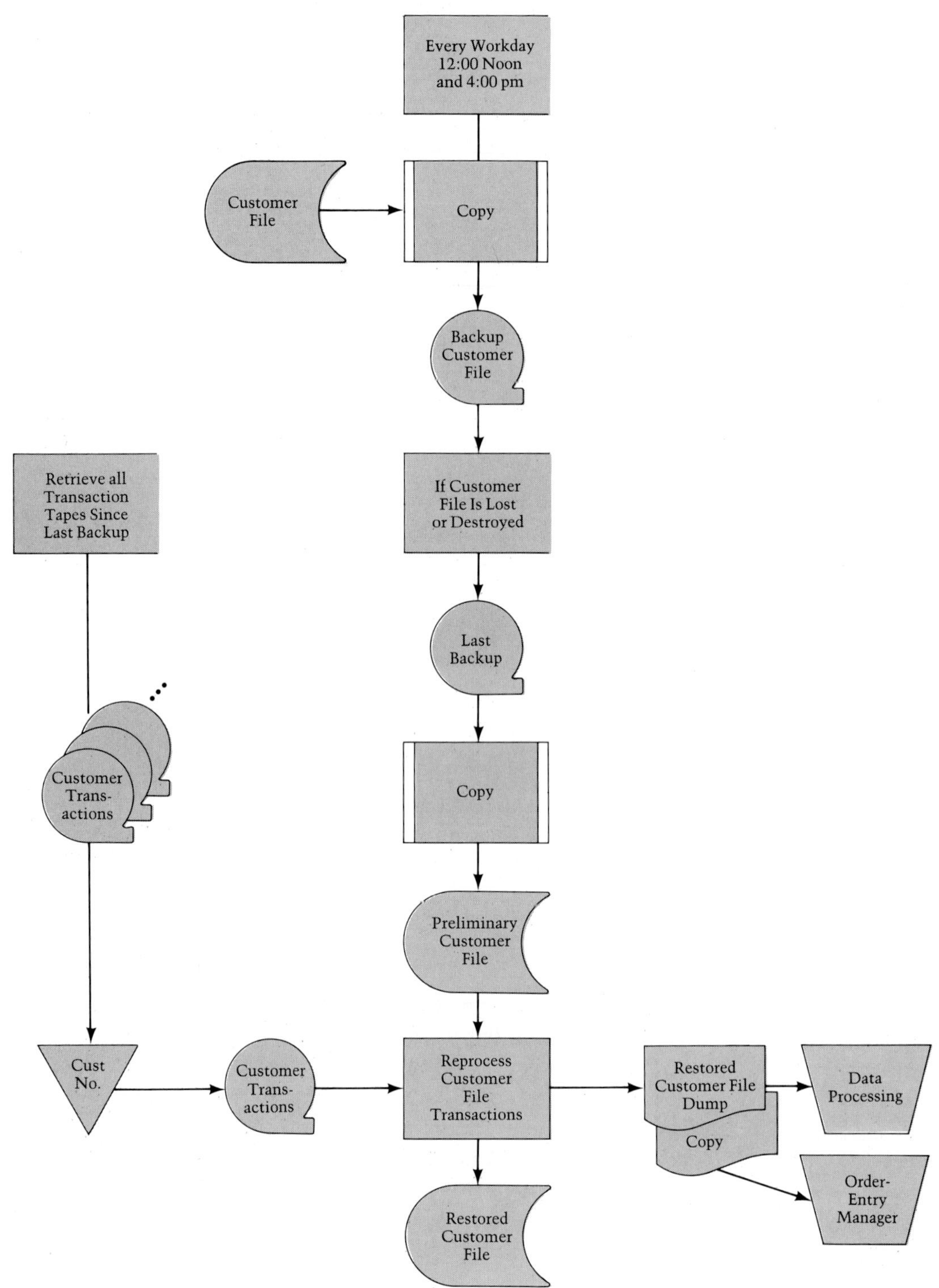

Every Workday
12:00 Noon
and 4:00 pm
Customer
File
Copy
Backup
Customer
File
Retrieve all
Transaction
Tapes Since
Last Backup
If Customer
File Is Lost
or Destroyed
Last
Backup
Customer
Trans-
actions
Copy
Preliminary
Customer
File
Cust
No.
Customer
Trans-
actions
Reprocess
Customer
File
Transactions
Restored
Customer File
Dump
Copy
Data
Processing
Order-
Entry
Manager
Restored
Customer
File

◀ Figure 15.20

Backup and recovery procedures. This is a typical flowchart for a backup and recovery procedure. Once again, the systems flowchart is relatively straightforward.

copy. Because this backup occurs weekly, to fully restore this file, we only need to reprocess those transactions that have taken place since the last backup. Similar backup and recovery procedures must be designed for every master and transaction file in the system.

SUMMARY

Methods and procedures define the sequence of events that produce outputs from inputs in a computer-based information system. A method is a way of doing something. Procedures are step-by-step plans for implementing a method. Data processing methods can be classified on two scales: degree of centralized or distributed processing and degree of batch or on-line processing.

In the not-too-distant past, all processing was centralized; that is, it was performed on the central computer. Today, the analyst must consider the possibility of distributed processing. In distributed processing, the workload is offloaded to satellite computer systems. But, because data may be needed in multiple locations, we consider linking the satellite computers into some form of network. There are several network architectures including *point-to-point networks, bus networks, star networks, hierarchical networks,* and *ring networks.* The analyst needs to be familiar with available networks and with the possibilities each network presents for distributed processing.

Batch processing and on-line processing alternatives are generally well known to most students and professionals. However, these two alternatives present the systems analyst with different requirements for internal control in systems. Internal controls must be documented in the methods and procedures for any system.

Systems flowcharts are a graphical tool used to depict methods and procedures. Although there is a national standard for systems flowchart symbols (ANSI), it is somewhat dated. Therefore, like us, you need to adopt your own departmental standards for drawing and using systems flowcharts. This chapter has presented suggestions for expanding the ANSI standard.

PROBLEMS AND EXERCISES

1. Explain the difference between batch, on-line, remote batch, and distributed methods of data processing. Define an input, and conceive a situation that might call for each of the three methods to be used.
2. Describe five different strategies for distributed processing. Make an appointment to visit a local data processing installation (alternative — study a case study in a distributed processing, network, or data communications textbook). Are they using microcomputers? If so, what networking strategy are they using or planning? If they aren't planning a network, find out why. There may be very good reasons. What data communications problems and issues are they concerned with at this time? What do they think will happen?
3. Draw a systems flowchart to depict the following methods and procedures:
   (a) Each morning, Monday through Friday, at 7:45, a program is executed to read the inventory file to identify products that are low in stock. A report is produced and delivered to the inventory purchasing clerk.
   (b) Customers visiting a small computer sales store frequently request price quotes at a computer terminal. A salesman at the store will execute a quote recording program. The program accepts data concerning the quote and checks an inventory file for availability, current prices, and other product data needed to respond to the quote. The quote is then calculated and placed in a quote file (ISAM). A hard copy of the quote is generated for the customer and salesman.
   (c) The Accounts Receivable Department fields phone calls from customers concerning disputes over invoices. Accounts Receivable uses a terminal to obtain information needed to resolve these disputes. An accounts receivable clerk may request information concerning a customer's account or an invoice.

   You may expand on these general descriptions as you desire.

4. A magazine publishing company receives magazine subscriptions through the mail. Subscriptions are routed to the Data-Entry Department for batch input. The resulting input tape (sorted by subscription number) is read by a program that updates a customer and subscription file. The program also produces a daily subscription register. Totals appearing on the register are compared with totals on a batch control slip. If the totals don't match, the discrepancies are resolved. Otherwise, the register is delivered to the Order-Entry Department supervisor. Prepare a systems flowchart that describes the methods and procedures previously described. Be sure the batch input procedures allow for complete editing and correction of subscriptions.

5. Prepare a systems flowchart to describe the backup and recovery procedures for the subscription file discussed in problem 4.

6. An on-line computer program is to input transactions, update two master files, and print five reports (including an external document). What are the implications of printing so many reports? What alternative procedures could be followed? Draw a systems flowchart for each alternative procedure.

7. How many computer files, including basic input and output files, does your computer system allow to be open at one time? What are the implications for design of methods and procedures? Draw general systems flowcharts to show how you would deal with a program that requires more files than can be open at one time.

8. What other symbols can be connected to the following symbols on a systems flowchart:
   (a) Computer program (rectangle)
   (b) Sort (diamond)
   (c) Source document or printed report
   (d) On-line input or keyboard
   (e) On-line output or screen
   (f) Data communications or upload or download arrow
   (g) Manual operation (trapezoid)
   (h) Disk file
   (i) Tape file
   (j) Extract (triangle)

9. A bounded data flow diagram indicates the computerized portion for system. The BDFD and the decisions made during output, file, and input design together aid in the construction of

systems flowcharts. However, it is quite common during fact-finding in the study phase to find systems flowcharts of an existing computerized system. The analyst may wish to convert the systems flowcharts into data flow diagrams to aid in verifying the system with data processing and (more importantly) users. Explain how systems flowcharts could easily be converted to data flow diagrams.

ANNOTATED REFERENCES AND SUGGESTED READINGS

Brill, Alan E. *Building Controls into Structured Systems.* New York: Yourdon Press, 1983. This book provides a comprehensive look at internal controls design, especially when using structured tools, such as data flow diagrams. The material covered is equally applicable when not using structured tools. This book is short and relatively easy to comprehend.

Fitzgerald, Jerry. *Internal Controls for Computerized Information Systems.* Redwood City, Calif.: Jerry Fitzgerald and Associates, 1978. This is our reference standard on the subject of internal controls. Jerry teaches a powerful matrix approach to designing internal controls.

Page-Jones, Meiler. *The Practical Guide to Structured Systems Design.* New York: Yourdon Press, 1980. The primary emphasis of this book is program design, not systems flowcharting. However, for those of you familiar with the Structured Systems Design methodology, Page-Jones shows that systems flowcharts and structure charts are not mutually exclusive. Structured systems design is introduced in the next chapter of this textbook.

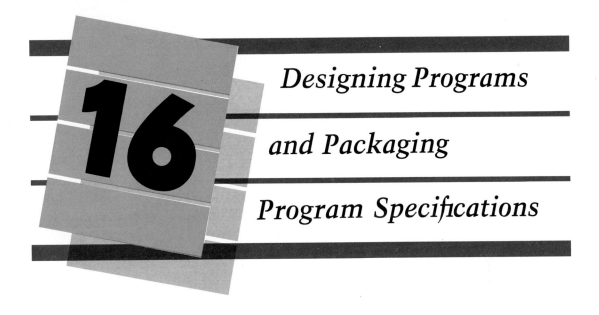

Minicase: Hayes Vending, Inc.

Richard Huffman, a programmer/analyst for Hayes Vending, Inc., a distribution center for vending machines in midnorthern Louisiana, had just sat down to lunch. Tom Ewing, senior partner in the firm, joined him.

Tom Hi, Dick! Long time, no see. What are you up to these days?

Dick Honestly? I'm frustrated! I had to take over the sales information system project that Judy left behind when she quit.

Tom I thought that thing was almost finished.

Dick Me too. But she didn't finish all of the programs.

Tom But she did do a good job of specifying all the required inputs and outputs. What's so tough about the programs?

Judy always preached about the benefits of structured programming. In fact, she taught me how to do it. Don't tell me she doesn't practice what she preaches!

Dick No, her code is very well structured. And her documentation is adequate. It's just that the programs seem so poorly designed.

Tom I realize I'm just a hacker, but what do you mean by 'poorly designed?'

Dick I don't know, exactly. Some of her subroutines are so long and complex that it's difficult to get a grasp on small enough pieces to test them for correctness. It seems like an all-or-nothing proposition. If I encounter a bug, I have to test large sections of code to zero in on the problem. Sometimes, the bug turns out to be in an entirely different subroutine!

Tom I guess I'm too used to small programs. Why didn't Judy break the system into smaller pieces?

Dick She did! The subroutines are evidence of that. But it almost seems like she generated the subroutines on the fly—as if to say, "Well, this piece of code is getting complex. I'd better put in a subroutine to finish it." She left me a rough draft of a structure chart, but I just don't understand the reasons she factored the system the way she did.

Tom That's the way I write programs. I start by trying to draw a flowchart on a single page—sort of the high-level flowchart. Then I factor the more complex processes into more detailed processes that I implement as subroutines. It sounds like that may be what Judy did.

Dick Maybe she did. But that strategy causes the lower-level subroutines to be very dependent on other routines. I frequently encounter bugs that get traced back to other seemingly unrelated routines. I'm just getting further behind schedule. I may just have to write the programs from scratch.

Tom Why don't you get some help. Rosemary just finished her project. Maybe she can help you. You could divide up the work and get it done faster.

Dick Divide up the work? I don't see how. Judy's program specifications are just one big document. I'm not completely sure which file and report specifications to match up to which modules. For that matter, I'm not sure the programs themselves are fully documented.

Tom I don't know what to tell you, Dick.

Discussion

1. If design specifications are thorough and complete and program code is well structured, how can the system still be difficult to construct?
2. How should subroutines in a program be conceived? How does Judy seem to have created them? What is the potential problem with creating subroutines on the fly (either during coding or during flowcharting)?
3. What effect does program and subroutine size have on testing?
4. What would Rosemary require in order to take on responsibility for some of the programs that haven't been written? What does any programmer need to be able to write a new program? How would you organize the necessary documentation of program requirements?

WHAT WILL YOU LEARN IN THIS CHAPTER?

In this chapter, you will learn how to design good programs. You will also learn how to package program design specifications. You will know that you understand how to design programs and package design specifications into a format suitable for programmers when you can:

1. Factor a program into manageable program modules around which complete specifications can be organized.
2. Use the IPO model to characterize the programmer's specification needs.
3. Associate each design documentation form presented in Part III of this book with the input, process, or output components of a computer program.

4. Determine which programs on a systems flowchart require detailed packaging.
5. Use structure charts and IPO charts to package a computer program and its specifications.

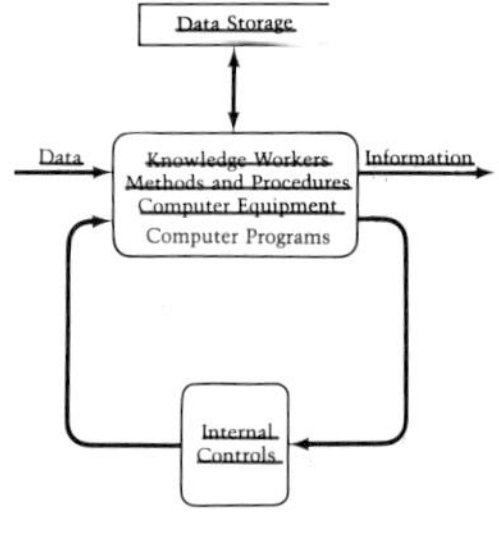

IPO Components

We're nearly finished with systems design. You've designed the inputs, outputs, files, terminal dialogue, methods, procedures, and controls. You've selected appropriate computer equipment and packaged software (which has hopefully been delivered and installed during systems design). What's left? As the title of this chapter suggests, program design and packaging. Computer programs are one of the fundamental components in your information system model (see margin).

Let's make sure you understand what we mean by program design and packaging. From your programming courses, you may think of program design as *algorithm* or *logic* design. That is NOT the subject of this chapter. We don't intend to reteach you how to draw structured program flowcharts, pseudocode, or construct box charts (sometimes called Nassi-Schneidermann charts). In our minds, that is clearly a subject for a programming textbook. Instead, we are concerned with how the programming specifications are presented to the computer programmer for implementation. To this end, we view program design as consisting of two components:

- *Modular design*—the decomposition of a program into manageable pieces.
- *Packaging*—the assembly of input, output, file, terminal dialogue, and processing specifications for each module.

The inclusion of this chapter is certain to be controversial. Rather than side-step the controversy, let's openly discuss it before we go on. Some readers are likely to interpret the material covered in this chapter as an invasion of the programmer's turf. It really varies from one data processing shop to another. Some shops insist that the analyst prepare detailed modular designs and program specifications (at a level close to pseudocode). Other shops believe that the analyst's job ends with general programming specifications, leaving modular design to the programmer. Depending on your opinion, you may want to omit this chapter. However, we recommend the chapter for the following reasons:

- Your career may take you to organizations or management that prefer each of the two opinions.
- The chapter helps tie the design specifications prepared in Chapters 11 through 15 to the program specifications that normally initiate the construction phase (discussed in detail in Chapter 17).
- In the absence of a company standard, you may want to consider a rigorous, personal standard for presenting specifications. Why? In Chapter 17, you will learn that the analyst is frequently engaged in a large number of activities during systems implementation. The more thorough and complete your programming specifications are, the less time you'll have to spend clarifying those specifications to the programmer. We can tell you from experience, that most program specifications are not this detailed and that the analyst wastes considerable time clarifying them and the programmer wastes considerable time redoing programs for which the specifications were misunderstood.

MODULAR DESIGN OF COMPUTER PROGRAMS

For those of you not familiar with modular design from your programming courses, we'll briefly review the concept. Large projects are most easily managed if they are broken into smaller pieces. You've seen us apply this concept with data flow diagrams. Computer programs can be similarly decomposed as depicted in Figure 16.1. What we did here was to recursively factor a large program into smaller and smaller pieces called modules. We will now study how this is accomplished.

Modular Decomposition of Programs

What is a module? It could be a subroutine or subprogram. And it could be a main program. On the other hand, it could be a unit of measure smaller than any of those. For instance, a module could be a PARAGRAPH in a COBOL program. So, what is a module? We will define a **module** as a group of executable instructions with a single point of entry and a single point of exit. Some modules exist to perform single functions. These include READ A RECORD, EDIT

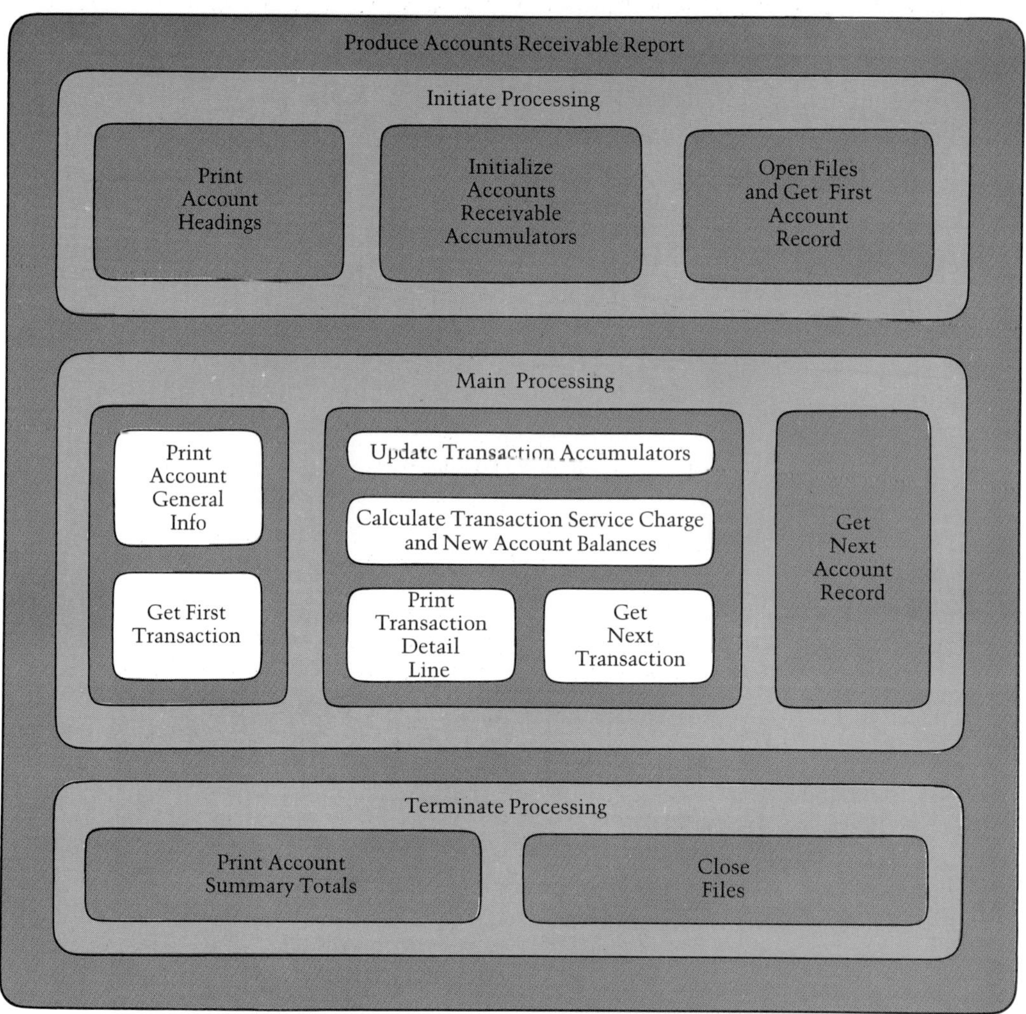

Figure 16.1

Modular design. This diagram is a useful way to depict the modular design approach, otherwise known as *Divide and Conquer.*

A RECORD, CALCULATE PAY, and ADD A RECORD TO A FILE, to name a few. Other modules exist to *supervise* or *drive* the function modules.

The length of a module is important. Evidence suggests that modules should consist of a relatively limited number of lines of executable instructions. Most experts suggest a number between twenty-four lines (the most typical display screen size) and sixty (the number of lines printed on an average page). Consequently, this guideline would suggest that any program that cannot be written in fewer than sixty lines of code should be decomposed into modules.

Tools for Modular Design There are two popular tools for depicting the modular design of programs. We'll use the simple example provided in Figure 16.1 to introduce these tools. The first tool we'll introduce is the Warnier/Orr bracket (see Figure 16.2). A **Warnier/Orr diagram** is nothing more than a hierarchy chart laid on its side. For this discussion, we want to focus on the tool itself, deferring our discussion of the Warnier/Orr methodology until the next section.

Brackets decompose modules into other lower-level modules that we'll call *submodules.* The Warnier/Orr diagram implies a sequence of execution that is read from top to bottom and left to right. A number in parentheses below a module indicates how many times that module executes (a *looping* concept). A plus sign between modules indicates that execution of those modules is mutually exclusive. In other words, each single execution of the calling module may call one or the other submodule (never both). Although we haven't seen it, a notation could easily be defined, say with an asterisk, to indicate that a module can call either or both submodules.

An alternative and somewhat more familiar tool is the structure chart. A **structure chart** (see Figure 16.3) is a treelike diagram. (We are purposely avoiding the term *hierarchy chart* so as not to confuse this chapter's use of the structure with that introduced in Chapter 7, Data Flow Diagrams.) Structure charts, by whatever other name you might know them, may be familiar to you from your introductory programming course.

Structure chart modules are depicted by rectangles. Modules are factored, from the top down, into submodules. Structure chart modules are presumed to execute in a top-to-bottom, left-to-right sequence. Structure charts can also illustrate looping (via the ringlike arrow).

We find Warnier/Orr diagrams easier to construct than structure charts (no need for a template). But structure charts are more familiar in the literature. Because it is more likely that you've encountered structure charts in your introductory programming course, we will use that notation throughout the remainder of this

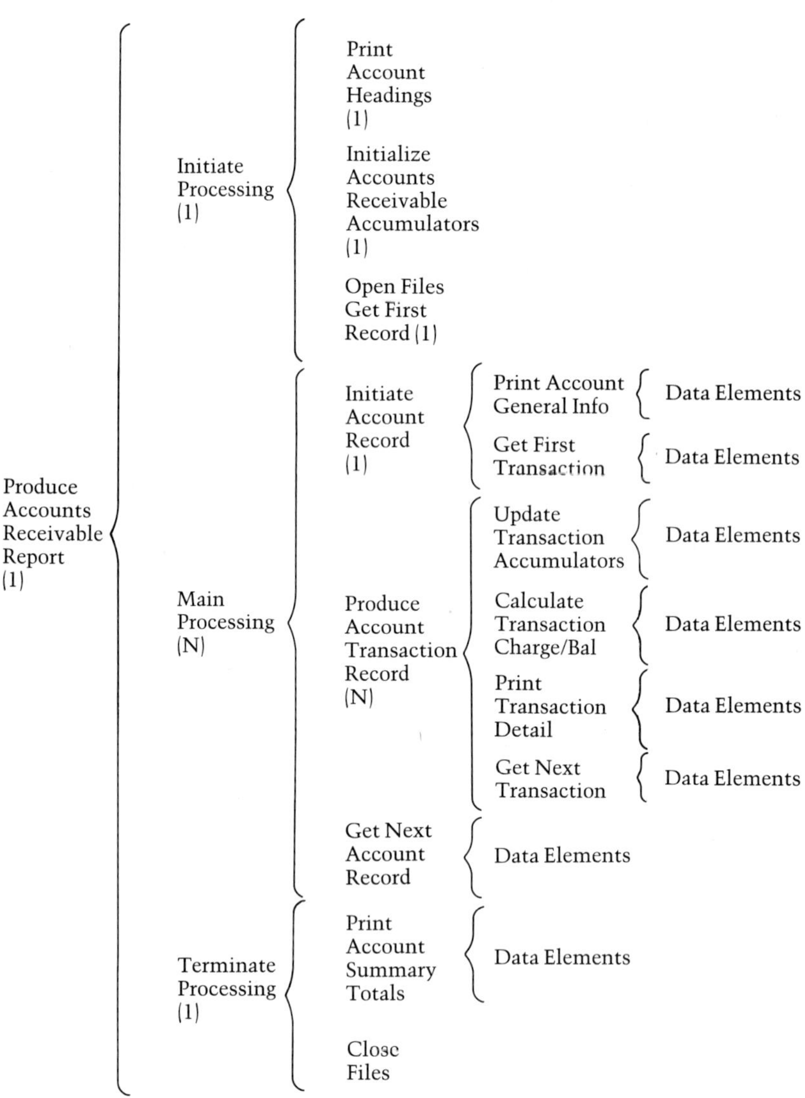

Figure 16.2

Warnier/Orr notation. Warnier/Orr brackets are a popular and simple-to-use modular design tool. Compare this notation with the diagram in Figure 16.1.

chapter. You can replace any of the structure charts we draw with an equivalent Warnier/Orr diagram. Let's move on to the strategies used to decompose a program (system) into modules.

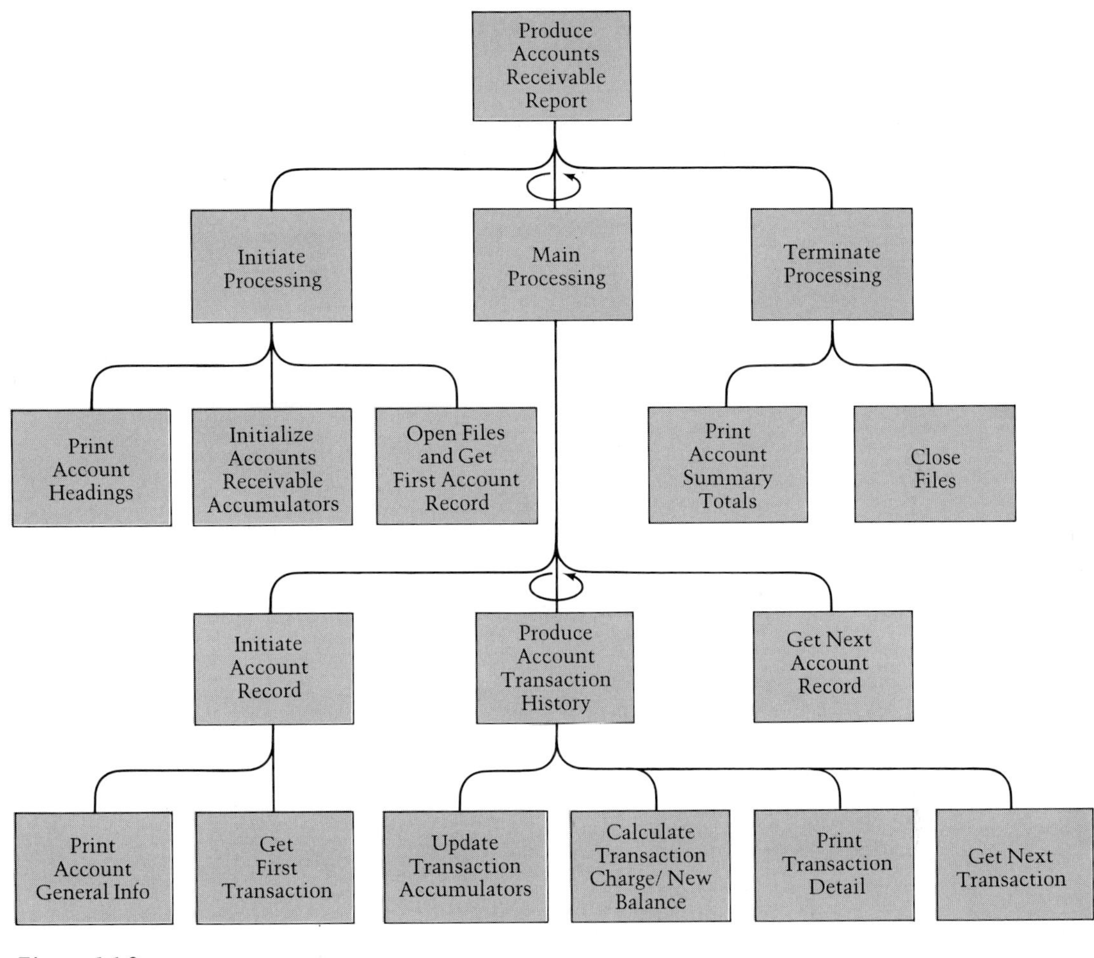

Figure 16.3

Structure chart notation. Structure charts are another popular tool for modular design. Compare this diagram with those in Figures 16.1 and 16.2.

Strategies for Modular Design Recall that structured design is a popular term for the decomposition of a program into modules. There are three popular strategies for structured design. We will review them briefly before we present an integrated strategy that we've found useful.

IBM's Hierarchy plus Input-Process-Output, called HIPO, was one of the earliest strategies for structured design. Using HIPO, the designer factors a program into logical functions, depicted as a structure chart (which they call a *vertical table of contents*). Each module is eventually documented with an IPO chart, which forces you to detail the inputs (these include inputs, file accesses, and subroutine parameter passing), processing requirements (narrative, pseudocode, or flowchart) and outputs (including reports, displays, file updates, and parameter passing). Although HIPO forces the decomposition of programs into modules, it doesn't really offer a strategy for doing so. Therefore, HIPO might be better thought of as a documentation tool than as a strategy. We'll show you how to take advantage of the HIPO documentation tool later in this chapter.

Ed Yourdon and Larry Constantine (Page-Jones, 1980) have developed what has become a popular strategy for determining an optimal structure chart for programs. Their technique is called *Structured Design* (a term we have already introduced), and it is based on the use of data flow diagrams. Essentially, you document programs with detailed logical data flow diagrams, study those diagrams, and convert the DFDs into *structure charts* (their term). They suggest two substrategies for developing the structure charts:

- *Transform analysis.* To make a long story short, **transform analysis** is an examination of the DFD to divide the processes into those that perform input and editing, those that do processing (such as calculations), and those that do output. Although we have greatly simplified the strategy, it is based on the IPO concept about which you have learned throughout this book.
- *Transaction analysis.* **Transaction analysis** is the examination of the DFD to identify processes which are distinct and therefore transaction centers. The resulting structure chart is factored into these transaction center modules (which may then be factored into IPO modules using transform analysis).

By using their strategy to divide a program into modules, you are able to end up with modules that are said to be *loosely coupled* and *highly cohesive.* Loosely coupled modules are less likely to be dependent on another (remember the problem Dick had in the Hayes Vending minicase?). Highly cohesive modules contain instructions that collectively work together to solve a specific task.

Another approach to developing an optimal modular structure has been suggested by Jean-Dominique Warnier and Ken Orr (Orr, 1977). This approach develops a program structure by working backward from the desired output data structure. This technique is called *Logical Design of Programs.* The output data structure is first defined using the Warnier/Orr notation. Then the input, file, and/or database structure is defined using a similar notation. Finally, a program structure is defined from these structures. The resulting program structure usually reflects input-process-output characteristics (or begin-process-terminate).

Both the Yourdon/Constantine and Warnier/Orr strategies have their die-hard advocates. We think the two strategies have much in common. Throughout this book, we have tried not to endorse any analysis or design methodology. This chapter will be no exception. Instead, we'd like to present a simplified strategy for modular design. The strategy is based on common sense and the fundamental principles that underly both the Yourdon/Constantine and the Warnier/Orr approaches.

How to Do Modular Design (A Simplified Approach)

Programs have been identified on both bounded data flow diagrams and systems flowcharts (Chapter 15). Given these programs, we want to break them into manageable modules around which program specifications will be written. Programmers can then build and test each module independently. Then modules can be integrated according to the structure chart and tested as a whole program. Now that you know what we're trying to accomplish, let's do it. We'll pay particular attention to how structure charts can be used to integrate large on-line programs because the trend appears to be toward such systems.

Step 1: Define the High-Level Structure Virtually all application programs can initially be broken down into three main functions: INITIATE PROCESSING, MAIN PROCESSING (the body of the program), and TERMINATE PROCESSING. Normally, the initiation and termination functions are performed once. The main processing function normally executes several times. Figure 16.4 can be used as a starting point for any normal program structure. These three essential functions are loosely based on Yourdon/Constantine's transform analysis strategy.

Adams, Wagner, and Boyer (1983) have cataloged a number of common functional modules that may be included in the INITIATE and TERMINATE PROCESSING functions. This is consistent with

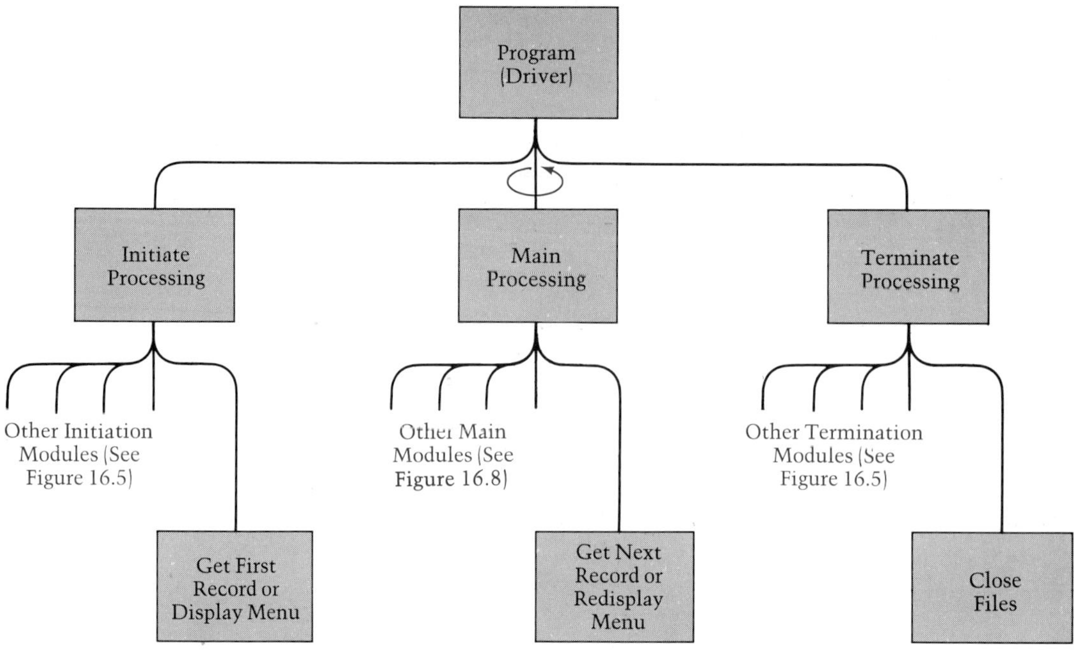

Figure 16.4

A de facto standard structure chart for most programs. Most programs can be initially factored into an INITIATE PROCESSING, MAIN PROCESSING, and TERMINATE PROCESSING structure. Those modules can be further factored using a number of popular strategies.

the concept of defining highly cohesive structures. These start-up and close-down functions are described in Figure 16.5. Notice in Figure 16.4, that the GET FIRST INPUT or RECORD function is almost always the last submodule of the INITIATE PROCESSING function. For an on-line system, this module might be labeled, DISPLAY MAIN MENU. Along the same lines, the STOP PROCESSING function is usually the last submodule of the TERMINATE PROCESSING.

What purpose does the MAIN PROGRAM module serve? It acts as a type of traffic cop, directing the execution of its subordinate modules. It executes the INITIATE PROCESSING module and begins executing the MAIN PROCESSING MODULE. When processing has been completely finished, it executes the TERMINATE PROCESSING module. That's it! For on-line systems, processing usually doesn't terminate — the main processing module is avail-

INITIATE PROCESSING FUNCTIONS:

BUILDING AND LOADING TABLES: Creating arrays to store tables, such as tax tables, actuary tables, and the like, and loading the data into those tables.

DEFINING CONSTANTS AND ACCUMULATORS: Constants are set in a dedicated module so those constants can be easily located if they need to be changed (for instance, SALES TAX PERCENT). Accumulators are used to count records and control totals during main processing.

OPENING FILES: Files must be opened before they can be read from or written to. It should be noted that some systems limit the number of files that can be open at any one time. If more files are needed than can be opened, then the program must be rewritten as multiple programs that pass intermediate results through temporary (scratch) files (which count as one open file).

FILE MERGING OR SORTING: This must be done before main processing can be done.

PRINTING REPORT HEADINGS: Why relegate report headings to a separate module? So they can be easily located if report headings need to be modified.

DISPLAYING (MAIN) MENU: For on-line systems, displaying the first menu and accepting the first choice from that menu is usually an initiation function.

GET FIRST INPUT RECORD: Read the first input record or file record to be processed.

TERMINATE PROCESSING FUNCTIONS:

CALCULATING CONTROL TOTALS: Performing arithmetic and statistical operations on totals accumulated during main processing functions.

PRINTING CONTROL TOTALS: Printing the accumulators and control totals maintained and calculated during main processing.

CLOSING FILES: The reverse of opening files. Disconnects the file from the program, thereby allowing other programs, which may have been locked out, to use those files.

Figure 16.5

Primitive functions performed by INITIATE and TERMINATE PROCESSING modules. This list (adapted from Adams, Wagner, and Boyer, 1984) suggests highly cohesive primitive modules that are typically controlled by an INITIATE or TERMINATE processing module. Any of these functions can be factored into primitive subsets to further improve cohesion and possibility for reuse.

able for execution until the system is no longer needed. At that time, the TERMINATE PROCESSING module is executed.

The remainder of our strategy will focus on how to factor the MAIN PROCESSING module.

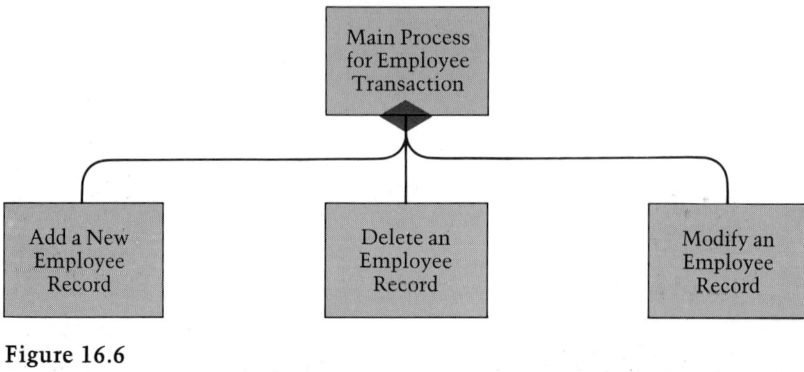

Figure 16.6

Transaction centers for a simple program. Generally, it is useful to factor a module into distinct submodules that act upon single transactions. These transactions centers are then said to be loosely coupled, that is, less likely to impact one another. The shaded diamond represents the selection of one or more modules based on *if-then-else* logic in the calling module.

Step 2: Identify Transaction Centers As a preface to factoring the MAIN PROCESSING module, the first question we like to ask is "Does this program have transaction centers?" This question is based on Yourdon/Constantine's transaction analysis strategy. What we are really asking is, "Does this program support multiple transactions?" If so, we will factor the MAIN PROCESSING module according to those transactions. The following are examples that would lend themselves to this strategy:

- A file maintenance program typically supports at least three transactions: ADD A NEW RECORD, DELETE A RECORD, and MODIFY A RECORD. Each transaction deserves its own module. Each transaction will cause the execution of one and only one of the transaction modules. For such a program, we would use the structure illustrated in Figure 16.6.
- An on-line system typically supports multiple levels of transactions. For instance, the main menu may offer three choices: EMPLOYEE FILE MAINTENANCE, PAYROLL TRANSACTION, and EMPLOYEE INQUIRY. Each of these subfunctions consists of multiple transactions. EMPLOYEE FILE MAINTENANCE could be factored as described in the preceding example. PAYROLL TRANSACTION could be factored into TIME CARD PROCESSING, SICK LEAVE PROCESSING, VACA-

TION PROCESSING, and so on. The resulting hierarchy chart might look something like Figure 16.7.

Although data flow diagrams may help you identify transaction centers, it depends on how detailed the analyst drew those data flow diagrams (for instance, many analysts won't factor the DFD process, MAINTAIN EMPLOYEE FILE, into three separate processes).

Finally, most transaction centers need to be further factored into their own INITIATE, PROCESS, and TERMINATE modules. For example, in Figure 16.7 we factored the PROCESS SICK LEAVE module into an initiate-process-terminate trio of submodules.

If the program you are trying to design cannot be factored into transactions (for instance, it supports a single transaction or only generates a single report), this step can be skipped.

Step 3: Factor the Initiate, Process, and Terminate Functions Into Primitive Functions At this point, we have factored our program into one or more iterations of INITIATE, PROCESS, and TERMINATE modules (*note:* we would have only one iteration if there were no multiple transaction centers). Now we can factor the initiate, process, and terminate modules into their primitive functions. The typical primitive modules for INITIATE and TERMINATE modules were listed in Figure 16.5. There are two strategies for factoring the PROCESS modules into primitives.

Most PROCESS modules can be factored into the primitive functions described in Figure 16.8. Once again, these primitive functions are generally considered to be highly cohesive. We should be able to write the logic of these modules with fifty or fewer statements of code. Along those lines, it may be appropriate to factor one of the simple functions from Figure 16.8 into submodules. For example, an EDIT ORDER module may be factored into EDIT GENERAL ORDER DATA, EDIT ORDERED PARTS, EDIT CUSTOMER DATA, and so on. The first strategy is demonstrated by the structure chart that appears in Figure 16.9 (p. 630).

The second strategy is based on the Warnier/Orr data structure approach. If the output consists of a natural hierarchy, we like to use the Warnier/Orr data structure approach to factor the process. This frequently happens with multiple control break outputs (a concept that should be familiar to students of programming). For instance, suppose our process module is supposed to produce a PART SALES SUMMARY REPORT. This report should contain

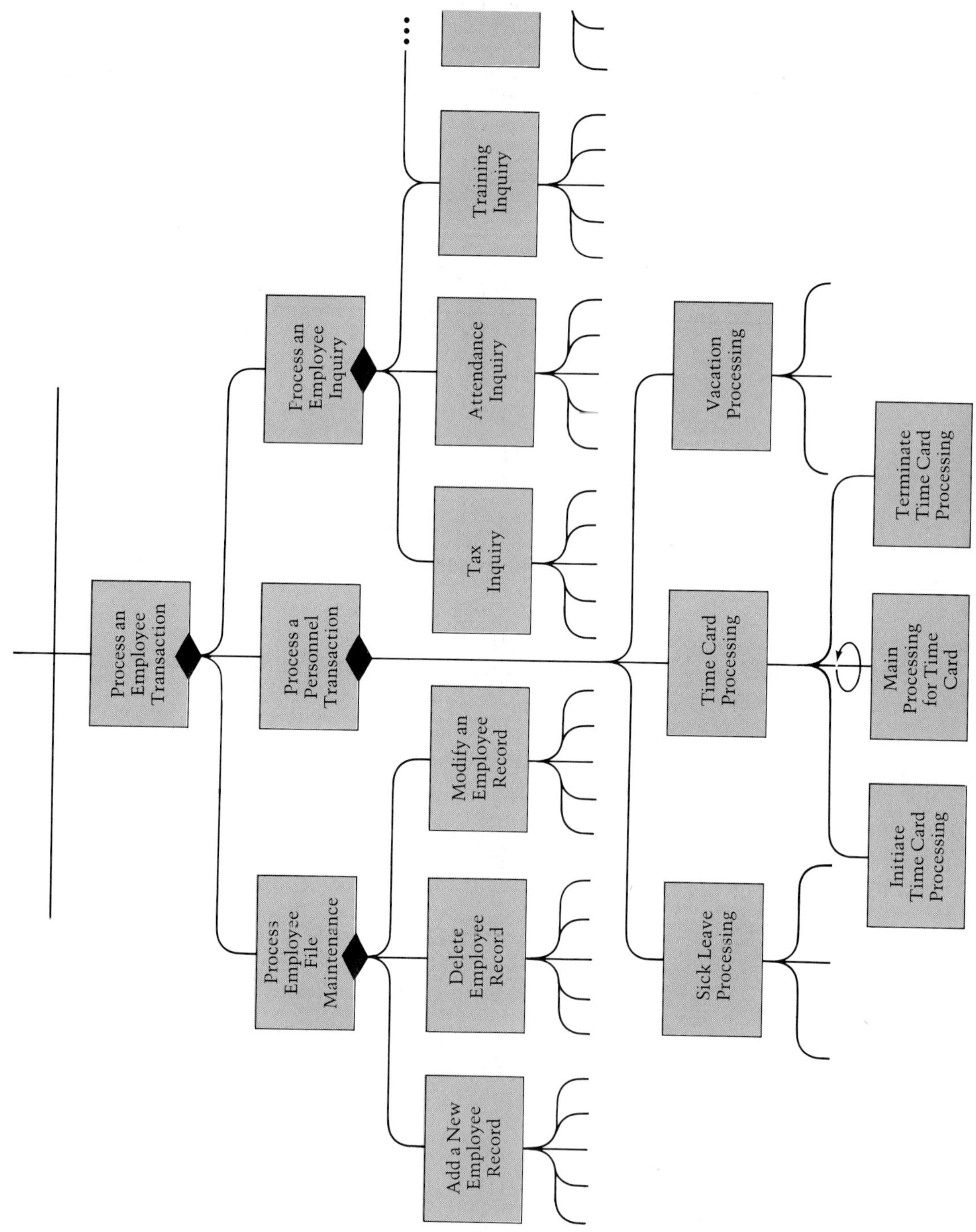

Process an Employee Transaction
Process Employee File Maintenance
Process a Personnel Transaction
Process an Employee Inquiry
Add a New Employee Record
Delete Employee Record
Modify an Employee Record
Tax Inquiry
Attendance Inquiry
Training Inquiry
Sick Leave Processing
Time Card Processing
Vacation Processing
Initiate Time Card Processing
Main Processing for Time Card
Terminate Time Card Processing

◀ **Figure 16.7**

On-line transaction centers. On-line systems are particularly suited to transaction analysis because their capabilities are called on demand and integrated through a high-level control program.

Figure 16.8 ▼

Primitive processes. This list (again adapted from Adams, Wagner, and Boyer, 1984) suggests primitive cohesive, MAIN PROCESSING functions. Again, these functions may have to be further factored to define small and reusable modules.

MAIN PROCESSING FUNCTIONS:

EDITING INPUT RECORDS: Performing picture, range, and completeness checks to make sure that data being input to the system for the first time is correct (this module will normally write to (or display) an errors report or file).

GETTING A SECONDARY RECORD: Reading an input or file record from a secondary source. For instance, if you are processing input ORDERS, you may have to retrieve a CUSTOMER RECORD for a credit check or retrieve PART records for an inventory check, all during main processing.

PERFORM CALCULATIONS: Performing arithmetic operations on data.

MAKING DECISIONS: Executing business policy decisions, such as credit checking, part availability, and discounting.

ACCUMULATING TOTALS: Where possible, totals should be accumulated in their own modules so those accumulators can be easily located and changed.

WRITING A DETAIL LINE: Recording a single detail line or transaction to a file or report that will contain many such detail lines.

WRITING A COMPLETE RECORD: Writing an entire record (as opposed to a detail line) to a report or file. For example, printing a paycheck, or updating a record in a master file.

GETTING THE NEXT RECORD: Retrieve or read the next record in the loop that drives the main processing routine.

REDISPLAY A MENU: Of options that are available in an on-line system.

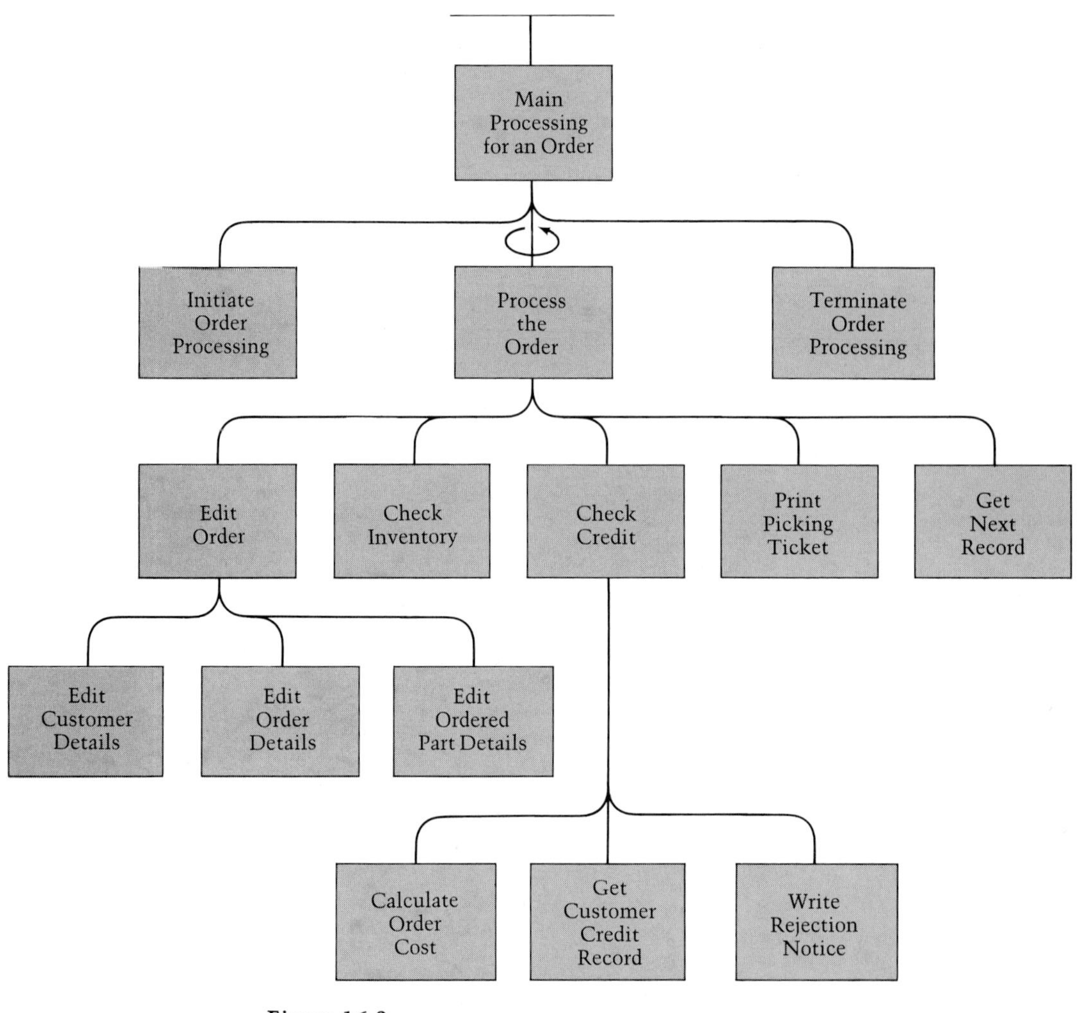

Figurc 16.9

Factoring MAIN PROCESSING into cohesive primitives. MAIN PROCESSING must eventually be factored down to loosely coupled, highly cohesive primitive modules.

detailed unit and dollar sales information for each part, each product line (consisting of multiple parts), and each warehouse zone (consisting of multiple product lines). We can factor the process module for this report into modules that correspond to the control breaks. This structure is illustrated in Figure 16.10. Notice that we added an INITIATE (to set accumulators) and TERMINATE (to

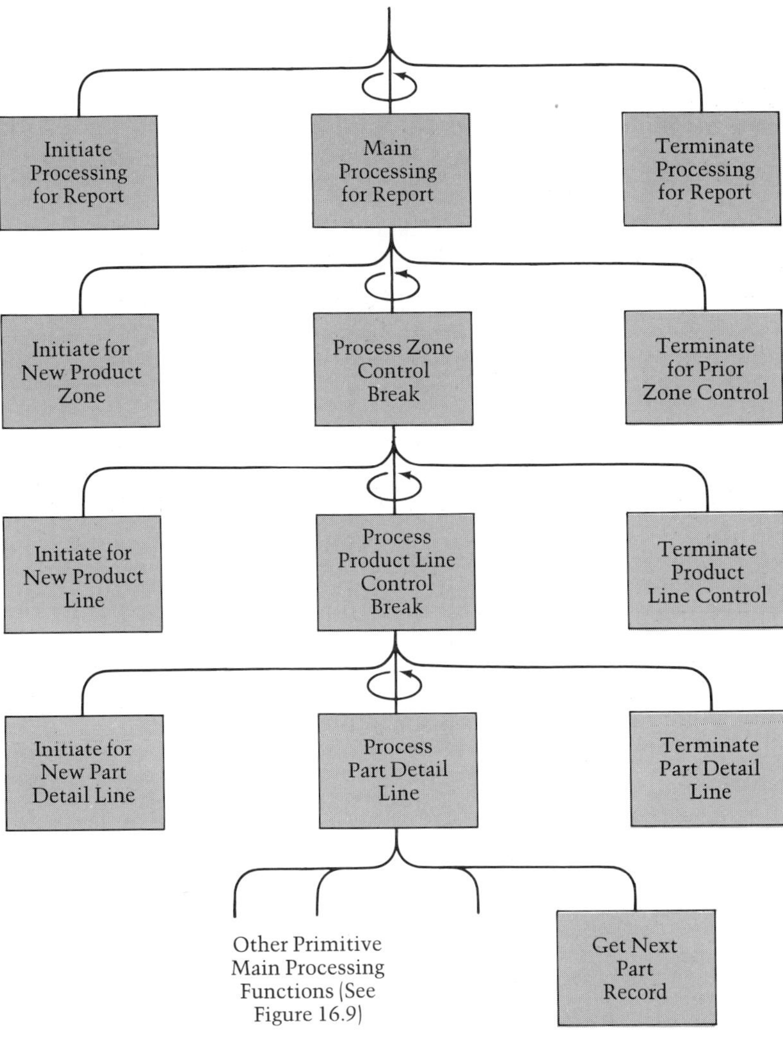

Figure 16.10

Data structure factoring. For programs that produce outputs with hierarchical data structure, the MAIN PROCESSING can be factored according to that hierarchy (control breaks). Each of these data-structure-oriented modules is flanked by modules that initiate and terminate the processing for that control break.

format and print control totals) module to each control break processing module. This structure chart makes it possible to implement the program with a single flag, "end of file," (thus loosely coupling the hierarchy of modules) and with much less code. The final process module, PROCESS PART DETAIL LINE, is factored into primitive tasks by using the first strategy, the primitive functions introduced in Figure 16.8.

And that, in an abbreviated form, is one possible strategy for program module design. We strongly urge you to study the full Warnier/Orr and Yourdon/Constantine strategies as part of your continuing education.

After performing modular design on all programs, we are ready to package programming specifications around the modular design.

PACKAGING PROGRAM SPECIFICATIONS

Using the design techniques presented in this unit, you have accumulated a good number of design specifications for the new system — perhaps you have separate stacks of documentation for the system outputs, files, inputs, terminal dialogue, systems flowcharts, and program modules. Now, put yourself in the shoes of the computer programmer. Are those specifications in a format that will help you write the programs? Not really. As a systems analyst, you are responsible for packaging that set of design documentation into a format suitable for the programmer.

As a direct result of modular design, you have a structure chart or, as IBM would call it, a **Vertical Table of Contents** (VTOC) for the computer programs to be written. We can now use IBM's *Hierarchy plus Input-Process-Output* (HIPO) technique to assemble and package program specifications around that VTOC.

What Does a Programmer Need in Order to Write Computer Programs?

You can't expect programmers to implement a correct program if they don't receive the necessary program specifications. You can avoid this problem by looking at packaging as salespeople look at their products. A good salesperson knows the product and knows how to sell it. In this section you're going to learn to look at a computer program as if it were a new product. Let's study the components of the program specifications package and see how the product can best be presented to knowledge workers and programmers.

The program specifications package is a collection of design documentation that clearly communicates the requirements for each computer program in the system. What exactly are the requirements associated with a computer program? All programs perform three types of tasks including input or reading of data, manipulation of input data, and output of data or information. In other words, all program tasks can be classified according to our IPO concept introduced in the previous chapters. This model will help us address the requirements for implementing a computer program.

Input Specifications As a systems analyst, you are responsible for providing complete specifications of all sources of input data for each program. To the computer programmer, the term *input* has a broad meaning. Although batch and on-line inputs are still important, *input* also refers to file accesses. The specifications for all these program inputs have been documented as follows:

1. Master, transaction, and scratch file specifications (Chapter 12) include:

   Expanded data dictionary entries

   Record layout charts

2. Batch input file specifications (Chapter 13) include:

   Source document layout

   Expanded data dictionary entries

   Input record layout charts

3. On-line input specifications (Chapters 13 and 14) include:

   Source document layout

   Expanded data dictionary entries

   Display layout charts

   Terminal dialogue charts

Processing Specifications All programs execute processing tasks (such as sorting, summarizing, and calculating) upon input data to produce outputs and information. These processing tasks are performed according to business policies and procedures. It is essential that the policies and procedures governing the processing tasks of a program be clearly explained to the programmer. A programmer can't implement a program that checks credit, for example, if credit policies are not clear, accurate, and complete.

How complete should the processing requirements be? How close should the analyst come to specifying code? Generally, procedure specifications should represent a more general explanation of how the tasks of a program are to be accomplished. Program logic is intended to be much more detailed. For example, a procedure specification instruction might state:

> Sort the DAILY ORDERS FILE in ascending order by CUSTOMER ORDER NUMBER.

Alternatively, we could provide the pseudocode logic for an internal sort (Figure 16.11). Some programmers might like this detailed specification very much. Others might be offended by such a precise description. Where should the systems analyst draw the line? Many organizations have adopted standards that dictate exactly what the systems analyst must provide the programmer. In the absence of standards, perhaps analysts will simply document critical business formulas and decision rules. On the other hand, most systems analysts are required to simply provide the programmer with a clear and *concise* statement of the program processing requirements. The specifications for computer processing requirements may be specified by:

Decision tables (covered in Chapter 9)
Structured English (covered in Chapter 9)

Output Specifications Along the same lines as *inputs*, the term *outputs* means more to the programmer than we have suggested in this unit. In addition to printouts, forms, and displays, outputs include updates to files. Output requirements include:

1. Printed output specifications (Chapter 11)
    - Expanded data dictionary entries
    - Printer spacing charts
2. On-line output specifications (Chapter 11)
    - Expanded data dictionary entries
    - Display layout charts
    - Terminal dialogue charts

Figure 16.11

Pseudocode. This is an example of pseudocode for a sorting requirement. The analyst should avoid this level of detail unless systems design standards call for it. This is the level of detail the programmer would use to design logic.

Initialize the ORDER SORT array subscript X to 1.

For each record in the DAILY ORDER FILE, do the following:

Store DAILY ORDER FILE record in ORDER SORT array at subscript X location.

Add 1 to subscript X.

Initialize the IS SORT COMPLETE FLAG to "NO".

Initialize the RECORDS TO SORT variable equal to the subscript X.

Initialize the SORT COUNTER variable to 1.

Repeat the following steps until the SORT COUNTER variable equals X − 1 or the SORT COMPLETE FLAG equals "YES":

Initialize SORT COMPLETE FLAG to "YES".

Subtract 1 from the RECORDS TO SORT variable.

Initialize the COMPARISON COUNTER to 1.

Repeat the following steps until the COMPARISON COUNTER is greater than the RECORDS TO SORT variable.

Calculate COMPARISON SUBSCRIPT using the following formula:

COMPARISON COUNTER + 1

If the CUSTOMER ORDER NUMBER for ORDER SORT array record at COMPARISON COUNTER location is less than the CUSTOMER ORDER NUMBER for ORDER SORT array record at COMPARISON SUBSCRIPT location, then:

Store ORDER SORT array record at location COMPARISON COUNTER in TEMPORARY STORAGE variable.

Store the ORDER SORT array record at location TEMPORARY STORAGE in ORDER SORT array at the COMPARISON COUNTER location.

Store the TEMPORARY STORAGE record in the ORDER SORT array at location COMPARISON COUNTER.

Set the IS SORT COMPLETED flag equal to "NO".

Add 1 to COMPARISON COUNTER variable.

Add 1 to SORT COUNTER variable.

Initialize the SORTED ORDER FILE COUNTER to 0.

For each record in the SORT ORDER array, do the following:

Store the SORT ORDER array record at the SORTED ORDER FILE COUNTER location in the SORTED ORDER FILE.

3. Master and transaction files updated specifications (Chapter 12)

   Expanded data dictionary entries

   Record layout charts

Packaging Program Specifications Using the HIPO Model

In this section, we will explain how to use systems flowcharts, structure charts (called a Vertical Table of Contents in HIPO) and a new tool, called *IPO charts,* to package program specifications. We'll begin by examining how systems flowcharts can be used to identify the specifications that are required for each program in a system. Then we'll examine the structure chart as an outline for packaging. Finally, we'll learn how the IPO chart can be used to organize the specifications for a program.

Packaging a Transaction Processing Program The systems flowchart can aid greatly in the packaging effort. How? It identifies programs to be packaged and documents all inputs and outputs for those programs. Recall that some programs can be used, as is, from the software library. These programs may not have to be packaged. Let's examine how we might use the systems flowchart to package the IPO requirements for a transaction processing program in our AAP case.

In Figure 16.12, we've reproduced a systems flowchart from Chapter 15. The program PROCESS NEW ORDER is actually a subprogram in an on-line system. The partial structure chart for the on-line system is illustrated in Figure 16.13. This structure will be used to organize our program specifications using the HIPO documentation technique.

HIPO stands for Hierarchy plus Input-Process-Output. HIPO refers to its hierarchy as a vertical table of contents. We have already done that step when we generated the structure chart in Figure

Figure 16.12 ►

Systems flowchart. A systems flowchart serves two purposes for program design. First, it identifies the programs to be designed. Second, it identifies the net inputs and outputs for that program. Notice the library programs. These programs don't normally have to be designed because they already exist.

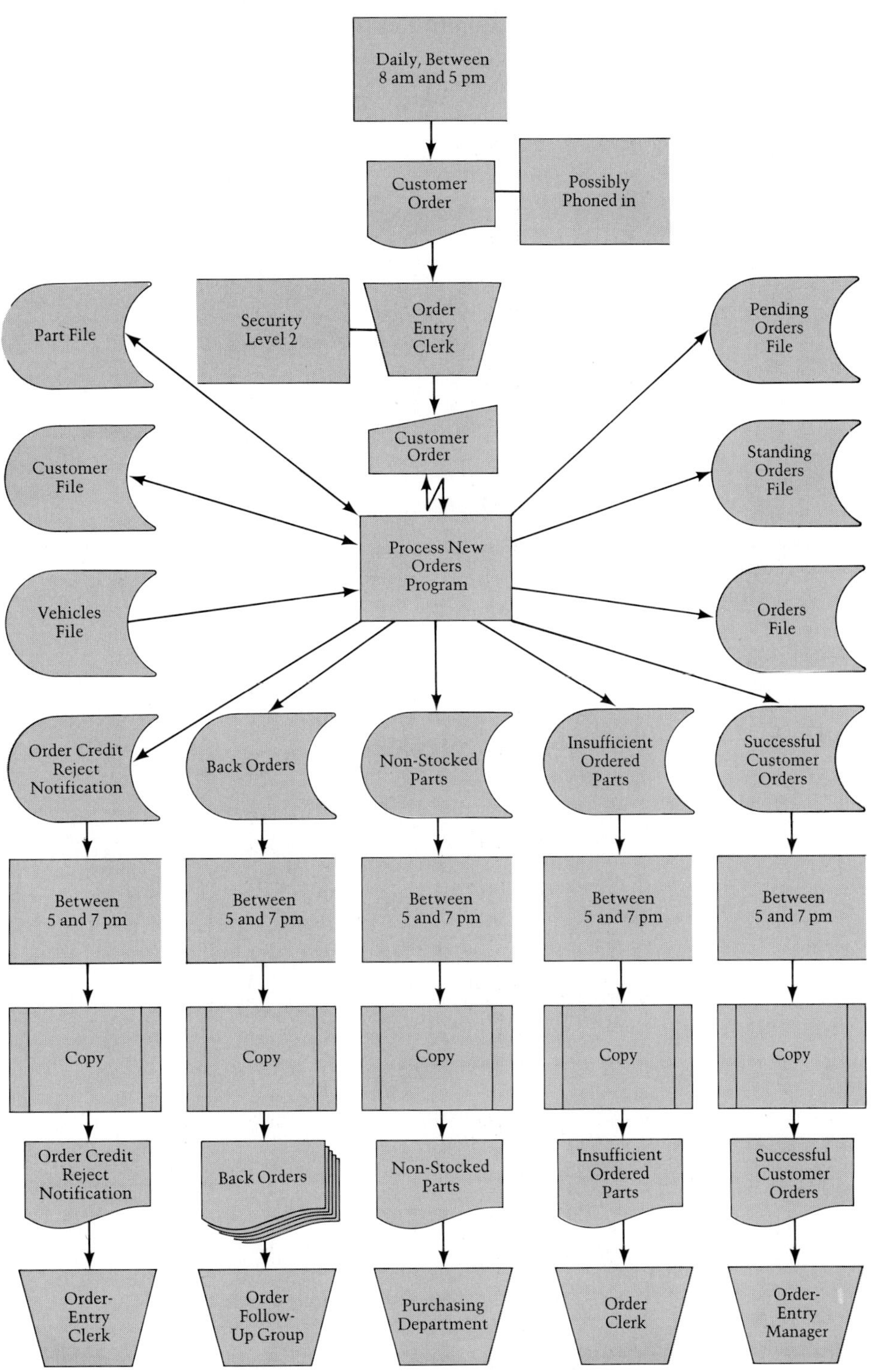
Daily, Between
8 am and 5 pm
Customer
Order
Possibly
Phoned in
Security
Level 2
Order
Entry
Clerk
Part File
Pending
Orders
File
Customer
File
Customer
Order
Standing
Orders
File
Process New
Orders
Program
Vehicles
File
Orders
File
Order Credit
Reject
Notification
Back Orders
Non-Stocked
Parts
Insufficient
Ordered
Parts
Successful
Customer
Orders
Between
5 and 7 pm
Between
5 and 7 pm
Between
5 and 7 pm
Between
5 and 7 pm
Between
5 and 7 pm
Copy
Copy
Copy
Copy
Copy
Order Credit
Reject
Notification
Back Orders
Non-Stocked
Parts
Insufficient
Ordered
Parts
Successful
Customer
Orders
Order-
Entry
Clerk
Order
Follow-
Up Group
Purchasing
Department
Order
Clerk
Order-
Entry
Manager

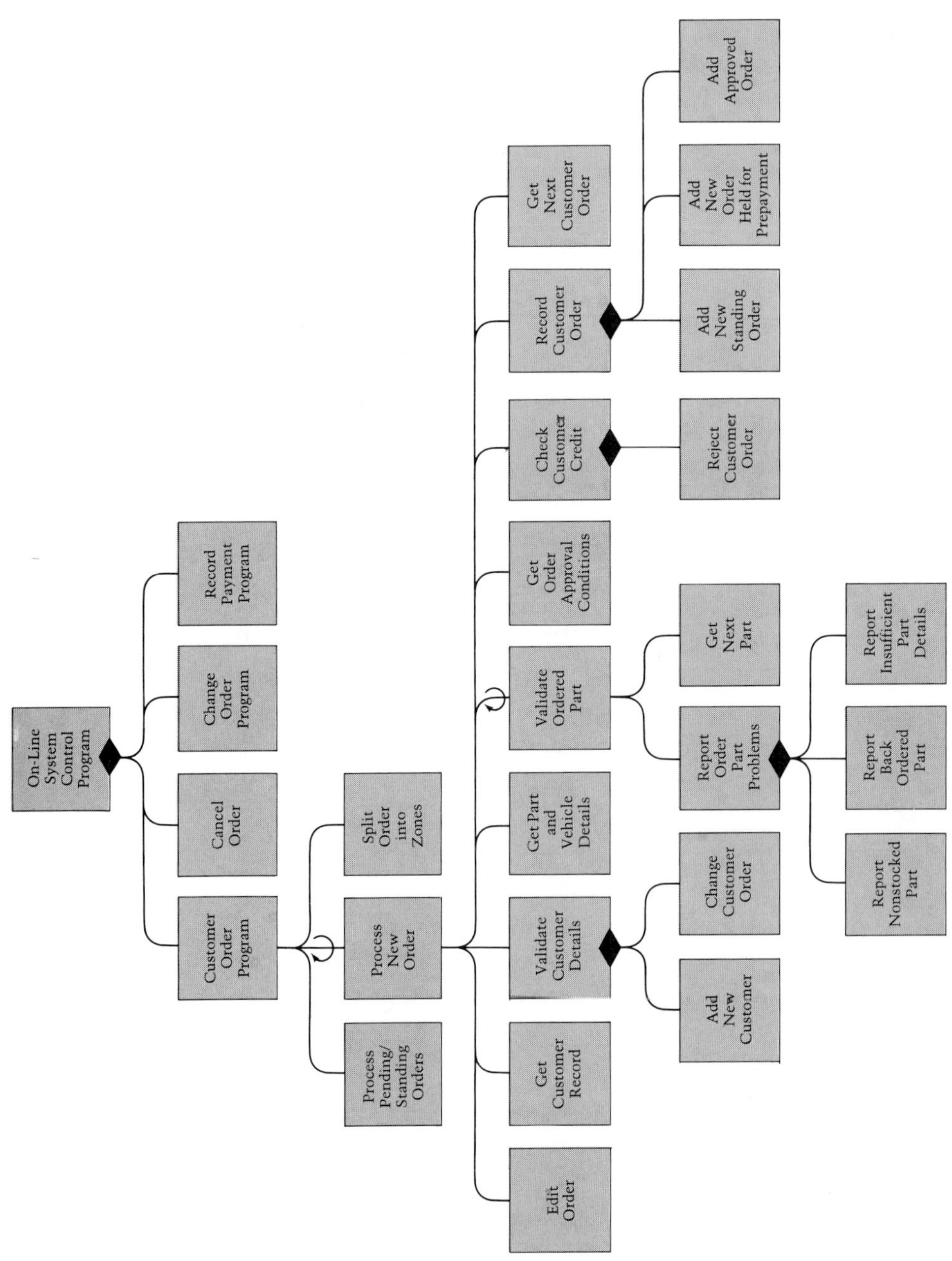
On-Line System Control Program
Customer Order Program
Cancel Order
Change Order Program
Record Payment Program
Process Pending/ Standing Orders
Process New Order
Split Order into Zones
Edit Order
Get Customer Record
Validate Customer Details
Get Part and Vehicle Details
Validate Ordered Part
Get Order Approval Conditions
Check Customer Credit
Record Customer Order
Get Next Customer Order
Add New Customer
Change Customer Order
Report Order Part Problems
Get Next Part
Reject Customer Order
Add New Standing Order
Add New Order Held for Prepayment
Add Approved Order
Report Nonstocked Part
Report Back Ordered Part
Report Insufficient Part Details

◀ **Figure 16.13**

Vertical table of contents. HIPO refers to structure charts as vertical tables of contents (VTOC) because they serve as an outline into their IPO charts.

16.13. The portion of the structure chart we are documenting for this example is highlighted. Notice that we factored the EDIT module into a series of sequentially executed submodules. You may ask, "Why not just stop factoring at the higher-level module? You wouldn't write each of those submodules as a separate subroutine, would you?" Actually, we would! Although those submodules *could* be implemented as paragraphs in a single subroutine, we would implement each as a separate subroutine for the following reasons:

- A single module would require significantly more than sixty lines of code (the theoretical maximum size of a manageable subroutine). Don't be fooled by the brevity of our procedure specification—it isn't code!
- By writing the modules as separate subroutines, the code may be reusable in this and other information systems. Reusable program code is becoming a popular standard in many data processing shops.
- Each of our primitive modules is truly performing a separate and distinct function.

Using true HIPO, you would specify each module in the structure chart. However, we need to be careful not to overspecify—many modules are relatively simple and are best specified by the programmer (for instance, initialization and termination modules). As analysts, our concern should be for those modules that transform inputs into outputs. Here the programmer, who may not be (as) familiar with the business policies and procedures, needs our help. Therefore, we confess to taking liberties with the HIPO approach. But our goal is to complete the program specification package as quickly as possible so that programming can begin. Productivity! Not busywork!

Figures 16.14(a) through (d) represent the IPO charts for the PROCESS NEW ORDER program. Like most complex programs, the IPO specification required several IPO charts. An IPO chart coordinates the detailed input, output, file, and dialogue specifica-

Figure 16.14(a) ►

IPO chart for the program as a whole. The IPO chart for the top module in a program is relatively simple. It provides some general information about the program and then describes the routine that manages the program.

tions you prepared in Chapters 11 through 14. The IPO chart is divided into three parts that correspond to our IPO concept. We call your attention to each of these zones on the chart and how they are used.

The input section of the chart serves two purposes. First, it is used to identify each source of input data to the program. Second, it is used to reference (point to) the detailed documentation you've collected for the inputs (for example, data dictionary entries, and layout charts). Notice that we use systems flowchart symbols in the input column. There is one notable difference, however. For on-line dialogue, we show all on-line inputs, including such items as a user's selection from a menu (recall that we only drew on-line symbols for *net* inputs and outputs on the systems flowcharts).

For each of these input symbols recorded in the input column, we provided a reference to the corresponding specifications we accumulated. Each of the design documents for a given program input should be assigned a figure number or some unique number that allows for referencing particular documents. Immediately below each input symbol in the input column of the IPO chart, we will record the reference number(s) of the corresponding input specification documents.

The output column of the IPO chart is similar to the input column. Again, we used systems flowchart symbols but we expanded the use of the display symbol to include displaying menus and error messages.

The process column serves two purposes. First, it is used to present general information about the program (see Figure 16.14a), such as programming language to be used, utilities and special-purpose software to be used (perhaps a teleprocessing monitor like CICS), equipment and operating system that are to be used, job control statements, security requirements, and any other worthwhile facts the programmer should know. If the program exists but needs to be modified, the process column should describe the modifications required, including any modifications to policies and procedures to be implemented.

PROGRAM ABSTRACT for PROCESS NEW ORDER (name of program)　Prepared by DOUG MATTHEWS　Date 4-1-86　Page 1 of 4

INPUT

This column would normally contain references to figure numbers for design specifications (e.g., layout charts, data dictionaries).

Input design specs for customer order

PROCESS

```
     This  program is to be available during the hours 8:00 A.M.  to 5:00 P.M.
on weekdays.  The program is an on-line program that may be accessible by  O/E
Clerks with a security level 2. The COBOL language should be used to implement
the program.


PROCESSING REQUIREMENTS:


Given the CUSTOMER ORDER data from the user, do the following:


EDIT ORDER

For all invalid CUSTOMER ORDER data supplied by user, do the following steps:
     Select the appropriate case:

       Case 1:  SALES ORDER NUMBER is invalid

            If  the SALES ORDER NUMBER is equivalent to the SALES ORDER NUMBER
            of any previously entered CUSTOMER ORDER then:
                 error   message  =  "Sales  order  number  was  assigned   to
                 previously entered sales order, please re-enter."

            If the SALES ORDER NUMBER fails the Modulus 11 check then:
                 error  message = "Sales order number  was  illegal,  possible
                 keying error, please re-enter."

       Case 2:  ORDER DATE is invalid

            Select appropriate case:

                 Case 2.1  ORDER DATE contains no values, then:
                      error  message = "The order date must be provided on all
                      orders,  please enter."

                 Case 2.2  ORDER DATE contains invalid values for MONTH,  DAY,
                 or YEAR then:
                      error message = "The order date is not valid, please re-
                      enter."

       Case 3:  Select appropriate case for BILLING ADDRESS:

                 Case 3.1:   BILL TO STREET ADDRESS,  BILL TO POST OFFICE  BOX
                 NUMBER,  BILL  TO  CITY,  BILL TO STATE,  or BILL TO  ZIPCODE
                 contains no values, then:
                      error message = "A complete billing address is  required
                      on all sales orders, please re-enter."

                Case 3.2:  BILL TO STATE contains invalid state code, then:
                     error message  = "Standard state codes  must be entered,
                     please re-enter."
```

OUTPUT

This column would normally contain references to figure numbers for design specifications (e.g., layout charts, data dictionaries).

Terminal dialogue design specs

Figure 16.14(b) ►

IPO chart (continued). The processing routines for the edit module have been consolidated into a single IPO chart (over two pages). Notice that each submodule is clearly marked.

The second purpose of the process column is to present policy and procedure requirements to the programmer. We like to use Structured English and decision tables to present such requirements; however, you could use alternative procedures or logic tools (such as program flowcharts). Also notice that we used arrows to tie the Structured English specification to the inputs and outputs. This notation immediately directs the programmer to the proper data dictionaries and layout charts for details.

Once again, some data processors may take exception to the pseudocode-like use of Structured English as a processing specification tool. They might argue that coding should be left to the programmer. As an alternative, you could replace the Structured English with a general narrative description of the requirements (possibly including decision tables). On the other hand, we'd like to remind you of the problems associated with the free-format English narrative. They were discussed in Chapter 9. We believe that programming specifications in Structured English result in fewer misunderstandings between the user, analyst, and programmer. As a result, the programs are implemented faster and are more likely to perform as expected. We are personally embarrassed to admit that some of our pre–Structured English specifications in programming assignments given to our students (which are usually less difficult than real world assignments) have resulted in needless misunderstandings and delays.

Due to size constraints on this book, we cannot provide you with all of these detailed design specifications. Instead, we refer you to Figure 16.14(d) for a summary of what documentation would be included with the IPO charts and how that documentation could be organized.

What if we were packaging the specifications for a batch version of the PROCESS NEW ORDER program? The on-line input symbol on the IPO chart would be replaced by the appropriate symbol for the batch input file. And instead of display layout charts, the data dictionaries and input record layout charts would be included in the program specifications package.

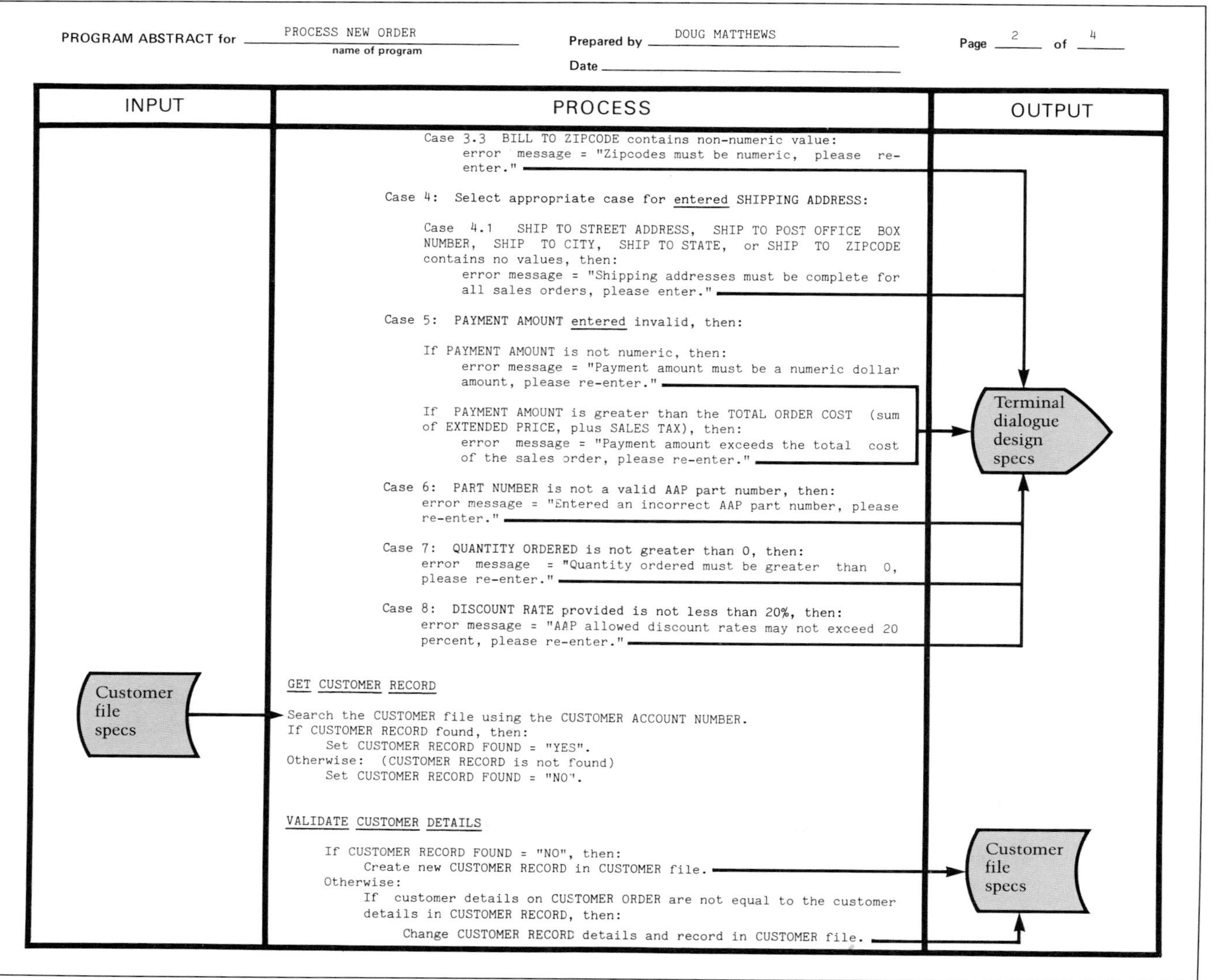

PROGRAM ABSTRACT for PROCESS NEW ORDER (name of program)   Prepared by DOUG MATTHEWS   Page 2 of 4

Date

INPUT	PROCESS	OUTPUT
	Case 3.3 BILL TO ZIPCODE contains non-numeric value: error message = "Zipcodes must be numeric, please re-enter." Case 4: Select appropriate case for <u>entered</u> SHIPPING ADDRESS: Case 4.1 SHIP TO STREET ADDRESS, SHIP TO POST OFFICE BOX NUMBER, SHIP TO CITY, SHIP TO STATE, or SHIP TO ZIPCODE contains no values, then: error message = "Shipping addresses must be complete for all sales orders, please enter." Case 5: PAYMENT AMOUNT <u>entered</u> invalid, then: If PAYMENT AMOUNT is not numeric, then: error message = "Payment amount must be a numeric dollar amount, please re-enter." If PAYMENT AMOUNT is greater than the TOTAL ORDER COST (sum of EXTENDED PRICE, plus SALES TAX), then: error message = "Payment amount exceeds the total cost of the sales order, please re-enter." Case 6: PART NUMBER is not a valid AAP part number, then: error message = "Entered an incorrect AAP part number, please re-enter." Case 7: QUANTITY ORDERED is not greater than 0, then: error message = "Quantity ordered must be greater than 0, please re-enter." Case 8: DISCOUNT RATE provided is not less than 20%, then: error message = "AAP allowed discount rates may not exceed 20 percent, please re-enter."	Terminal dialogue design specs
Customer file specs	<u>GET CUSTOMER RECORD</u> Search the CUSTOMER file using the CUSTOMER ACCOUNT NUMBER. If CUSTOMER RECORD found, then: Set CUSTOMER RECORD FOUND = "YES". Otherwise: (CUSTOMER RECORD is not found) Set CUSTOMER RECORD FOUND = "NO".	
	<u>VALIDATE CUSTOMER DETAILS</u> If CUSTOMER RECORD FOUND = "NO", then: Create new CUSTOMER RECORD in CUSTOMER file. Otherwise: If customer details on CUSTOMER ORDER are not equal to the customer details in CUSTOMER RECORD, then: Change CUSTOMER RECORD details and record in CUSTOMER file.	Customer file specs

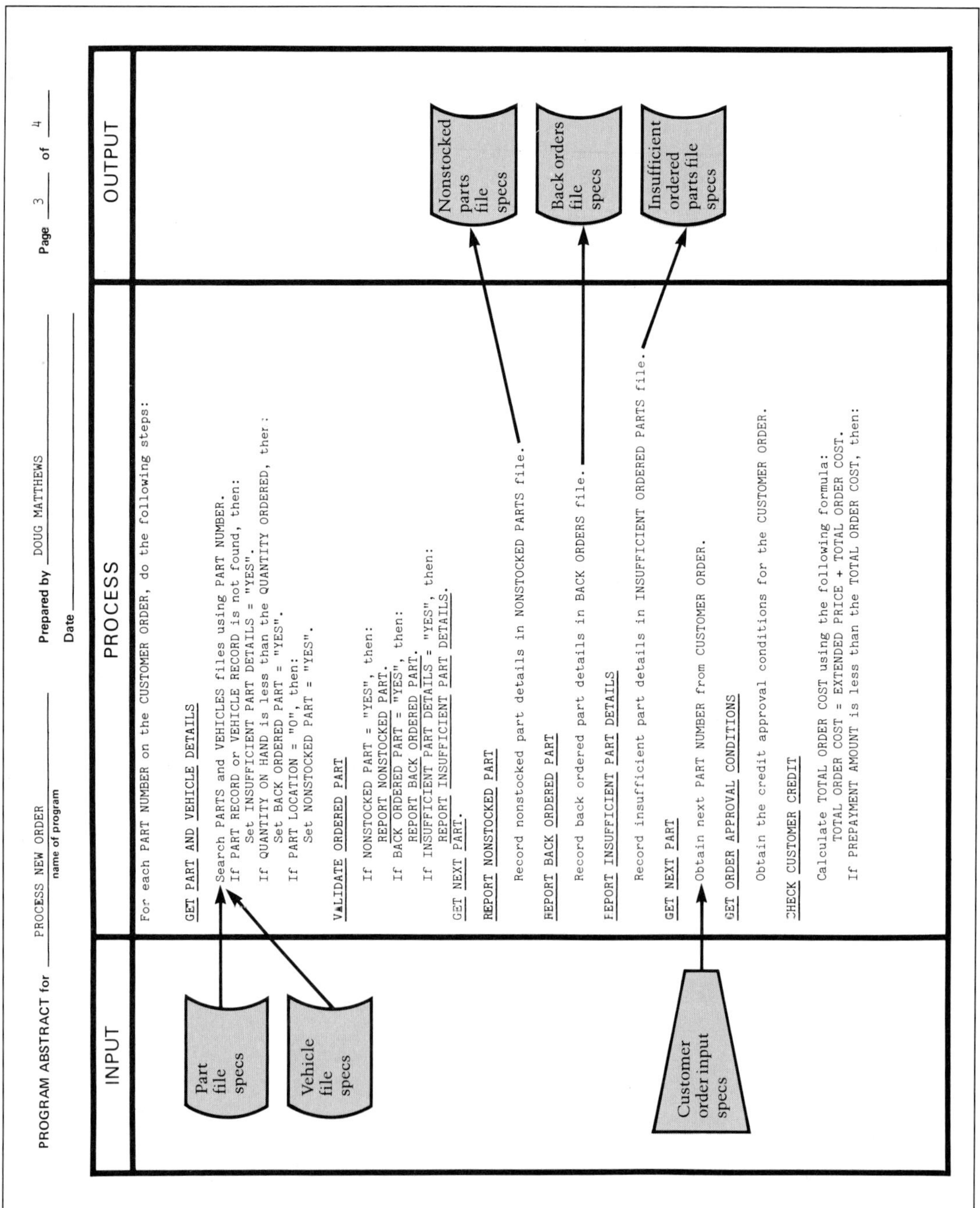

Figure 16.14(c)

IPO chart (continued).

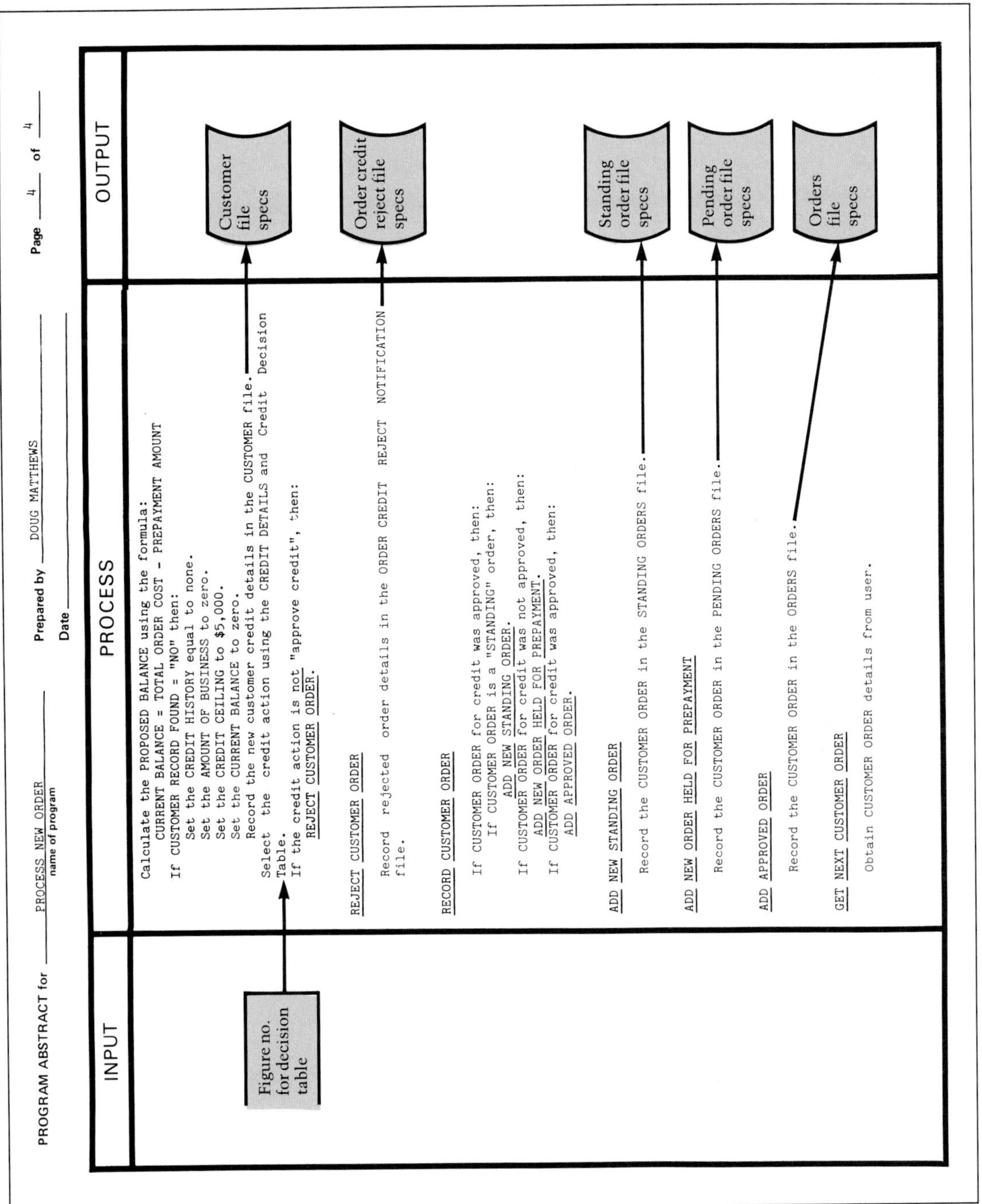

Figure 16.14(d)

IPO chart (continued).

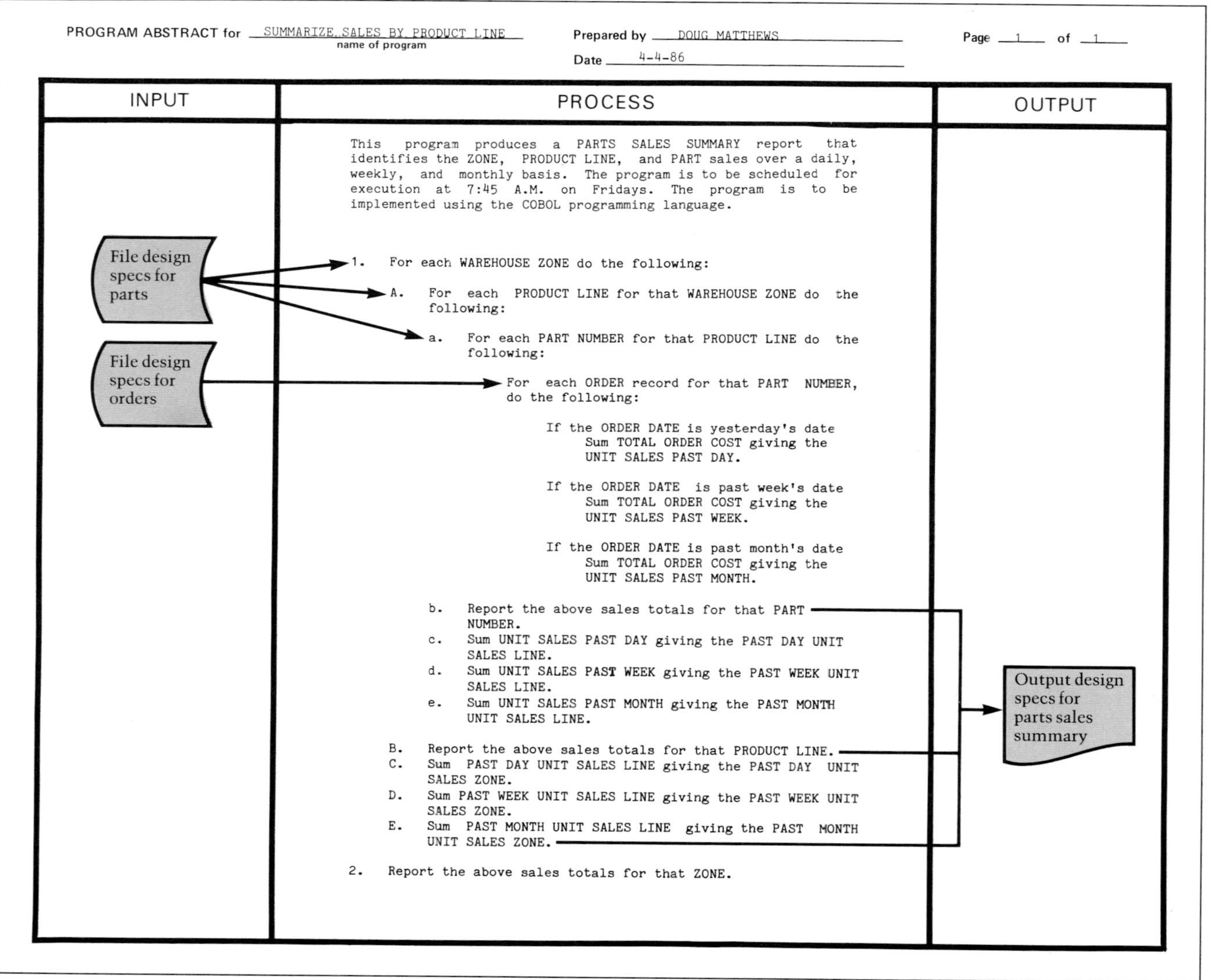

PROGRAM ABSTRACT for SUMMARIZE SALES BY PRODUCT LINE (name of program)

Prepared by DOUG MATTHEWS

Date 4-4-86

Page 1 of 1

INPUT	PROCESS	OUTPUT
File design specs for parts File design specs for orders	This program produces a PARTS SALES SUMMARY report that identifies the ZONE, PRODUCT LINE, and PART sales over a daily, weekly, and monthly basis. The program is to be scheduled for execution at 7:45 A.M. on Fridays. The program is to be implemented using the COBOL programming language.	Output design specs for parts sales summary

```
1.  For each WAREHOUSE ZONE do the following:
    A.  For each PRODUCT LINE for that WAREHOUSE ZONE do the
        following:
        a.  For each PART NUMBER for that PRODUCT LINE do the
            following:
              For each ORDER record for that PART NUMBER,
              do the following:

                If the ORDER DATE is yesterday's date
                    Sum TOTAL ORDER COST giving the
                    UNIT SALES PAST DAY.

                If the ORDER DATE is past week's date
                    Sum TOTAL ORDER COST giving the
                    UNIT SALES PAST WEEK.

                If the ORDER DATE is past month's date
                    Sum TOTAL ORDER COST giving the
                    UNIT SALES PAST MONTH.
        b.  Report the above sales totals for that PART
            NUMBER.
        c.  Sum UNIT SALES PAST DAY giving the PAST DAY UNIT
            SALES LINE.
        d.  Sum UNIT SALES PAST WEEK giving the PAST WEEK UNIT
            SALES LINE.
        e.  Sum UNIT SALES PAST MONTH giving the PAST MONTH
            UNIT SALES LINE.
    B.  Report the above sales totals for that PRODUCT LINE.
    C.  Sum PAST DAY UNIT SALES LINE giving the PAST DAY UNIT
        SALES ZONE.
    D.  Sum PAST WEEK UNIT SALES LINE giving the PAST WEEK UNIT
        SALES ZONE.
    E.  Sum PAST MONTH UNIT SALES LINE giving the PAST MONTH
        UNIT SALES ZONE.
2.  Report the above sales totals for that ZONE.
```

◀ **Figure 16.15**

IPO chart for a typical reporting program.

Packaging a Management Reporting Program Figure 16.15 is an IPO chart for the SUMMARIZE SALES BY PRODUCT LINE management report program. Notice that the IPO chart for this program is much simpler than the one for a transaction-processing program. This is typical. The total package is similar to the one we did for transaction processing. The primary difference between the two program specifications packages is that the SUMMARIZE SALES BY PRODUCT LINE program generates a printed report. Therefore, the appropriate specifications for this output must be obtained and included in the packet (data dictionaries and printer spacing charts).

Packaging a Decision Support Program The HIPO documentation for a typical decision support program, QUERY PART, is illustrated in Figures 16.16 and 16.17. The IPO chart is self-explanatory.

This concludes our discussion of program packaging. As you have learned, this design task reorganizes the design documentation that you learned to develop in Chapters 11 – 15. Try packaging a sample computer program.

SUMMARY

The systems analyst's role in computer program design includes module design and packaging of design specifications. A module is defined as single entry – single exit group of instructions that performs a single function. To deal with complexity of logic, programmers tend to break programs into modules. A better strategy is to break programs into code to deal with *functions.*

There are two popular tools for documenting modular structure, Warnier/Orr bracket charts and structure charts. Although often sold as distinct tools, they are actually quite similar. There are also two strategies for modular design. The Yourdon/Constantine approach suggests that modules be defined by studying the flow of data between primitive functions. The Warnier/Orr approach sug-

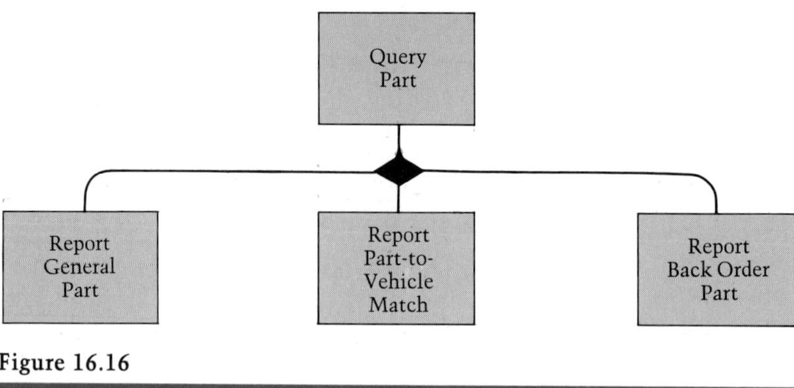

Figure 16.16

VTOC for a typical decision support inquiry program.

gests that modules be defined by studying the data structure of the outputs and inputs. This chapter presented a hybrid approach based on the two strategies.

Structure charts and Warnier/Orr charts adequately factor each program into manageable modules that can be assigned to programmers. IBM's Hierarchy plus Input-Process-Output (HIPO) provides a documentation tool for packaging detailed input, processing, and output details around the structure chart. In addition to the structure chart and input-process-output charts, the analyst must assemble the various data dictionaries, spacing charts, layouts, and systems flowcharts needed to present a complete program specification for the programmer.

PROBLEMS AND EXERCISES

1. Obtain a copy of the documentation for a completed programming assignment. Study the program's source code to identify all referenced modules. Using a Warnier/Orr diagram and a structure chart, document the existing modular structure implemented by the program.
2. Study the processing requirements for the program you used for problem 1. Using the modular design approach suggested in this chapter, develop a new structure chart for the program. Compare the structure chart with the one derived in problem 1. Which would you prefer to work from as a programmer? Why?

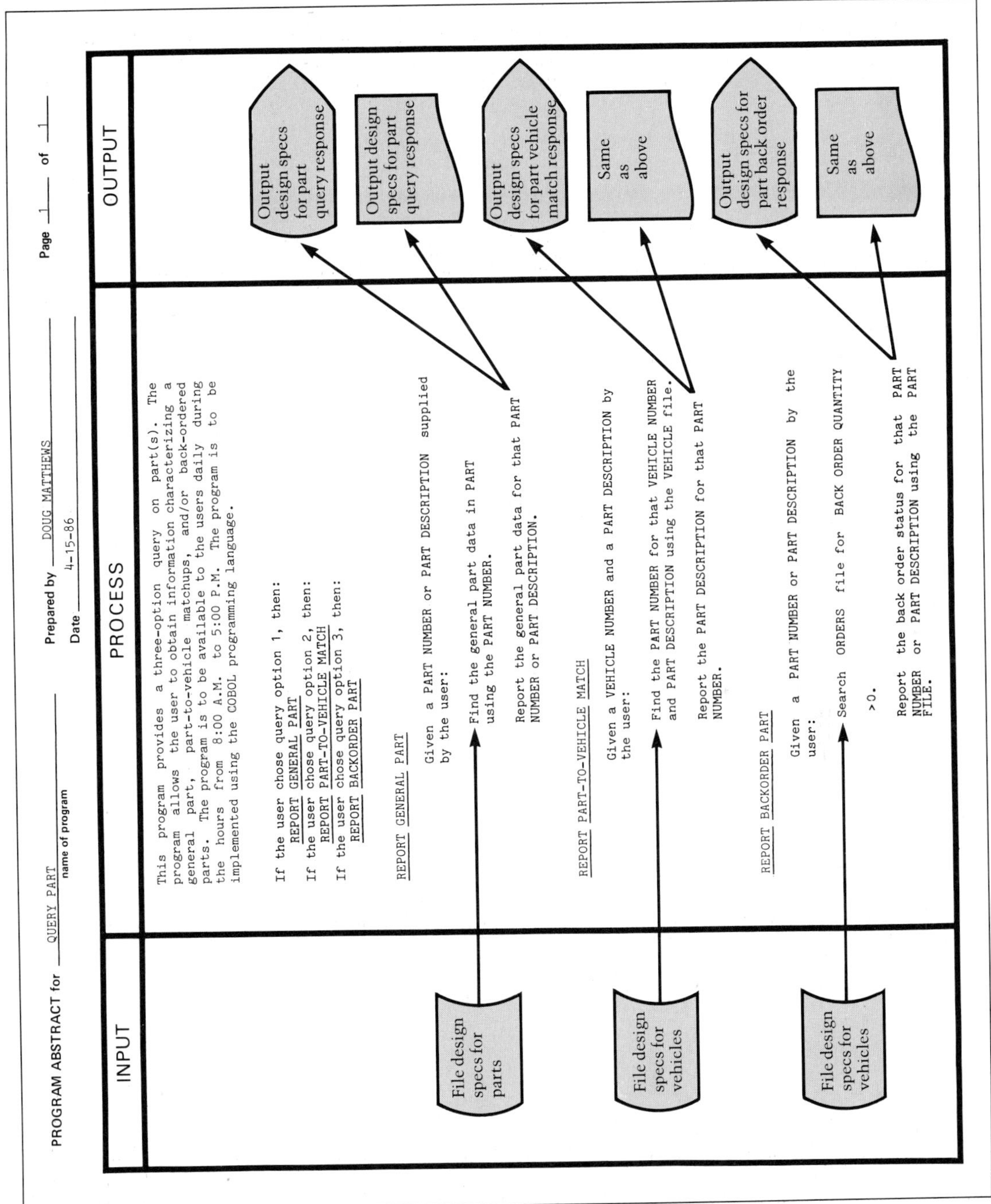

Figure 16.17

IPO chart for the decision support example.

The Next Generation

Automatic Code Generators — Will the Programmer Become Obsolete?

A continuing theme in these "Next Generation" features is the emergence of productivity tools for systems development. One of the great frustrations of the systems analyst occurs when carefully prepared program specifications don't get translated into the computer programs that were originally envisioned. This chapter has focused on tools and techniques that reorganize design specifications in a fashion suitable for programmers. Although it is true that improperly packaged and incomplete specifications are the cause of many program inadequacies, we don't intend to imply that the tools and techniques discussed in this chapter will eliminate the problem, although they will help. Will a future generation of tools and techniques promise to eliminate the problem? Perhaps!

It has long been suggested that programming, being a logical process, could be automated. In other words, we may be able to write programs that input (and insist upon!) complete specifications and generate and test computer programs — all in a fraction of the time required by human programmers. And there are a few products that support this concept.

In this book, we have frequently referred to fourth-generation languages. You might consider them the answer to our problem. But although these end-user languages are good and getting better, they are not suitable for all information systems. They may be limited in *what* they can do. And they are frequently inefficient when compared with their third-generation language counterparts (such as COBOL, using conventional file organization techniques). Why? Prototypes are based on small files. When fully loaded files are installed and multiple users start accessing the system, the throughput and response time becomes unacceptable. Therefore, many prototype systems developed using fourth-generation languages are rewritten in languages such as COBOL after the prototype has been approved by users. Thus we want to address an alternate question: Is there any way to improve productivity when using such languages as COBOL, BASIC, FORTRAN, PL/I, and PASCAL?

There are in the class we speak of. Higher Order Software (HOS), Inc. sells a product called *USE.IT*, which automates program design. The package forces you to recursively factor a program into binary (two) functions and subfunctions. The resulting structure can be translated by *USE.IT* into executable program code that HOS claims can be mathematically proven to be bug-free. Other products use structured design techniques to develop a program from a general idea by using structured design techniques, such as Warnier/Orr. These programs can also generate usable code. We encountered a simpler approach at one Fortune 500 company. They have studied programs in their environment and developed programs that generate skeleton PL/I code for functions they know to be needed in multiple applications.

In any case, we can expect to see more products of this type. They will become more sophisticated and will generate even more efficient program code. The impact on programmers is clear. We'll still need programmers to maintain operational systems and to enhance and customize the code from these program generators, but we will clearly need fewer programmers. But that's no problem — we'll need more and better analysts because these program generators will be dependent on clear and complete program specifications. ■

3. Some typical initiate, processing, and terminate functions were presented in Figures 16.5 and 16.8. Can you identify other processing functions that might be included in the lists? How would you classify them—as initiate, processing, or terminate functions? Explain why.
4. Prepare a systems flowchart for the program in problem one. Use the structure chart (from problem two) and the systems flowchart to prepare an input-process-output chart(s) to package the program.
5. What value would an existing structure chart and input-process-output chart of an existing program be to a systems analyst during the study phase?
6. What value would an existing structure chart and input-process-output chart for a program be to a programmer who has to maintain the program?
7. What programs appearing on a systems flowchart does the systems analyst need to package? What correlations can be drawn between the systems flowchart and the input-process-output chart?
8. What are thc transaction centers in the following program?

   An on-line program allows a user to perform inquiries to obtain information concerning customer accounts, orders, invoices, and products. The user is allowed to obtain general information concerning an order or information about specific orders that have been placed on back order. The user who wishes to obtain information concerning orders placed on back order may request information describing orders that have been back ordered for less than one week, back ordered for more than one week but less than two weeks, or back ordered for more than a two-week period. The user may also perform inquiries to retrieve general information about a specific part and information concerning back ordered parts.

ANNOTATED REFERENCES AND SUGGESTED READINGS

Adams, David R., Gerald E. Wagner, and Terrence J. Boyer. *Computer Information Systems: An Introduction.* Cincinnati, Ohio:

South-Western Publishing, 1983. We are indebted to this book's suggestion that most programs can be factored into initiate, main process, and terminate functions (Chapter 8). We adapted this approach to provide a high-level framework into which the various modular design strategies can be integrated.

Boehm, Barry. "Software Engineering." *IEEE Transactions on Computers,* Vol. C-25, December 1976. This paper, a classic, described the logarithmic relationship between time and the cost to correct an error in the systems specification.

Orr, Kenneth T. *Structured Systems Development.* New York: Yourdon Press, 1977. Although somewhat dated, this is still our favorite book on the Warnier/Orr method of modular design. It is short, easy to read, and contains numerous examples. It also contains an easy-to-read, albeit somewhat negative, discussion of the HIPO documentation technique.

Page-Jones, Meiler. *A Practical Guide to Structured Systems Design.* New York: Yourdon Press, 1980. This is our favorite book on the Yourdon-Constantine method of modular design, a methodology called *Structured Systems Design.* It is easy to read and contains numerous examples of both transform and transaction analysis. The concepts of coupling and cohesion are also covered in greater detail. This book is must reading for both analysts and programmers.

Analysts in Action

Implementation of the New System

Cheryl and Doug have completed the design of the new order-entry system. Now they must supervise implementation of the new system.

Episode 8

Three months have passed since the design specifications for the new order-entry system were approved. During the past three months, Beverly's programming team has been writing and testing the computer programs. Meanwhile Cheryl and Doug have been writing comprehensive user and operations manuals. We begin this episode in the conference room where Cheryl has assembled key users, management, and computer operations personnel. Doug is leading this meeting.

"I want to thank you all for coming. This meeting should be brief. Before I begin, I'm supposed to remind you that the company barbeque is this weekend. We're all supposed to meet at shelter B in the amusement park. And all of us in this room have very good reason to celebrate. The moment we've been waiting for is nearly at hand. I want to review our progress as we get ready to convert to the new order-entry system."

After a brief applause, Doug continued. "This is a chart of our schedule and progress (Figure 1). Each bar represents a task. The shading you can see on some of the bars indicates work that has been completed. As you can see, we're nearly done with the programming and testing tasks. And when those tasks are complete, we'll be converting to the new system.

"The first training sessions begin next Monday. The order-entry clerks are scheduled to attend class from 8 to 9 A.M. each day next week. Joey and Madge and the secretarial staff will hold down the fort during the classes."

Joey interrupted, "Doug, what exactly is involved in the first training session? I see from the chart, that the system still won't be quite finished."

Doug replied, "Good question. The first training session is centered around the user's manual and demonstration. The transaction processing and query programs, which are finished, will be demonstrated to the clerks. Until the second training session, there will be limited hands-on training."

Noting that Joey's question had been answered, Doug continued. "Files will be loaded or converted beginning a week from Monday. This will take one and a half weeks."

Joey interrupted again. "I don't get it! What do you mean the files will be loaded and converted? And why so long to do it?"

Cheryl sensed some frustration and joined the conversation. "You see, Joey, up to now, we've been testing the programs on small test files, and we've been using representative rather than real data. Before we place your system into operation, we have to get the files loaded with your actual data. For instance, we've got to get all your customer file index cards loaded into computer files. And we have to do that to all the other new computer ▶

Figure 1

A typical project management tool.

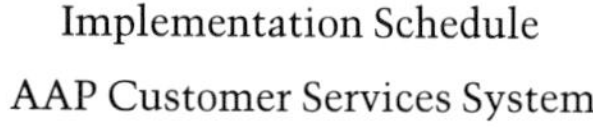

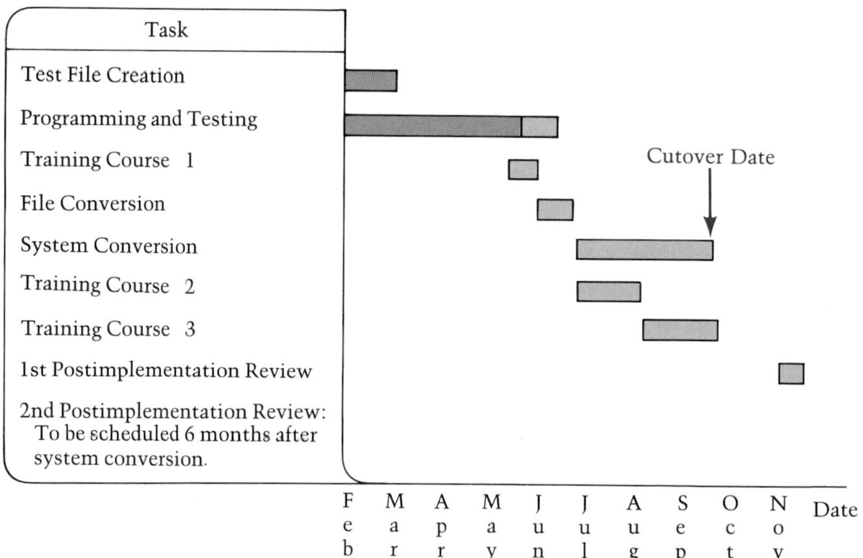

files that are currently manual. There are a lot of records to be input and checked for accuracy. And that takes time."

Joey smiled and replied, "I had no idea. Of course it will take a while. Do you think one and a half weeks is enough?"

"Yes," answered Cheryl. "We've studied the sizes of your files and the the types of data to be input. We're buying temporary data-entry help from a local service bureau. One and a half weeks should do it."

Doug continued reviewing the schedule. "The big day is two and a half weeks away. That's when we convert to the new system."

"Just like that?" asked Madge. "What if it doesn't work perfectly?"

Doug responded, "We won't completely cut over to the new system right away. Instead, we're going to operate the new system and the old system in parallel until we are sure the new system works properly."

"How long?" asked Joey.

"We've budgeted one month of parallel operation. During that month, you will process all transactions twice, the old way and the new way. It's not double work. Most of the work in the new system is performed by the computer. If you discover any discrepancies or errors, you should notify Cheryl or myself immediately. Our programming team will go to work immediately to correct any errors. As you can see, we plan to cut over to the new system at the end of September." ►

Madge asked, "What if we find opportunities to improve the system? Not errors, just improvements?"

Doug answered, "Well, we are obviously going to give priority to correcting errors and omissions. However, if suggested improvements are simple to do, we'll do them. Otherwise, we'll record them into an enhancements request to be acted on later."

Joey asked, "What if the system works perfectly right off the bat? Can we stop the parallel processing early?"

"We'd rather not" answered Doug. "We want to be certain before we ditch the old system completely. Besides, the cut over corresponds to the beginning of a new fiscal quarter. That's ideal for the reporting features of the system."

Joey responded, "Is this how you did the implementation of the purchasing system?"

"Yes," answered Doug.

"Doug, I see a second training session on your chart." said Madge.

Doug replied, "Yes, those sessions begin the day before the parallel processing begins. By that time, the new CRT terminals will have been delivered and installed. The second training session includes hands-on practice using several sample transactions that Cheryl developed. Also, the second training session includes in-office consulting for three days. Cheryl and I will provide this training and consulting."

Joey interrupted. "What's the third training session?"

Doug responded, "That's the training session for managers and supervisors. Secretaries are also invited. During these sessions, you'll learn not only the transaction-processing and query procedures but also the management-reporting and advanced decision support features of the system."

Joey replied, "Now that's what I'm waiting for!"

Doug continued, "Finally, you'll notice that two months after the system has been operating by itself, we've scheduled a review meeting to discuss problems, limitations, and enhancements. We don't want to leave any loose ends. Are there any questions?"

When nobody asked any questions, Joey stood up and said, "Well, I, for one, am tickled to death to see this project near completion. It looks like every possibility has been considered. Again, Cheryl, Doug: We appreciate all your efforts on our behalf. I say, let's go for it!"

Where Do We Go from Here?

This episode has introduced several post analysis and design considerations that are normally managed by the systems analyst. For a more detailed survey of systems implementation, read Chapter 17.

Observing Cheryl and Doug we recognize two particularly important skills that must be exercised during systems implementation—communication and project management. You can learn about effective communication skills by reading Part IV, Module C: "Communication Skills for the Systems Analyst." Finally, an equally important skill is project management. You can learn about project management in, Module A: "Project Management." ■

17 How to Perform Systems Implementation

Minicase: Transport Pipe Company (revisited)

In Chapters 6 and 10, we sat in on two job performance reviews with Ken Hayes, MIS manager at Transport Pipe Company, and Tim Stallard, one of Ken's employees. During these two interviews, we have seen Tim's career being directed toward systems analysis and design. Six months have passed since Tim was promoted to programmer/analyst. And once again it's time for his semiannual job performance review. So let's listen in.

"Another six months!," exclaimed Ken. "It hardly seems that long since your last job performance review."

"Time flies!" replied Tim. "I personally feel very good about my progress over the last six months. I'm especially proud of my improved writing skills. The college courses are helping. I hope you agree."

"Absolutely!" answered Ken. "More than any technical skills, your ability to communicate will determine your long-term career growth. Let's look at your progress in other areas. Yes, you've been supervising the MRP project implementation for the last few months. This is your first real experience with the entire implementation process, right?"

Tim responded, "Yes. You know, I was a programmer for three years. I thought I knew everything there was to know about systems implementation. But this project has taught me different."

"How's that?" asked Ken.

"The computer programming tasks have gone smoothly. In fact, we finished testing the entire system of programs six weeks ahead of schedule."

Ken interrupted, "I don't mean to interrupt but I just want to reaffirm the role your design specifications played in accelerating the computer programming tasks. Bob has told me repeatedly that he had never seen such thorough and complete design specifications. The programmers seem to know exactly what to do."

"Thanks, Ken. That really makes me feel good. It takes a lot of time to prepare design specifications like that, but I think that it really pays off during implementation. Now, what was I going to say? Oh yes. Even though the programming and testing were completed ahead of schedule, the system still hasn't been placed into operation; it's two weeks late."

Ken replied, "That means you lost the six-week buffer plus another two weeks. What happened?"

"Well," answered Tim, "I'm to blame. I just didn't know enough about the nonprogramming activities of systems implementation. First, I underestimated the difficulties of training. My first-draft training manual made too many assumptions about computer familiarity. My users didn't understand the instructions, and I had to rewrite the manual. I also decided to conduct some training classes for the users. My instructional delivery was terrible, to put it mildly. I guess I never really considered the possibility that, as a systems analyst, I'd have to be a teacher. I think I owe a few apologies to some of my former instructors. Do you have any idea how much time goes into preparing for a class?"

Ken smiled. "Yes, especially when you're technically oriented and your audience isn't."

Tim continued, "Anyway, that cost me more time than I had anticipated. But there are still other implementation problems that have to be solved. And I didn't budget time for them!"

"Like what?" asked Ken.

"Like getting data into the new files. We have to enter several thousand new records. And to top it off, management is insisting that we operate the new system in parallel with the old system for at least two months. Then, and only then, will they be willing to allow the old system to be discarded."

"Well, Tim, I think you're learning a lot. Obviously, we threw you to the wolves on this project. But I needed Bob's [Tim's mentor] cxperience and attention elsewhere. I knew when I pulled Bob off the project that it could introduce delays—I call it the *rookie factor.* Under normal circumstances, I would never have let you work on this alone. But you're doing a good job and you're learning. We have to take the circumstances into consideration. But you'll obviously feel somc heat from your users because the implementation is behind schedule, and I want you to deal with that on your own. I think you can handle it. But don't hestiate to call on Bob or me for advice. Let's talk about some training and job goals for the next six months. What do you think . . ."

Discussion

1. Above and beyond programming, what tasks do you think make up systems implementation? Can you think of any tasks that weren't described in this minicase?
2. Why is training so difficult? How do you feel about the prospects of becoming a "teacher?" How long do you think it takes to prepare for one hour of classroom instruction? What tasks do you think would be involved in preparing a lesson plan?
3. A 3,000 record master file must be created for a new system. Each record consists of fifteen fields. The record length is 200 bytes. How long do you suppose it would take to create that file? If necessary, use your own typing speed as a performance gauge. What factors would effect how long it may take to get the file up and running?
4. What assumption did Tim make about transition from the old system to the new system? Why was it wrong? Can you think of any circumstances under which it would be correct?

WHAT WILL YOU LEARN IN THIS CHAPTER?

In this chapter you will learn about two systems implementation phases: (1) the construction of the new information system and (2) the delivery of the new information system. You will know that you understand the systems implementation process when you can:

1. Define *systems implementation* and relate the term to the construction and delivery phases of the life cycle.
2. Describe the construction and delivery phases of the life cycle in terms of:
   (a) Purpose and objectives
   (b) Each dimension of the information system pyramid
   (c) Tasks and activities that must or may be performed
   (d) Skills you need to master to properly perform the phase
3. Explain how the time spent on systems implementation can be managed.

What is *systems implementation?* When we asked that question about *systems analysis* and *systems design*, we consulted Webster's Dictionary for an answer. We are interested in the noun *implement*, which is defined as follows:

> **im·ple·ment** . . . 1. to carry into effect; fulfill; accomplish 2. to provide the means for the carrying out of . . .
> (From *Webster's New World Dictionary of the American Language, Second College Edition*, Simon & Schuster, a Division of Gulf & Western Corporation, 1980. Used with permission.)

For our purposes, **systems implementation** is the fulfillment or carrying out of the design specifications to put the new information system into operation. In this chapter, we will study systems implementation.

We will examine two systems implementation phases: the construction of the new information system and the delivery of the new information system. Figure 17.1 illustrates these phases in terms of the systems development life cycle. For each of these two phases, we will study the *purpose* and *objectives*, specific *tasks* and *activities* that should be performed, and important *skills* to be mastered. As we did in Chapters 6 and 10, we will carefully build on the concepts and models that you learned in Part I. We will also build on the your knowledge of the systems analysis process (Chapter 6) and the sys-

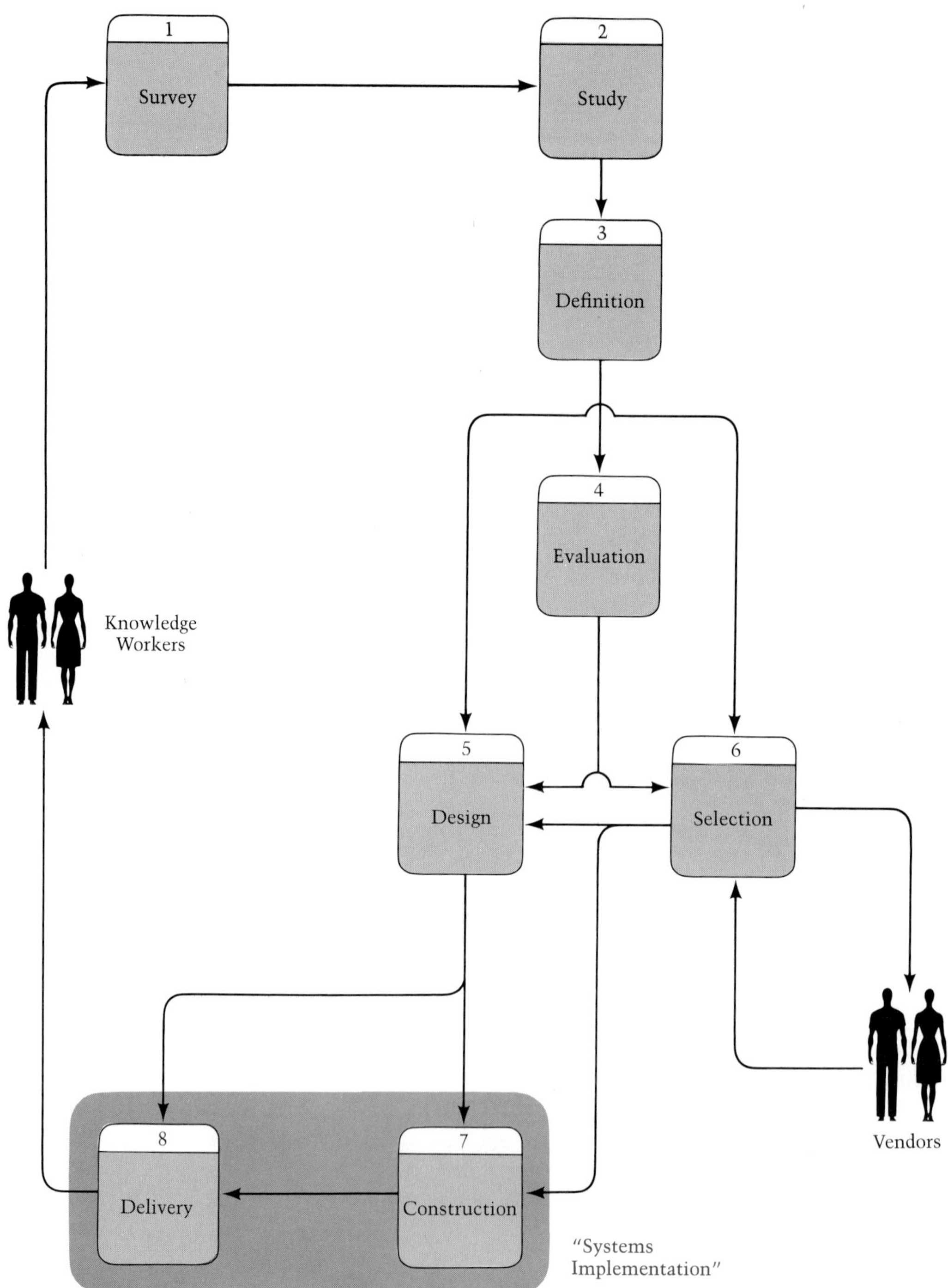
1
Survey
2
Study
3
Definition
4
Evaluation
Knowledge
Workers
5
Design
6
Selection
Vendors
8
Delivery
7
Construction
"Systems
Implementation"

◀ **Figure 17.1**

The systems implementation process. Systems implementation is defined as the construction and delivery phases of your system development life cycle.

tems design process (Chapter 10). Finally, we'll survey some of the project management implications of systems implementation.

You might be wondering why a chapter on *systems implementation* is included in a *systems analysis and design* book. First and foremost, implementation is part of the systems development life cycle you have been studying throughout this book. Second, as a systems analyst, you can expect to directly involved in many, if not all, of the implementation activities. Finally, we want you to understand the close working relationship between the systems analyst and the computer programmer.

HOW TO CONSTRUCT THE NEW INFORMATION SYSTEM

Construction of the new information system is a phase that is familiar to most of you. This is the phase in which most of the computer programming for the system will occur. Why not just call it *programming*? Because there's more to building the final system than computer programming! Although that may or may not surprise you, you'll soon understand the full implications of the construction phase.

Purpose and Objectives of the Construction Phase

The purpose of the **construction phase** in the life cycle is to build a working information system from the design specifications prepared during the design phase. To achieve the purpose of the construction phase, we must accomplish the following objectives:

- Construct, modify, or install the software and hardware components of the information system.
- Construct a system that fulfills the user requirements for transaction processing, management reporting, and decision support.

- In some modern environments, directly involve knowledge workers in the construction of their own systems.

Once again, we have defined these objectives around the dimensions of your information system model. Let's examine each of these objectives in greater detail.

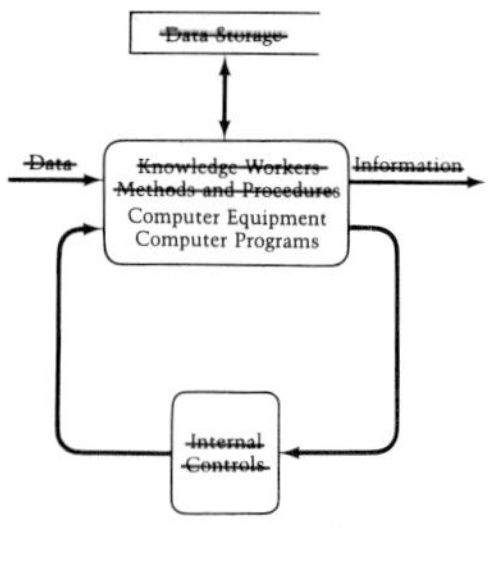

IPO Components

Information Systems Components to Be Constructed What do we construct? We construct the hardware and software components of the new system (see margin). Actually, *construct* may not be the best term for what happens during this phase. *Construct* implies building from scratch. Although many programs are built from scratch, others may actually be modified to fulfill new requirements. And still other software is installed. This is particularly true of purchased software. Those packages may have to be customized, but it beats writing the programs from scratch.

Furthermore, hardware components are not constructed. New hardware was chosen during the selection phase of our life cycle. During the construction phase, this hardware is installed so that the programmers can utilize it to construct the system. Note that the programmers may have to learn how to use new hardware and software packages before they can construct or modify the system.

Still, the most familiar and time-consuming activity is computer programming and maintenance. For that reason, we will stick with the *construction* label. Do any other elements in the IPO components model have to be constructed or installed? Absolutely! Preprinted forms conceived during the design phase must be physically printed. This is usually accomplished through a specialized forms manufacturer. Along similar lines, stocks of supplies may have to be built up; for instance, diskettes, tapes, logbooks, and furniture.

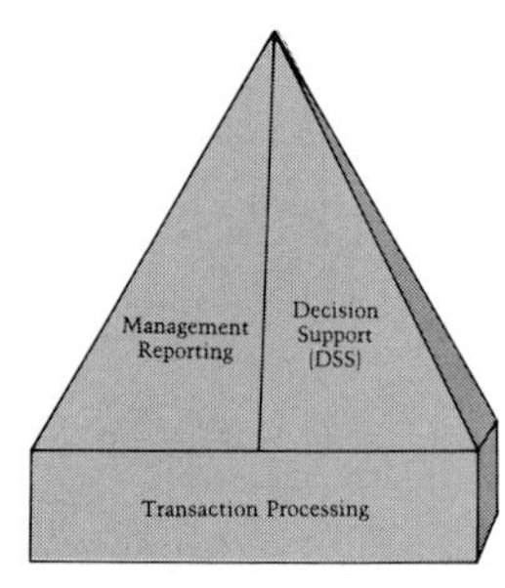

Information System Functions

Information Systems Functions and Their Importance During the Construction Phase It is very important that the programmers not stray from the design specifications without the analyst's approval. Why? Because, the design specifications were prepared to fulfill user requirements (reproduced in the margin). A change in these specifications could throw the system out of synchronization with the user's requirements. The computer programmer often has little or no direct contact with those users. Therefore, during the construction phase, the analyst is primarily concerned that the information system fulfills the transaction-processing, management-reporting, and decision support capabilities specified during the definition and design phases.

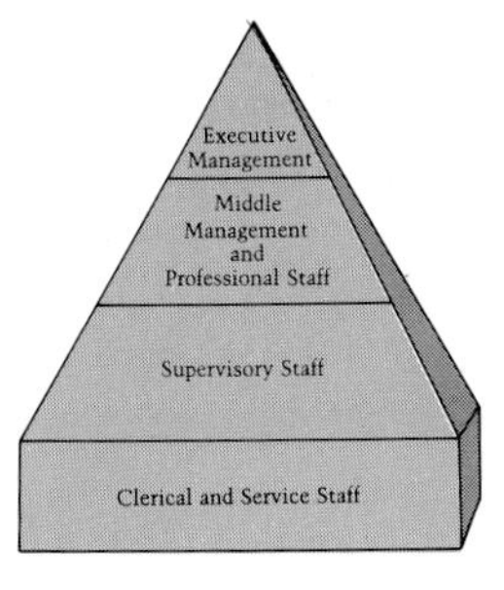

Knowledge Workers

Knowledge-Worker Involvement During the Construction Phase You have already learned the importance of knowledge-worker (see margin) involvement during the study, definition, evaluation, selection, and design phases of our life cycle. What about the construction phase? For most systems development, computer programmers will work alone to develop, debug, and test computer programs to fulfill design specifications. But, as we've said on several occasions in this book, a new class of friendly programming languages is emerging. These fourth-generation programming languages, hereafter called 4GLs, are generally considered to be more user friendly. The net result will be twofold:

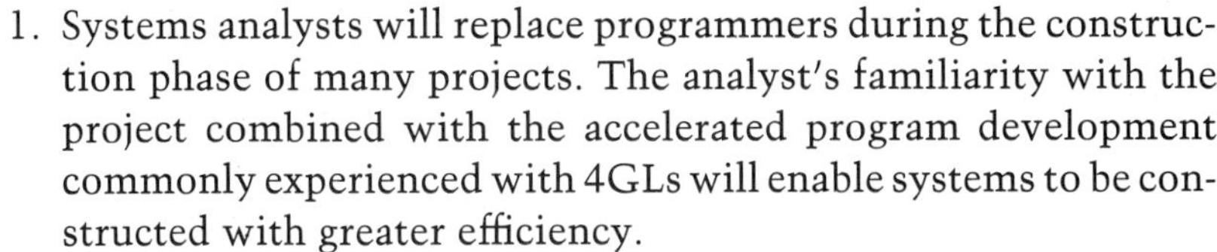

1. Systems analysts will replace programmers during the construction phase of many projects. The analyst's familiarity with the project combined with the accelerated program development commonly experienced with 4GLs will enable systems to be constructed with greater efficiency.
2. End users will become directly involved in the construction phase. Although analysts and programmers will implement the more difficult transaction and file maintenance programs, the end users will be able to construct the management-reporting and decision support programs. All 4GLs offer easy-to-learn and easy-to-use report generators and query facilities that can be directly applied by end users.

How to Complete the Construction Phase

In this section, we want to identify and discuss the specific tasks, documentation, and skills required for the construction phase. Figure 17.2 illustrates the construction phase tasks and documentation in greater detail. By now, the notation should be familiar. The process symbols are tasks, and the data flows are documentation. As we further examine each task and its key documents, we will identify those skills you need to develop to perform the task. Some of these tasks are specific to computer programming. Although we will identify those tasks and their associated skills, we will direct you to your programming curriculum for training in these subjects. We

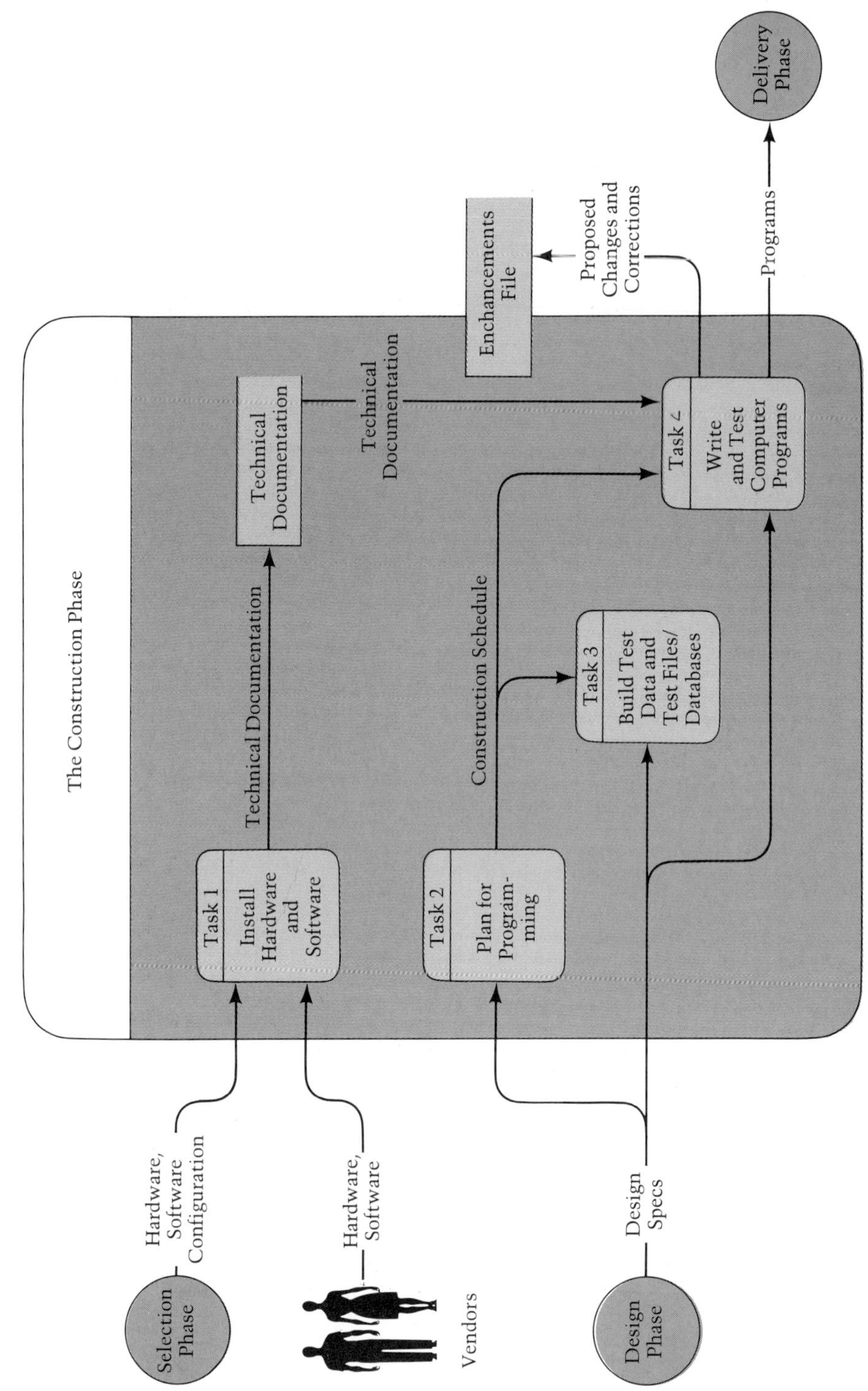
The Construction Phase
Selection Phase
Hardware, Software Configuration
Vendors
Hardware, Software
Design Phase
Design Specs
Task 1
Install Hardware and Software
Technical Documentation
Technical Documentation
Technical Documentation
Task 2
Plan for Program-ming
Construction Schedule
Task 3
Build Test Data and Test Files/ Databases
Task 4
Write and Test Computer Programs
Enchancements File
Proposed Changes and Corrections
Programs
Delivery Phase

◄ **Figure 17.2**

Construction phase tasks. The construction phase can be broken down into the tasks suggested on this diagram. The arrows depict documentation. Notice the enhancements file. It is created during this phase to begin collecting ideas for improving the system — ***without*** **delaying the implementation.**

want only to place computer programming into the context of the systems development life cycle, of which it is a part.

Task 1: Install Hardware and Software (if necessary) Recall from Chapter 10 that the new information system may be built around new or upgraded technology that was ordered during the selection phase. A net output of the selection phase, the hardware/software configuration for the new system is a net input to a construction phase task, install hardware and software. Installation is frequently a two-step process.

The first step may be site preparation. New equipment may require a special environment (for instance, air conditioning, furniture, printing rooms). While the hardware/software order is being filled, the analyst can work with computer center management or end user management to prepare the site for installation of the technology. An example should drive this point home.

A new on-line system may specify that there will be an IBM 3270 terminal on each clerk's desk. Now is the time to plan for that delivery. The 3270 is a rather large terminal, and each clerk must make space for it. It is possible that now is the time to consider specialized furniture that can ergonomically handle the terminal and its cable connections. Telephone lines may need to be installed if the computer is at a remote site. In the computer center itself, a new controller may have to be installed to handle the new terminals. This controller will take up space. Where should it be located? These are issues to be decided before the equipment is delivered.

The second step is to install the delivered hardware and software. Hardware is normally installed and tested by the vendor (even microcomputer stores frequently offer this service). Software may or may not be installed by the vendor. In any case, specialists called *systems programmers* often become involved in the installation, testing, and modification of such software as operating systems, database management systems, word processors, spreadsheets, telecommunications software, and other general purpose software packages.

Of course, if the new information system requires no new or additional technology, then the selection phase and this task are not necessary. Although site preparation and installation are not typically performed by systems analysts, they are included here as a construction phase task because construction cannot proceed without the required technology. On the other hand, the installation of new hardware and software usually goes hand in hand with the need to train programmers and analysts about how to use the new technology.

Task 2: Plan for Programming Recall that an implementation plan was generated as the final task of the design phase. The implementation plan, included in the design specifications, specified systems test data and a schedule for the construction and delivery phases. This plan is rarely detailed enough to begin constructing the new system. Therefore, our next task is to plan the programming effort. The refined plan should include the following:

- *Review of the design specification.* One major controversy that should be addressed is the freezing of the design specifications. By **freezing,** we mean that changes to the design specifications are discouraged or prohibited. Why? With no discouragement against changes, users will continually be permitted to identify something they forgot or some new need or idea, and the system may never be constructed and delivered. On the other hand, some experts dispute the idea of freezing the specifications. They argue that such an action is artificial and not consistent with our goal to serve the user. Both sides are right! We suggest that you tentatively freeze the document. If changes are proposed, ask yourself a simple question: "Is this a critical change that will make or break the system, or is it an enhancement that could be added later?" Critical changes require the specifications document to be modified. Do it! If the change isn't critical, log the change in an enhancements file. We'll discuss this file later.

- *Organization of the programming team.* Most large programming projects require a team effort. One popular organization strategy is the use of **chief programmer teams.** This team is managed by the chief programmer, a highly proficient and experienced programmer who assumes overall responsibility for the program design strategy, standards, and construction. The chief programmer oversees all coding and testing activities and helps out with the most difficult aspects of the programs. Other team members include a backup chief programmer, program librarian, programmers, and specialists. The backup programmer is able to assume the chief programmer's role as well as to perform normal programming activities. The program librarian maintains the program documentation and program library. The programmers, often selected because of specialized programming skills relevant to the project, code and test the programs. Specialists offer unique skills pertinent to the project (such as database techniques or telecommunications background).

Where does the analyst fit in? That depends on the organization. Sometimes the analyst is the project manager to whom the chief programmer reports. Other times, the analyst is a consultant to the chief programming team, possibly as one of the specialists reporting to the chief programmer. Chief programming teams are formed and disbanded with each successive project.

- *Development of a detailed construction phase plan.* You don't just start programming. Most design specifications include numerous programs. Which programs should be written first? Many systems are built in **versions.** The first version implements the most critical aspects of the system, so that a version can be placed into operation before the system has been completely constructed. Another appropriate approach is to construct transaction-processing programs first. Implement these programs in the same sequence as that in which they would have to be run (NEW ORDER PROCESSING before ORDER CANCELLATION before BILLING and so on). Then implement management-reporting and decision support programs according to their relative importance. General file maintenance and backup and recovery programs are written last.

People planning and scheduling are project management skills that every systems analyst should develop and master.

Task 3: Build Test Data and Test Files and Databases Building test files and databases is a task unfamiliar to many students who have little or no data processing experience. They are accustomed to having an instructor provide them with the test data and files. This task must immediately precede other programming activities because files and databases are the resource shared by the computer programs to be written. Test files and databases are constructed quickly using valid test data that conforms to data dictionary values specified during systems analysis and design. The files should be large enough to test various transactions and report capabilities but small enough so they can be quickly created and tested. These are not final files or databases, and the data should be representative but not necessarily real. Test files and databases are usually constructed by using editors and software utilities that are available on most computers.

To learn to appreciate this skill, commit yourself to initially preparing your own test data and test files when you receive your next programming assignment.

Task 4: Write and Test Computer Programs The major activity of the construction phase is the writing and testing of computer programs. And this is the activity with which many of you have the most experience. This book is not intended as a programming course. However, we'd like to summarize at least one appropriate computer program development cycle for comparison with our systems development life cycle. The difference between good, mediocre, and poor programmers is usually their degree of discipline in writing programs. An appropriate program development life cycle is illustrated in Figure 17.3.

This particular program development life cycle begins with a review of program structure. By program structure, we mean the top-down, modular factoring of the program. According to this book's systems development life cycle, program structure was specified during systems design (Chapters 10 and 16). Some data processing shops insist that top-down, modular design is the programmer's responsibility. When that is the case, this first step could be changed from *review* to *design.*

Figure 17.3 ▶

A program development life cycle. Just as there are for the systems development life cycle, there are many versions of a program development life cycle. This is one example. This approach suggests a top-down strategy. The high-level modules are built first.

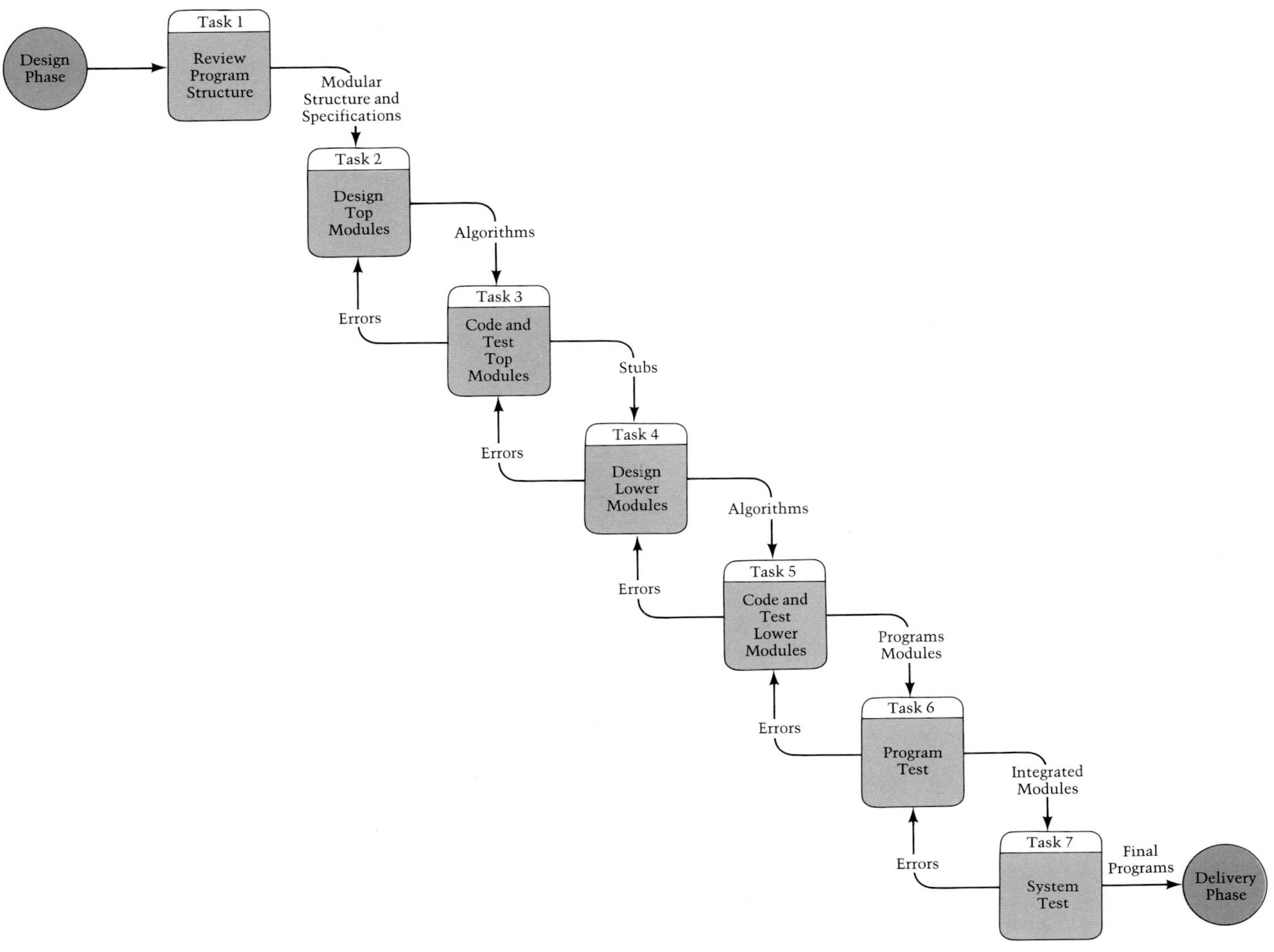
Design Phase
Task 1
Review Program Structure
Modular Structure and Specifications
Task 2
Design Top Modules
Algorithms
Errors
Task 3
Code and Test Top Modules
Stubs
Errors
Task 4
Design Lower Modules
Algorithms
Errors
Task 5
Code and Test Lower Modules
Programs Modules
Errors
Task 6
Program Test
Integrated Modules
Errors
Task 7
System Test
Final Programs
Delivery Phase

The program development life cycle depicted in Figure 17.3 suggests a top-down implementation—that is, modules are designed, coded, and tested beginning with the top module. The upper-level modules *drive* the lower level modules. Each module goes through three stages of development: algorithm design, coding, and testing. As modules are completed, they are integrated and tested. Eventually, the entire program is completed and tested as a whole. Each program for the new system goes through this cycle. After all of the programs have been individually coded and tested, the entire set of all programs that have been developed for the system are integrated and tested as a system.

Testing is an interesting skill that is often overlooked in academic courses on computer programming. If modules are coded top-down, they should be tested and debugged top-down *and as they are written.* Testing is not an activity to be deferred until after the program has been completely written! There are three levels of testing to be performed:

1. *Stub testing.* Stub testing is the test performed on individual modules (whether they be main program, subroutine, subprogram, block, or paragraph). How can you test a higher-level module before coding its lower level modules? Easy! You simulate the lower-level modules. These lower-level modules are often called *stubs.* Stub modules are subroutines, paragraphs, and the like that contain no logic. Perhaps all they do is print that they have been correctly called, and then control goes back to the parent module.
2. *Unit or program testing.* All of the modules that have been coded and stub tested are tested as an integrated unit. Eventually, all modules will have been implemented, and that unit equals the program itself. Unit testing uses the test data that were created during the design phase.
3. *System testing.* Just because each program works properly, it doesn't mean that the programs work *together* properly. The integrated set of programs should be run through a systems test to make sure that one program properly accepts, as input, the output of the other programs.

We'll talk about additional tests when we discuss the delivery phase. Computer programming activities are frequently governed by data processing standards. These standards dictate program design, coding, testing, and documentation rules that are intended to promote a consistent style within all information systems. These standards are often subject to design and code walkthroughs that check the program for conformance to standards (as well as logic and design errors). Some data processing shops have a Quality Assurance Department staffed by specialists who check program documentation (and systems analysis and design documentation) for conformance to standards.

Programming skills and structured programming are beyond the scope of this book. As we conclude this section, we'd like to leave you with two opinions. You cannot be an effective systems analyst without computer programming experience—that experience helps you appreciate the importance of thorough systems design. Finally, the use of structured programming techniques results in programs that are easier to write, read, and (especially!) maintain. Learn structured programming, and learn how to prepare design specifications that are thorough. This will allow the programmers time to apply structured programming techniques!

Finally, we remind you that the construction of computer programs may be replaced or supplemented by the installation of purchased software. These packages were chosen during the selection phase. Now they may have to be modified or customized to fulfill your user and design requirements (specified in earlier phases). This modification to the construction phase is illustrated in Figure 17.4. Task 5 is the installation of the applications software package and task 6 is the modification of the software package.

HOW TO DELIVER THE NEW INFORMATION SYSTEM INTO OPERATION

Now we come to the last phase in our life cycle: Deliver the new information system. The analyst is the principal figure in the delivery phase, regardless of his or her role in the construction phase. Let's set the stage for this concluding phase. From the definition and evaluation phases, we know what parts of the new system are manual and what parts are computerized. From the design phase, we know how all inputs, outputs, and procedures are implemented. And from the construction phase, we have working hardware and

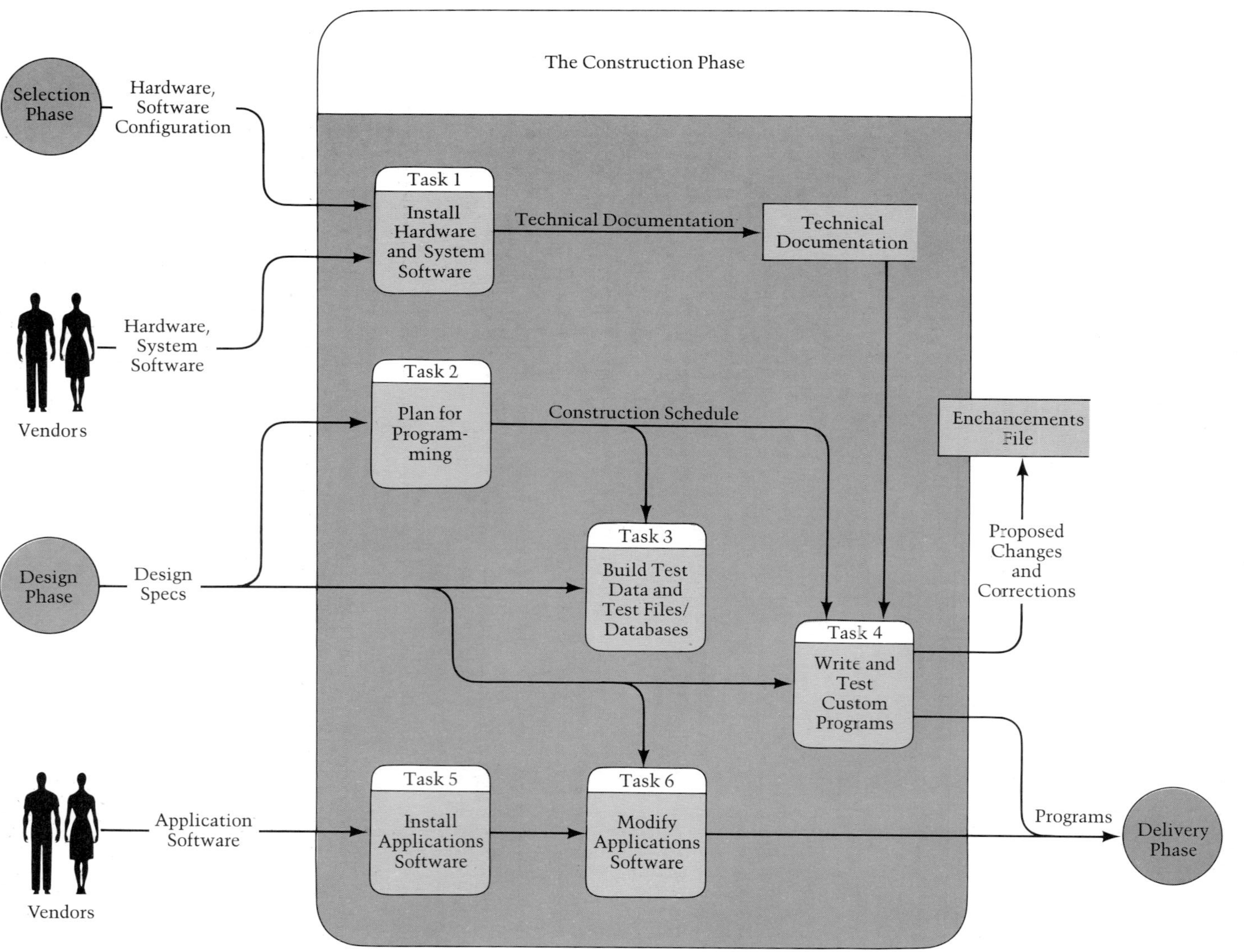

The Construction Phase
Selection Phase
Hardware, Software Configuration
Vendors
Hardware, System Software
Design Phase
Design Specs
Vendors
Application Software
Task 1
Install Hardware and System Software
Technical Documentation
Technical Documentation
Task 2
Plan for Program- ming
Construction Schedule
Task 3
Build Test Data and Test Files/ Databases
Task 4
Write and Test Custom Programs
Enchancements File
Proposed Changes and Corrections
Task 5
Install Applications Software
Task 6
Modify Applications Software
Programs
Delivery Phase

◄ **Figure 17.4**

A modified construction phase. This version of construction phase tasks reflects the installation and modification of software packages (as opposed to writing programs in-house).

software to support the new system. Now we must put the new system into operation.

Purpose and Objectives of the Delivery Phase

The purpose of the delivery phase is to smoothly convert from the old information system to the new information system. To achieve the purpose of the delivery phase, we must accomplish the following objectives:

- Train and assist knowledge workers in the use of the new system.
- Determine how well the new system fulfills its business mission as defined earlier in the project.
- Place the integrated hardware, software, people, methods, procedures, and data stores into operation, and ensure that they are performing properly to generate information from data.

Here we take a more detailed look at each of these objectives.

Knowledge-Worker Involvement in the Delivery Phase The system is *for* the user! Knowledge-worker involvement is important in the delivery phase because the users (see margin) will inherit your successes and failures from this phase. Fortunately, user involvement during this phase is rarely overlooked. The most important aspect of user involvement in the delivery phase is training and advising of the users. They must be trained to use equipment and to follow the procedures required by the new system. But no matter how good the training is, your users will become confused at times. Or perhaps they will find mistakes or limitations (an inevitable product despite the best of analysis, design, and implementation techniques). The analyst will help the users through the learning period until they become more familiar and comfortable with the new system.

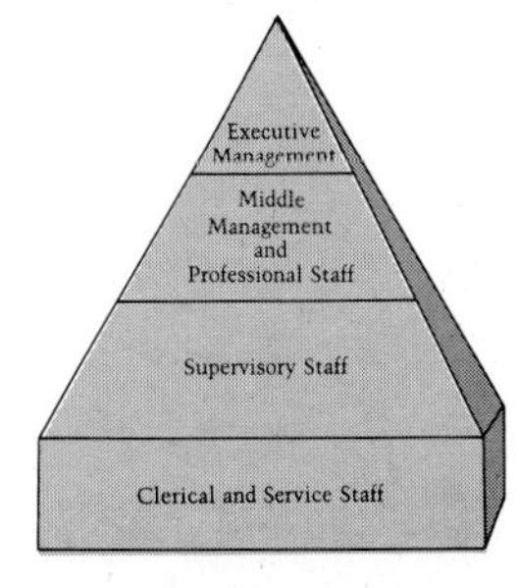

Knowledge Workers

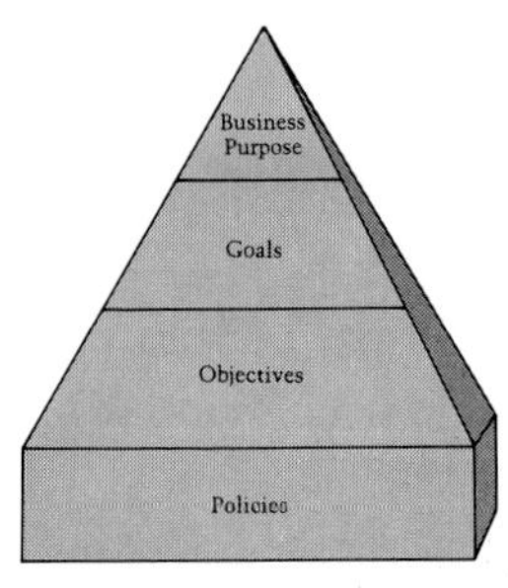

Business Mission

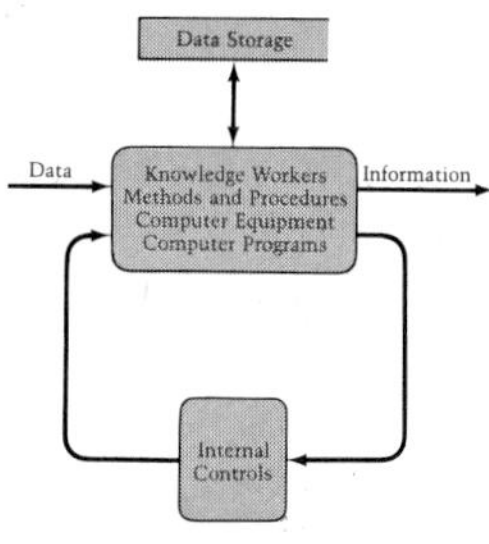

IPO Components

The Business Mission and the New System At the end of the delivery phase, the analyst should grade the system. How should the system be graded? A number of criteria are possible. Did the system cost more or less than its budgeted development cost? Although this may affect the payback period for the system, the costs cannot be recovered. Did the system come in on schedule? This is good for a pat on the back; but if you didn't meet the deadline, you cannot get schedule overruns back. What's done is done! You can only learn from your mistakes. The best criterion was, and still is, does the system fulfill the business mission (see margin). The system's grade relative to this criterion will determine the lifetime costs and usefulness of the system. If the system is successful, you will spend less time and money to fix it!

Information Systems Components and the Delivery Phase As was the case with all other phases, the IPO components (see margin) are the most visible dimension of the information system. In this case, "what you see is what you get." By now, we shouldn't have to detail these components — you know them well. Instead, we address the two most critical components:

1. *People.* Jobs and responsibilities change. Some jobs are created. Others are eliminated or totally redefined. The training implications were addressed earlier in this section.
2. *Methods and procedures.* The ways in which people perform their jobs are changing. The conversion from the old system to the new system must be carefully addressed. This applies not only to data processing methods and procedures but also to manual methods and procedures.

The key point is that the new system represents *change,* possibly dramatic. You should expect apprehension on the part of some of the users involved. No matter how involved and enthusiastic the users have been, people are naturally apprehensive about change. The current system, however flawed it may be, represents something that the users understand — and familiarity breeds content. If you've done a good job of analysis, design, and implementation, user apprehension will not last long, and your reputation will be secure. Just remember, when you do something right, people don't always remember it (at least not for long). But when you do something wrong, people tend *not* to forget. Teachers and analysts know this better than most people.

How to Complete the Delivery Phase

Now we can discuss the specific tasks, documentation, and skills that make up the delivery phase. The basic activities of the delivery phase are illustrated in Figure 17.5. Let's look at each activity in greater detail.

Task 1: Install Files and Databases During the construction phase, you built test files and test databases. But to place the system into operation, you need fully loaded files and databases. Therefore, the first task we'll survey is installation of files and databases. At first, this activity may seem trivial. But consider the implications of loading a typical file, say, CUSTOMER ACCOUNT. Tens or hundreds of thousands of records may have to be loaded. Each must be input, edited, and confirmed before the file is ready to be placed into operation.

For manual files that are being converted to computer files or databases, the basic method is simplified because you have already written file or database maintenance programs to add, delete, and modify records. The only problem is overhead. You have to load every record! Each record must be edited, processed, and confirmed via an update report. Data entry and validation will take a lot of overtime.

For existing computer files or databases that are being restructured, the procedure is more complicated. A special program must be written to read the old file and write to the new file, using the new structure. Then, if new fields were added to any of the records, additional programs must be written to initialize those fields (although you may be able to use the file maintenance programs mentioned in the previous paragraph). File conversion is an activity performed by data-entry personnel and computer programmers, not systems analysts.

As a systems analyst, you should calculate file and database sizes and estimate the time required to perform the task of installing them. The task itself is usually performed by data-entry personnel because users cannot release themselves for enough time to complete this task. Sometimes, temporary help must be hired for this one-time installation effort.

Task 2: Train Users to Use the New System A task more typically performed by systems analyst is to train users to use the new system. There are at least two fundamental training requirements: (1)

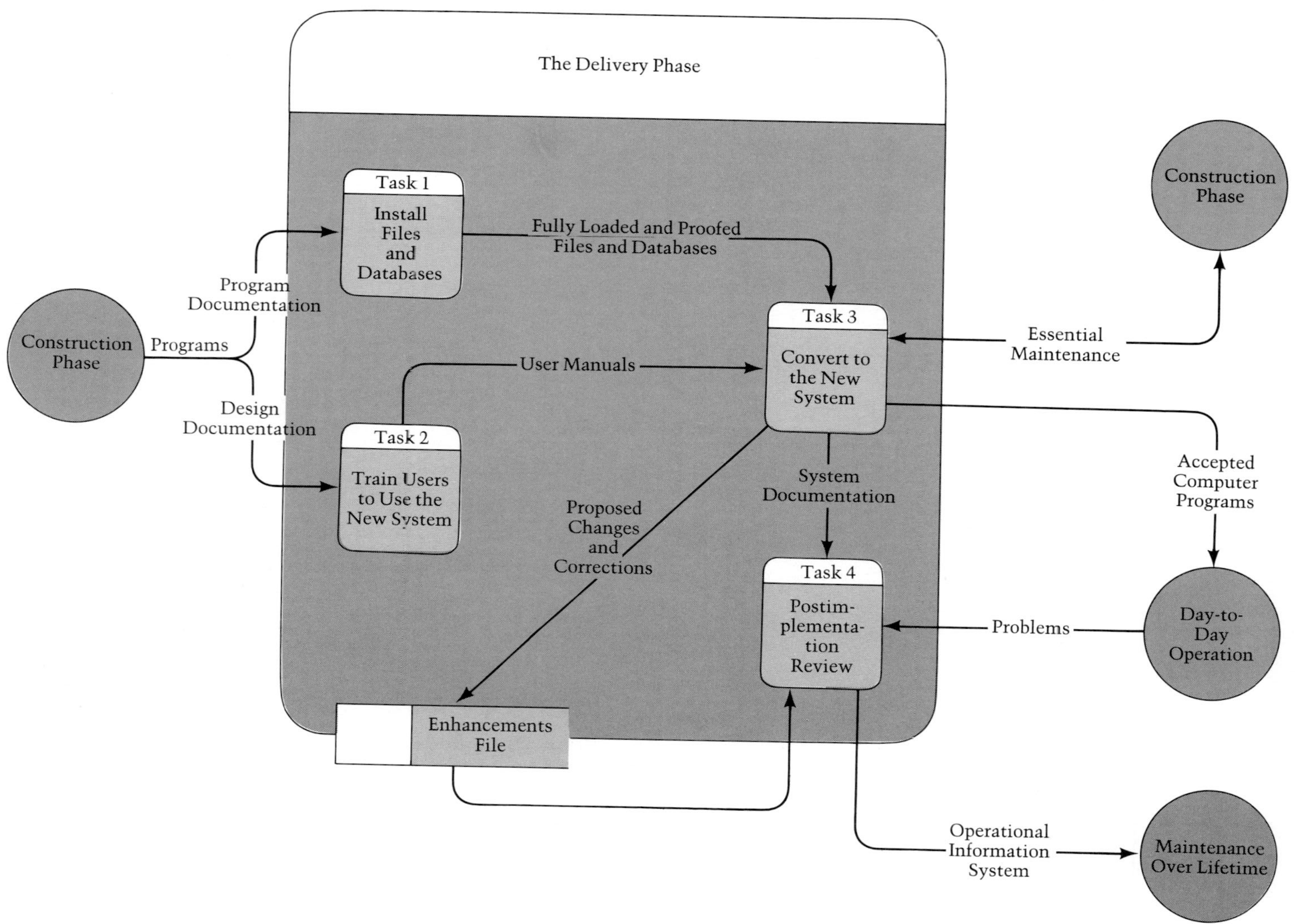

The Delivery Phase
Construction Phase
Programs
Program Documentation
Design Documentation
Task 1
Install Files and Databases
Task 2
Train Users to Use the New System
Fully Loaded and Proofed Files and Databases
User Manuals
Task 3
Convert to the New System
Proposed Changes and Corrections
Enhancements File
System Documentation
Task 4
Postimplementation Review
Construction Phase
Essential Maintenance
Accepted Computer Programs
Day-to-Day Operation
Problems
Operational Information System
Maintenance Over Lifetime

◄ **Figure 17.5**

Delivery phase tasks. The delivery phase can be broken down into the tasks suggested on this diagram. As usual, the arrows depict documentation.

training manuals and (2) the training itself. Many organizations hire special systems analysts who do nothing but write user documentation and training guides. If you have a skill for writing clearly, then the demand for your services is out there! Figure 17.6 is a typical outline for a training manual. The golden rule should apply for user manual writing: "Write unto others as you would have them write unto you." You are not a business expert. Don't expect the reader to be a technical expert. Every possible situation and its proper procedure must be documented.

The actual training is built around the user manuals. Training can be performed one-on-one. However, group training is generally preferred. It is a better use of your time and it encourages group learning possibilities. Think about your education for a moment. Isn't it true that you really learn more from your fellow students and colleagues than from your instructors. Instructors facilitate learning and instruction, but you master specific skills through practice with large groups because, with them, common problems and issues can be addressed more effectively. Take advantage of the ripple effect of education. The first group of trainees can then train several other groups.

Related to user manuals and training is the complementary preparation of computer operations manuals and training. These manuals instruct computer operators on how to carry out data processing procedures as documented in systems flowcharts.

Once again, written and oral communications skills are critical. Familiarity with organizational behavior and psychology may also prove helpful. The delivery phase represents *change,* and people have a natural tendency to resist change or look for fault in change. There is comfort in the status quo — even if the current system is fraught with problems.

Task 3: Convert to the New System Conversion to the new system from the old system is a significant milestone. After conversion, the ownership of the system *officially* transfers from the analysts and programmers to the users. There are four conversion or installation strategies commonly used:

TRAINING MANUAL/USERS GUIDE OUTLINE

I. Introduction

II. Manual

  A. The manual system (a detailed explanation of peoples' jobs and standard operating procedures for the new system)

  B. The computer system (how it fits into the overall workflow)

    1. Terminal/keyboard familiarization

    2. First-time users

      a. Getting started

      b. Lessons

  C. Reference manual (for nonbeginners)

III. Appendices

  A. Error messages

Figure 17.6

An outline for a training manual. A good training manual or procedures manual can prevent many problems during the lifetime of a system. This is an outline for one such manual.

1. *Abrupt cutover.* On a specific date, usually a date that coincides with an official business period (such as month, quarter, or fiscal year), the old system is terminated and the new system is placed into operation. This is a high-risk approach because there may still be major problems that won't be uncovered until the system has been in operation for at least one business period. On the other hand, there are no transition costs. Abrupt cutover may be necessary if, for instance, a governmental mandate or business policy becomes effective on a specific date and the system couldn't be implemented prior to that time.
2. *Parallel conversion.* Under this approach, both the old and new systems are operated for some period of time. This is done to ensure that all major problems in the new system have been solved before the old system is discarded. The final cutover may be either abrupt (usually at the end of one business period) or gradual (as portions of the new system are deemed adequate). Obviously, this strategy minimizes the risk of major flaws in the

new system causing irreparable harm to the business. But it also means that the cost of running two systems over some period of time must be incurred. Because running two editions of the same system on the computer could place an unreasonable demand on computing resources, this may only be possible if the old system is largely manual.

3. *Location conversion.* When the same system will be used in numerous geographical locations, it is usually converted at one location (using either abrupt or parallel conversion). As soon as that site has approved the system, it can be farmed to the other sites. Other sites can be cut over abruptly because major errors have been fixed. Furthermore, other sites benefit from the learning experiences of the first test site. Incidentally, the first production test site is often called a *beta test site.*
4. *Staged conversion.* Like location conversion, staged conversion is a variation on the abrupt and parallel conversions. A staged conversion is based on the version concept introduced earlier. Each successive version of the new system is converted as it is developed. Each version may be converted using the abrupt, parallel, or location strategies.

What happens during the systems conversion? Yes, training may occur, but we factored training out as a separate task that should begin well before systems conversion. The major activity is the **systems acceptance test.** At this point, we should differentiate between what we called a *systems test* earlier in the chapter and the *systems acceptance test* performed here. The systems test was performed by programmers using test data. The systems acceptance test is performed by users using real data over an extended period of time. The systems acceptance test should be extensive. There are three levels of acceptance testing:

1. *Verification testing* runs the system in a simulated environment using simulated data. This simulated test is sometimes called *alpha testing.* The simulated test is primarily looking for errors and omissions regarding user and design specifications that were specified in the earlier phases but not fulfilled during construction.
2. *Validation testing* runs the system in a live environment using real data. This is sometimes called *beta testing.* During this validation, we are testing a number of items including:

- *Systems performance.* Is the throughput and response time for processing adequate to meet a normal processing workload? If not, some programs may have to be rewritten to improve efficiency, or processing hardware may have to be replaced or upgraded to handle the additional workload.
- *Peak workload processing performance.* Can the system handle the workload during peak processing periods? If not, we may have to improve hardware and/or software to increase efficiency or rethink our scheduling of processing — that is, consider doing some of the less critical processing during nonpeak periods.
- *Human engineering test.* Is the system as easy to learn and use as anticipated? If not, is it adequate? Can enhancements to human engineering be deferred until after the system has been placed into operation?
- *Methods and procedures test.* During conversion, the methods and procedures for the new system will be put to its first real test. Methods and procedures may have to be modified if they prove to be awkward and inefficient from the users' standpoint.
- *Backup and recovery testing.* Now that we have full-sized computer files and databases with real data, we should test all backup and recovery procedures. Simulate a data loss disaster, and test the time required to recover from that disaster. Also, do a before-and-after comparison of the data to ensure that data was properly recovered. It is crucial to test these procedures — don't wait until the first disaster to find an error in the recovery procedures.

3. *EDP (Electronic Data Processing) Audit Testing* certifies that the system is free of errors and ready to be placed into operation. Not all organizations require an EDP audit. But many firms have an independent EDP Audit or Quality Assurance staff that must certify a system's acceptability and documentation before that system is placed into final operation. There are independent companies that perform systems and software certification for clients' organizations.

The systems acceptance test is the final opportunity for users, management, and data processing operations management to accept or reject the system. Hopefully, the analysts and programmers are well aware of the criteria for acceptance before this stage. Well-established systems objectives, systems requirements, and data processing and EDP audit policies are important if rework is to be minimized or eliminated.

As users and management uncover errors, the programs and procedures may have to be slightly modified. It might be useful to have regular maintenance programmers (essential existing system support specialists, as one company calls them) perform these modifications. This will enable us to test the quality of the program documentation while the programs are fresh in the minds of the original programmers.

As the system conversion progresses, users will undoubtedly suggest enhancements. These enhancements should be added to the enhancements file we introduced earlier in the chapter.

As a point of review, let's summarize the complete documentation that has accumulated during the entire project and then discuss the value of that documentation.

- *Project management data.* Charts containing data describing both the planned schedule and costs as well as the actual time used and the costs incurred during systems development should be maintained as a valuable reference to assist future analysts in making better estimates.
- *Study phase documentation.* The DFDs and study phase report are only of historical interest because the old system has now been replaced with a new, improved system. Why keep that documentation? First, it documents improvements made to the system. Second, it provides valuable training and reference material on the use of the systems analysis and design tools and techniques.
- *Requirements statement and design specifications.* This is the major project workbook for the new system. It contains DFDs for the new system, systems flowcharts, and a complete data dictionary that includes both the data structure of all inputs, outputs, and files and the layout charts for those components. It also contains the minispecs and program specifications for the new system. There are two very important benefits to be derived from the project workbook:

    1. Maintenance Programmers can use this workbook as a starting point for making minor modifications to the system. Ideally, modifications should be logged into the workbook so that the workbook becomes a *living document.*

The Next Generation *Getting a Handle on Systems Development Documentation*

During the course of systems analysis, design, and implementation, we assemble a great deal of documentation that needs to be maintained for the benefit of those who will maintain, enhance, and eventually replace the new system. Contrary to popular belief, prototyping will not signal the end for all systems development documentation —it will merely reduce that documentation. Getting a grip on the volume of documentation generated during the project can be very difficult and frustrating. But help is on the way. In Chapter 6, we introduced the concept of a systems analyst productivity workstation. In this feature, we'd like to review and expand on that concept.

By way of review, a systems analyst productivity workstation is a microcomputer-based set of software tools intended to enhance analyst productivity and integrate the myriad of documentation associated with a project. Examples include Index Technology's *Excelerator* and Nastec's *Case 2000,* both of which run on IBM Personal Computers. These products include CAD/CAM graphics systems for drawing data flow diagrams, systems flowcharts, program flowcharts, program structure charts, Warnier/Orr charts, database models such as entity relationship diagrams, and the like. That, in and of itself, is a productivity aid because these diagrams are subject to constant modification and redrawing. The workstations make changing the diagram no more difficult than using a word processor to change a document.

These workstations may also include project management tools, spreadsheets for performing cost/benefit analyses, word processors for writing reports, and screen and report design facilities that simplify some of our systems design tasks.

But the real power of the workstation is the integration of all these tools (including the graphics) with a central data dictionary to organize project details. Let's say you're looking at a data flow diagram on the screen. You see a data flow you want ▶

2. When the system becomes obsolete or a candidate for major redesign, the SDLC is greatly accelerated because the workbook literally represents the study of the current system. This is especially true if the documentation has been kept up to date.

- *Systems proposal.* Recall that this report culminated the evaluation phase. The systems proposal records your recommendations, which can be especially important if management decided *not* to follow them. It also serves as a historical document that may help future analysts make better feasibility estimates.

The Next Generation (continued)

to know more about. Place the cursor on the data flow in question, select the correct function, and presto—the screen displays the data structure composition for that data flow. In that data structure you see an element you don't understand, so you place the cursor on that element, select a function, and again—the screen displays facts about that element: its size, attributes, and legitimate values. Finally, you know the data flow to be an on-line input. Select the proper function and the workstation takes you to a screen design and prototyping facility that allows you to see exactly how to implement that function. This ability to integrate systems analysis and design documentation and retrieve it in various reports and queries will revolutionize systems analysts' productivity.

The future? The workstations will get even better. Perhaps fourth-generation languages, such as *FOCUS* and *RAMIS,* can be integrated into the workstation, making it easier to generate prototypes off the integrated documentation. Perhaps the workstations will be able to generate their own efficient program code in languages such as COBOL. But most important, the project dictionaries will likely be merged through networking technology to maintain a central data dictionary for all systems.

And future workstations will include very sophisticated (by today's standards) analyzers that help the systems analyst spot incompleteness, inconsistencies, redundancies, human engineering errors, and the like. Wouldn't it be nice to have an analyzer to tell you that you have a balancing error (Chapter 7) in your DFDs. Or perhaps the analyzer could tell you that you can't possibly generate a particular output from the inputs shown on the DFD (by checking the data flows against their associated data dictionary entries). Admittedly, this is a utopian view of the future. And it won't happen overnight. But we believe it will happen in our lifetime. ■

- *Program documentation.* We won't get into a discussion of programming etiquettes or documentation standards! Suffice it to say, program-run books should be included in the systems documentation. The run books should include the structure charts, logic charts, code, test data, and test runs. Many organizations impose rigid standards on program documentation.
- *User manuals and computer operations manuals.* These were discussed earlier in this chapter. As enhancements and modifications to the system are implemented, user manuals should be updated.

Task 4: Postimplementation Review The final task of the delivery phase is the postimplementation review. This task is sometimes called the *systems audit.* The review is intended to accomplish two goals:

1. Evaluate the operational information system that was developed.
2. Evaluate the systems development procedures to determine how the project could have been improved.

This is the easiest phase to skip. And that would be a major mistake. True, there are other projects waiting to be started or finished. But you have to learn to look at the long-term benefits of the task. How will you ever do a better job of systems analysis and design if you don't evaluate your current performance?

Evaluation of the new information system should not be done until some period of time after the conversion has been completed. The following elements should be reviewed:

- Does the new information system fulfill the goals and objectives identified and refined early in the project?
- Does the system adequately support the transaction-processing, management-reporting, and decision support requirements of the business?
- Are the projected benefits being realized?
- How do the users feel about the new system? How can user relations be improved for future projects?
- Should any of the proposed enhancements to the system be addressed immediately? Enhancements should be prioritized.
- Are the internal controls adequate?

Ideally, these questions should be addressed twice. The first review should occur as soon as possible after the system has been placed into operation. Why? At this point, everything is fresh in everybody's mind. The second review should occur after some reasonable operating period has elapsed — say, six months after delivery. Answers to the same questions may be very different after the newness of the system has worn off. Isn't that true of cars, houses, and other durable goods?

Evaluation of the systems development procedures should address the following:

- *Did the system come in under budget?* If not, why not? How could estimating procedures be improved? What factors should be taken into consideration when making future estimates?
- *Did the system come in on time?* If not, why not? How can estimating procedures be improved? How can procedures be improved to accelerate systems development efforts without sacrificing quality?
- *How did each person perform during the project?* What skills could be improved? What skill will be improved on the next project?
- *How did the project leader perform?* What leadership traits and skills could be improved? What improvement will the project leader address on the next project?

As you can see, the review process is a question and answer session intended to benefit future projects.

HOW TO MANAGE THE TIME SPENT ON IMPLEMENTATION

We'll conclude this survey of the systems implementation process with a brief discussion of project management implications for the two implementation phases. First, we will determine how much time should be spent on systems implementation. Then we will discuss the sequencing and overlapping opportunities for the tasks that make up its two phases.

How Much Time Should Be Spent on Systems Implementation?

The amount of time that should be spent on implementation is a function of the following factors:

- The size of the project (as was the case with the analysis and design phases).

- The quality and completeness of the design specifications and the requirements statement.
- The techniques used to write computer programs (for instance, prototyping or structured design and programming).
- The type of systems conversion used (for example, abrupt, parallel).

The second factor—quality and completeness of the design specifications and the requirements statement— is particularly important. Considerable empirical evidence suggests that the cost of fixing errors grows exponentially during the phases of systems development (Boehm, 1976). For instance, an error that would cost $8 to fix in the study phase could cost $60 to fix in the design phase, $300 to fix in the construction phase, and $9,000 to fix after construction. Given the sharp inflationary trend in analyst and programmer salaries since Boehm's research was published, these costs are not overstated! Thus, the quality of the work done in each phase dramatically effects all subsequent phases and the lifetime costs of the system.

At one time, it was not unusual for systems implementation to consume 75% or more of the total project schedule. But improvements in programming methods (for example, structured programming and structured design) have reduced these requirements. However, programmers still found themselves spending 60% or more of the total schedule time for implementation. Why? Because systems analysis and design methods were so poor. Programmers constantly found themselves backtracking to fulfill new requirements and design specifications not documented by the analysts. But with the advent of improved analysis and design tools and techniques, the implementation effort can be reduced to 20–30% of the total schedule. Still, many firms continue to experience 50% ratios, largely attributed to shortcuts taken during systems analysis and design.

What effect will prototyping have on the time spent? If the prototyping trend continues (and we think it will), we could see a reversal of the trend toward less time on the implementation phases. This is because prototyping is construction intensive. But the increased time spent on construction is often offset by a dramatically reduced time requirement for the analysis and design processes—particularly design, which is consolidated with construction when prototyping! The net result is much faster systems development and better systems.

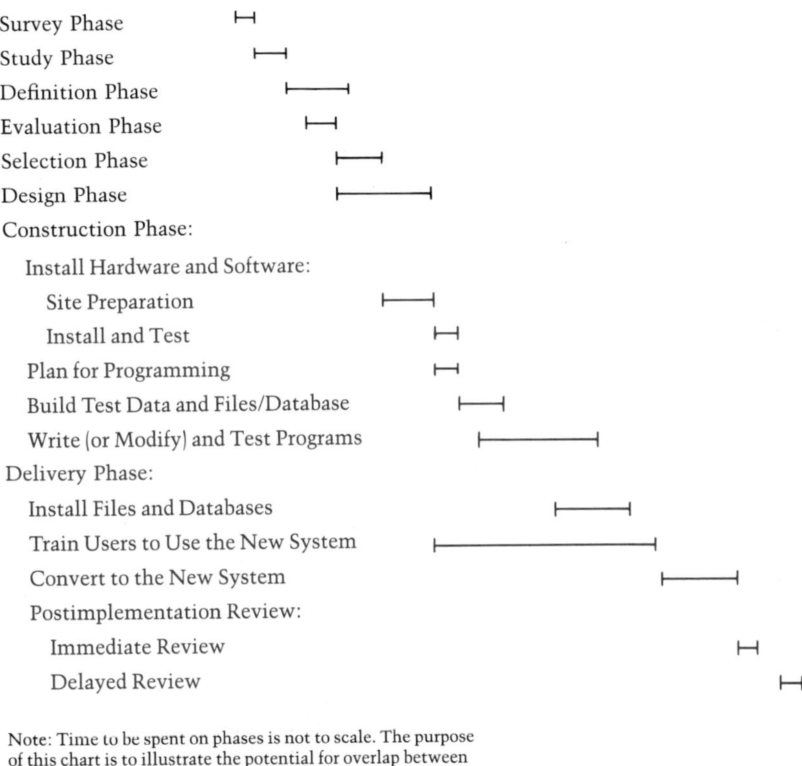

Figure 17.7

Overlapping the construction and delivery tasks. This Gantt chart illustrates the opportunities for overlapping the tasks of the construction and delivery phases. The chart also shows the relationship of the construction and delivery phases relative to the other phases of systems development.

To What Degree Can the Phases and Tasks Be Overlapped?

The sequencing of tasks within the construction and delivery phases was presented in the DFDs in Figures 17.2 and 17.5. The construction phase must be completed before the delivery phase begins because the delivery phase places the system into operation.

The Gantt chart in Figure 17.7 demonstrates overlapping opportunities as well as some sequencing constraints in addition to the one just mentioned. For instance, notice that the implementation phase tasks are generally started only after the design has been frozen (with the qualifications discussed earlier in this chapter). But also notice that site preparation and hardware/software installation may begin before the design is complete. Notice, too, that many of the implementation tasks are completed in parallel (for instance, programming and training). Vertical bars indicate sequencing constraints that limit the overlapping opportunities.

Notice that we added a new phase to the life cycle in the Gantt chart, the maintenance phase. After the system has been placed into operation, it will be in the maintenance phase for the remainder of its useful life, probably for years. During the maintenance phase, modifications will be made to fine tune the system's performance, correct errors missed during the systems acceptance test, and make enhancements to the system (new reports, new queries, and the like). At some time, management will probably decide that the system needs to be overhauled and redesigned to correct major problems or to exploit new opportunities. At that point, the systems development phases will be started all over again.

SUMMARY

Systems implementation is the process whereby a new information system is placed into operation. Systems implementation consists of two phases: construction and delivery.

The purpose of the construction phase is to create the hardware and software elements for the new system. For the hardware elements, this may involve site preparation and installation. Site preparation includes both planning space for equipment and creating a favorable environment (such as temperature, humidity, and noise control). Installation includes taking delivery of new equipment, placing the equipment into operation, and making sure the equipment is functioning properly. For software elements, the construction phase includes computer programming. Not all programs are created from scratch. Some programs are modified. And those programs that were purchased (instead of being built in-house) are installed, tested, and if necessary, modified.

The purpose of the delivery phase is to place the new system into operation. Delivery includes user training, computer staff training, file conversion and loading, and systems conversion. Of these, training is the most important; systems conversion is the most time-consuming. Systems conversion is the process whereby a smooth transition is made from the current information system to the newly constructed information system. Strategies for systems conversion include *abrupt cutover, parallel conversion, site conversion,* and *staged conversion.* After the new system has been placed into operation, both the system and the project should be reviewed. Postimplementation reviews identify improvements—to both the system and the systems development process.

The amount of time spent on systems implementation has gradually decreased, reflecting the overall improvement in the systems analysis and design methods that precede the implementation phases. Implementation should consume no more than 25 to 30 percent of the total project schedule. Many of the construction and delivery phase tasks can be completed in parallel; however, construction must be completed before delivery can progress to its own conclusion.

PROBLEMS AND EXERCISES

1. How can a successful and thorough systems analysis and design be ruined by a poor systems implementation? How can poor systems analysis or design ruin a smooth implementation? For both questions, list some implementation consequences.
2. What skills are important during systems implementation? Create an itemized list. Identify computer, business, and general education courses that would help you develop or improve those skills.
3. How does your information systems pyramid model aid in systems implementation? Examine each face of the pyramid, and address issues and relevance to the systems implementation phases: construction and delivery.
4. What products of the systems design phases are used in the systems implementation phases? Why are they important? How are they used? What would happen if they were incomplete or inaccurate?
5. What are the end products of the construction and delivery

phases? Explain the purpose and content of each of those products?

6. Explain how time spent on systems implementation can best be managed. Take a computer program or system that you constructed for a programming course. Put together a complete schedule to deliver that program or system. Write your schedule in the format of a memo to management. (Remember, management has a limited knowledge of computer vocabulary.)
7. What implications do the use of fourth-generation languages have upon the construction phase?
8. How would the construction phase differ if the computer software for supporting the system was purchased?
9. Why should a systems analyst perform a postimplementation review? What types of benefits can be derived? Why do you really need two reviews?
10. What are four strategies commonly used to convert over to a new system? Describe situations for which each approach would be most preferred and required.

ANNOTATED REFERENCES AND SUGGESTED READINGS

Boehm, Barry. "Software Engineering." *IEEE Transactions on Computers.* Vol. C-25, December, 1976. This classic paper demonstrated the importance of catching errors and omissions before programming begins.

Metzger, Philip W. *Managing a Programming Project.* Second Edition, Englewood Cliffs, N.J.: Prentice-Hall, 1981. This excellent book covers, in considerable detail, what we refer to as the construction and delivery phases. It is one of the few books to place emphasis solely on the implementation process.

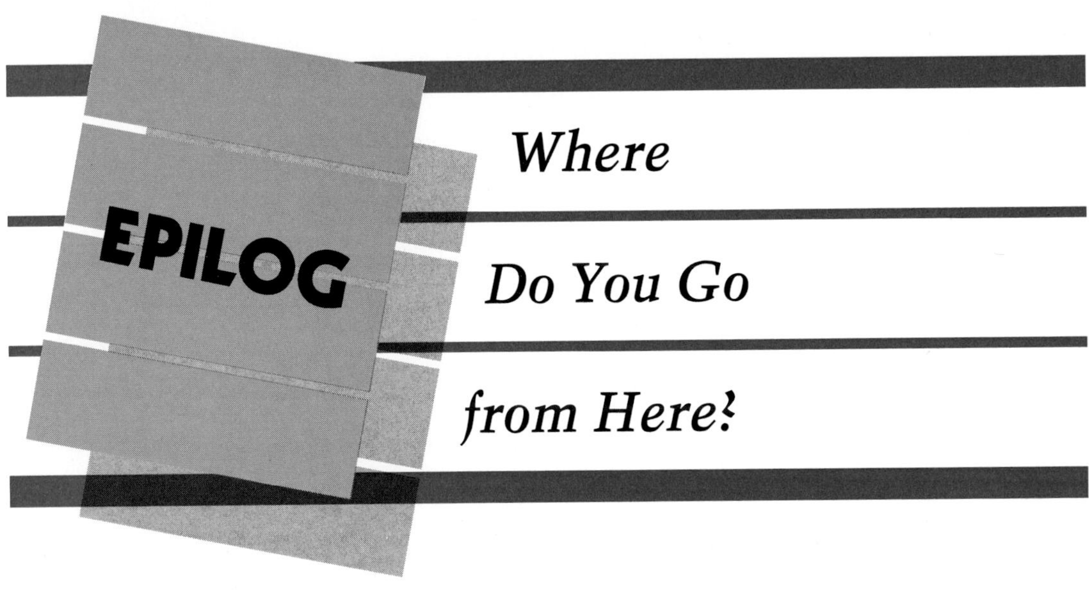

Where Do You Go from Here?

So now you're ready to go out there and successfully perform systems analysis and design. Don't fool yourselves! Remember, you don't become a proficient programmer, accountant, or manager by reading a book. We wish it were that easy, but it isn't. Like most authors, we'd like to say so much more than we have. But size and cost are issues for any book! Before we leave you to *practice* your new-found skills, we should review what we've learned and discuss where you should direct your continuing education to become a better analyst.

WHAT HAVE YOU LEARNED IN THIS BOOK?

As systems analysts, you will be responsible for studying the problems and needs of an organization to determine how people, methods, procedures, and computer technology can best accomplish improvements. And when computer technology is used, you will be responsible for the efficient capture of data from its business source, the flow of that data to the computer, the processing and

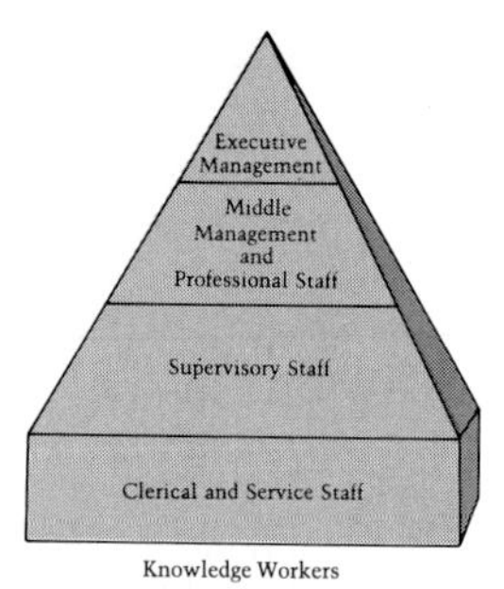

Knowledge Workers

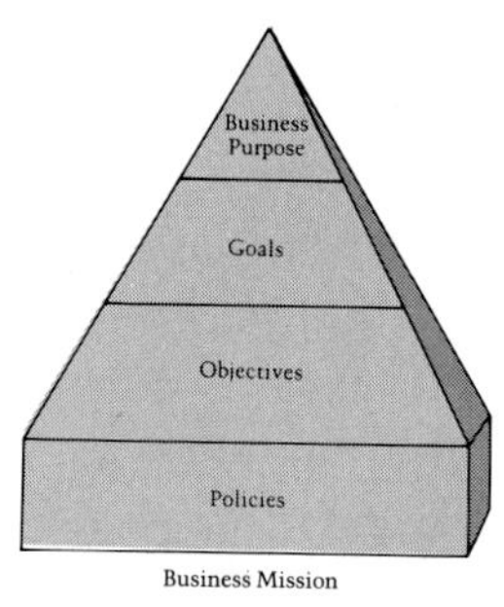

Business Mission

storage of that data by the computer, and the flow of useful information back to the business users. From this book, you have received a solid foundation in two skill sets that were introduced in Chapter 1:

- Concepts and principles of systems analysis and design.
- Tools and techniques of systems analysis and design.

Concepts and Principles

Two conceptual frameworks were introduced in Part I and used throughout this book. First, the pyramid model of an information system provided you with four important dimensions (depicted in the margins) that you should not forget when performing systems analysis and design:

1. We are building information systems to serve the needs of our knowledge workers (or users). Different knowledge workers serve different roles in the business, and we must strive to understand their jobs and responsibilities.
2. Organizations are driven by a business mission that consists of a purpose, goals, objectives, and policies. Because information systems are a subsystem of the business system, we must understand the business mission before we can build information systems that support that mission.
3. Modern information systems provide three information functions: transaction processing, management reporting (MIS), and decision support (DSS). These functions are highly integrated in modern systems.
4. Information systems should function like well-oiled machines that consist of components interacting according to an input-process-output pattern. These components include data, people, methods and procedures, data storage, computer equipment, and computer software. Each component must be designed by the analyst.

The second conceptual framework used throughout the book was the systems development life cycle. This life cycle is used by analysts to build information systems. The generalized life cycle suggested in this book consists of three basic processes and seven phases:

1. The systems analysis process consists of three phases:
   (a) The study of the current information system
   (b) The definition of user requirements for an improved information system
   (c) The evaluation of alternative solutions that fulfill the requirements
2. The systems design process has two phases:
   (d) The selection of computer technology to support the new information system
   (e) The design of the computer components of the information system (such as inputs and outputs)
3. The systems implementation process has two phases:
   (f) The construction of the new information system (including computer programming)
   (g) The delivery of the new information system

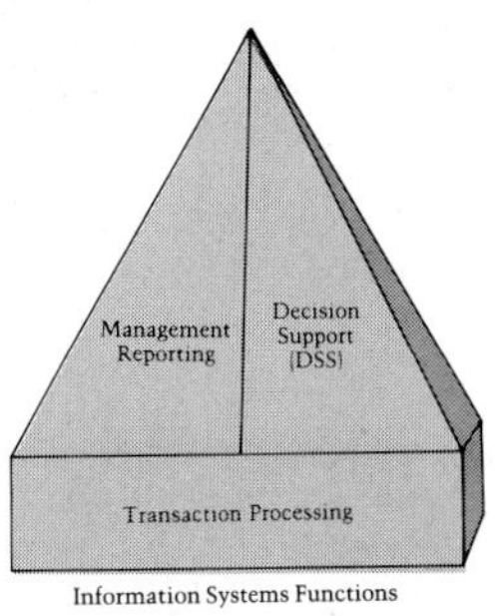

Information Systems Functions

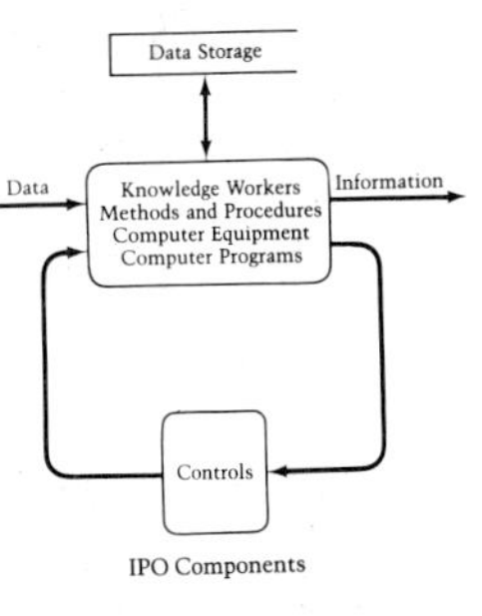

IPO Components

The conceptual frameworks provided for systems analysis and design are relatively stable. We know that your practical side has probably placed emphasis on the specific skills covered in this book. But don't lose sight of the forest for the trees. When you get confused about where you're going or how you should get there, don't start looking for the tool until you understand the situation. Go back to the conceptual frameworks. Where are you in the life cycle? What is your perspective relative to the information system model? The frameworks will help you communicate what you're doing to those less familiar with information systems and systems development. Tables 1 through 4 may help. They describe the analyst's perspective for each phase relative to a dimension in the pyramid model. If you study these tables, you'll notice that they summarize what you learned in Chapters 6, 10, and 17.

Tools and Techniques

We've given you a tool box for systems analysis and design. It's not a supersophisticated tool box. But it does include your basic hammer, screwdrivers, wrenches, and rulers; in other words, the fundamental tools and skills required for systems analysis and design. In the next section, we're going to give you some suggestions for adding to your tool box. Eventually, you'll have a craftsman's collection of tools to support your profession. But first, let's review what you've got in your handyman's tool box:

Table 1 The Knowledge Worker Perspective During Systems Development. The systems analyst must have a clear understanding of the involvement of knowledge workers during all phases of the systems development life cycle.

	Clerical and Service Staff	Supervisory Staff	Middle Management and Professional Staff	Executive Management and Staff
1. Study Phase	During the study phase, the systems analyst needs to identify *all* the knowledge workers who work in the system or administer the system. The analyst should follow the reporting and evaluation relationships all the way up or down the pyramid for the system being studied. What is each individual's interest in this system? What does each person do in or for the system?			
2. Definition Phase	During the definition phase, the analyst should actively involve all of the knowledge workers identified during the study phase. Each knowledge worker, at his or her level in the pyramid structure, should be given the opportunity to define his or her requirements. Participation can be encouraged by refraining from discussion of how the computer will be used and by focusing on what the user wants and why. The *why* often reveals better opportunities. Always ask why.			
3. Evaluation Phase	During the evaluation phase, the analyst should leave the final decision for design alternatives to the knowledge workers. The analyst should document the alternatives and present the technical, operational, and economic feasibility data to the knowledge workers. The analyst can make recommendations, but the decision should be left to the user. The exception to the rule is when the user selects an infeasible solution. Then the analyst should intervene to prevent an infeasible solution from going through the remainder of the life cycle.			
4. Selection Phase	The knowledge workers may not feel technically comfortable with hardware selection decisions. Still, the recommended solution should be pre			

The tools listed to the right include those tools taught in the modules that follow this chapter. Ideally, you have been reading and skimming those modules as you covered each chapter in this book.

- A basic repertoire of fact-finding techniques that can be used to collect facts from your knowledge workers
- Data flow diagrams that can be used to model the flow of data and information through an information system
- A data dictionary syntax that can be used to document the data structure of any data flow, data store, input, or output
- Structured English and decision tables for describing business policies and procedures and computer program requirements
- A few fundamentals of interpersonal communications skills that will ultimately determine your success as a systems analyst

Table 1 *(continued)*

	Clerical and Service Staff	Supervisory Staff	Middle Management and Professional Staff	Executive Management and Staff
Selection Phase (continued)	sented to management in a manner consistent with all other financial investment decisions in the organization. With respect to software selection, knowledge workers should be involved to the extent that they are in the best position to determine whether the system is easy to use and whether the reports or terminal dialogue meet their needs.			
5. Design Phase	The design phase may be computer-oriented; however, during the design phase, important human-engineering decisions will be made. The format and layout of all reports, inputs, and terminal dialogue must meet with the approval of those knowledge workers who will have to live with the system.			
6. Construction Phase	Most knowledge workers have little interest in computer programming. Therefore, this phase is often done with little knowledge-worker participation. As Chapter 1 suggested, this situation is changing in environments that have fourth-generation programming languages available (e.g. FOCUS, RAMIS). These languages are easy to learn, and users frequently find they can write their own programs. The systems analyst often acts as a consultant to programming by knowledge workers.			
7. Delivery Phase	During this phase, knowledge-worker involvement is extremely important. The users need to be brought up-to-speed with the new system. Training and user manual writing are key interfaces to be considered. *The Bottom Line: Knowledge workers (users) should be actively involved in most or all phases of systems development.*			

- Some simple cost/benefit analysis tools that will help evaluate the feasibility of proposed solutions
- Output design forms and charts for specifying the design of computer-generated outputs
- File design forms and charts for specifying the design of computer files
- Input design forms and charts for specifying the design of computer inputs
- Dialogue charts for specifying the logic of a terminal dialogue session

Table 2 The Business Mission Perspective During Systems Development. The systems analyst must maintain perspective of the business mission during each phase of the systems development life cycle.

	Purpose, Goals, Objectives, Policies
1. Study Phase	During the study phase, the systems analyst should identify all of the goals and objectives that are driving the current system. The analyst should try to determine if the objectives are helping achieve the goals. Policies should be identified and analyzed as to whether they are consistent with the objectives. The key during the study phase is to look for inconsistencies between goals, objectives, and policies.
2. Definition Phase	The definition of any new system should be driven by the expectations of the business as defined by goals and objectives. The goals and objectives of the business function may need to be expanded or modified. Furthermore, goals and objectives for the project itself should be defined. The computer should not be expressly included in any goal or objective because computing should only be viewed as a means to an end. The tasks to be performed by the new system should be consistent with the goals and objectives of the business and the project.
3. Evaluation Phase	Each alternative solution should be evaluated for operational feasibility against the goals and objectives defined for the business and project. Each task should be evaluated by users to get a general feeling of how acceptable they find that proposed task.
4. Selection Phase	During the selection of hardware and software, it is important to check alternative vendor proposals for consistency with goals and objectives. Tasks to be performed by software packages must be evaluated for consistency with the objectives they should support.
5. Design Phase	A primary concern of the design phase is to not get sidetracked. The design should continue to fulfill the goals, objectives, and tasks set forth in the definition phase. Many objectives are performance, control, or security oriented. These objectives can only be fulfilled *during* the design phase.
6. Construction Phase	The systems analyst has hopefully invested considerable effort in the definition, evaluation, and design phase to maintain integrity with respect to goals and objectives. The analyst should evaluate the construction activities to ensure that the computer programs fulfill the expectations of the requirements and design specifications.
7. Delivery Phase	The ultimate acceptance test for any new system is "does this new system fulfill the goals, objectives, and policies specified by the business?" *The Bottom Line: Purpose, Goals, Objectives, and Policies are the final determination of a life cycle's success or failure.*

- Systems flowcharts for specifying the detailed methods and procedures for data processing components of an information system
- Structure charts (or Warnier/Orr charts) and IPO charts for organizing systems design documentation into distinct computer program specifications for each computer program in an information system
- PERT and Gantt charts for project management

That's quite a tool chest! Hopefully you won't try to screw a nail. In other words, you should now understand that you need to select the proper tool for the proper situation. Table 5 summarizes the documentation value of each tool relative to the IPO components of an information system. And Table 6 gives you an interesting and new perspective on the tools you've studied. The matrix shows a wide variety of possible uses for different tools in the different phases of the systems development life cycle. Some of the tools suggest alternate uses of the tools, uses that are different from the techniques you learned in this book.

But don't let tools run the show. Bertrand Russell, a famous scholar, once stated, "There must be an ideal world, a sort of mathematician's paradise where everything happens as it does in textbooks." In other words, you have to be flexible enough to adapt the tools to the constraints and environment that you work in. No tool works as perfectly as we sometimes imply in a textbook! Try them. Adapt them. Experience is the best teacher of these tools and techniques.

That's enough of a review of the tools and techniques you've learned in this book. As a *career*-minded professional, you want to know where you should focus your continuing education in systems analysis and design.

WHAT DO YOU STILL NEED TO LEARN?

In Chapter 1, we outlined some of the general skills a systems analyst requires to be proficient. Those skills include:

- A working knowledge of data processing techniques and computer programming

Table 3 The Information System Functions Perspective During Systems Development. The systems analyst must maintain a clear perspective on the information systems functions during all phases of the systems development life cycle.

	Transaction Processing	Management Reporting	Decision Support (DSS)
1. Study Phase	During the study phase, the analyst should identify both the transactions currently processed and any problems that exist with processing those transactions. The current auditing requirements should be investigated.	During the study phase the analyst should identify all the information currently being used by knowledge workers. Emphasis should be placed on learning how the information (computer-generated or manual) is used and specific problems with that information (untimely, incomplete, inaccurate, format, etc.)	During the study phase the analyst should study the structured decisions made by the knowledge workers. The analyst would also do well to identify data being collected by knowledge workers for no specific reason—that data is frequently used for unstructured decision making.
2. Definition Phase	During the definition phase, the analyst should define the transactions that need to be processed by the new system. These transactions may be identical to those processed by the current system; however, the data captured, the information generated, or the processing required may differ.	During the definition phase, the analyst should define all the information requirements that the user can specifically address. Be sure to ask why the information is needed. The answer may suggest that different information would be more appropriate.	During the definition phase, the analyst should identify all of the data which may be pertinent to the decision-making processes of the knowledge workers. That data needs to be captured and stored (if it isn't already reflected in the transaction processing requirements).

- At least a working knowledge of one or more typical business functions (for example, accounting, marketing, operations)
- The insight and creativity to solve problems

Table 3 *(continued)*

	Transaction Processing	Management Reporting	Decision Support (DSS)
3. Evaluation Phase	During the evaluation phase, the analyst should evaluate the operational feasibility of each alternative method for processing transactions (e.g. batch, on-line). Technical and economic feasibility are important, but operational acceptability is crucial.	During the evaluation phase, the analyst can evaluate alternative information media (e.g. tabular reports versus graphical displays, on-line versus batch, etc.)	During the evaluation phase, the analyst should evaluate alternative decision support aids (e.g. query languages, report writers, simulators, etc.)
4. Selection Phase	During the selection phase, the analyst must select the hardware/software that best fulfills the transaction processing, management reporting, and decision support requirements of the new system.		
5. Design Phase	The important issue during the design phase is "does the design fulfill the requirements and the issues expressed in the preceding phases?" Layout and format of knowledge-worker reports and forms are very important.		
6. Construction Phase	The important issue during the construction phase is the fulfillment of the design phase specifications.		
7. Delivery Phase	Transaction processing should be evaluated to ensure that the new system fulfills expectations.	Management reports should be reviewed for acceptability.	Decision support should be reviewed to determine if required information is available for decisions.

- The ability to communicate, both orally and in writing
- Interpersonal skills
- Formal systems analysis and design skills

Table 4 The Information System Components Perspective During Systems Development. The systems analyst must maintain a clear perspective of the information systems components during each phase of the systems development life cycle.

	People	Methods and Procedures	Data Storage	Computer Equipment	Computer Programs
1. Study Phase	(see Table 1, pp. 694–695)	Identify and analyze existing data processing methods and manual procedures.	Identify existing files (including manual files) and databases.	Identify and analyze existing computer equipment and the support provided by that equipment.	Identify and analyze existing computer programs and how well they support current needs.
2. Definition Phase	(see Table 1)	*Ignore data processing methods!* Focus on defining the procedures necessary to fulfill business needs.	*Ignore computer file and database concerns.* If a file or database can't meet needs, it shouldn't be built! Define data needs and the natural structure of that data.	*Ignore completely!*	*Ignore completely!*
3. Evaluation Phase	Evaluate alternative person/machine boundaries. Study alternatives that lie between the extremes of a completely manual and a fully automated system.	*Now evaluate different data processing methods!* Look at batch and on-line methods.	Evaluate conventional file and database alternatives.	Evaluate the ability of existing equipment to support each alternative. If new equipment is needed, specify the need so a selection phase can be initiated to meet the need.	Evaluate the "construct in-house" versus "buy" decision. If you decided to buy, a selection phase will be needed.
4. Selection Phase	(see Table 1)	If necessary, selected methods can be communicated to vendors because they were defined in the evaluation phase.	Specify requirements if storage technology is to be selected. This may have been done in the definition phase.	Select the equipment that best fulfills requirements. Appropriate demonstrations and tests should be conducted before the equipment is selected.	Select the software that best fulfills requirements. Appropriate demonstrations and tests should be conducted before the software is selected.
5. Design Phase	Design manual procedures necessary to support the system. Also, see Table 1.	Design detailed flow and control of activities for the new system. Prepare complete programming specifications for activities to be automated.	Design files and database. Specify access methods and organization of files.	*No implications.*	Prepare complete programming specifications for every computer program to be written or modified.
6. Construction Phase and Delivery Phase	(see Table 1)	Train users on new procedures. Convert system to new methods.	Convert files and databases.	Install equipment.	Write and test programs. Modify purchased programs and install.

Relative to career planning and continuing education, we'd like to focus on the last three skill sets in the list. It is in these three areas that you will find the most opportunities for continuing education specific to systems analysis and design.

Development of Communications Skills

Let's discuss communications skills first. No other set of skills will play a bigger role in your success or failure! That's right! Many students and new analysts quickly become frustrated by the apparent inadequacies of the tools and techniques that they learned in courses and books. But it's too often true that the tools and techniques are not at fault. Instead, the analyst is having trouble communicating with the user or the vendor or the manager or the programmer. Good tools do not make up for poor communications skills. Some experts argue that good tools are so dependent on communications skills that poor communications skills make the tools look much worse than they are. You need special and continuing education in the interpersonal communications field. Specifically, we recommend that you seek training in the following areas:

- How to write business reports and communiques
- How to write technical reports
- How to write specialized data processing documents, such as user manuals, operations manuals, requests for proposals, and simple contracts
- How to run meetings and walkthroughs
- How to sell ideas and solutions to users and vendors
- How to present technical information to nontechnical audiences

Module C surveys some of these skills. However, a short module just won't suffice. There are courses and new books specifically oriented toward developing and refining these skills for the systems analyst. Seek out this training. More than any of the other skills we talk about in this epilogue, communications skills are the most important component of your systems analysis and design career.

Table 5 Does the Tool or Technique Document the Information System? This table can be used to determine the effectiveness of a tool or technique (listed in the left-most column) in documenting each information system component. The table can also be used to quickly compare the effectiveness of all the tools and techniques for a specific information system component.

Tool or Technique	Data	Computer Equipment	Computer Programs	Knowledge Workers	Methods and Procedures	Data Storage	Information
Data Flow Diagrams	Yes, at high level	On PDFDs	On PDFDs	On PDFDS	On PDFDs	Yes, at general level	Yes, at high level
Data Dictionary	Yes, in detail	No	No	No	No	Yes, in detail	Yes, in detail
Structured English and Decision Tables	No, but it references data thru DD	No	Yes, can be used for logic	No	Yes	No, but tells how used	No, but it references information through DD
Output Design Tools	No, output is information	Somewhat	No	Through human engineering	Internal controls	No	Yes, in detail
File Design Tools	No	Somewhat	Somewhat	No	Internal controls	Yes, in detail	No
Input Design Tools	Yes, in detail	Somewhat	Somewhat	Through human engineering	Internal controls	No	No

Developing Interpersonal Skills

This set of skills is closely related to communications skills. A person may exhibit adequate communication skills but not know how to work with people. Working with people is the essence of systems analysis and design. Recall that we proclaimed people the most important component in the modern information system. Relative to the development of interpersonal skills, we suggest that you need to learn the following:

Table 5 *(continued)*

Tool or Technique	Data	Computer Equipment	Computer Programs	Knowledge Workers	Methods and Procedures	Data Storage	Information
Terminal Dialogue Design Tools	Yes, in detail	Somewhat	Somewhat	Through human engineering	Internal controls	No	Yes, in detail
Systems Flowcharts	Yes, at general level	Somewhat	General level	Interface to computer	Yes	Yes, at general level	Yes, at general level
Structure Charts and IPO Charts	Yes	Possible	Yes	No	Yes	Yes	Yes
PERT and Gantt Charts	No	No	No	No	No	No	No
Fact-Finding Techniques	Yes	Yes	Yes	Yes	Yes	Yes	Yes
Interpersonal Communications	Yes	Yes	Yes	Yes	Yes	Yes	Yes
Cost/Benefit Analysis	Yes	Yes	Yes	Yes	Yes	Yes	Yes

- How to get users actively involved in the systems development life cycle
- How to motivate people to cooperate; what people like and dislike
- How to brainstorm as part of a group
- How to deal with problem behaviors, such as distrust, fear, overzealousness, impatience, and sabotage

Table 6 How the Tools or Techniques Are Used in the Systems Development Life Cycle. This table can be used to determine how a specific tool or technique is used during each phase of the SDLC. Alternatively, appropriate tools and techniques that may be used during a particular phase of the SDLC can also be quickly identified using the table.

	Phase						
Tool or Technique	Survey/ Study	Definition	Evaluation	Selection	Design	Construct	Delivery
Data Flow Diagrams	Document current system	Document user requirements	Document alternative solutions	Tell vendors what you need	Document new system	Not applicable	Train users
Data Dictionary	Maybe to document current system	Document user requirements	Not applicable	Maybe tell vendors what you need	Expanded DD, Part III of this book	Document programs and files/ database	Train users
Structured English and Decision Tables	Document current system and decisions	Document user requirements	Not applicable	Not applicable	Document program logic	Document program logic	Write user manuals
Output Design Tools	May exist for current outputs	Not applicable	Not applicable	May exist for vendor products	Document computer outputs	Communicate outputs to programmers	Not friendly
File Design Tools	May exist for current files	Not applicable	Not applicable	May exist for vendor products	Document computer files	Communicate files to programmers	Convert files
Input Design Tools	May exist for current inputs	Not applicable	Not applicable	May exist for vendor products	Document computer inputs	Communicate inputs to programmers	Not friendly
Dialogue Design Tools	May exist for current dialogue	Not applicable	May exist for vendor products	Document computer dialogue	Communicate dialogue to programmers	Demonstrate dialogue	

Table 6 *(continued)*

Tool or Technique	Phase: Survey/ Study	Definition	Evaluation	Selection	Design	Construct	Delivery
Systems Flowcharts	May exist for current system	Not applicable	Alternative to DFD to document solutions	May exist for vendor products	Document methods and procedures	Communicate with programmers	Train computer operators
Structure Charts and IPO Charts	May exist for current system	Not applicable	Not applicable	May exist for vendor products	Package program specs	Communicate with programmer	Maintain computer programs
PERT and Gantt Charts	To manage the entire system development life cycle						
Fact-Finding Techniques	Learn about current system	Learn about user requirements	Identify alternatives	Collect facts from vendors	Get user opinions	Not applicable	Evaluate new system
Interpersonal Communications	Reports, presentations, walk-throughs	Reports, presentations, walk-throughs	Proposal to management	Request for proposals	Reports, presentations, and walk-throughs	Clarify instructions to programmers	Training, user manuals
Cost/Benefit Analysis	Assess cost of problems	Assess benefits of requirements	*Justify a proposed system*	Evaluate vendor products	Re-evaluate feasibility	Not applicable	Evaluate original estimates

- How to help people cope with change (People naturally fear and avoid change.)
- How to lead and manage people

The list isn't exhaustive, but you should note the common denominator: people skills! More and more courses and books to develop these skills are becoming available with each passing day.

Developing Systems Analysis and Design Skills

And of course, there is much more to learn about systems analysis and design itself. Let's begin with the most notable omission in this book, methodologies. In Chapters 1 and 5, methodologies were defined as specific strategies for applying specific tools and techniques in a disciplined manner to develop systems. We intentionally supported no methodology in this book because it's too easy to become a blind devotee of one methodology. Many of the tools in this book are an integral part of one or more methodologies. However, you have learned to look at tools independent of methodology. As new methodologies and tools become available, we hope you will be inclined to look for opportunities to share the tools and techniques of one methodology with another.

We recommend the following methodologies for your study:

- Structured systems analysis and design
- Information engineering (also called *information modeling* and *database modeling*)
- Prototyping

All of these were highlighted in the text or in the "Next Generation" features. Prototyping, in particular, appears to be a methodology of destiny geared toward improving both analyst and programmer productivity. Whatever the current pros and cons of prototyping, we believe that productivity will become the watchword of the next decade — the economy will force that issue. As for structured analysis and design and information engineering, there is an ever-growing list of courses and books on these subjects. Learn these methodologies.

What about tools and techniques? Are there any specific tools, techniques, or skills that you still need to learn? Yes! First, we should note that you will likely encounter new tools and techniques in new methodologies as they emerge. But beyond that, we offer the following suggestions:

- *Project management.* We briefly introduced this topic in Module A. It deserves much more emphasis. We assume you want to be successful. If you become successful, you will likely be asked to manage projects. To do this effectively, you will need to develop specific skills for organizing systems projects, assigning personnel, managing personnel, budgeting, controlling costs, and much more. It's more than managing people. It's managing an entire project!
- *Feasibility analysis.* Most of us have trouble developing this skill. Experience helps, but there are numerous guidelines and tools that can be used to develop expertise in estimating operational, technical, and economic feasibility.
- *Database.* We're throwing this one in just in case you didn't read Module E, "Database: The Alternative to Files." It is becoming difficult to distinguish precisely where the systems analyst's responsibilities end and where the database expert's responsibilities begin. Different organizations assign different responsibilities. In any case, as the number of database applications increase, the everyday systems analyst must understand the technology and its implications for systems analysis and design.
- *Hardware and software selection.* Many alumni tell us that their first job assignments involved the evaluation and selection of hardware and software. Hardware and software selection normally receives little attention in schools. For that matter, many professionals are uncomfortable or uncertain of this important decision-making process. There *is* help out there. Courses and books are available to teach strategies, tools, and techniques for soliciting proposals, dealing with vendors, evaluating products, and justifying recommendations to management.
- *Data communications.* Making computers talk to one another is one of the exciting technologies as we go to press. If the popularity of microcomputers continues to grow (and in all likelihood, it will), then distributed processing will be the standard, and information system networks will also be common.

Again, this list certainly isn't exhaustive. You have to keep up on your reading of periodicals to keep your continuing education wish-list up to date.

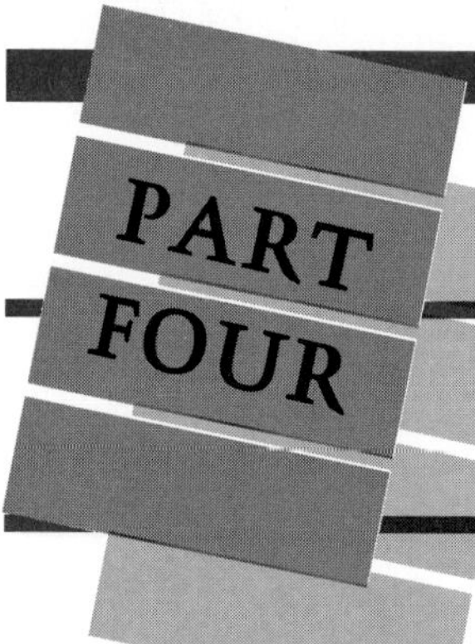

Skills that Overlap Systems Analysis, Design, and Implementation

The modules of Part IV are not appendixes! *We want to state that fact right up front so there is no confusion. There are a number of skills and issues that are important to all three major systems development phases: systems analysis, systems design, and systems implementation. We feel strongly that these comprehensive skills are more important than any specific tool or technique you learn from this book. So why are they at the end of the book?*

If we had placed these modules *(a name chosen to distinguish them from the* chapters *that you've been reading) in either the analysis unit (Part II) or the design and implementation unit (Part III), it would have understated their value relative to the unit that didn't contain the material. On the other hand, these modules do require some prerequisite knowledge—specifically, Chapters 1 through 5 and possibly certain chapters in Parts II and III. By locating these modules at the end of the book, we give you and your instructor the flexibility of introducing and reviewing them at your own preferred locations (after specific chapters). Each module begins by describing the prerequisite chapters in Parts II and III (Part I is assumed for all modules).*

We cannot understate the value of these modules. The material presented will have a greater impact on your success as a systems analyst than any other material in this book. *The modules teach skills that make the concepts, tools, and techniques presented in Parts I, II, and III much easier to apply to real problems.*

Module A introduces project management concepts, tools, and techniques. All projects are dependent on the planning, control, and leadership principles that are surveyed. Some tools are also introduced. Module B surveys fact-finding techniques. No analysis or design task can be completed without using these techniques to collect facts from the users and managers—facts about the current system, opinions and ideas, and facts about requirements. Module C presents interpersonal communications skills for the analyst. You will learn how to run team meetings, verify facts and requirements, make formal presentations, and write reports. Module D introduces feasibility analysis and cost/benefit analysis techniques. These techniques are practiced throughout the systems development life cycle, not just at the beginning of a project! Your ability to defend project proposals depends on these techniques. Finally, Module E presents databases as an alternative to files. The growing impact of database technology on information systems projects cannot be ignored. This module only surveys the implications. We encourage you to pursue additional knowledge in this important area.

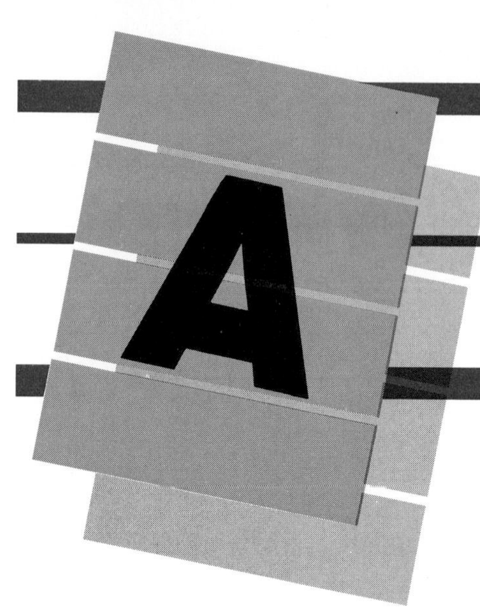

Project Management

WHEN SHOULD YOU READ THIS MODULE?

This module will prove most valuable if read after *any* of the following chapters:

- Chapter 5, "A Systems Development Life Cycle"—The life cycle itself is a project management tool.
- Chapter 6, "How to Perform a Systems Analysis"—Even if you've already read this module, a review may help you place the systems analysis tasks into perspective.
- Chapter 10, "How to Perform a Systems Design"—Again, even if you've already read this module, a review will place the content of Chapter 10 into perspective.
- Chapter 17, "How to Perform Systems Implementation"—A review would again be appropriate.

Most of you are familiar with Murphy's Law, which suggests that if anything can go wrong, it will. Murphy's Law motivated numerous pearls of wit and wisdom about projects, machines, and people and why things go wrong. Among these gems we encounter *Spark's Ten Rules for the Project Manager* (Bloch, 1977, pp. 58–59):

1. *Strive to look tremendously important.*
2. *Attempt to be seen with important people.*
3. *Speak with authority; however, only expound on the obvious and proven facts.*
4. *Don't engage in arguments, but if cornered, ask an irrelevant question and lean back with a satisfied grin while your opponent tries to figure out what's going on—Then quickly change the subject.*
5. *Listen intently while others are arguing the problem. Pounce on a trite statement and bury them with it.*
6. *If a subordinate asks you a pertinent question, look at him as if he had lost his senses. When he looks down, paraphrase the question back at him.*
7. *Obtain a brilliant assignment, but keep out of sight and out of the limelight.*
8. *Walk at a fast pace when out of the office—this keeps questions from subordinates and superiors at a minimum.*
9. *Always keep the office door closed. This puts visitors on the defensive and also makes it look as if you are always in an important conference.*
10. *Give all orders verbally. Never write anything down that might go into a "Pearl Harbor File."*

Murphology is fun. Unfortunately, the many amusing laws, postulates, and theorems were conceived from our failures as project and people managers. And although it's fun to laugh at our mistakes and shortcomings, we should never take them so lightly that we accept them as facts of life. Why? Because, in addition to basic analysis and design responsibilities, the systems analyst frequently assumes a project management role. The project manager is usually a senior systems analyst who must plan, staff, and control the project's many tasks.

The purpose of this module is to introduce you to project management. Because project management is applied during systems analysis, systems design, and systems implementation, we decided to place it in this supplementary module. You will learn about the importance of project management as well as guidelines, tools, and techniques for managing projects.

WHAT IS PROJECT MANAGEMENT?

For the systems project, **project management** is the process of directing the development of an acceptable system at a minimum cost within a specified timeframe. Although the tools and techniques of systems analysis and design play a critical role in achieving successful systems, these methods are not sufficient on their own. Project mismanagement can deter or render ineffective the best of analysis and design methods. What goes wrong in systems projects? What role does mismanagement play in these failures? How can the project manager avoid such failures? We'll answer these questions in this section.

What Goes Wrong in Systems Projects?

We can develop an appreciation for the importance of project management by studying the mistakes of other project managers. Failures and limited successes far outnumber very successful information systems. Why's that? True, many systems analysts and data processors are unfamiliar with or undisciplined in the tools and techniques of systems analysis and design. But that only partially explains the shortcomings of systems projects. Many projects suffer from poor leadership and management. Witness the following case.

The Anatomy of an Unsuccessful Project Let's listen in on a post-implementation review for an information systems project:

> **Jim** Sharon, I want to discuss the registration system project your team completed last month. Now that the system has been operational for a few weeks, we need to evaluate the performance of you and your team. Frankly, Sharon, I'm a little disappointed.
>
> **Sharon** Me too! I don't know what happened! We used the standard methodology and tools, but we still have problems.
>
> **Jim** Well, I've talked to several of the analysts, programmers, and users on the project, and I've drawn a few conclusions. Obviously, the users are less than satisfied with the system. Sharon, you took some shortcuts in the methodology, didn't you?

Sharon We had to, Jim! We got behind schedule. We didn't have time to follow the methodology to the letter.

Jim But now we have to do major parts of the system over. If you didn't have time to do it right, where will you find time to do it over?

You see, Sharon, systems development is more than tools, techniques, and methodologies. It's also a management process. In addition to missing the boat on user requirements, I note two other problems. And both of them are management problems. The system was over budget and late. The projected budget of $35,000 was exceeded by 42 percent. The project was delivered thirteen weeks behind schedule. Most of the delays and cost overruns occurred during programming. The programmers tell me that the delays were caused by rework of analysis and design specifications. Is this true?

Sharon Yes, for the most part.

Jim Once again, those delays were likely caused by the shortcuts taken earlier. The shortcuts you took during analysis and design were intended to get you back on schedule. Instead, they got you further behind schedule when you got into the programming phase.

Sharon I see that now. But the project grew. How would you have dealt with the schedule slippage during analysis?

Jim If I were you, I would have reevaluated the scope of the project when I first saw it changing. In this case, either project scope should have been reduced or project resources (schedule and budget) should have been increased.

Don't be so glum! We all make mistakes. I had this very conversation with my boss seven years ago. You're going to be a good project manager. That's why I've decided to send you to this project management course and workshop . . .

This case highlights the three common results of mismanaged projects:

- Unfulfilled or unidentified requirements and needs
- Cost overruns
- Late delivery

These problems are not always caused by project mismanagement, but mismanagement certainly plays a role in such problems.

Project Management Causes of Failed Projects What project management failures cause unfulfilled requirements and needs, cost overruns, and late deliveries? Before we get into project mismanagement causes, let's recognize that one possible cause of the aforementioned problems could be inadequate systems analysis and design tools and techniques. But for purposes of this module, we will focus on causes that can be traced to project management.

In Sharon's registration project, user requirements and needs were not fulfilled because shortcuts had been taken during the project. The systems development life cycle (discussed in Chapters 5, 6, 10, and 17) provides a basic plan for a systems project. Each phase and activity is an important part of that plan. For all parts to work together, the life cycle must be monitored and managed!

Another common cause of unfulfilled requirements is lack of or imprecise targets. The problem in systems projects is that, during the early phases, the scope of the project is rarely precise. And for many projects, the scope is never precisely defined. If the project leader fails to recognize this problem, the project team is frequently forced to make late changes to specifications and programs. As a result, the system doesn't fulfill requirements and needs. And to further compound the problem, unless you know where you are going, you can't estimate how long it will take to get there and how much it will cost. That brings us to budget overruns.

What causes projects to exceed their budgets? One of the major problems with cost overruns is that many methodologies or project plans call for an unreasonably precise estimate of costs before the project begins. These estimates are made after a quick and dirty preliminary study or feasibility study. Think about it! Can you accurately estimate project costs before making a detailed study of the current system or defining user requirements? Can you estimate the costs of computer programming before a detailed systems design has been completed? It's not likely. The cost estimates of a project will change as you get further into the systems development process.

Poor estimating techniques are another cause of cost overruns. We suspect that many systems analysts estimate by making the best calculated estimate (*guess-timate?*) and then doubling that number. Hardly a scientific approach, right? There are better approaches available; some useful techniques are discussed in Module D.

And finally, cost overruns are often caused by schedule delays. What causes the delays? Once again, we can point to premature estimates as a problem. These early estimates are based on the initial scope of the project. Because systems analysts (and data processing professionals in general) are eternal optimists, they often quote optimistic schedules and fail to modify those schedules as the true scope of the project becomes apparent.

Because many managers and analysts are often poor time managers, project schedules slip slowly but steadily. "So we've lost a day or two! It's no big deal. We can make it up later." This may be true, but then again, it might not. This attitude fails to recognize the fact that in the systems development life cycle certain tasks are dependent on other tasks. Because of this dependence, a one-day slip can set the whole schedule back. And when those one-day delays pile up, we inevitably find ourselves working fifteen-hour days at the end of the project.

Another cause of missed schedules is what Fred Brooks (1975) has described as the *mythical man-month.* As the project gets behind schedule, the project leaders frequently try to solve the problem by assigning more people to the project team. It just doesn't work! There is no linear relationship between time and number of personnel. The addition of personnel creates more communications and political interfaces. The result? The project gets even further behind schedule.

You've probably noticed that the causes of failed projects are related. For instance, missed requirements may cause schedule slippages that, in turn, cause cost overruns. You might ask why somebody isn't able to recognize these problems and correct them. Somebody should. And that person is supposed to be the project manager or leader. Which brings us to a major cause of project failure: lack of management and leadership. Good computer programmers don't always go on to become good analysts. Similarly, good analysts don't automatically perform well as managers and leaders. To be a good project manager, the analyst must possess or develop skills in the basic functions of management.

Basic Functions of the Project Manager

The project manager is *not* just a senior analyst who happens to be in charge. As Sharon found out, a project manager must apply a set of skills different from those applied by the analyst. What skills must the project manager possess or learn? The basic functions of a manager or leader have been studied and refined by management theorists for many years. These basic functions include planning, staffing, organizing, directing, and controlling.

Planning Project Tasks and Staffing the Project Team A good manager always has a plan. The manager estimates resource requirements and formulates a plan to deliver the target system. This is based on the manager's understanding of the requirements of the target system at that point in its development. A basic plan for developing an information system is provided by the systems development life cycle. Many firms have their own standard life cycles, and some firms have standards for the methods and tools to be used.

Each task required to complete the project must be planned. How much time will each require? How many people will be needed? How much will the task cost? What tasks must be completed before other tasks are started? Can some of the tasks be overlapped? These are all planning issues. Some of these issues can be resolved with a tool called the PERT chart, which is discussed later in this module.

Project managers frequently select analysts and programmers for the project team. The project manager should carefully consider the business and technical expertise that may be needed to successfully finish the project. The key is to match the personnel to the required tasks that have been identified as part of project planning.

Organizing and Scheduling the Project Effort Given the project plan and the project team, the project manager is responsible for organizing and scheduling the project. Members of the project team should understand their own individual roles and responsibilities as well as their reporting relationship to the project manager.

The project schedule should be developed with an understanding of task time requirements, personnel assignments, and intertask dependencies. Many projects present a deadline or requested delivery date. The project manager must determine whether a workable schedule can be built around such deadlines. If not, the deadlines must be delayed or the project scope must be trimmed. We will soon discuss a project-scheduling tool called the Gantt chart.

Directing and Controlling the Project Once the project has begun, the project manager becomes a leader. As leader, the manager directs the team's activities and evaluates progress. Therefore, every project manager must demonstrate such people management skills as motivating, rewarding, advising, coordinating, delegating, and appraising team members. Additionally, the manager must frequently report progress to superiors.

Perhaps the most difficult and important function of the manager is controlling the project. Few plans will be executed without problems and delays. We've already discussed the causes and effects of unsuccessful projects. The project manager's job is to monitor tasks, schedules, and costs in order to control those elements. If the project scope is increasing, the project manager is faced with a decision: Should the scope be reduced so the original schedule and budget will be met, or should the schedule and budget be revised? The project manager must be able to present the alternatives and their implications on the budget and schedule to the steering committee or management.

Space permitting, we could easily write several chapters on these project management functions. But space doesn't permit. However, we will introduce some of the more popular project management tools that are used to assist project managers.

PROJECT MANAGEMENT TOOLS AND TECHNIQUES

Two popular tools used by project managers are PERT charts and Gantt charts. PERT charts are useful for project planning; Gantt charts, for project scheduling and progress reporting. Today, computer software is being used to construct both of these types of charts and to provide the project manager with rapid and useful information.

PERT Charts: A Planning and Control Tool

PERT (which stands for *Project Evaluation and Control Technique*) was developed in the late 1950s to plan and control large weapons development projects for the United States Navy. It was developed to make clear the interdependence of project tasks when projects are being scheduled. Essentially, PERT is a graphical networking technique; this can be a useful tool because pictures often say more than words. Let's take a closer look at PERT charts, what they are, how to draw them, and how to use them.

PERT Definitions and Symbols On PERT charts, projects can be organized in terms of events and tasks. An event represents a point in time, such as the start or completion of a task (or several tasks). A variety of symbols (circles, squares, and the like) have been used to depict events on PERT charts. For our discussion, we will use circles, often called *nodes* (see Figure A.1) to represent an event. Each node is divided into three sections. The left half of the node includes an event identification number. This number is usually keyed to a legend that explicitly defines the event. The upper and lower right-hand quarters of the node are used to record the earliest and latest completion times for the event. Instead of dates, time is counted from TIME = 0 where 0 corresponds to the date on which the project is started. Every PERT chart has one beginning node that represents the start of the project and one end node that represents the completion of the project.

On a PERT chart, a task is depicted by an arrow between nodes. The task identification letter and the expected duration of the task are recorded on the arrow. Look at the arrow between event 1 and event 2 in Figure A.1. The direction of the arrow indicates that event 1 must be completed prior to event 2. The expected duration of the task resulting in the completion of event 2 is four days. A dashed arrow is special. It represents a dependency between events. However, because there is no activity to be performed, there is no duration between the events. This is called a *dummy task.*

The classical approach to PERT presents one major problem when applied to information systems development. In the classical approach, a node represents the start *or* finish of a task or series of tasks. Consider the simple PERT chart presented in Figure A.2. It's a PERT chart for our high-level systems development life cycle (Chapter 5). Do you see the problem?

Classical PERT charting implies that the definition phase must be completed *before* either the evaluation phase or the design phase can be started. This, however, is not the case. Although neither the evaluation nor design phase can be considered complete before the definition phase has been completed, both evaluation and design can begin *while* the definition phase is in progress. Classical PERT was developed to support projects that are often completed using an assembly line approach. This does not include information systems!

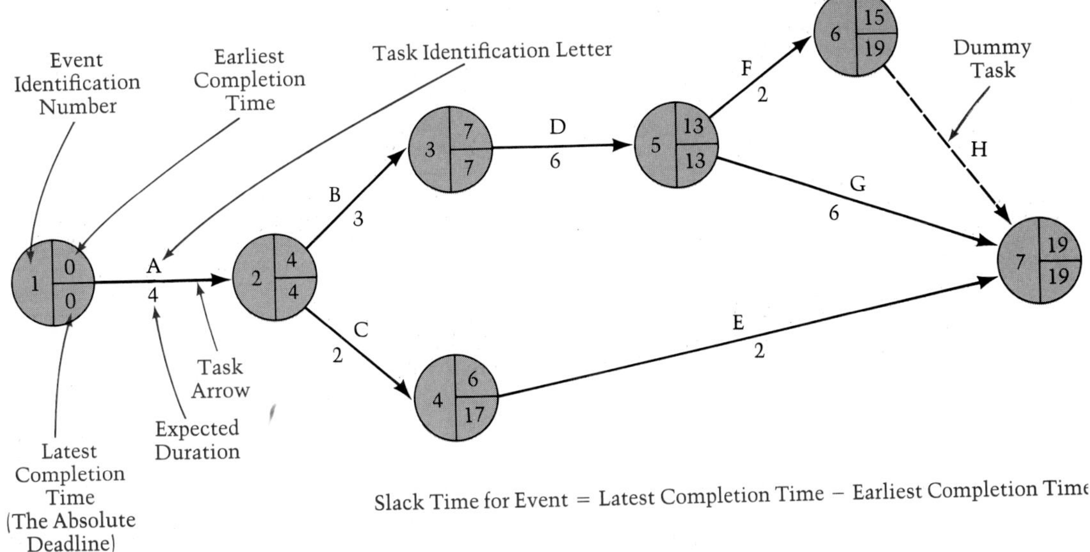

Figure A.1

PERT notation. A PERT chart depicts events and tasks. Nodes represent events. Arrows represent tasks. Each event node includes an ID number, an earliest completion time, and a latest completion time. Each task arrow includes an ID letter and an expected duration time estimate. A dashed arrow represents a dummy task showing a dependency between tasks although no time is required.

The tasks of systems development can overlap; it is only the *completion* of tasks that must occur in sequence. Don't assume that the next task cannot start until the prior task has been completed.

Estimating Project Time Requirements and Deriving the PERT Chart Before drawing a PERT chart, you must estimate the time needed for each project task. The PERT chart will be used to indicate the estimated earliest finish and latest finish time for each event and the expected duration of each project task. Although these times are often expressed in terms of *person-days,* this approach is not recommended. Why? Because there is no proven linear relationship between project completion time and the number of people assigned to a project team. Many systems projects that were late have been further delayed by assigning additional personnel to them. Because two people can do a job in four days is no reason to

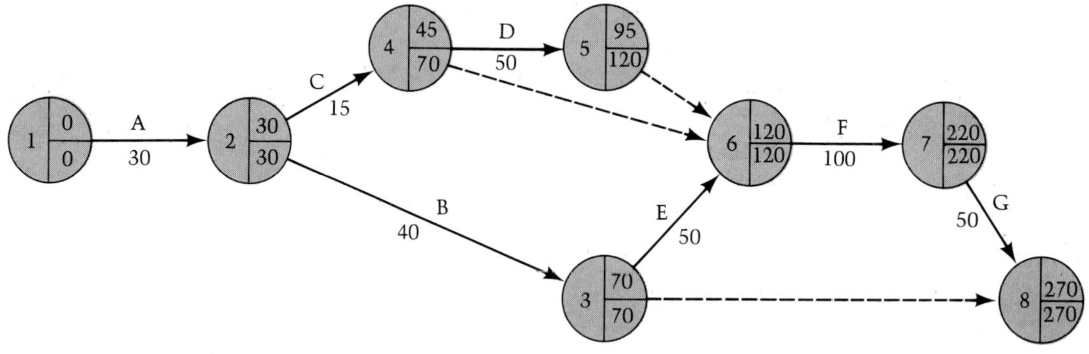

Event	Description	Task	Description
1	Project Approved	N/A	N/A
2	Study Phase Report	A	Study the Current System
3	Requirements Statement	B	Define User Requirements
4	New System Proposal Report	C	Evaluate Alternative Solutions
5	Hardware/Software Ordered	D	Select Computer Technology
6	Design Specs Report	E	Design the New System
7	Programs Tested and Debugged	F	Construct the New System
8	Post Implementation Review	G	Deliver the System

Figure A.2

Sample PERT chart for SDLC. This simple PERT chart depicts interphase dependencies between tasks in the systems development life cycle (SDLC). Each node, often called a milestone, represents the *completion* of a phase. PERT charts depict the sequence for completing tasks. They do not, however, depict the potential for overlapping phases and tasks.

Factors That Affect Time Estimates

- **Size of Project Team**
- **Experience of Team Members**
- **Number of Users and Managers**
- **Attitudes of Users**
- **Management Committment**
- **Availability of Users and Managers**
- **Other Projects in Progress**

assume that four people can do the same job in two days. We suggest that time be expressed in *calendar days*, given the number of people assigned to the task. A calendar day is independent of the number of people assigned to the task.

Unfortunately, we cannot offer you a set of formulas to use to derive time requirements for any task. You must estimate these project time requirements. By *estimate* we don't mean that you simply make something up. A good systems analyst project manager draws on experience and data from previous projects. Some factors that might influence estimates are listed in the margin.

Many organizations have developed internal standards for deriving project time estimates in a more structured manner. These standards may involve examining a task in terms of its difficulty, skill requirements, and other identifiable factors. Alternatively, you could make an optimistic estimate and then adjust that estimate quantifiably by applying weighting factors to various criteria, such as the size of the team, the number of users with whom you have to interact, the availability of those users, and so on (Weinberg, 1979). Each weighting factor may either increase or decrease the estimate. As we go through this discussion, we'll try to give you some guidelines for estimating. When you begin to make estimates, seek the counsel of more experienced analysts (the more the better) until you are comfortable with the process.

Let's assume we're to derive the project time requirements and draw a PERT chart for a typical programming project. The project involves constructing a large program to update an employee master file. The project manager has identified seven program routines that are to be delegated to programmers for coding, testing, and debugging. The project planning table in Figure A.3 was used to derive the project time requirements and construct a PERT chart. Five steps are required:

1. *Make a list of all project tasks and events.* The first two columns in Figure A.3 provide a description and identification letter for each task. The completion of a task is assigned an event identification number, which is entered into the third column.
2. *Determine intertask dependencies.* For each task, record the tasks that must be completed before and after the task in question is completed (columns four and five).
3. *Estimate the duration of each task.* This can be determined as follows:
   (a) Estimate the minimum amount of time it would take to perform the task. We'll call this the optimistic time (OT). The optimistic time estimate assumes that even the most likely interruptions or delays (such as occasional employee illnesses) will not happen.
   (b) Estimate the maximum amount of time it would take to perform the task. We'll call this the pessimistic time (PT). The pessimistic time estimate assumes that anything that can go wrong will go wrong. All possible interruptions or delays (such as labor strikes, illnesses, training, inaccurate specification of requirements, equipment delivery delays, and underestimation of the systems complexity) are assumed to be inevitable.

TASK ID.	TASK DESCRIPTION	EVENT ID. NUMBER	PRECEDING EVENT	SUCCEEDING EVENT	EXPECTED DURATION	EARLIEST FINISH	LATEST FINISH
A	CODE, TEST, AND DEBUG ROUTINE "A010 UPDATE MASTER FILE"	2	1	3	3	3	3
B	CODE, TEST, AND DEBUG ROUTINE "B010 INITIATE PROCESSING"	3	2	4	2	5	5
C	CODE, TEST, AND DEBUG ROUTINE "B020 PROCESS TRANSACTION"	4	3	5,6,7,8	2	7	7
D	CODE, TEST, AND DEBUG ROUTINE "C210 ADD EMPLOYEE RECORD"	5	4	8	7	14	14
E	CODE, TEST, AND DEBUG ROUTINE "C220 MODIFY EMPLOYEE RECORD"	6	4	8	6	13	14
F	CODE, TEST, AND DEBUG ROUTINE "C230 DELETE EMPLOYEE RECORD"	7	4	8	3	10	14
G	CODE, TEST, AND DEBUG ROUTINE "B030 TERMINATE PROCESSING"	8	4	8	2	14	14
H	COLLECTIVELY TEST AND DEBUG PROGRAM	9	8	NONE	5	19	19

Figure A.3

Project planning table. A project planning table is used to prepare data for drawing a PERT chart. The table will also serve as a legend for the chart.

(c) Estimate the most likely amount of time that will be needed to perform the task (MLT). Don't just take the median of the optimistic and pessimistic times. Attempt to identify interruptions or delays that are likely to occur (such as occasional employee illnesses, inexperienced personnel, and occasional training).

(d) Calculate the expected duration (ED) as follows:

$$ED = \frac{OT + (4 \times MLT) + PT}{6}$$

This commonly used formula provides a weighted average of the various estimates. The formula is based on historical experience and may be modified to reflect project history in any firm. Expected duration is recorded in column six of the table shown in Figure A.3.

4. *Derive the earliest and latest completion times (ECT and LCT) for each task* as follows:
   (a) The ECT for event n is equal to the largest ECT for the preceding events (column four) plus the estimated duration time for the task culminating in event n. For the first event, the ECT is equal to zero.
   (b) The LCT (also called the absolute deadline) for event n is equal to the smallest LCT for succeeding events minus the estimated duration time for the task culminating in event n. For the last event, the LCT equals the ECT.

   The data in our table provides considerable planning and control assistance to the project manager.

5. Draw the PERT chart. The PERT chart includes sequencing and identification for all tasks and events along with their time estimates. Notice that our PERT chart (Figure A.4) contains three dummy tasks (represented by the dotted arrows). This means that events 5, 6, and 7 must occur before event 8. However, there is no associated time factor between the three events and event 8.

An alternative approach to deriving PERT charts is *backward scheduling.* The backward scheduling approach schedules activities starting with a proposed task or project completion date and working backward to schedule the tasks that must come before it. This approach is particularly useful when determining the feasibility of a proposed completion date. If all tasks preceding the prescribed date cannot be scheduled for completion prior to the current date, then

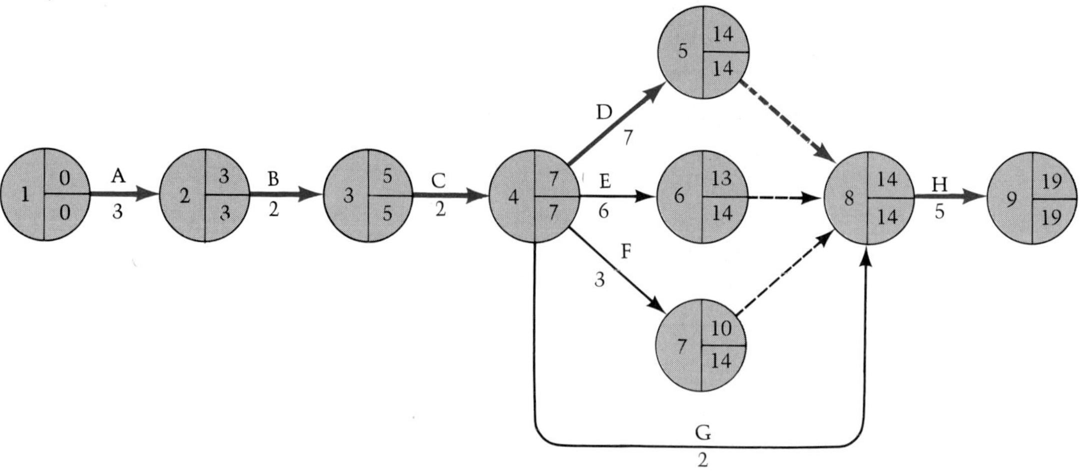

Figure A.4

Completed PERT chart. This is the PERT chart for the project planning table completed in Figure A.3. The bold arrows identify the critical path, those tasks for which there is no slack time.

the proposed completion date must be moved forward or the scope of the project must be decreased.

The Critical Path in a PERT Network Why are some of the solid arrows in Figure A.4 bolder than the others? This series of arrows represents the critical path. The **critical path** is a sequence of dependent project tasks that have the largest sum of estimated durations. It is the path that has no slack time built in. The slack time available for any task is equal to the difference between the earliest and latest completion times. If the earliest and latest completion times are equal, the task is on the critical path.

If any task on the critical path gets behind schedule, the whole project is thrown off schedule. Consequently, each task appearing on the critical path is referred to as a *critical task.* The critical path of the PERT chart for the programming project in Figure A.4 consists of tasks A, B, C, D, and H. This path represents the expected completion time for the project. Critical tasks must be monitored closely by the project manager.

To find the critical path on a project's PERT chart, begin by identifying all the alternate paths or routes that exist from event 1 to the final event. For example, Figure A.4 contains four paths:

Path One: A – B – C – D – dummy task – H

Path Two: A – B – C – E – dummy task – H

Path Three: A – B – C – F – dummy task – H

Path Four: A – B – C – G – H

After all paths have been identified, calculate the total expected duration time for each path. The total expected duration time for a path is equivalent to the sum of the expected duration times for each task in the path. For example:

Path One: $3 + 2 + 2 + 7 + 0 + 5 = 19$

Path Two: $3 + 2 + 2 + 6 + 0 + 5 = 18$

Path Three: $3 + 2 + 2 + 3 + 0 + 5 = 15$

Path Four: $3 + 2 + 2 + 2 + 5 = 14$

You can now identify the critical path as the one having the longest total expected duration time. In our example, path one is the critical path and indicates the expected time for completing programming project is nineteen days. But, what if task G in path four had an expected duration time of seven days? We would then have two critical paths containing tasks that the project manager would have to monitor closely!

Using PERT for Planning and Control Project managers find PERT charts particularly useful for communicating schedules of large systems projects to superiors. However, the primary uses and advantages of the PERT chart lie in its ability to assist in the planning and controlling of projects. In planning, the PERT chart aids in determining the estimated time required to complete a given project, deriving actual project dates, and in allocating resources.

As a control tool, the PERT chart helps the manager identify current and possible future problems. Particular attention should be paid to the critical path of a project. When a project manager identifies a critical task that is running behind schedule and is in danger of upsetting the entire project schedule, alternative courses of action are examined. Corrective measures, such as the shuffling of manpower resources, might be taken. These manpower resources are likely to be temporarily taken away from a noncritical task that is currently running smoothly. These noncritical tasks normally offer some *slack time* for the project.

Gantt Charts: A Scheduling and Evaluation Tool

The **Gantt chart** is a simple time-charting tool that was developed by Henry L. Gantt in 1917. Gantt charts, which are still popular today, are effective for project scheduling and progress evaluation. Like PERT charts, the Gantt chart is graphical. The popularity of Gantt charts stems from their simplicity: They are easy to learn, read, prepare, and use. Let's study this project management tool in more detail.

Gantt Chart Definitions and Symbols The Gantt chart is a simple bar chart (see Figure A.5). Each bar represents a project task. *Task* has the same meaning in both PERT and Gantt charts. Within a Gantt chart, the horizontal axis represents time. Because Gantt charts are used to schedule tasks, the horizontal axis should include dates. The tasks are listed vertically in the left-hand column. And that's all there is to the Gantt chart.

Notice that our Gantt charts clearly depict the overlap of scheduled tasks. Because systems development tasks frequently overlap, this is a major advantage. But also notice that Gantt charts fail to clearly show the dependency of one task on another. That is a major strength of PERT charts. Let's briefly discuss the scheduling and evaluation uses of Gantt charts.

How to Use a Gantt Chart for Scheduling It's easy to use a Gantt chart to generate a schedule. First, identify the tasks that must be scheduled. (If you prepared a PERT chart first, this step would already have been completed.) Next, determine the duration of each task. You learned an appropriate time-estimating technique and formula in the preceding section. If you haven't already prepared a PERT chart, you should at least determine the interdependencies between tasks. Gantt charts cannot clearly show such dependencies, and it is imperative that the schedule recognize them. Now you are ready to schedule the tasks.

List each activity in the left-hand column of the Gantt chart. Record dates corresponding to the duration of the project on the horizontal axis of the chart. Determine starting and completion dates for each task. Careful! The start of any task may be dependent on at least the partial completion of a previous task. Additionally, the completion of a task is frequently dependent on the completion of a prior task. A simple example is in order.

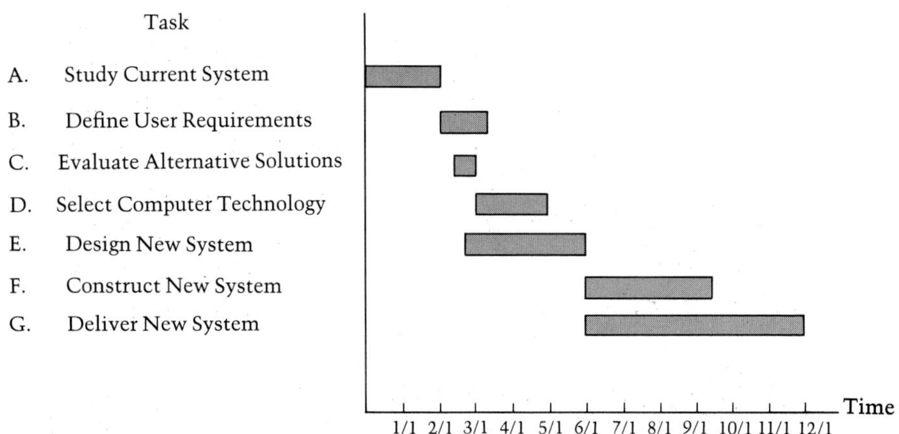

Figure A.5

Sample Gantt chart for SDLC. This is a sample Gantt chart for the systems development life cycle (SDLC). Each bar represents a phase or task. The task is described in the left-hand column. The horizontal axis represents a calendar of dates.

Figure A.5 presents a Gantt chart for our high-level systems development life cycle. It offers some useful information that the PERT chart (Figure A.2) could not. Notice that the start of the definition phase appears to be dependent on the completion of the study phase. On the other hand, the evaluation phase is scheduled to begin after the definition phase has started but before that phase is completed. In fact, the definition phase overlaps the entire evaluation phase.

If you compare the Gantt and PERT charts for the systems development life cycle, you will see that the sequence for *completing* phases (PERT) is maintained in the Gantt chart. Thus the preparation of a PERT chart can significantly aid the preparation of a Gantt chart.

Using Gantt Charts to Evaluate Progress One of the project manager's frequent responsibilities is to report project progress to superiors. Gantt charts frequently find their way into progress reports because they can conveniently compare the original schedule with actual performance. To report progress we must expand our Gantt charting conventions. If a task has been completed, completely

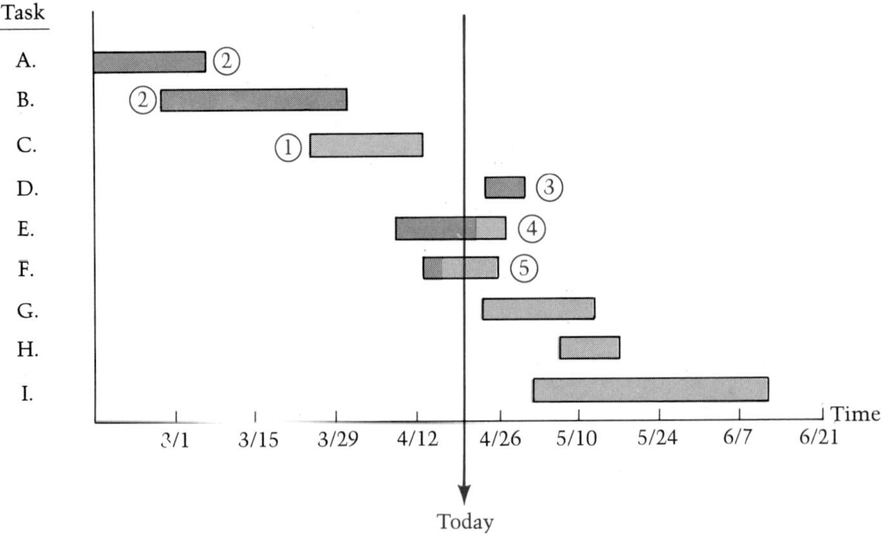

Figure A.6

Progress reporting with Gantt charts. Gantt charts can be annotated to clearly depict project progress. The bold vertical line represents today's date. Task bars are shaded in to reflect progress. Any unshaded bar to the left of today's date is behind schedule.

shade in the bar corresponding to that task. If a task is partially completed, partially shade in the bar. The percentage of the bar that is shaded should correspond to the percentage of the task completed. Unshaded bars represent tasks that have not begun. Next, draw a bold vertical line that is perpendicular to the horizontal axis and that intersects the current date. You can now evaluate project progress.

Let's look at the sample Gantt chart presented in Figure A.6. The unshaded bar to the left of the current date (see ① on Figure A.6) is very much off schedule. This task is supposed to be completed but hasn't even been started. Completely shaded bars to the left of the current date (labeled ② on the figure) represent tasks that have been completed on schedule. Completely shaded bars to the right of the current date (labeled ③) represent tasks that have been completed ahead of schedule. Tasks that are currently in progress have to be evaluated relative to their shaded portions. If the shaded portion extends to or past the current date (see ④ on the figure), that task is on or ahead of schedule. Otherwise, the task is behind schedule (see

⑤). You should see that, with a little practice, the Gantt chart can convey project progress at a glance.

A Comparison of the PERT and Gantt Charting Techniques

PERT and Gantt charting are frequently presented as mutually exclusive project management tools. PERT is usually recommended for larger projects with high intertask dependency. Gantt is recommended for simpler projects. But PERT and Gantt charting should not be considered as alternative project management approaches. All systems development projects have some intertask dependency. And all projects also offer opportunities for task overlapping. Therefore, we recommend that PERT and Gantt charts be used in a complementary manner to plan, schedule, evaluate, and control systems development projects.

PERT would normally be used before Gantt because intertask dependencies, task duration times, and critical path must be determined prior to formal scheduling of tasks. Then the data from the PERT chart are used to prepare the Gantt chart, allowing the project manager to take advantage of overlapping opportunities while not violating intertask dependencies. Project progress can then be recorded on the Gantt chart. And if any task falls behind schedule, the project manager can refer to the PERT chart to determine the impact of the delay and alternative changes that might be made in the schedule.

SUMMARY

In addition to systems analysis and design responsibilities, a systems analyst frequently assumes a project management role. Project mismanagement frequently leads to missed user requirements, cost overruns, and late delivery. The causes of these problems include shortcuts during systems development, imprecise targets, premature cost estimates, poor estimating techniques, poor time management, and lack of leadership. It is the project manager's responsibility to avoid these pitfalls and successfully complete the project on time and within budget. The project manager's basic functions include planning project tasks, staffing the project team, organizing and scheduling the project effort, directing the project team, and controlling project progress.

There are two major tools frequently used by analysts to plan, schedule, and control systems development projects. PERT charts graphically depict project tasks and events and show the dependency of tasks on one another. They also depict the time requirements for each task. Gantt charts graphically depict project tasks to show a project schedule. Gantt charts allow the project manager to show the overlapping of tasks in a project. They are also useful for depicting project progress. PERT and Gantt charts complement one another to provide the manager with an integrated planning, scheduling, evaluation, and control environment. This environment is being further enhanced by the availability of computer software to support these project management tools.

PROBLEMS AND EXERCISES

1. What are some causes of mismanaged projects that result in missed requirements and needs, cost overruns, and late delivery? Explain how these problems that result from mismanaged projects are related.
2. Systems analysts have a tendency to assign additional people to a project that is running behind schedule. What are some of the potential problems of such an action?
3. What are the basic functions of a project manager? Briefly explain how these functions are applied during a systems development project.
4. Explain the advantages and disadvantages of a PERT chart and of a Gantt chart. Explain how each tool can be best used by a project manager.
5. Why shouldn't estimated project time requirements be stated in terms of person-days?
6. Calculate the expected duration for the following tasks:

Task ID Letter	*Optimistic Time (OT)*	*Pessimistic Time (PT)*	*Most Likely Time (MLT)*
A	3	6	4
B	1	3	2
C	4	7	6
D	2	5	3

7. Derive the earliest and latest completion times (ECT and LCT) for each of the following:

Task ID Letter	*Event ID Number*	*Preceding Event*	*Succeeding Event*	*Expected Duration*
A	2	1	3	2
B	3	2	4	3
C	4	3	5,6	4
D	5	4	7	5
E	6	4	7	4
F	7	5,6	8,9	3
G	8	7	10	6
H	9	7	10	5
I	10	8,9	None	6

8. Draw the PERT chart described in problem 7. Be sure to include sequencing and identification for all tasks and events along with their time estimates. What is the critical path? What is the total expected duration time represented by the critical path?

9. Make a list of the tasks you performed on your last programming assignment. Alternatively, make a list of the tasks required to complete your next programming assignment. Develop a PERT chart to depict the tasks and events and the dependency of tasks on one another. What is the critical path? How can the PERT chart aid in planning and scheduling the programming assignment?

10. Derive a Gantt chart to graphically depict the project schedule and overlapping of tasks for the programming assignment you chose for problem 9. How can the Gantt chart be used to evaluate any progress that is being, or has been, made?

11. Draw a PERT chart for the curriculum in which you are enrolled. Be sure to consider the prerequisites for all courses.

12. Draw a Gantt chart for your plan of study to get your degree. Annotate the graph to indicate your progress toward your degree or job objectives.

ANNOTATED REFERENCES AND SUGGESTED READINGS

Bloch, Arthur. *Murphy's Law and Other Reasons Why Things Go Wrong.* Los Angeles, Calif.: Price/Stern/Sloan, 1977. This ninety-six page paperback includes hundreds of humorous laws, theorems, and postulates about projects, people, machines, management, and anything else that can go wrong. It's a nice diversion that can help place the realities of project management into perspective.

Brooks, Fred. *The Mythical Man-Month.* Reading, Mass.: Addison-Wesley, 1975. A classic set of essays on software engineering, also known as systems analysis, design, and implementation. Emphasis is on managing complex projects.

Gildersleeve, Thomas. *Data Processing Project Management.* New York: Van Nostrand Reinhold, 1974. An entire book on project management! No coverage of PERT/CPM, Gantt, or any other tool, but an excellent book on personpower and resource management.

London, Keith. *The People Side of Systems.* New York: McGraw-Hill, 1976. Chapter 8, "Handling a Project Team," does an excellent job of teaching the people and leadership aspects of project management.

Senn, James A. *Analysis and Design of Information Systems.* New York: McGraw-Hill, 1984. Although his treatment of PERT/CPM and Gantt charting is of an introductory nature (like ours), we are indebted to Senn for his PERT/CPM symbol notation, which we emulated in this book.

Weinberg, Victor. *Structured Analysis.* New York: Yourdon Press, 1979. Chapter 11 contains some valuable guidelines and strategies for estimating. Although Weinberg uses his weighting strategy to adjust *costs* according to various factors, we have suggested that scheme would work equally well on *time* estimates.

Wiest, Jerome D., and Ferdinand K. Levy. *A Management Guide to PERT-CPM: With GERT-PDM, DCPM and Other Networks.* 2d ed. Englewood Cliffs, N.J.: Prentice-Hall, 1977. A good source for more on PERT/CPM and other project planning and control networks.

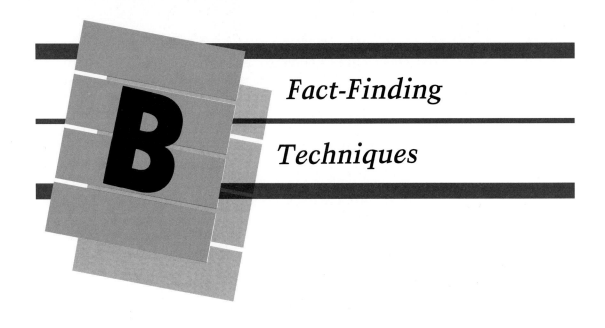

Fact-Finding Techniques

WHEN SHOULD YOU READ THIS MODULE?

You should study this module after reading *any* of the following chapters:

- Chapter 6, "How to Perform a Systems Analysis" — All of the fact-finding techniques (sampling, observation, questionnaires, and interviews) are applicable to the survey, study, definition, and evaluation phases.
- Chapter 10, "How to Perform a Systems Design" — Fact finding is important when designing report formats, terminal dialogue preferences, and data input methods.
- Chapter 17, "How to Perform Systems Implementation" — Fact finding is particularly important during acceptance testing and postimplementation review.

WARNING! The use of the tools and techniques presented in this book could be hazardous to your career!

Have we got your attention? Applying the tools and techniques of systems analysis and design in the classroom is easy. Applying those same tools and techniques in the real world may not work . . . that is, if they are not complemented by effective methods for collecting facts. Tools document facts, and conclusions are drawn from facts. If you can't collect the facts, you can't use the tools. Fact-finding skills must be learned and practiced.

As a systems analyst, you need an organized method of collecting facts. Especially, you need to develop a detective mentality, to be able to discern relevant facts! The purpose of this module is to present fact-finding techniques, also known as information-gathering and data collection techniques. Although an entire textbook could be devoted to fact-finding techniques and strategies, no introductory systems course would be complete without the following survey.

FUNDAMENTALS OF FACT FINDING

Before we leap headfirst into specific fact-finding methods, let's make sure we understand what we are trying to accomplish. The tools of systems analysis and design are used to *document* facts about an existing or proposed information system. These facts are in the domain of the business application and its knowledge workers. Therefore, you must collect those facts in order to effectively apply the documentation tools and techniques. When should you use fact-finding techniques? What kinds of facts should you collect? And how will you collect those facts?

What Facts Does the Systems Analyst Need to Collect, and When?

There are many occasions for fact finding during the systems development life cycle (discussed in Chapter 5). The most notable time is during each systems analysis phase (Chapter 6). During the *study phase,* the analyst must learn and understand the existing information system. During the *definition phase,* the analyst collects facts about user requirements and priorities. As the project proceeds into the *evaluation phase,* the analyst must solicit facts about alternative technical solutions and user preferences for computer solutions. And after systems design (Chapter 10) gets underway, the analyst must collect facts about report formats, terminal dialogue preferences, and input methods. Also, during systems implementation (Chapter 17), fact finding is particularly necessary in the *postimplementation review* whereby the operational system and the project development process are evaluated. Thus we can see that fact finding is an essential skill.

What types of facts must be collected? It would certainly help if we had a framework to help us determine what facts need to be collected, no matter what project we are working on. Fortunately, you have such a framework. Throughout the systems development process, we are looking at an existing or proposed information system. In Chapters 2 and 3, you learned that any information system problem can be examined in four dimensions. Those four dimensions were depicted as the four faces of our pyramid model, which appears throughout this book. As it turns out, the facts that describe any information system also correspond nicely with the dimensions of that pyramid model (see margin).

Information System Pyramid Model Dimensions

- Knowledge Workers
- Business Mission
- Information System Functions
- IPO Components

What Fact-Finding Methods Are Available?

Now that we have a framework for our fact-finding activities, we can introduce four common fact-finding techniques:

1. Sampling of existing documentation, forms, and files
2. Observation of the work environment
3. Questionnaires
4. Interviews

An understanding of each of these techniques is essential to your success. An analyst usually applies several of these techniques during a single systems project. To be able to select the most suitable technique for use in any given situation, you will have to learn the advantages and disadvantages of each of our four fact-finding techniques.

TECHNIQUES FOR SAMPLING EXISTING DOCUMENTATION, FORMS, AND FILES

Particularly when you are studying an existing system, you can develop a pretty good feel for the system by studying existing documentation, forms, and files. Because it would be impractical to study every occurrence of every form, analysts normally use sampling techniques to get a large enough cross section to determine what can happen in the system. A good analyst always gets facts first from existing documentation rather than from people.

Collecting Facts from Existing Documentation

What kind of documents can teach you about a system? The first document the analyst should seek out is the *organization chart.* What's the next step? One possibility is to trace the history that led to the project. To accomplish this, you may want to collect and review documents that describe the problem. These include:

- Interoffice memoranda, studies, minutes, suggestion box notes, customer complaints, and reports that document the problem area
- Accounting records, performance reviews, work measurement reviews, and other scheduled operating reports
- Data processing project requests, past and present

In addition to documents that describe the problem, there are usually documents that describe the business function being studied or designed. These documents may include:

- The company's mission statement and strategic plan
- Formal objectives for the organization subunits being studied
- Policy manuals that may place constraints on any proposed system
- Standard operating procedures (SOPs), job outlines, or task instructions for specific day-to-day operations
- Completed forms that represent actual transactions at various points in the processing cycle
- Manual and computerized files
- Manual and computerized reports

Don't forget to check for documentation of previous systems studies and designs performed by systems analysts and consultants. This documentation may include:

- Various types of flowcharts and flow diagrams

- Data dictionaries
- Design documentation (such as inputs, outputs, and files)
- Program documentation
- Computer operations manuals and training manuals

All documentation collected should be analyzed to determine how up-to-date it is. Don't discard outdated documentation. Just keep in mind that additional fact finding will be needed to verify or update the facts collected. As you review existing documents, take notes, draw pictures, and use systems analysis and design tools to model what you are learning about or proposing for the system.

Document and File Sampling Techniques

Sampling is the process of collecting sample documents, forms, and records. When studying documents or records from a file, study enough samples to identify all the possible processing conditions and exceptions. How do you determine if the sample size is large enough to be representative? You use statistical sampling techniques.

How to Determine Sample Size The size of the sample depends on how representative you want the sample to be. There is a simple and reliable formula for determining sample size:

$$\text{sample size} = 0.25 \times (\text{ certainty factor } / \text{ acceptable error })^2$$

The certainty factor depends on how certain you want to be that the data sampled will not include variations not in the sample. The certainty factor is calculated from tables (available in many industrial engineering texts); a partial example follows:

Desired Certainty	*Certainty Factor*
95%	1.960
90%	1.645
80%	1.281

Suppose you want 90 percent certainty that a sample of invoices will contain no unsampled variations. Your sample size, SS, is calculated as follows:

$$SS = 0.25\ (\ 1.645\ /\ 0.10\ )^2 = 68$$

We need to sample sixty-eight invoices to get the desired accuracy.

Selecting the Sample How do we choose our sixty-eight invoices? Two commonly used sampling techniques are randomization and stratification. In randomization, there is no predetermined pattern or plan for selecting sample data. Therefore, we just randomly choose sixty-eight invoices. The stratification technique is a systematic approach for selecting sample data. This technique attempts to reduce the variance of the estimates by spreading out the sampling (for example, choosing documents or records by formula) and by avoiding very high or low estimates.

For computerized files, stratification sampling can be executed by writing a sample program. For instance, suppose our invoices were on a computer file that had a volume of approximately 250,000 invoices. Recall that our sample size needs to include sixty-eight invoices. We will simply write a program that prints every 3,676th record (= 250,000 / 68). This is an example of stratification sampling on a computer file. For manual files and documents, we could execute a similar scheme.

OBSERVATION OF THE WORK ENVIRONMENT

Observation is one of the most effective data collection techniques for obtaining an understanding of a system. In **observation,** the systems analyst either participates in or watches a person perform activities to obtain facts about the system. This technique is often used when the validity of data collected through other methods is in question or when the complexity of certain aspects of the system prevents a clear explanation by the knowledge workers.

Collecting Facts by Observing People at Work

Even with a well-conceived observation plan, the systems analyst is not assured that fact finding will be successful. You should become aware of the pros and cons of the technique of observation. Advantages and disadvantages include:

Advantages

1. Data gathered by observation tend to be highly reliable. Some-

times, observations are conducted to check the validity of data obtained directly from individuals.

2. The systems analyst is able to see exactly what is being done. Complex tasks are sometimes difficult to clearly explain in words. Through observation, the systems analyst can identify tasks that have been missed or inaccurately described by other fact-finding techniques. Also, the analyst can obtain data describing the physical environment of the task (for example, physical layout, traffic, lighting, noise level).
3. Observation is relatively inexpensive compared with other fact-finding techniques. Other techniques usually require substantially more employee release time and copying expenses.
4. Observation allows the systems analyst to do work measurements.

Disadvantages

1. Because people usually feel uncomfortable when being watched, they may unwittingly perform differently when being observed.
2. The work being observed may not involve the level of difficulty or volume normally experienced during that time period.
3. Some system activities may take place at odd times causing scheduling inconvenience for the systems analyst.
4. The tasks being observed are subject to various types of interruptions.
5. Some tasks may not always be performed in the manner in which they are observed by the systems analyst. For example, the systems analyst might have observed how a company filled several customer orders. However, the procedures the systems analyst observed may have been those steps used to fill a number of regular customer orders. If any of those orders had been special orders (such as an order for goods not normally kept in stock) the systems analyst would have observed a different set of procedures being executed.
6. If people have been performing tasks in a manner that violates standard operating procedures, they may temporarily perform their jobs correctly while you are observing them. In other words, people may let you see what they want you to see.

Guidelines for Observation

How does the systems analyst obtain facts through observation? Does one simply arrive at the site of observation and begin recording everything that's viewed? Of course not. Much preparation should take place in advance. The analyst must determine how data will actually be captured. Will it be necessary to have special forms on which to quickly record data? Will the individual(s) being observed be bothered by having someone watch and record their actions? When are the low, normal, and peak periods of operations for the task to be observed? The systems analyst must identify the ideal time to observe a particular aspect of the system.

Observation should first be conducted when the workload is normal. Afterward, observations can be made during peak periods to gather information for measuring the effects caused by the increased volume. The systems analyst might also obtain samples of documents or forms that will be used by those being observed. As you can see, a great deal of planning and preparation must be done up front.

The sampling techniques discussed earlier are also useful for observation. In this case, the technique is called *work sampling.* **Work sampling** involves a large number of observations taken at random intervals. This technique is less threatening to the people being observed because the observation period is not continuous. When using work sampling, you need to predefine the operations of the job to be observed. Then calculate a sample size as you did for document and file sampling. Make that many random observations, being careful to observe activities at different times of the day. By counting the number of occurrences of each operation during the observations, you will get a feel for how employees spend their days.

With proper planning completed, the actual observation can be done. Effective observation is difficult to carry out. Experience is the best teacher; however, the following guidelines may help you develop your observation skills:

DO

1. Determine the who, what, where, when, why, and how of the observation.
2. Obtain permission from appropriate supervisors or managers.

3. Inform those who will be observed of the purpose of the observation.
4. Keep a low profile.
5. Take notes during or immediately following the observation.
6. Review observation notes with appropriate individuals.

DON'T

1. Interrupt the individuals at work.
2. Focus heavily on trivial activities.
3. Make assumptions.

QUESTIONNAIRES

The **questionnaire** is a special-purpose document that allows the analyst to collect information and opinions from respondents. The document can be mass-produced and distributed to respondents, who can then complete the questionnaire on their own time. Questionnaires allow the analyst to collect facts from a large number of people while maintaining uniform responses. When dealing with the large audience, no other fact-finding technique can tabulate the same facts as efficiently.

Collect Facts by Using Questionnaires

The use of questionnaires has been heavily criticized and is often avoided by systems analysts. Why? Many systems analysts claim that the responses lack reliable, valid, and useful information. But questionnaires can be an effective method for fact gathering, and many of these criticisms can be attributed to their inappropriate use by systems analysts. Before using questionnaires, you should first understand the pros and cons associated with their use.

Advantages

1. Most questionnaires can be answered quickly. People can complete and return questionnaires at their convenience.

2. Questionnaires provide a relatively inexpensive means for gathering data from a large number of individuals.
3. Questionnaires allow individuals to maintain anonymity. Therefore, individuals are more likely to provide the real facts, rather than telling you what they think their boss would want them to.
4. Responses can be tabulated and analyzed quickly.

Disadvantages

1. The number of respondents is often low.
2. There's no guarantee that an individual will answer or expand upon all of the questions.
3. Questionnaires tend to be inflexible. There's no opportunity for the systems analyst to obtain voluntary information from individuals or to reword questions that may have been misinterpreted.
4. It's not possible for the systems analyst to observe and analyze the respondent's body language.
5. There is no immediate opportunity to clarify a vague or incomplete answer to any question.
6. Good questionnaires are difficult to prepare.

Types of Questionnaires

There are two formats for questionnaires, free format and fixed format. A free-format questionnaire offers the respondent greater latitude in the answer. A question is asked, and the respondent records the answer in the space provided after the question. Examples of free format questions are:

1. What reports do you currently receive and how are they used?
2. Are there any problems with these reports (for example, are they inaccurate, is there insufficient information, or are they difficult to read and/or use)? If so, please explain.

Obviously, such responses may be difficult to tabulate. However, the analyst receives much more data about the opinions and attitudes of the respondents. It is possible that the respondent's answer may not match the question. In order to ensure good responses in free format questionnaires, the analyst should:

- Phrase the question in simple sentences and not use words (such as *good*) that can be interpreted differently by different respondents
- Ask questions that can be answered with three or fewer sentences (Otherwise, the questionnaire may take up more time than the respondent is willing to sacrifice)

A fixed-format questionnaire contains questions that require specific responses from individuals. Given any question, the respondent must choose from the available answers. This makes the results much easier to tabulate. On the other hand, the respondent cannot provide additional information that might prove valuable. There are three types of fixed-format questions:

1. *Multiple choice,* in which the respondent is given a question and several answers. The respondent should be told if more than one answer may be selected. Some multiple choice questions allow for very brief free-format responses when none of the standard answers apply. Examples of multiple choice, fixed-format questions are:

   Do you feel that back orders occur too frequently?
   ☐ YES ☐ NO

   Is the current accounts receivable report that you receive useful?
   ☐ YES ☐ NO If no, please explain.

2. *Rating,* in which the respondent is given a statement and asked to use supplied responses to state an opinion. To prevent built-in bias, there should be an equal number of positive and negative ratings. The following is an example of a rating fixed-format question:

   The implementation of quantity discounts would cause an increase in customer orders.
   ☐ strongly agree
   ☐ agree
   ☐ no opinion
   ☐ disagree
   ☐ strongly disagree

3. *Ranking*, in which the respondent is given a question and several possible answers, which are to be ranked in order of preference or experience. An example of a ranking fixed-format question is:

   Rank the following transaction according to the amount of time you spend processing them:
   ______% new customer orders
   ______% order cancellations
   ______% order modifications
   ______% payments

Developing a Questionnaire

Good questionnaires are designed. If you write your questionnaires without designing it first, your chances of success are limited. The following procedure is effective:

1. Determine what facts and opinions must be collected and from whom you should get them. If the number of people is large, consider using a smaller, randomly selected group of respondents.
2. Based on the needed facts and opinions, determine whether free- or fixed-format questions will produce the best answers. A combination format that permits optional free-format clarification of fixed-format responses is often used.
3. Write the questions. Examine them for construction errors and possible misinterpretations. Make sure that the questions don't offer your personal bias or opinions. Edit the questions.
4. Test the questions on a small sample of respondents. If your respondents had problems with them or if the answers were not useful, edit the questions.
5. Duplicate and distribute the questionnaire.

INTERVIEWS

The personal interview is generally recognized as the most important and often used fact-finding technique. **Interviews** provide systems analysts the opportunity to collect information from individuals, face-to-face. Interviewing can be used to achieve any of the goals listed in the margin. There are two roles assumed in an interview. The systems analyst is the interviewer, responsible for organizing and conducting the interview. The user, manager, or advisor is the interviewee, who is asked to respond to a series of questions. Unfortunately, many systems analysts are poor interviewers. In this section, you will learn how to conduct proper interviews.

Interview Goals

- Fact Finding
- Fact Verification
- Clarification
- Generate Enthusiasm
- Get User Involved
- Identify Requirements
- Solicit Ideas and Opinions

Collecting Facts by Interviewing People

The most important element of an information system is people. And more than anything else, *people want to be in on things.* No other fact-finding technique places as much emphasis on people as interviews. But people have different values, priorities, opinions, motivations, and personalities. Therefore, to use the interviewing technique, you must possess good human relations skills for dealing effectively with different types of people. And like other fact-finding techniques, interviewing isn't the best method for all situations. Interviewing has its advantages and disadvantages, which should be weighed against those of other fact-finding techniques for every fact-finding situation.

Advantages

1. Interviews give the analyst an opportunity to motivate the interviewee to respond freely and openly to questions. By establishing a rapport, the systems analyst is able to give the interviewee a feeling of actively contributing to the systems project.
2. Interviews allow the systems analyst to probe for more feedback from the interviewee.
3. Interviews permit the systems analyst to adapt or reword questions for each individual.
4. Interviews give the analyst an opportunity to observe the interviewee's nonverbal communication. A good systems analyst may be able to obtain information by observing the interviewee's body movements and facial expressions as well as by listening to verbal replies to questions.

Disadvantages

1. Interviewing is a very time-consuming, and therefore costly, fact-finding approach.

2. Success of interviews is highly dependent upon the systems analyst's human relations skills.
3. Interviewing may be impractical due to the location of interviewees.

Interview Types and Techniques

There are two types of interviews, unstructured and structured. In the *unstructured interview,* the interviewer conducts the interview with only a general goal or subject in mind and few, if any, specific questions. The interviewer counts on the interviewee to provide a framework and direct the conversation. This type of interview frequently gets off the track, and the analyst must be prepared to redirect the interview back to the main goal or subject. For this reason, unstructured interviews don't usually work well for systems analysis and design.

In the *structured interview,* the interviewer has a specific set of questions to ask of the interviewee. Depending on the interviewee's responses, the interviewer will direct additional questions to obtain clarification or amplification. Some of these questions may be planned and others spontaneous. Questions may be either open-ended or closed-ended. *Open-ended questions* allow the interviewee to respond in any way that seems appropriate. An example of an open-ended question is "Why are you dissatisfied with the report of uncollectable accounts?" *Closed-ended questions* restrict answers to either specific choices or short, direct responses. An example of such a question might be "Are you receiving the report of uncollectable accounts on time?" or "Does the report of uncollectable accounts contain accurate information?" Realistically, most questions fall between the two extremes.

How to Conduct an Interview

Your success as a systems analyst is at least partially dependent upon your ability to interview. A successful interview will involve selecting appropriate individuals to interview, preparing extensively for the interview, conducting the interview properly, and following up on the interview. Here we examine each of these aspects in more detail. Let's assume that you've identified the need for an interview and you have determined exactly what kinds of facts and opinions you need.

Select Interviewees Who should you interview? You should interview the knowledge workers of the information system you are studying. A formal organizational chart will help you identify these individuals and their responsibilities. You should attempt to learn as much as possible about each individual prior to the interview. Attempt to learn what their strengths, fears, biases, and motivations might be. The interview can then be geared to take the characteristics of the individual into account.

Always make an appointment with the interviewee. Never just drop in. Limit the appointment to somewhere between a half hour and an hour. The higher the management level of the interviewee, the less time you should schedule. If the interviewee is a clerical, service, or blue-collar worker, get the supervisor's permission before scheduling the interview. Be certain that the location you want for the interview will be available during the time the interview is scheduled. Never conduct an interview in the presence of your office mates or the interviewee's peers.

Prepare for the Interview Preparation is the key to a successful interview. An interviewee can easily detect an unprepared interviewer. In fact, the interviewee may very much resent the lack of preparation because it is a waste of valuable time. When the appointment is made, the interviewee should be notified about the subject of the interview. To ensure that all pertinent aspects of the subject are covered, the analyst should prepare an interview guide.

An **interview guide** is a checklist of specific questions the interviewer will ask the interviewee. It may also contain follow-up questions that will only be asked if the answers to other questions warrant the additional answers. A sample interview guide is presented in Figure B.1. Questions should be carefully chosen and phrased. Most questions begin with the standard *who, what, when, where, why,* and *how much* type of wording. Avoid the following types of questions:

- *Loaded questions,* such as "Do we have to have both of these columns on the report?" The question conveys the interviewee's personal opinion on the issue.
- *Leading questions,* such as "You're not going to use this OPERATOR CODE, are you?" The question leads the interviewee to respond "No, of course not", regardless of actual opinion.
- *Bias questions,* such as "How many codes do we need for

INTERVIEW AGENDA

INTERVIEWEE: Jeff Bentley, Accounts Receivable Manager
DATE: Tuesday, March 22, 1986
TIME: 1:30 P.M.
PLACE: Room 223, Admin. Bldg.
SUBJECT: Current Credit Checking Policy

1-2 min. Open the interview.

Introduce ourselves.
Thank Mr. Bentley for the use of his valuable time.
State the purpose of the interview--to obtain an understanding of the existing credit checking policies.

5 min. What conditions determine whether a customer's order is approved for credit?

5 min. What are the possible decisions or actions that might be taken once these conditions have been evaluated?

3 min. How are customers notified when credit is not approved for their order?

1 min. After a new order is approved for credit and placed in the file containing orders that can be filled, a customer might request a modification be made to the order. Would the order have to go through credit approval again if the new total order cost exceeds the original cost?

1 min. Who are the individuals that perform the credit checks?

1-3 min. May I have permission to talk to those individuals to learn specifically how they carry out the credit checking process?

If so:

When would be an appropriate time to meet with each of them?

1 min. Conclude the interview:

Thank Mr. Bentley for his cooperation and assure him that he will be receiving a copy of what transpired during the interview.

21 minutes
+ 9 minutes for follow-up questions and redirection

30 minutes allotted for interview (1:30 P.M.-2:00 P.M.)

◀ **Figure B.1**

Sample interview guide. The sample interview guide represents an agenda that a systems analyst might use to obtain facts about a company's existing credit approval policy. Notice that the agenda is carefully laid out, with specific time allocated to each question. Note, too, that time has been reserved for follow-up questions and redirecting the interview.

FOOD-CLASSIFICATION in the INVENTORY FILE? I think twenty ought to cover it." Why bias the interviewee's answer with your own?

Additional guidelines for questions are provided in the margin. You should especially avoid threatening or critical questions. The purpose of the interview is to investigate, not to evaluate or criticize.

Guidelines for Interview Questions

1. Use clear and concise language.
2. Don't include your opinion as part of questions.
3. Avoid long or compound questions.
4. Avoid threatening questions.
5. Don't use *you* when you mean *a group of people* (such as a department or the people who work in that office).

Conduct the Interview The actual interview can be characterized as consisting of three phases: the opening, body, and conclusion. The opening is intended to influence or motivate the interviewee to participate and communicate by establishing an ideal environment. When establishing an environment of mutual trust and respect, you should identify the purpose and length of the interview and explain how the gathered data will be used. Several ways to effectively begin an interview are:

1. Summarize the apparent problem, and explain how the problem was discovered.
2. Offer an incentive or reward for participation.
3. Ask the interviewee for advice or assistance.

The body of an interview represents the most time-consuming phase. During this phase, you obtain the interviewee's responses to your list of questions. Listen closely and observe the interviewee. Take notes concerning both verbal and nonverbal responses from the interviewee. It's very important for you to keep the interview on track. Anticipate the need to adapt the interview to the interviewee. Often questions can be bypassed if they have been answered earlier in part of an answer to another question, or they can be deleted if determined to be irrelevant, based on what you've already learned during the interview. Finally, probe for more facts when necessary.

Conducting the Interview

DO

1. Be courteous.
2. Listen carefully.
3. Maintain control.
4. Probe.
5. Observe mannerisms and nonverbal communication.
6. Be patient.
7. Keep interviewee at ease.
8. Maintain self-control.

DON'T

1. Continue an interview unnecessarily.
2. Assume an answer is finished or leading nowhere.
3. Reveal verbal and nonverbal cues.
4. Use jargon.
5. Reveal your personal biases.
6. Talk instead of listening.
7. Assume anything about the topic and the interviewee.

During the conclusion of an interview, you should express your appreciation and provide answers to any questions posed by the interviewee. The conclusion is very important for maintaining rapport and trust with the interviewee.

The importance of human relations skills in interviewing cannot be overemphasized. These skills must be exercised throughout the interview. In the margin, you will find a set of rules that should be followed during an interview.

Follow-Up on the Interview To help maintain a good rapport and trust with interviewees, you should send them a memo that summarizes the interview. This memo should remind interviewees of their contributions to the systems project and allow them the opportunity to clarify any misinterpretations that you may have derived during the interview. In addition, the interviewees should be given the opportunity to offer additional information they may have failed to bring out during the interview.

A FACT-FINDING STRATEGY

At the beginning of this module, we suggested that an analyst needs an *organized* method for collecting facts. An inexperienced analyst will frequently jump right into interviews. "Go to the people. That's where the real facts are!" Wrong! This attitude fails to recognize an important fact of life: people must complete their day-to-day jobs! Your job is not their main responsibility. Now you may be thinking, "But I thought you've been saying that the system is for people and that direct user involvement in systems development is essential! Aren't you contradicting yourselves?"

Not at all! Time is money. To waste your users' time is to waste your company's money. To make the most of the time you spend with users, don't jump right into interviews. Instead, first collect all the facts you can by using methods other than asking people. Consider the following step-by-step strategy:

1. *Learn all you can from existing documents, forms, reports, and files.* You'll be surprised how much of the system becomes clear without any people contact.
2. *If appropriate, observe the system in action.* Agree not to ask

questions. Just watch and take notes or draw pictures. Make sure that the workers know that you're not evaluating individuals. Otherwise, they may perform in a more efficient manner than normal.

3. *Given the facts you've already collected, design and distribute questionnaires to clear up things you don't fully understand.* This is also a good time to solicit opinions on problems and limitations. Questionnaires do require your users to give up some of their time. But *they* choose when to best make that sacrifice.
4. *Now conduct your interviews.* Because you have already collected most of the pertinent facts by low-user-contact methods, you can use the interview to verify and clarify the most difficult issues and problems. You are unlikely to waste user time as you gather information you could have obtained in other ways.

This strategy is not sacred. Although a fact-finding strategy should be developed for every pertinent phase of systems development, every project is unique. Sometimes, observation and questionnaires may be inappropriate. But the idea should always be to collect as many facts as possible before using interviews.

Before we close this discussion, you are reminded that collecting facts, as an activity by itself, is not sufficient. You must verify the facts that have been collected. You can do this in one of two ways. First, you can verify facts collected by one fact-finding technique by using an alternative fact-finding technique. For instance, you could verify the results of a questionnaire by observing the system in action. Second, you can verify facts by documenting them using the tools and techniques presented in Parts II and III of this book. Then you can meet with your users to review that documentation. Techniques for presenting facts, documentation, and conclusions are presented in Module C.

SUMMARY

Effective fact-finding techniques are crucial to the application of systems analysis and design methods during systems projects. Fact finding is performed during the study, definition, evaluation, design, and implementation phases of the systems development life cycle. To support development activities, the analyst must collect facts about the knowledge workers, the business, data and information resources, and information system components. There are four common fact-finding techniques: sampling, observation, questionnaires, and interviews.

The sampling of existing documents and files can provide many facts and details with little or no direct personal communication. The analyst should collect historical documents, business operations manuals and forms, and data processing documents. In order to ensure that an adequate number of documents have been studied, analysts often use sampling techniques. These techniques help the analyst collect a representative subset of the documents and minimize the chance of not identifying exceptional events. Observation is a fact-finding technique in which the analyst studies people doing their jobs. To minimize the chance that the observation time is not representative of normal workloads, the analyst can use work sampling to randomly collect observation data. Questionnaires are used to collect similar facts from a large number of individuals. Questionnaires can be either free format or fixed format.

Interviews are the most popular but time-consuming fact-finding technique. When interviewing, the analyst meets individually with people to gather information. Most systems analysis and design interviews are structured, meaning that the analyst has prepared a specific set of questions prior to the interview. After determining the need for an interview, the analyst arranges for appointments with the interviewees, carefully prepares the interview questions, conducts the interviews, and summarizes the results. Because interviews are time-consuming, the analyst should collect as many facts as possible by using the other fact-finding methods.

PROBLEMS AND EXERCISES

1. Explain how the information system pyramid model can serve as a framework in determining what facts need to be collected during systems development.
2. Explain how an organization chart can aid in planning for fact finding. What are some of the potential drawbacks to using an existing organization chart?

3. A systems analyst wants to study documents stored in a large metal file cabinet. The cabinet contains several hundred records describing product warranty claims. The analyst wishes to study a sample of the records in the file and to be 95 percent certain (certainty factor = 1.960) that the data from which the sample is taken will not include variations not in the sample. How many sample records should the analyst retrieve to get this desired accuracy?
4. For the sample size in problem 3, explain two specific strategies for selecting the samples.
5. Describe how you would use form and/or file sampling in the following phases. If you think sampling would be inappropriate for any of these phases, explain why.
   (a) Study of the current system
   (b) Definition of user requirements
   (c) Evaluation of alternative solutions
   (d) Selection of computer equipment and software
   (e) Design of the new information system
   (f) Construction of the new information system
   (g) Delivery of the new information system
6. Repeat question 5 for the technique of observation.
7. Make a list of things that might affect your work performance when you are being observed performing your job. What could an observer do to eliminate these concerns or problems?
8. Repeat question 5 for the questionnaire technique.
9. Give two examples of free-format questions and two examples of each of the following types of fixed-format questions:
   (a) multiple choice
   (b) rating
   (c) ranking
10. Repeat question 5 for the interviewing technique.
11. Explain the difference between a structured and unstructured interview. When is each type of interview appropriately used?
12. Prepare a sample interview guide to use in obtaining from your academic advisor facts describing course registration policies and procedures.
13. Mr. Art Roads is the Accounts Receivables Manager. You have been assigned to do a study of Mr. Roads's current billing sys-

tem and need to solicit facts from his subordinates. Mr. Roads has expressed his concern that, although he wishes to support you in your fact-finding efforts, his people are extremely busy and must get their jobs done. Write a memo to Mr. Roads describing a fact-finding strategy you could follow to maximize your fact finding while minimizing the release time required for his subordinates.

ANNOTATED REFERENCES AND SUGGESTED READINGS

Berdie, Douglas R., and John F. Anderson. *Questionnaires: Design and Use.* Metuchen, N.J.: Scarecrow Press, 1974. A practical guide to the construction of questionnaires. Particularly useful because of its short length and illustrative examples.

Davis, William S. *Systems Analysis and Design.* Reading, Mass.: Addison-Wesley, 1983. Provides useful pointers for preparing and conducting interviews.

Fitzgerald, Jerry, Ardra F. Fitzgerald, and Warren D. Stallings, Jr. *Fundamentals of Systems Analysis.* 2d ed. New York: Wiley, 1981. A good survey text for the systems analyst. Chapter 6, "Understanding the Existing System," does a good job of presenting fact-finding techniques in the light of the study phase.

Gildersleeve, Thomas R. *Successful Data Processing Systems Analysis.* Englewood Cliffs, N.J.: Prentice-Hall, 1978. Chapter 4, "Interviewing in Systems Work," provides a comprehensive look at interviewing specifically for the systems analyst. A thorough sample interview is scripted and analyzed in this chapter.

London, Keith R. *The People Side of Systems.* New York: McGraw-Hill, 1976. Chapter 5, "Investigation versus Inquisition," provides a very good people-oriented look at fact finding, with considerable emphasis on interviewing.

Lord, Kenniston W., Jr., and James B. Steiner. *CDP Review Manual: A Data Processing Handbook.* 2d ed. New York: Van Nostrand Reinhold, 1978. Chapter 8, "Systems Analysis and Design," provides a more comprehensive comparison of the merits and demerits of each fact-finding technique. This material is intended to prepare data processors for the Certificate in Data Processing examinations, one of which covers Systems Analysis and Design.

Salvendy, G., ed. *Handbook of Industrial Engineering.* New York: Wiley, 1974. A comprehensive handbook for industrial engineers; systems analysts are, in a way, a type of industrial engineer. Excellent coverage on sampling and work measurement.

Stewart, Charles J., and Cash, William B., Jr. *Interviewing: Principles and Practices.* 2d ed. Dubuque, Iowa: Brown, 1978. Popular college textbook that provides broad exposure to interviewing techniques, many of which are applicable to systems analysis and design.

Weinberg, Gerald M. *Rethinking Systems Analysis and Design.* Boston: Little, Brown, 1982. Chapter 3, "Observation," and Chapter 4, "Interviewing," are both excellent reading. Gerald Weinberg's interesting style and thought process should be read by every analyst. The fables, stories, and anecdotes blend well into this insightful book.

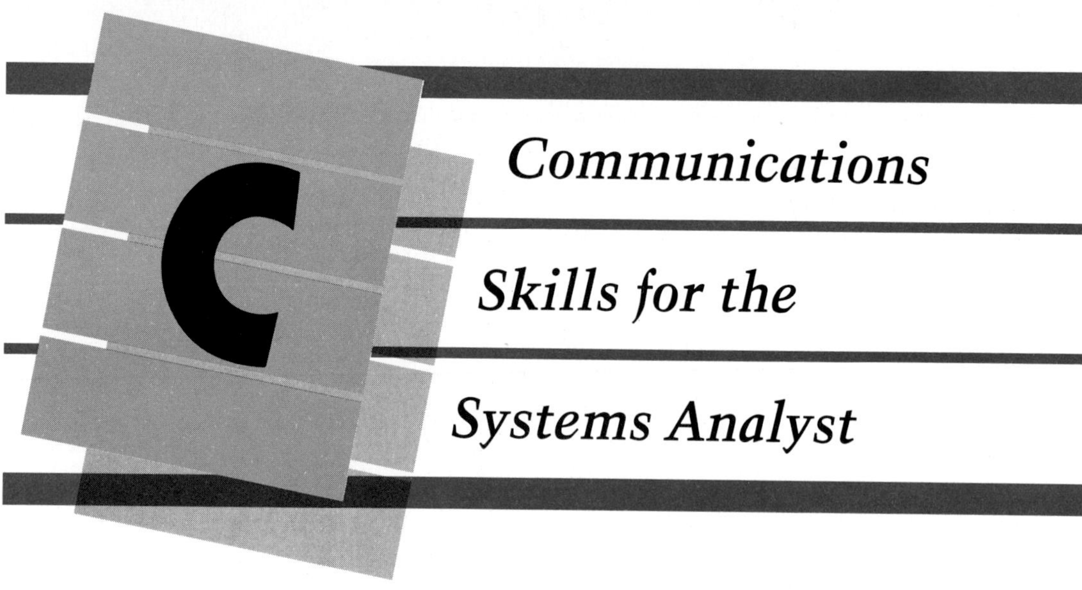

Communications Skills for the Systems Analyst

WHEN SHOULD YOU READ THIS MODULE?

You should study this module after reading *any* of the following chapters:

- Chapter 6, "How to Perform a Systems Analysis"—All of the communications skills discussed in this module—meetings, walkthroughs, presentations, and reports—are applicable to the survey, study, definition, and evaluation phases.
- Chapter 10, "How to Perform a Systems Design"—All of the communications skills in the module are applicable to the design and selection phase. During systems design, communication becomes more difficult because it is at this point that technical issues are introduced.
- Chapter 17, "How to Perform Systems Implementation"—All communications skills discussed in this module are applicable to programmers and analysts who construct and deliver the information system.

Once upon a time all the world spoke a single language and used the same words. As men journeyed in the east, they came upon a plain in the land of Shinar and settled there. They said to one another, "Come, let us make bricks and bake them hard"; they used bricks for stone and bitumen for mortar. "Come," they said, "let us build ourselves a city and a tower with its top in the heavens, and make a name for ourselves; or we shall ever be dispersed all over the earth." Then the Lord came down to see the city and tower which mortal men had built, and he said, "Here they are, one people with a single language, and now they have started to do this; henceforward nothing they have a mind to do will be beyond their reach. Come, let us go down there and confuse their speech, so that they will not understand what they say to one another." So the Lord dispersed them from there all over the earth, and they left off building the city. That is why it is called Babel, because the Lord there made a babble of the language of all the world; from that place the Lord scattered men all over the face of the earth.
[Genesis 11:1–9] (From *The New English Bible.* © The Delegates of the Oxford University Press and The Syndics of the Cambridge Press 1961, 1970. Reprinted by permission.)

The story of the Tower of Babel is the story of the creation of communications problems in the world. And where God left off, we have further complicated the problem. The Tower of Babel failed for the same reason many information systems projects fail, a breakdown of communications. Information systems projects are frequently plagued by communications barriers that we erect between ourselves and the users. The business world has its own language to describe forms, methods, procedures, financial data, and the like. And the data processing industry has its own language of acronyms, terms, buzzwords, and procedures. As was the case in the Tower of Babel project, a communications gap has developed between the user and data processor.

The systems analyst is supposed to bridge this communications gap. A typical project enlists the participation of a diverse audience, both technical and nontechnical. The purpose of this module is to survey interpersonal communications skills, the cornerstone of successful systems development. Because communications skills are vital in all phases of systems development, we chose to locate this survey in a module rather than in any one section of the book.

COMMUNICATING WITH PEOPLE

Because systems are built for people and by people, understanding people is an appropriate introduction to communications skills. With whom does the analyst communicate? What words influence these people?

Three Audiences for Interpersonal Communication During Projects

For years, English and communications scholars have told us that the secret of effective oral and written communications is to know your audience. Who is the communications audience during the systems development project? We can identify at least three distinct groups:

1. The *project team,* consisting of your colleagues—other analysts, programmers, and data processing specialists.
2. Your *users,* the people whose day-to-day jobs will be most affected, directly or indirectly, by the new system.
3. *Management,* who in addition to being users, will approve system expenditures and eventually own the new system.

You should recognize all of these audiences as knowledge workers. Each audience has different levels of technical expertise, different perspectives on the system, and different expectations. Users and management, in particular, present special problems. These people have day-to-day responsibilities and time constraints. Before communicating with any of them, ask yourself the following questions:

- What are the responsibilities of, and how might the new system affect, this person?
- What is the attitude of this person toward the existing or target system? Enthusiasm? Skepticism? Hostility? Apathy?
- What kind of information about the project does this person really need? Want?
- How busy is this person? How much time and attention can I reasonably hope to get?

Use of Words: Turn-Ons and Turn-Offs

We communicate with words, oral and written. How important are words? Ask any politician. The wrong words at the wrong time, no matter what the intention, and the next election is history. But that's just politics, right? No. All businesses are political. And words are important, especially to the systems analyst, who must carefully communicate with a diverse group of users, managers, and technicians. What words affect the attitudes and decisions of your audience?

On an upbeat note, let's first talk about terms (words and phrases) that turn on users and managers. Leslie Matthies (1976) a noted author and consultant in the systems development field, has identified two categories of terms that influence managers: benefit terms and loss terms. Both can be used to sell ideas. Benefit terms sell themselves. Examples include *increase productivity, reduce inventory, improve customer relations, increase sales, increase profit margin,* and *reduce risk.* The list goes on and on. Loss terms can be used to sell proposed changes. Managers will accept ideas that eliminate loss terms. Examples of loss terms include: *high costs, out-of-stock inventory, higher credit losses, increased processing errors, higher taxes, delays,* and *waste.* Again, the list is nearly endless. Benefit and loss terms can be used to sell ideas.

Are there other turn-on words or phrases? Yes! People like to feel they are part of the systems development effort. Avoid using the first person *I*. They also like words of appreciation for their time and effort — systems development is your job, not theirs; and they are helping you. Make their names and department names a vivid part of any presentation. Most of all, people want respect. Words should be carefully chosen to show respect for people's feelings, knowledge, and skills.

Now, what about turn-off words or phrases? These can kill projects by changing the attitudes and opinions of management. Let's start with the oldest turn-off, the use of jargon. Jargon is important to the analyst and technician because it helps us communicate with the computing industry and our colleagues. But jargon has no place in the business user's world. Avoid such terms as *JCL, EBCDIC, CPU, ROM,* and *DOS* — leave your acronyms in the DP offices, and this includes the jargon you've learned in this book. Instead of saying "This is a *DFD* of your materials handling system," try saying "This is a *picture of the work and data flow* in your materials handling operation."

Other red-flag terms include those that attack people's performance or threaten their job. Before you candidly state that the current system is ridiculously inefficient and cumbersome, consider the possibility that a user who had much influence in its development and approval may be in your audience. Consider threats to job security when you get ready to propose elimination of job steps. In other words, be diplomatic and tactful when you speak.

The remainder of this module will survey specific interpersonal communications techniques, specifically:

- Meetings, presentations, and walkthroughs
- Written reports

MEETINGS, PRESENTATIONS, AND WALKTHROUGHS

During the course of a systems project, many team meetings are held. A **meeting** is intended to accomplish an objective as a result of discussion under leadership. Some possible objectives are listed under "Meeting Purposes" in the margin. The ability to coordinate or participate in a meeting is critical to the success of any project. In this section, we'll discuss how to run a meeting and then give extra attention to two special types of meetings: formal presentations and project walkthroughs.

How to Run a Group Meeting

Meeting Purposes

- Problem Definition
- Brainstorming Ideas
- Problem Solving
- Conflict Resolution
- Progress Analysis
- Gather Facts
- Merge Facts

Most meetings are poorly organized and conducted. Meetings are an expensive use of time because they consume time that could be spent on other productive work. The more individuals involved in a meeting, the more the meeting costs. Because meetings are essential, we must strive to offset the costs by maximizing benefits (in terms of project progress) realized during the meeting. It is not difficult to run a meeting if you are well organized. Without good organization, however, the meeting may prove chaotic or worthless to the participants. When planning and conducting meetings, try following the procedure outlined here.

1. Determine the Need for and Purpose of the Meeting Why do you need a meeting? Every meeting should have a well-defined purpose that can be communicated to its participants. Meetings without a well-defined purpose are rarely productive. The purpose of every meeting should be attainable within sixty to ninety minutes because longer meetings tend to become unproductive. However, when necessary, longer meetings are possible as long as they are divided into well-defined submeetings that are separated by breaks so people can catch up on their normal responsibilities. But it must be remembered that longer meetings are more likely to conflict with the participants' day-to-day responsibilities. The effect on the job can be as if everyone took vacation time on the same day.

2. Schedule the Meeting and Arrange for Facilities After deciding the purpose of the meeting, determine who should attend. (But take note: The larger the number of participants, the less the amount of work likely to be completed.) The participants are chosen to ensure that the purpose of the meeting will be attained. Given the number of participants, the meeting can now be scheduled. The date and time for the meeting will be subject to availability of the meeting room and the prior commitments of the participants. Morning meetings are generally better than afternoon meetings because the participants are fresh and not yet caught up in the workday's problems. It is best to avoid scheduling meetings at the following times: late afternoon (people are becoming anxious to go home), before lunch, before holidays, and on the same day as other meetings for the same participants.

The meeting location is important. The checklist in the margin identifies important factors to consider when selecting a meeting location. Seating arrangement is particularly important. If leader–group interaction is required, the group should face the leader but not necessarily other members of the group. If group–group interaction is needed, the team members, including the leader, should all face one another. Make sure that any necessary visual aids (flipchart, overhead projector, chalk, and so forth) are also scheduled for the room.

Meeting Location Factors

- Size of Room
- Lighting
- Noise from Outside Room
- Seating Arrangement
- Temperature
- Audiovisual Needs

Write up an agenda for the meeting and distribute it well in advance. The agenda confirms the date, time, location, and duration of the meeting. It also states the meeting's purpose and offers a tentative timetable for discussion and questions. If participants should bring specific materials with them or review specific documents prior to the meeting, specify this in the agenda. Finally, the agenda may include any supplements (for example, reports, documentation, memoranda) that the participants will need to scan or study prior to or during the meeting.

3. Conduct the Meeting Try to start on time, but do not begin the meeting until everyone is present. If any important participant is more than fifteen minutes late, then consider canceling the meeting. Try to start on time. Once the meeting has started, try to discourage interruptions and delays (such as phone calls). Have enough copies of any handouts for all participants. Get off to a good start by listing or reviewing the agenda so that the discussion items become group property. Then, cover each item on the agenda according to the timetable developed when the meeting was scheduled. The group leader should ensure that no person dominates or is left out of the discussion. Decisions should be made by consensus opinion or majority vote. One rule is always in order: *Stay on the agenda and end on time!* If you do not finish discussing all items on the agenda, schedule another meeting.

Brainstorming can be an effective technique for generating ideas during group meetings. Contrary to what you might believe, brainstorming is a formal technique. It requires discipline. That's right! Here's how it works:

1. One person is appointed to record ideas. This person should use a flipchart, chalkboard, or overhead projector that can be viewed by the entire group.
2. Within a specified time period, team members call out their ideas as quickly as they can think of them. *No idea is considered absurd or infeasible,* and the recorder or leader must insist that no idea be evaluated, analyzed, or otherwise critiqued at this point. Go for quantity of ideas.

   Alternatively, ideas can be generated by having each team member jot down a number of ideas. The ideas are then recorded after all members are finished.
3. After all ideas have been recorded, then and only then, should they be analyzed.

4. Follow up the Meeting As soon as possible after it is over, the minutes of the meeting should be published. The minutes are a brief, written summary of what happened during the meeting—items discussed, decisions made, and items for future consideration. The minutes are usually prepared by the *recording secretary,* a team member designated by the group leader.

How to Make a Formal, Oral Presentation

Presentation Uses

- Sell New System
- Sell New Ideas
- Sell Change
- Head off Criticism
- Address Concerns
- Verify Conclusions
- Clarify Facts
- Report Progress

Presentations are special meetings used to sell new ideas and gain approval for new systems. They may also be used for any of the purposes listed in the margin. In many cases, oral presentations set up or supplement a more detailed written presentation. Effective and successful presentations require three critical ingredients: preparation, preparation, and preparation. We're not trying to be funny. The time allotted to presentations is frequently brief; therefore, organization and format are critical issues. You cannot *wing it* and expect acceptance.

Presentations offer the advantage of impact through immediacy and spontaneity. The audience can respond to the presenter who can use emphasis, timed pauses, and body language to convey messages not possible with the written word. Are there any disadvantages to the oral presentation? Yes, the material presented is easily forgotten because the words are spoken and the visual aids are transient. That's why presentations are often followed by a written report, either summary or detailed.

Preparing for the Oral Presentation As is the case for most communication, it is particularly important to know your audience. This is especially true when your presentation is trying to sell new ideas and a new system. As Machiavelli wrote in his classic book, *The Prince:*

> There is nothing more difficult to carry out, nor more dangerous to handle, than to initiate a new order of things. For the reformer has enemies in all who profit by the old order, and only lukewarm defenders in all those who would profit from the new order, this lukewarmness arising partly from fear of their adversaries—and partly from the incredulity of mankind, who do not believe in anything new until they have had actual experience of it. (From Machiavelli, Niccolo, trans. Luigi Ricci: *The Prince and the Discourses,* 1940, 1950, Random House, Inc. Reprinted by permission of Oxford University Press.)

People are predisposed against change. There is comfort in the way things are today. To effectively present and sell change, you must be confident in your ideas and have the facts to back them up. Preparation is the key!

First, define your expectations of the presentation (for instance, that you are seeking approval to continue the project, that you are trying to confirm facts, and so forth). A presentation is a summary of your ideas and proposals — directed toward your expectations.

Executives are usually put off by excessive detail. To avoid this, your presentation should be carefully organized around the allotted time (usually thirty to sixty minutes). Although each presentation differs, you might try the following organization and time allocation:

I. Introduction (one-sixth of total time available)
   A. Problem statement
   B. Work completed to date

II. Main part of the presentation (two-thirds of total time available)
   A. Summary of existing system problems and limitations
   B. Summary description of the proposed system
   C. Feasibility analysis
   D. Proposed schedule to complete project

III. Questions and concerns from the audience (time here is not to be included in the time allotted for presentation and conclusion. It is determined by those asking the questions and voicing their concerns)

IV. Conclusion (one-sixth of total time available)
   A. Summary of proposal
   B. Call to action (request for whatever authority you require to continue system development)

What else can you do to prepare for the presentation? Because of the limited time, use visual aids (predrawn flipcharts, overhead slides, and the like) to support your position. Just as a written paragraph does, each visual aid should convey a single idea. When preparing pictures or words, use the guidelines shown in Figure C.1. To hold your audience's attention, consider distributing photocopies

Figure C.1 ►

Guidelines for visual aids. Properly prepared and carefully selected visual aids both enhance and expedite a presentation. (Copyright Keith London. Reproduced by permission of Curtis Brown, Ltd.)

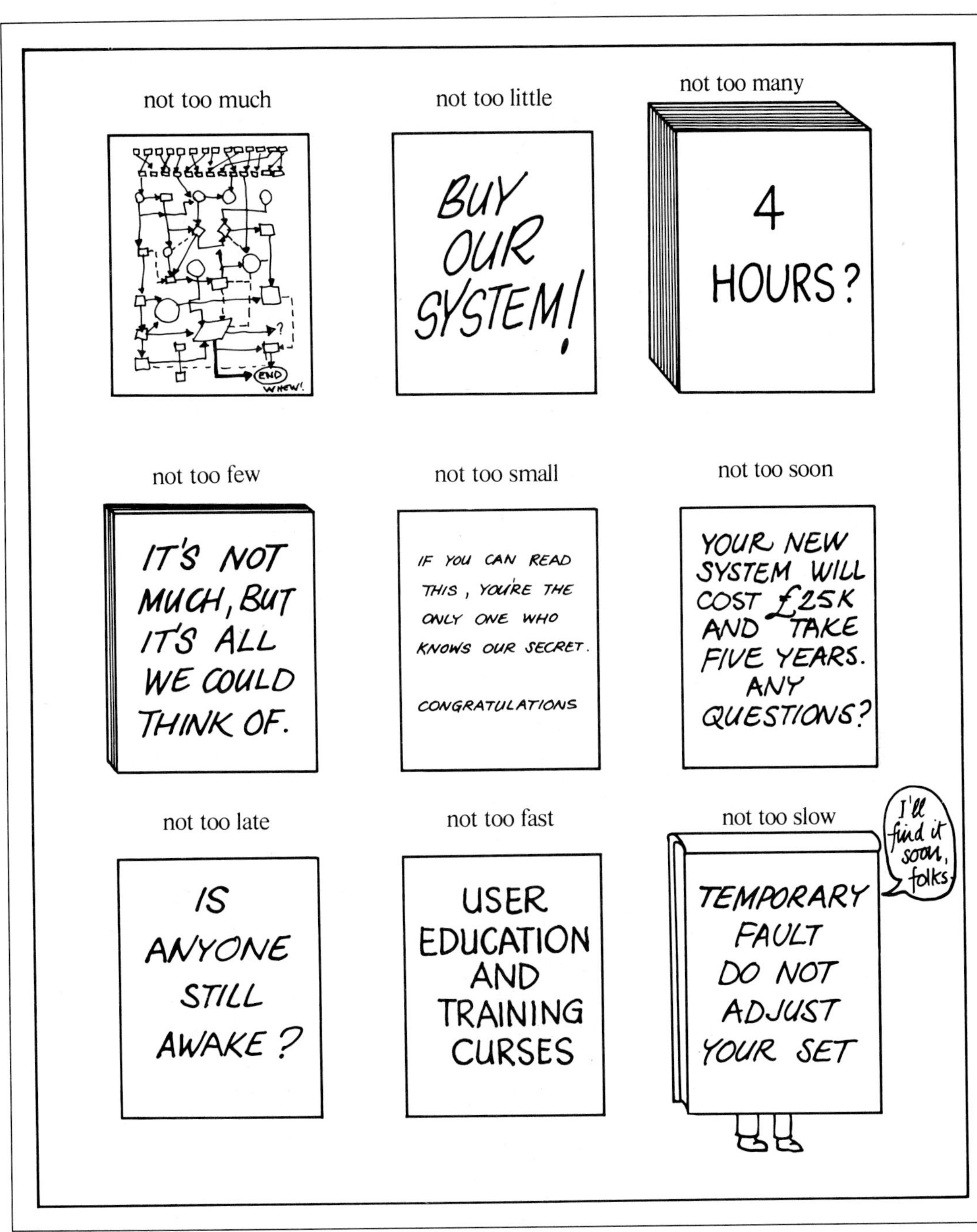
not too much
END
WHEW!
not too little
BUY OUR SYSTEM!
not too many
4 HOURS?
not too few
IT'S NOT MUCH, BUT IT'S ALL WE COULD THINK OF.
not too small
IF YOU CAN READ THIS, YOU'RE THE ONLY ONE WHO KNOWS OUR SECRET.
CONGRATULATIONS
not too soon
YOUR NEW SYSTEM WILL COST £25K AND TAKE FIVE YEARS. ANY QUESTIONS?
not too late
IS ANYONE STILL AWAKE?
not too fast
USER EDUCATION AND TRAINING CURSES
not too slow
TEMPORARY FAULT DO NOT ADJUST YOUR SET
I'll find it soon, folks.

of the visual aids at the start of the presentation. This way, the audience doesn't have to take as many notes.

Finally, practice the presentation in front of the most critical audience you can assemble. Play your own *Devil's Advocate,* or better yet, get somebody else to raise criticisms and objections. Practice your responses to these issues.

Conducting the Presentation If you are well prepared, the presentation is 80 percent complete. Here are a few additional guidelines that may benefit the actual presentation:

- *Dress professionally.* The way you dress influences people. John T. Malloy's books, *Dress for Success* and *The Woman's Dress for Success Book,* are excellent reading for both wardrobe advice and the results of studies regarding the effect of clothing on management.
- *Avoid the word* I when making the presentation. Use *you* and *we* to assign ownership of the proposed system to management (which is as it should be).
- *Maintain eye contact with the group and keep an air of confidence.* If you don't convince management that you believe in your proposal, why should they believe in it?
- *Be aware of your own mannerisms.* Some of the most common mannerisms include: talking too much with your hands, pacing, repeatedly saying "you know" or "Okay." Although mannerisms alone don't contradict the message, they can distract the audience.

Documentation That Can Be Verified Through Walkthroughs

- Data Flow Diagrams
- *Small* Data Dictionaries
- Policies and Procedures
- Systems Flowcharts
- Output Designs
- Input Designs
- File and Data Base Designs
- Terminal Dialogue Designs
- Program Structure Charts
- Program Flowcharts
- Program Test Data
- Program Code
- Program Documentation
- User Manuals

Walkthroughs: A Peer Group Review Technique

The **walkthrough,** another type of meeting, is a peer group review of systems development documentation. Walkthroughs may be used to verify virtually any type of detailed documentation (some of these are listed for you in the margin). Why does peer group review tend to identify errors that go unnoticed by the analyst who prepared the documentation? Consider, if you will, the last paper or report you wrote. You probably gave that report to a colleague or teacher to review. And that colleague or teacher caught obvious errors that you didn't, right? Why didn't you catch them? Because you (like any author) have mental blocks that prevent you from discovering errors in your own products.

Who Participates in the Walkthrough A walkthrough group should consist of seven or fewer participants. All parties in the walkthrough should be treated as equals. The analyst who prepared the documentation to be reviewed should present that documentation to the group during the walkthrough. Another analyst or key user is appointed as *coordinator* of the walkthrough. The coordinator schedules the walkthrough and ensures that each participant gets the documentation well before the meeting date. The coordinator also makes sure that the walkthrough is properly conducted and mediates disputes and problems that arise during the walkthrough. The coordinator has the authority to ask participants to stop a disagreement and move on. Finally, the coordinator designates a *recorder* to take notes during the walkthrough.

The remaining participants include users, analysts, or specialists who evaluate the documentation. These reviewers may also assume roles. For example, some reviewers may evaluate the accuracy of the documentation while other reviewers comment on quality, standards, and technical issues. Participants must be willing to devote time to details. However, walkthroughs should never last more than ninety minutes. Our experience indicates that users particularly enjoy walkthroughs because such meetings encourage a sense of personal importance in the project.

How to Conduct a Walkthrough All participants must agree to follow the same set of rules and procedures. Also, the participants must agree to review the *documentation;* this should not be done by the person who prepared the documentation. The basic purpose of the walkthrough is error *detection,* not error *correction.* The analyst who is presenting the documentation should seek only whatever clarification is needed to be able to correct the errors. This maximizes the use of time! The analysts should not argue with the reviewers' comments. A defensive posture inhibits constructive criticism. The coordinator is responsible for seeing that these rules are properly outlined and followed. Reviewers should be encouraged to offer at least one positive and one negative comment in order to guarantee that the walkthrough is not superficial.

After the walkthrough, the coordinator asks the reviewers for a recommendation. There are three possible alternatives:

1. Accept the documentation in its present form.
2. Accept the documentation with the revisions noted.

3. Request another walkthrough because a large number of errors were found or because criticisms created controversy.

The walkthrough should be promptly followed by a report from the coordinator. The report contains a management summary that states what was reviewed, when the walkthrough occurred, who attended, and the final verdict. A sample set of forms used for walkthroughs in a real company are displayed in Figures C.2 and C.3.

WRITTEN REPORTS

The business and technical report is the primary method used by analysts to communicate information about a systems development project. The purpose of the report is to either inform or persuade, possibly both. In these few pages, it is not possible to provide a comprehensive discussion of report writing. But because people make judgements about who we are and what we can accomplish based on our writing ability, we can offer some motivation for further study and some guidelines for current practice.

Business and Technical Reports for Systems Development

What types of formal reports are written by the systems analyst? Content outlines for several reports can be found in Chapters 6, 10, and 17, which place those reports into the context of the systems development life cycle phases. But an overview (or review) is appropriate here.

Systems Analysis Reports The first major phase of the life cycle is the *study of the current system.* After completing this phase, the analyst normally prepares a report to verify with users their understanding of the current system and analysis of problems, limita-

Figure C.2 ▶

Walkthrough form (page 1). [Courtesy of Cummins Diesel Engine, Columbus, IN]. This standardized walkthrough form can be completed by the recorder, duplicated, and distributed to all meeting participants as a record of the walkthrough.

WALKTHROUGH ACTION LIST - SCRIBE'S REPORT

Co-ordinator	Scribe	Date
Project	Segment	

✓ = fixed	Issues raised in review

FORM 5590-0679N

WALKTHROUGH REPORT

Co-ordinator	Project
Segment for Review	

Co-ordinator's checklist:

1. Confirm with developer that material is ready and stable ____________________

2. Issue invitations, assign responsibilities, distribute materials

Date ____________ Time ____________ Duration ____________

Place ____________________

Responsibilities		Participants	Can attend	Received materials?

Agenda:

____ 1. All participants agree to follow the SAME set of rules.

____ 2. New segment: walk-through of material

____ Old segment: item-by-item checkoff of previous action list

____ 3. Creation of new action list (contributions by each participant)

____ 4. Group decision

____ 5. Deliver copy of this form to project management.

Decision:

____ Accept product as-is

____ Revise (no further walkthrough)

____ Revise and schedule another walkthrough

Signatures		

Form 5589-0679N

tions, and constraints in that system. This report might be titled a "Study and Analysis of the Current <insert name> System."

The second phase of the life cycle, *define user requirements,* results in a specification document called a *requirements statement.* The requirements statement, often large and complex, is rarely written up as a report to users and management. It is best reviewed in walkthroughs (in small pieces) with users and maintained as a reference for analysts and programmers.

The next formal report, the **system proposal,** is generated after the *evaluation of alternative solutions* phase has been completed. This report combines an outline of the user requirements from the definition phase with the detailed feasibility analysis of alternative solutions that fulfill those requirements. The report concludes with a recommended or proposed solution. This report is normally preceded or followed by an oral presentation to those managers and executives who will decide on the proposal.

Systems Design Reports The *design phase* results in detailed design specifications that are often organized into a technical design report. This report is quite detailed and is primarily intended for data processing professionals. It tends to be quite a large report because it contains numerous forms and charts.

The *selection phase* of system development is only undertaken if the new system requires the purchase of new hardware or software. Several reports can be generated during this phase. The most important report, the **request for proposals** is used to communicate requirements to prospective vendors who may respond with specific proposals. Especially when the selection decision involves significant expenditures, the analyst may have to write a report that defends the recommended proposal to management.

Systems Implementation Reports Perhaps the most important report of them all is written during the *construction* and *delivery* phases. Actually, it isn't a report; it's a manual — specifically, it's a user's manual and reference guide. This document explains how to use the computer system (such as what keys to push, how to react to certain messages, and where to get help). How well this manual is

◄ **Figure C.3**

Walkthrough form (page 2).

written will frequently determine how many phone calls you'll get over the months that follow the conversion to the new system. In addition to computer manuals, the analyst may rewrite the standard operating procedures for the system. A standard operating procedure explains both the noncomputer and computer tasks and policies for the new system.

Size of a Written Report

Unfortunately, the written report is the most abused method used by analysts to communicate with users. We have a tendency to generate large, voluminous reports that look impressive. Sometimes such reports are necessary, but many times they're not. If you lay a 300-page technical report on a manager's desk, you can expect that the manager will skim it but not read it—and you can be almost certain it won't be studied carefully!

Report size is an interesting issue. After many bad experiences, we have learned to use the following guidelines to restrict report size:

To executive level managers—one or two pages

To middle level managers—three to five pages

To supervisory level managers—less than ten pages

To clerk level personnel—less than fifty pages

It is possible to organize a larger report to include subreports for managers who are at different levels. These subreports are usually included as early sections in the report and summarize the report, focusing on the bottom line—What's wrong; what do you suggest or want?

Organizing the Written Report

There is a general pattern to organizing any report. Every report consists of primary and secondary elements. **Primary elements** present the information. **Secondary elements** package the report so the reader can easily identify the report and its primary elements. Secondary elements also add professional polish to the report.

Primary Elements As indicated in Figure C.4, the primary elements can be organized in one of two formats: factual and adminis-

FACTUAL FORMAT	ADMINISTRATIVE FORMAT
I. Introduction	I. Introduction
II. Methods and Procedures	II. Conclusions and Recommendations
III. Facts and Details	III. Summary and Discussion of Facts and Details
IV. Discussion and Analysis of Facts and Details	IV. Methods and Procedures
V. Recommendations	V. Final Conclusion
VI. Conclusion	VI. Appendixes with Facts and Details

Figure C.4

Alternative formats for reports. The factual format is used to place emphasis on details. The administrative format is used to place emphasis on conclusions and recommendations.

trative. The *factual format* is very traditional and is best suited to readers who are as interested in facts and details as in conclusions. This is the format we would use to specify detailed requirements and design specifications to users. On the other hand, the factual format is not appropriate for most managers and executives.

The *administrative format* is a modern, result-oriented format preferred by many managers and executives. This format is designed for readers who are interested in results, not facts. Notice that it presents conclusions or recommendations first. Any reader can read the report straight through, until the point at which the level of detail exceeds their interest.

Both formats include common elements. The *introduction* should include four components: purpose of the report, statement of the problem, scope of the project, and a narrative explanation of the contents of the report (sequential). The *methods and procedures* section should briefly explain how the information contained in the report was developed (for example how the study was performed or how the new system was designed). The bulk of the report will be in the *facts* section. This section should be named to describe the type of factual data to be presented (for example, "Existing System Description," "Analysis of Alternative Solutions," or

"Design Specifications"). The *conclusion* should briefly summarize the report, verifying the problem statement, findings, and recommendations.

Secondary Elements Figure C.5 shows the secondary, or packaging, elements (of the report) and their relationship to the primary elements. Many of these elements are self-explanatory. We briefly discuss here those that may not. No report should be distributed without a *letter of transmittal* to the recipient. This letter should be clearly visible, not inside the cover of the report. A letter of transmittal states what type of action is needed on the report. It can also call attention to any features of the project or report that deserve special attention. In addition, it is an appropriate place to acknowledge the help you've received from various people.

The *abstract* or *executive summary* is the one- or two-page capsule summary of the entire report. It helps readers decide if the report contains information they need to know. It can also serve as the highest level summary report. Virtually every manager reads these summaries. Most managers will read on, possibly skipping the detailed facts and appendixes.

Writing the Business or Technical Report

This is not a writing textbook. Do avail yourselves of every opportunity to improve your writing skills (through business and technical writing classes, books, audiovisual courses, and seminars). Writing can greatly influence career paths in any profession. Figure C.6 illustrates the proper procedure for writing a formal report. Some of the guidelines follow:

- *Paragraphs should convey a single idea.* They should flow nicely, one to the next. Poor paragraph structure can almost always be traced to outlining deficiencies.
- *Sentences should not be too complex.* The average sentence length should not exceed twenty words. Independent studies suggest that sentences longer than twenty words are more difficult to read and understand.
- *Write in the active voice.* The passive voice, with its use of the verb *to be* (including such words as *is, was,* and *were*), becomes wordy and boring when used consistently.

Letter of Transmittal

Title Page

Table of Contents

List of Figures, Illustrations, and Tables

Abstract or Executive Summary

(The primary elements—the body of the report, in either the factual or administrative format—are presented in this portion of the report.)

Appendixes

Figure C.5

Secondary elements of a report. Secondary elements are used to package the report. The same secondary elements are common to both the factual and administrative formats. Secondary elements exhibit organization and professionalism.

- *Eliminate jargon* (for example, say "picture of your business requirements" not "DFD"; replace "DBMS" by "Data Base Management Systems software"), *big words, and deadwood* (for example, substitute *so* for *accordingly;* try *useful* instead of *advantageous;* use *clearly* instead of *it is clear that*).

Get yourself a copy of *Elements of Style* by William Strunk, Jr., and E. B. White. This classic little paperback may set an all-time record in value/cost ratio. Just barely bigger than a pocket-sized book, it is a virtual goldmine. And anything we might suggest about grammar and style can't be said any more clearly than the way it's said in *Elements of Style.*

SUMMARY

Because the systems analyst is expected to bridge the language barrier between business users and data processing technicians, communications skills have become an important part of the analyst's tool kit. Three distinct groups of people are part of the analyst's

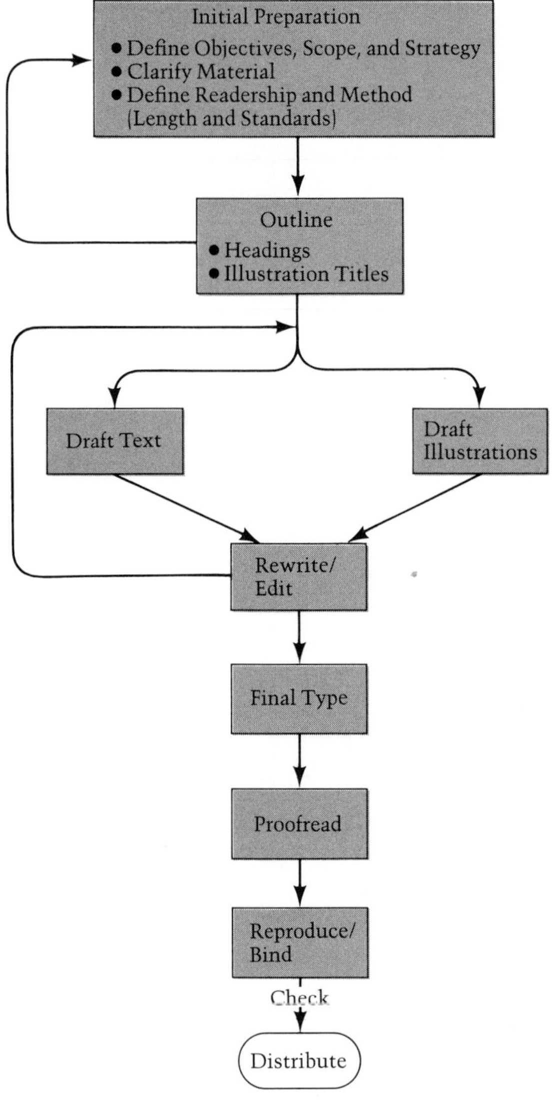

Figure C.6

How to write a report. (Copyright Keith London. Reproduced by permission of Curtis Brown, Ltd.)

audience: colleagues, users, and management. Before directing any communication to any of these audiences, the analyst should profile the audience.

Systems analysts can expect to spend a considerable amount of time in meetings. To maximize the use of meeting time, the analyst should follow the following steps: determine the purpose of the meeting, schedule the meeting at an appropriate time and arrange for adequate facilities, conduct the meeting according to a pre-established agenda, and follow up on meeting results. If the meeting is intended to generate ideas, brainstorming is an effective technique. Oral presentations are a special type of meeting at which a person presents conclusions, ideas, or proposals to an interested audience. Preparation is the key to effective presentations. Walkthroughs are peer group evaluation meetings that seek to identify (but not correct) errors in systems development documentation.

Written reports are the most common communication vehicle used by analysts. Reports consist of primary and secondary elements. Primary elements contain factual information. Secondary elements package the report for ease of use. Reports may be organized by either the factual or administrative format. The factual format presents details before conclusions; the administrative format reverses that order. Managers like the administrative format because it is result-oriented and gets right to the bottom-line question, "What's next?"

PROBLEMS AND EXERCISES

1. The secret of effective oral and written communications is to know your audience. What are some of the things you would want to know about your audience prior to making a formal presentation to them? How could this knowledge be used to your advantage in formulating a presentation?
2. Identify the audience (or audiences) for each of the following systems development reports (*note:* chapter references are provided so you can skip those reports you haven't covered):
   (a) Feasibility survey (Chapter 6)
   (b) Study and analysis of the current information system (Chapter 6)
   (c) Requirements statement (Chapter 6)
   (d) Systems proposal (Chapter 6)
   (e) Design specifications for the new information system (Chapter 10)

(f) Request for proposals for hardware and software (Chapter 10)
(g) Analysis for proposals for hardware and software (Chapter 10)
(h) Program runbook (Chapter 17)
(i) User guide or training manual (Chapter 17)
(j) Postimplementation review (Chapter 17)
(k) Project progress report (Module A)
(l) Walkthrough report (Module B)
(m) Interview report (Module B)

3. Get permission to attend a board meeting or subcommittee meeting of a local organization (such as the Data Processing Management Association or the Association of Computing Machinery), school committee, or some other business meeting. Observe how the meeting is run by the leader. What was the purpose of the meeting? Did the purpose of the meeting appear to be understood by all participants? Why? Did the meeting start and end on time? If not, what caused the delay(s). Was the meeting room reserved ahead of time? Did the room provide a comfortable atmosphere? Were there any problems with the meeting location? Was an agenda distributed prior to or during the meeting? Did the leader follow the agenda during the meeting? Were arrangements made for the minutes of the meeting to be published and distributed to appropriate individuals?
4. Analyze a team meeting for a team project to which you've been assigned. Use the criteria listed for question 3.
5. While attending the next lecture in each of your classes, observe the instructor's presentation of class material. Make a note of and learn from the techniques the professor uses to clearly deliver difficult material. If you feel comfortable about discussing the lecture with your professor, discuss your findings.
6. Arrange a formal walkthrough of one of your systems analysis and design assignments. Try to include your instructor and a few students. Prepare a walkthrough report.
7. In a current programming class, discuss the possibility of formal walkthroughs on one programming assignment. You'll need to secure permission so that your instructor will not consider the walkthrough cheating. Conduct walkthroughs as soon as you've completed the program design and immediately after

coding (but before you compile or interpret the program). Analyze the impact the walkthroughs had on your productivity by comparing the number of compiles that you required to finish the assignment against the number of compiles that programmers who didn't use walkthroughs required.

8. Can word processing software packages aid your development of written communication skills? How?
9. Why do formal presentations usually accompany written reports?
10. Systems analysts have a tendency to generate written reports that are much too large for managers to read. How would you handle a size problem with a technical report?
11. What are some ways you might improve your written communications skills? Identify specific courses that may help you improve your skills.
12. Try to obtain a systems development report outline or table of contents from a data processing shop. Was the report organized using the factual format or the administrative format? Do you think everybody in the audience for the report read that report? Why or why not? Reorganize the outline or table of contents into an alternative format. Be sure to include secondary elements, even if they weren't included in the original report.
13. Take one of the report outlines in Chapters 6, 10, or 17 and prepare formal outlines that include primary and secondary elements for both the factual and administrative formats.

ANNOTATED REFERENCES AND SUGGESTED READINGS

Gallagher, William J. *Writing the Business and Technical Report.* Boston, Mass.: CBI Publishing, 1978. A good professional development book for managers and professionals in any field.

Gildersleeve, Thomas R. *Successful Data Processing Systems Analysis.* Englewood Cliffs, N.J.: Prentice-Hall, 1978. Tom doesn't talk too much about tools in his books—that's why we like him! Chapter 5 discusses presentations, and Chapter 10 discusses interpersonal relations. They are worthwhile additional readings for any analyst.

London, Keith. *The People Side of Systems.* New York: McGraw-Hill, 1976. Chapters 9 through 12 provide an excellent treatment of presentations, reports, group meetings, and special illustrative techniques. Perhaps the best concentrated unit on communications skills in any systems textbook we've seen.

Machiavelli, Niccolo. *The Prince and Discourses.* New York: Random House, 1950. Who says the classics aren't practical reading for professionals? This classic book is considered must reading by students in management and business schools. Because it documents the power and political struggles that exist in both nations and organizations, it is equally valuable to the systems analyst.

Malloy, John T. *Dress for Success.* New York: Warner, 1975. Based on this best-selling book, John Malloy has been labeled "America's first wardrobe engineer." This book (and its sequel for women) teaches men how to dress for power and prestige. The guidelines are based on research conducted by Malloy.

Malloy, John T. *The Woman's Dress for Success Book.* New York: Warner, 1975. The working woman's version of Malloy's successful book on how to dress for power and respect.

Matthies, Leslie H. *The Management System: Systems Are for People.* New York: Wiley, 1976. Chapter 10 in Matthies' book is all about how to present and sell a new system to management. Some concepts we use were initially presented in this book.

Smith, Randi Sigmund. *Written Communication for Data Processing.* New York: Van Nostrand Reinhold, 1976. An excellent book on written communications for DP professionals — not just reports, but memos and letters too!

Strunk, William, Jr., and E. B. White. *The Elements of Style.* New York: McMillan, 1979. What we have here is a half-inch-thick handbook that summarizes everything most of us have forgotten from elementary school, high school, and college grammar classes. Many colleges require their students to have a copy. And we personally recommend that you keep that copy, at least until the English language becomes extinct.

Stuart, Ann. *Writing and Analyzing Effective Computer System Documentation.* New York: Holt, Rinehart, & Winston, 1984. At last! A book to students about writing in the data processing environment. And a good book at that. Must reading!

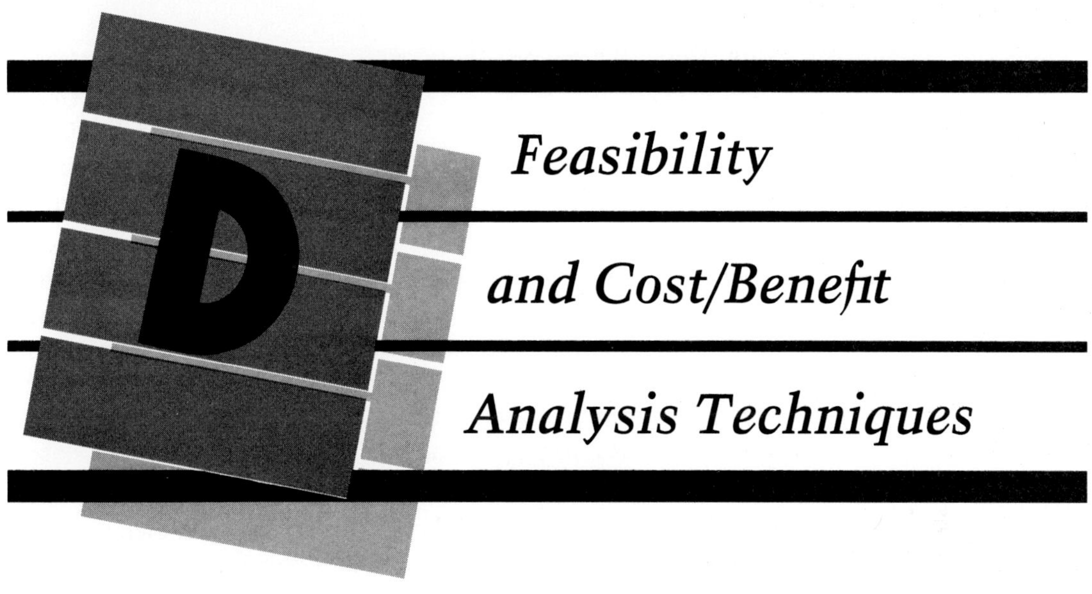

D Feasibility and Cost/Benefit Analysis Techniques

WHEN SHOULD YOU READ THIS MODULE?

This module will be most valuable if studied after *any* of the following chapters have been studied:

- Chapter 6, "How to Perform a Systems Analysis"—Feasibility analysis is an integral part of three systems analysis phases: survey, study, and evaluation.
- Chapter 10, "How to Perform Systems Design"—Feasibility is reassessed during the design and selection phases.

"As you can see, we've designed a system that can fulfill all the needs you specified earlier in the project. Furthermore, this on-line system is very easy to learn and friendly to use. That concludes my presentation," Frank said. "Are there any questions?"

Benjamin Pierce, senior manager responded, "That was quite a presentation, Frank. And the system is every bit as good as you claim. But how much is this going to cost me?"

"To develop the system, we estimate that it will cost $45,000. And the system will cost approximately $4,500 per year to operate. That includes an annual allowance for minor maintenance."

"And how much have we spent up to this point?" asked Ben.

"About $12,000 for analysis and design," answered Frank. "But that money can't be recovered, so we shouldn't consider it in our decision on whether to proceed."

Ben's tone turned more serious. "I agree that the project shouldn't be continued or canceled solely on the basis of the money spent so far. However, I disagree that the money is irrelevant. If the project is continued, I should think that the new system would eventually pay for itself. By my calculation, development costs would total $57,000. And if the system will incur another $4,500 expenses per year, how long until it pays for itself?"

Frank answered, "You'll start receiving benefits immediately."

Ben countered, "But how many months or years will pass before the lifetime benefits surpass the lifetime costs?" There was a moderate silence after which Ben continued, "Look, I have the money you need to develop and operate this system. But I also have managers who are asking for new equipment and for facilities upgrades. Why should I give you the money and deny it to them?"

Frank seemed confused, "I don't understand. This system fulfills the needs that *you* and your staff specified, Ben."

Ben replied, "Frank, you are a marvelous computer professional. You understand my business workflow and needs. And you can design some of the best computer solutions to those needs that I've ever seen. But you've got a lot to learn about business."

Computer applications are expanding at a record pace, and now more than ever, management expects data processing to pay for itself. Information systems are a capital expenditure that must be justified, just as marketing must justify a new product and manufacturing must justify a new production plant. Will an investment return more money than it will cost? Are there other investments that will return even more money? In our opening scenario, Frank didn't pay attention to the fact that business is driven by economics — profits! Dollars and cents! Frank *knows* this, and so do you; but we all easily forget that point when it comes to our fascination with the computer and the potential it holds for information systems in business.

This module deals with cost/benefit analysis and other feasibility issues of interest to the systems analyst. Few topics are more important! Feasibility analysis isn't really *systems analysis,* and it isn't really *systems design* either. Indeed, we consider feasibility analysis to be an ongoing activity of the systems development life cycle (SDLC).

WHAT IS FEASIBILITY AND WHEN DO YOU EVALUATE IT?

Let's get right down to business. **Feasibility** is a measure of how beneficial the development of an information system would be to an organization. **Feasibility analysis** is the process by which feasibility is measured. Feasibility analysis should be performed throughout the systems development life cycle. We call this a creeping commitment approach to feasibility. The scope and complexity of an apparently feasible project can change after the current problems are fully understood or after the users' needs have been defined in detail or after technical requirements are established. Thus, a project that is feasible at one stage of systems development may become less feasible or infeasible at a later checkpoint.

Feasibility Checkpoints in a Project

If you study your company's project standards or SDLC, you'll probably see a feasibility study, if it exists, but not the ongoing feasibility analysis. But look closer! You'll probably see *go/no go* checkpoints or *management review* checkpoints. These checkpoints identify specific times during systems development at which feasibility is reevaluated. A project can be canceled, or resource estimates can be changed at such a time. Where are these checkpoints in a typical project?

Feasibility checkpoints can be installed into any systems development life cycle you are using. Figure D.1 shows checkpoints added to our life cycle. The checkpoints are represented by diamonds. The diamonds indicate management decisions to be made after a phase is complete. A project may be canceled or revised at any checkpoint, despite whatever resources have been spent thus far. This idea may bother you at first. Your natural inclination would be to justify continuing the project on the basis that you've already spent time and money. But the resources you have already spent

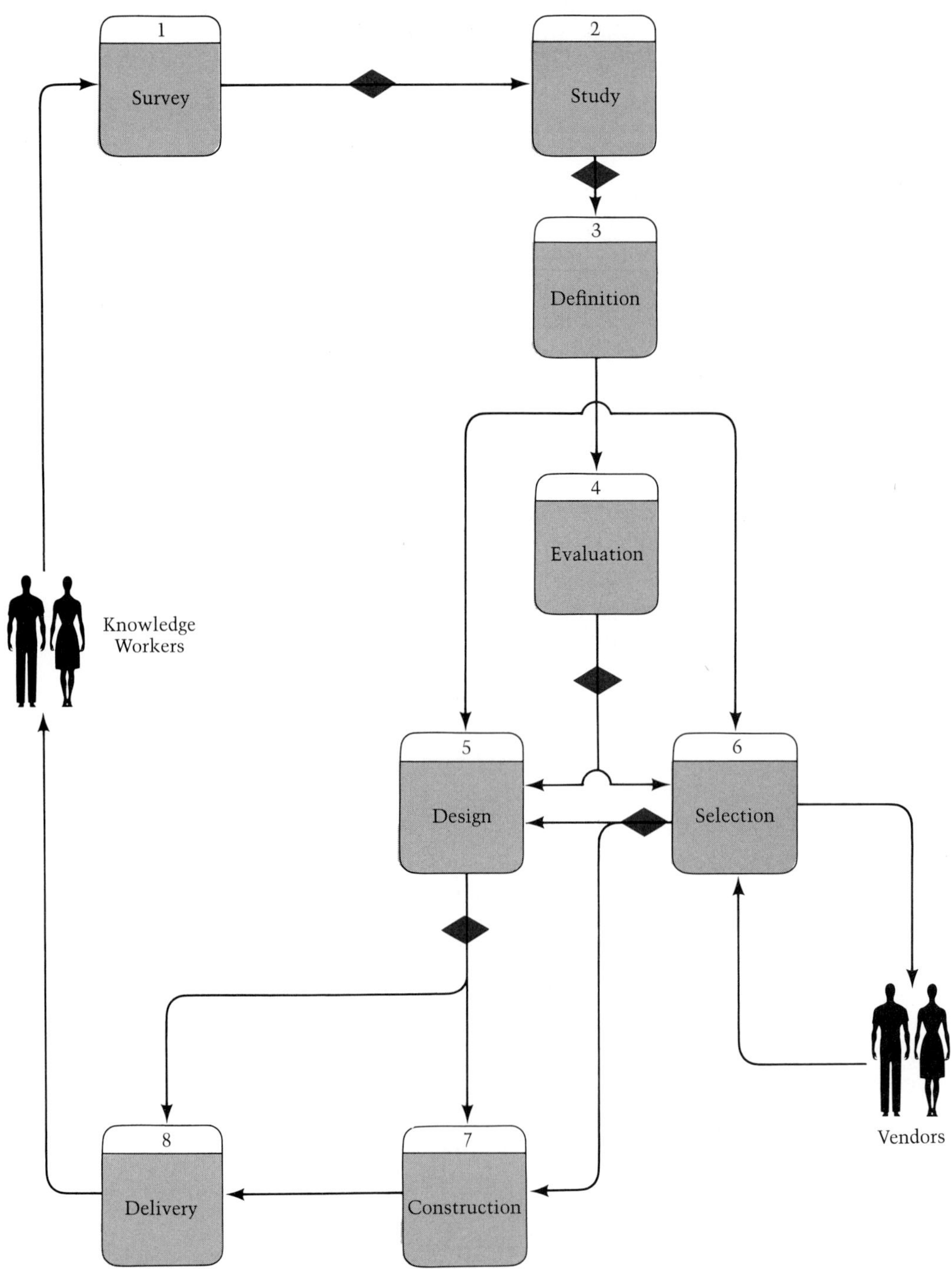
1
Survey
2
Study
3
Definition
4
Evaluation
5
Design
6
Selection
7
Construction
8
Delivery
Knowledge
Workers
Vendors

◄ Figure D.1

Feasibility checkpoints in the systems development life cycle. This is our familiar SDLC with checkpoints (indicated by diamonds) for feasibility analysis. At any checkpoint, analysts and management reevaluate feasibility and determine whether to cancel, revise, or continue the project. This approach is called creeping commitment.

cannot be recovered. They're *sunk!* A fundamental principle of management is never to throw good money after bad money. If the project is now infeasible, minimize your losses — cancel or revise the project! Let's briefly survey these checkpoints because each has a different perspective on feasibility.

The Survey Phase Checkpoint We conduct our first feasibility analysis during the survey phase. This is the feasibility study that was introduced earlier. At this early stage of the project, feasibility is rarely more than a measure of the *urgency of the problem* and a *first cut estimate of development costs.* Do these problems or opportunities warrant the cost of a detailed study of the current system? Realistically, feasibility can't be accurately measured until the problems (study phase) and requirements (definition phase) are better understood.

Study Phase Checkpoint Our next checkpoint occurs after a study of the current system has been completed. Because the problem(s) is better understood, the analysts can make *better* estimates of development costs and the value of solving the problems. The value of solving a problem is equivalent to the cost of that problem. For example, if inventory carrying costs are $35,000 over budget, then the potential benefit of solving that inventory problem is at least $35,000. However, development costs are still *guesstimates* since specific user requirements (definition phase) and technical solutions (design phase) haven't been specified.

Evaluation Phase Checkpoint In some SDLCs and books, the evaluation phase IS the feasibility study. Certainly, the evaluation phase is the most detailed feasibility analysis checkpoint since it is during this phase that alternative solutions are defined and a target computer-based solution is selected.

Problems and general requirements are defined prior to the evaluation phase. During the evaluation phase, alternative solutions are defined in terms of their input and output methods, storage requirements and methods, computer hardware and software requirements, processing methods, and people implications. The following solutions present the typical range of options that can be defined by the analyst:

1. Do nothing! Leave the current system alone. To ensure that any other option(s) will prove superior to the current system, this option should always be considered.
2. Implement noncomputer changes to the manual methods and procedures currently being used. This includes streamlining activities, reducing duplicate and unnecessary tasks, reorganizing office layouts, and eliminating redundant and unnecessary forms, among others.
3. Modify, enhance, or supplement an existing computer system.
4. Purchase a packaged applications software system.
5. Design and construct a custom applications software system.

Of course, an alternative may be a variation on or combination of these themes.

After defining these options (discussed in Chapter 6), each option is analyzed for operational, technical, and economic feasibility. This chapter will examine these three classes of feasibility criteria. One alternative is chosen, and that solution is passed along to the design and selection phases of our project.

Selection Phase Checkpoint Because the selection of computer equipment and software involves economic decisions that usually require sizable outlays of cash, it shouldn't surprise you that feasibility analysis is required before a hardware or software contract is extended to the vendor. It should be pointed out that the selection phase (covered more extensively in Chapter 10) may be consolidated into the evaluation phase because hardware/software selection may have a significant impact on the feasibility of the solutions being considered.

Design Phase Checkpoint A final checkpoint is installed after the new system has been designed. The detailed design specifications have been completed. Therefore, the complexity of the solution is well understood. Because computer programming (Construct the New System) and implementation (Deliver the New System) are the most time-consuming and expensive phases, the checkpoint after design gives us one last chance to update our project estimates and reëvaluate feasibility.

Three Tests for Project Feasibility

So far, we've defined feasibility and determined when to perform a feasibility analysis. Most analysts have agreed that there are three categories of feasibility tests:

1. **Operational feasibility** is a measure of how well the solution of problems or a specific alternative solution will work in the organization. Also, a measure of how people feel about the system.
2. **Technical feasibility** is a measure of the practicality of a specific technical solution and of the availability of technical resources.
3. **Economic feasibility** is a measure of the cost-effectiveness of a project or solution (this is often called a cost/benefit analysis).

In the remainder of this module we will focus on each of these feasibility criteria.

MEASURING PROJECT FEASIBILITY

Recall the scenario that introduced this module. Based on the dialogue that began this module, Frank's proposed system was very likely operationally and technically feasible. The people seemed to like the system because it filled their requirements. And Frank was unlikely to propose a technical solution he couldn't implement. Operational and technical feasibility criteria measure the worthiness of a problem or solution. Operational feasibility is people oriented. Technical feasibility is computer oriented.

But economic feasibility was questioned by the manager who had to make the financial decisions. Economic feasibility deals with the costs and benefits of the information system. The proposed project may very well have been economically feasible, but we can't tell because Frank didn't analyze costs and benefits. Actually, few systems are infeasible, as in *not* feasible. Instead, different options tend to be *more* or *less* feasible than others. Let's take a closer look at the three feasibility criteria.

Operational Feasibility Criteria

Operational feasibility criteria measure the urgency of the problem (survey and study phases) or the acceptability of a solution (evaluation, selection, and design phases). How do you measure operational feasibility? There are two aspects of operational feasibility to be considered:

1. Is the problem worth solving *or* will the solution to the problem work?
2. How do the users and management feel about the problem (solution)?

Is the Problem Worth Solving or Will the Solution to the Problem Work? Do you recall the PIECES framework for identifying problems that was discussed in Chapter 4? PIECES can be used as the basis for analyzing the urgency of a problem or the effectiveness of a solution. The following is a list of the PIECES issues accompanied by some of the questions that address them.

- **P** *Performance.* Does the system provide adequate throughput and response time? (*Note: the term* system, *used throughout this discussion, may refer either to the existing system or to a proposed system solution.*)
- **I** *Information.* Does the system provide users and managers with timely, pertinent, accurate, and usefully formatted information?
- **E** *Economy.* No, we are not prematurely jumping into economic feasibility! The question here is, "Does the system offer adequate service level and capacity to reduce the costs of business or increase the profits of the business?"
- **C** *Control.* Does the system offer adequate controls to insure against fraud and embezzlement and to guarantee the accuracy and security of data and information?
- **E** *Efficiency.* Does the system make maximum use of avail-

able resources, including people, time, flow of forms, minimum processing delays, and the like?

S *Services.* Does the system provide desirable and reliable service to those who need it? Is the system flexible and expandable?

How Do the Users and Managers Feel About the Problem (Solution)? It's not only important to evaluate whether a system *can* work. We must also evaluate whether a system *will* work. A workable solution might fail because of user or management resistance. The following questions address this concern:

- Does management support the system?
- How do the users feel about their role in the new system?
- What users or managers may resist or not use the system? People tend to resist change. Can this problem be overcome? If so, how?
- How will the working environment of the users change? Can or will users and management adapt to the change?

Technical Feasibility Criteria

Technical feasibility can only be evaluated after those phases during which technical issues are resolved, namely, after the evaluation and design phases of our life cycle, have been completed. Today, very little is technically impossible. Consequently, technical feasibility looks at what is *practical* and *reasonable.* Technical feasibility addresses three major issues:

1. Is the proposed technology or solution practical?
2. Do we currently possess the necessary technology?
3. Do we possess the necessary technical expertise, and is the schedule reasonable?

Is the Proposed Technology or Solution Practical? The technology for any defined solution is normally available. The question is, whether that technology is mature enough that it can be easily applied to our problems. Some firms like to use state-of-the-art technology. But most firms prefer to use mature and proven technology. A mature technology has a larger customer base for obtaining advice concerning problems and improvements.

Do We Currently Possess the Necessary Technology? Assuming that the solution's required technology is practical, we must next ask ourselves, "Is the technology available in our data processing shop?" If the technology is available, we must ask if we have the capacity. For instance, "will our current printer be able to handle the new reports and forms required of a new system?"

If the answer to either of these questions is no, then we must ask ourselves, "Can we get this technology?" The technology may be practical and available, and yes, we need it. But we simply may not be able to afford it at this time. Although this argument borders on economic feasibility, it is truly technical feasibility. If we can't afford the technology, then the alternative that requires the technology is not practical and is technically infeasible.

Do We Possess the Necessary Technical Expertise and Is the Schedule Reasonable? This consideration of technical feasibility is often forgotten during feasibility analysis. We may have the technology, but that doesn't mean we have the skills required to properly apply that technology. For instance, we may have a database management system (DBMS). However, the analysts and programmers available for the project may not know that DBMS well enough to properly apply it. True, all data processing professionals can learn new technologies. But that learning curve will impact the technical feasibility of the project; specifically, it will impact the schedule.

Given our technical expertise, are the project deadlines reasonable? Some projects are initiated with specific deadlines. You need to determine whether the deadlines are mandatory or desirable. For instance, a project to develop a system to meet new government reporting regulations may have a deadline that coincides with when the new reports must be initiated. Penalties associated with missing such a deadline may make meeting it mandatory. If the deadlines are desirable rather than mandatory, the analyst can propose alternative schedules. It is preferable (unless the deadline is absolutely mandatory) to deliver a properly functioning information system two months late rather than to deliver an error-prone, useless information system on time! Missed schedules are bad. Inadequate systems are worse! It's a choice between the lesser of two evils.

Economic Feasibility Criteria

The bottom line in many projects is economic feasibility. During the early phases of the project, economic feasibility analysis amounts to little more than judging whether the possible benefits of solving the problem are worthwhile. Costs are practically impossible to estimate at that stage because the user's requirements and alternative technical solutions have not been identified. However, as soon as specific requirements and solutions have been identified, the analyst can weigh the costs and benefits of each alternative. This is called a cost/benefit analysis. Here we will examine how costs and benefits are estimated, after which we will present cost/benefit analysis techniques.

What Benefits Will the System Provide? Because benefits or potential benefits become known prior to costs, we'll discuss benefits first. Benefits normally increase profits or decrease costs, both highly desirable characteristics of a new information system.

To as great a degree as possible, benefits should be quantified in dollars and cents. Benefits that can be easily quantified are called **tangible benefits. Tangible benefits** are usually measured in terms of monthly or annual savings or of profit to the firm. For example, consider the following scenario:

> During the course of processing student housing applications, we discover that considerable data is being redundantly typed and filed. An analysis reveals that the same data is typed seven times requiring an average of 44 additional minutes of clerical work per application. The office processes 1,500 applications per year. That means a total of 66,000 minutes or 1,100 hours of redundant work per year. If the average salary of a secretary is $6 per hour, the cost of this problem and the benefit of solving the problem is $6,600 per year.

Alternatively, tangible benefits might be measured in terms of unit cost savings or profit. For instance, an alternative inventory valuation scheme may reduce inventory carrying cost by $0.32 per unit of inventory. Some examples of tangible benefits are listed in the margin.

Other benefits are intangible. **Intangible benefits** are those benefits believed to be difficult or impossible to quantify. Unless these benefits are at least identified, it is entirely possible that many projects would not be feasible. Examples of intangible benefits are listed in the margin.

Unfortunately, if a benefit cannot be quantified, it is difficult to accept the validity of an associated cost/benefit analysis. Why? Be-

Tangible Benefits

- Fewer Processing Errors
- Increased Throughput
- Decreased Response Time
- Elimination of Job Steps
- Reduced Expenses
- Increased Sales
- Faster Turnaround
- Better Credit
- Reduced Credit Losses

Intangible Benefits

- Improved Customer Goodwill
- Improved Employee Morale
- Improved Employee Job Satisfaction
- Better Service to Community
- Better Decision Making

cause that analysis is based on incomplete data. Some analysts dispute the existence of intangible benefits. They argue that all benefits are quantifiable; some are just more difficult than others. Suppose, for example, improved customer goodwill is listed as a possible intangible benefit. Can we quantify goodwill? You might try the following analysis:

1. What is the result of customer "badwill?" The answer: the customer will submit fewer (or no) orders.
2. To what degree will a customer reduce orders? Your user may find it difficult to specifically quantify this impact. But you could try to have the user estimate the possibilities (or invent an estimate to which the user can react). For instance:
   - There is a 50 percent (.50) chance that the regular customer would send a few orders (fewer than 10 percent of all their orders) to competitors to test their performance.
   - There is a 20 percent (.20) chance that the regular customer would send as many as half their orders (.50) to competitors, particularly those orders we are historically slow to fulfill.
   - There is a 10 percent (.10) chance that a regular customer would send us an order only as a last resort. That would reduce that customer's normal business with us to 10 percent of their current volume (90% or .90 loss).
   - There is a 5 percent (.05) chance that a regular customer would choose not to do business with us at all (100% or 1.00 loss).
3. We can calculate an estimated business loss as follows:

$$\begin{aligned}\text{loss} &= .50 \times (\ .10 \text{ loss of business})\\ &+ .20 \times (\ .50 \text{ loss of business})\\ &+ .10 \times (\ .90 \text{ loss of business})\\ &\underline{+ .05 \times (1.00 \text{ loss of business})}\\ &= .29 = 29\% \text{ loss of business}\end{aligned}$$

4. If the average customer does \$40,000/year of business, then we can expect to lose 29 percent or \$11,600 of that business. If we have 500 customers, this can be expected to amount to a total of \$5,800,000.
5. Present this analysis to management, and use it as a *starting point* for quantifying the benefit.

How Much Will the System Cost? Costs fall into two categories. There are costs associated with developing the system. And there are costs associated with operating a system. The former can be estimated from the outset of a project and should be refined at the end of each phase of the project. The latter can only be estimated once specific computer-based solutions have been defined (during the evaluation phase or later). Let's take a closer look at the costs of information systems.

The costs of developing an information system can be classified according to the phase in which they occur. Systems development costs are usually one-time costs that will not reoccur after the project has been completed. Many organizations have standard cost categories that must be evaluated. In the absence of such categories, the following lists should help:

- *Personnel costs*—the salaries of systems analysts, programmers, consultants, data-entry personnel, computer operators, secretaries, and the like that work on the project. Because many of these individuals spend time on many projects, their salaries should be prorated to reflect the time spent on the projects being estimated.
- *Computer usage*—Computer time will be used for one or more of the following sorts of activities: programming, testing, conversion, word processing, maintaining a project data dictionary, prototyping, loading new data files, and the like. If a computing center charges for usage of computer resources, the cost should be estimated.
- *Training*—If computer personnel or users have to be trained, the training courses may incur expenses. Packaged training courses may be charged out on a flat fee per site, a student fee (such as $395 per student), or an hourly fee (such as $75 per class hour).
- *Supply, duplication, and equipment costs.*
- *Cost of any new computer equipment and software.*

Sample development costs for a typical solution are displayed in Figure D.2.

Almost nobody forgets systems development budgets when itemizing costs. On the other hand, it is easy to forget that a system will incur costs after it has been placed into operation. The lifetime

Estimated Costs for the On-Line System Alternative

DEVELOPMENT COSTS:	
Personnel:	
2 Systems analysts (400 hours/ea @ $35.00/hr)	$28,000
4 Programmers (250 hours/ea @ $25.00/hr)	25,000
1 Operator (50 hours @ $10.00/hr)	500
1 Secretary (75 hours @ $6.00/hr)	450
3 Data entry clerks (during file conversion --40 hours/ea @ $5.00/hr)	600
Computer usage:	
500 hours @ $25.00	12,500
Supplies and expense:	
Training (database--3 persons @ $395/person)	1,185
Training users (15 hours @ $10.00/hr)	1,500
Duplication	300
New equipment:	
2 Personal computers configured to emulate a terminal--also include printers	14,000
5 CRT terminals	2,500
7 New desks for office personnel	1,400
ANNUAL OPERATING COSTS (not incurred in existing system)	
Personnel:	
Systems analysts (maintenance--80 hours/year @ $35.00/hr)	2,800
Programmers (maintenance--200 hours/year @ $25.00/hr)	5,000
1 additional office clerk--2,000 hours/year @ $6.00/hr	12,000
Computer usage:	
2,000 hours/year @ $45.00/hr--includes overhead	90,000
Supplies and expenses:	
Prorated renewal of database software license	1,000
Preprinted forms (15,000/year @ .22/form)	3,300

Figure D.2

Costs for a proposed system solution. The costs for a proposed information system should be itemized into development costs and operating costs.

benefits must recover both the developmental and operating costs. Unlike systems development costs, operating costs tend to reoccur throughout the lifetime of the system. The costs of operating a system over its useful lifetime can be classified as fixed and variable.

Fixed costs occur at regular intervals but at relatively fixed rates. Examples of fixed operating costs include:

- Lease payments and software license payments
- Prorated salaries of data processing operators and support personnel (although salaries tend to rise, the rise is gradual and tends not to change dramatically from month to month)

Variable costs occur in proportion to some usage factor. Examples include:

- Costs of computer usage (CPU time used, terminal connect time used, storage used) varies with the workload.
- Supplies (preprinted forms, printer paper used, punched cards, floppy disks, magnetic tapes, and other expendables) vary with the workload.
- Prorated overhead costs, such as utilities, maintenance, and telephone service. Overhead expenses can be allocated throughout the lifetime of the system using standard and common techniques of cost accounting.

Sample operating cost estimates for a solution are displayed in Figure D.2. After determining the costs and benefits for a possible solution, you can perform the cost/benefit analysis. Cost/benefit analysis techniques will be discussed shortly.

The Bottom Line

You have learned that any alternative solution can be evaluated according to three criteria: operational, technical, and economic feasibility. How do you pick the best solution? It's not always easy. Operational and economic issues often conflict. For example, the solution that provides the best operational impact to the users may also be the most expensive and, therefore, the least economically feasible. The final decision can only be made by sitting down with users, reviewing the data, and choosing the best overall alternative.

COST/BENEFIT ANALYSIS TECHNIQUES

Once you have itemized costs and benefits at any specific stage of a project, you can perform a **cost/benefit analysis** to determine if the project is (still) cost-effective. By cost-effective, we mean that the resulting information system's lifetime costs are exceeded by that system's lifetime benefits. If a proposed system is not cost-effective, the system will cause the business to *lose* money during its lifetime. Obviously, a project to develop that system should be immediately canceled or modified in scope. Yes, the costs incurred so far represent a net loss, but that loss is minimized by canceling the project.

There are three common cost/benefit techniques, payback analysis, return-on-investment analysis, and present value analysis. These methods can be made to overlap. A discussion of each follows.

Payback Analysis

Payback analysis is a simple and popular method for determining if and when an investment will pay for itself. Because systems development costs are incurred long before benefits begin to accrue, it will take some period of time for the benefits to overtake the costs. And after implementation, you will incur additional operating expenses that must be recovered. Payback analysis determines how much time will elapse before accrued benefits overtake accrued and continuing costs. This period of time is called the *payback period.*

In Figure D.3, we see an information system that will be developed at a cost of $100,000. The estimated net operating costs for each of the next 6 years are also recorded in the table. Now look at the estimated net benefits over the same 6 operating years. What is the payback period? Notice that the lifetime costs are increasing over the 6-year period because operating costs are being incurred. But also notice that the lifetime benefits are accruing at a much faster pace. Lifetime benefits will overtake the lifetime costs between years 3 and 4. We can estimate that the breakeven will occur at 3.9 years after the system has been placed into operation. Is this information system a good or bad investment?

It depends! Many companies have a payback period guideline for all investments. In the absence of such a guideline, you need to

PAYBACK ANALYSIS

CASH FLOW DESCRIPTION	YEAR 0	YEAR 1	YEAR 2	YEAR 3	YEAR 4	YEAR 5	YEAR 6
Development Costs	100,000						
Operating Costs*		4,000	4,500	5,000	6,000	7,000	8,000
Cumulative Lifetime Costs	100,000	104,000	108,500	113,500	119,500	126,500	134,500
Benefits		25,000	30,000	35,000	50,000	60,000	70,000
Cumulative Lifetime Benefits		25,000	55,000	90,000	140,000	200,000	270,000

PAYBACK PERIOD

*adjusted for inflation and growth

Figure D.3

Payback analysis for a project. In payback analysis, you determine how much time will pass before the lifetime benefits exceed the lifetime costs. In this example, benefits will pass costs between years 3 and 4.

determine a reasonable guideline before you determine the payback period. Suppose the guideline states that all investments must have a payback period of less than or equal to 5 years. Because our example has a payback period of 3.9 years, it is a good investment. If the payback period for the system were more than 5 years, the information system would be a bad investment.

One disadvantage of the payback analysis is that it only shows whether the solution is good or bad. It does not clearly demonstrate *how* good or bad the solution is. For this reason, payback analysis can't be used to compare alternatives. Why? Other alternatives may pay back more slowly but may pay back more over the total lifetime of the system. To overcome this disadvantage, you can use the return-on-investment analysis method.

Return-on-Investment Analysis

Return-on-investment (ROI) **analysis** is a technique for comparing the lifetime profitability of alternative solutions or projects. The

ROI for a solution or project is a percentage rate that measures the relationship between the amount the business gets back from an investment and the amount invested. The ROI for a potential solution or project is calculated as follows:

$$\text{ROI} = \frac{\text{estimated lifetime benefits} - \text{estimated lifetime costs}}{\text{estimated lifetime costs}}$$

Let's calculate the ROI for the same system solution we used in our discussion of payback analysis. The estimated lifetime benefits minus estimated lifetime costs equals \$135,500 (270,000 − 134,500). Therefore, the ROI is

$$\text{ROI} = 135{,}500 \,/\, 134{,}500 = 100.74\,\% \qquad \text{(lifetime, } \textit{not} \text{ annual)}$$

This solution can be compared with alternative solutions. The solution offering the highest ROI is the best alternative. However, as was the case with payback analysis, the business may set a minimum acceptable ROI for all investments. If none of the alternative solutions meet or exceed that minimum standard, then none of the alternatives are economically feasible.

Does ROI have any disadvantages? Yes! The rate of return calculated is an *average* rate of return. The actual rate of return may vary during the lifetime. For instance, the solution may have a much lower rate of return in the earlier years than in the later years, or vice versa. ROI doesn't consider this time factor. And neither payback analysis nor ROI, as presented, considers the time value of money. What is the time value of money?

Present Value Analysis

All of the techniques covered so far ignore an important reality of the financial world, the *time value of money.* A dollar today is worth more than a dollar one year from now. Why? Because you could invest a dollar today and, through accrued interest, have more than one dollar a year from now. Thus, you'd rather have that dollar today than in one year. That's why your creditors want you to pay your bills promptly—they can't invest what they don't have. The same principle can be applied to costs and benefits *before* a cost/benefit analysis is performed.

Some of the costs of a system will be accrued after implementation. Additionally, all benefits of the new system will be accrued in the future. Before cost/benefit analysis, these costs should be brought back to *present value dollars.* For instance, suppose we are going to realize a benefit of $20,000 two years from now. What is the present value of that $20,000 benefit? The present value of the benefit is the amount of money we would need to invest today to have $20,000 two years from now. If the current return on our investments is running about 10 percent, an investment of $16,528 today would give us our $20,000 in two years (we'll show how to calculate this later). Therefore, the present value of the estimated benefit is $16,528—that $16,528 is just as good today as a promise to give you $20,000 two years from now.

Why go to all this trouble? Because projects are often compared against other projects that have different lifetimes. Time value analysis techniques have become the preferred cost/benefit methods for most managers. By time-adjusting costs and benefits, you can improve both the payback and return-on-investment analysis techniques. Better still, time value adjustments can be used with a technique called *present value analysis* to determine the true dollar worth of alternative solutions or projects. Here's how it works.

To perform **present value analysis,** you first determine the costs and benefits for each year of the system's lifetime. The estimated systems development costs are accumulated in year 0, the date the system is placed into operation. Figure D.4 shows the costs and benefits over the lifetime for a typical project. Next, we need to bring all of the costs and benefits back to present dollar values.

The present value of a dollar in year n depends on something typically called a *discount rate.* The discount rate is a percentage similar to interest rates that you earn on your savings account. In present value analysis, the discount rate for a business is the *opportunity cost* of being able to invest money in other projects (including the possibility of investing in the stock market, money market funds, bonds, and the like). This discount rate also represents what the company considers an acceptable return on their investments. Let's say that the discount rate for our sample company is 12 percent.

The present value of a dollar at any time in the future can be calculated using the following formula:

$$PV_n = \frac{1}{(1+i)^n}$$

where

PRESENT VALUE ANALYSIS

CASH FLOW DESCRIPTION	YEAR 0	YEAR 1	YEAR 2	YEAR 3	YEAR 4	YEAR 5	YEAR 6
Development Costs	100,000						
Operating Costs		4,000	4,500	5,000	6,000	7,000	8,000
Discount Rate @ 12%	1.000	.893	.797	.712	.636	.567	.507
Present Value	100,000	3,572	3,587	3,560	3,816	3,969	4,056
TOTAL COSTS							122,560
Benefits		25,000	30,000	35,000	50,000	60,000	70,000
Discount Rate @ 12%		.893	.797	.712	.636	.567	.507
Present Value		22,325	23,910	24,920	31,800	34,020	35,490
TOTAL BENEFITS							169,465
NET PRESENT VALUE							46,905

Figure D.4

Present value analysis for a project. Using present value analysis, you can determine the profitability, in today's dollars, of any project. Present value analysis is the preferred evaluation technique of most financial managers.

PV_n is the present value of \$1.00, n years from now
i is the discount rate

Therefore, the present value of a dollar two years from now is

$$PV_2 = \frac{1}{(1 + .12)^2} = 0.797$$

Does that bother you? We stated earlier that a dollar today is worth more than a dollar a year from now. But it looks as if it is worth less, no? This is an illusion. If you have 79.7 cents today, that is still better than having 79.7 cents two years from now. How much better? Exactly 20.3 cents better since that 79.7 cents would grow into one dollar in two years.

To determine the present value of any cost or benefit in year 2, you simply multiply 0.797 times the estimated cost or benefit. For example, the estimated operating expense in year 2 is \$4,500. The

PRESENT VALUE OF A DOLLAR

Periods	...	8%	10%	12%	14%	...
1		0.926	0.909	0.893	0.877	
2		0.857	0.826	0.797	0.769	
3		0.794	0.751	0.712	0.675	
4		0.735	0.683	0.636	0.592	
5		0.681	0.621	0.567	0.519	
6		0.630	0.564	0.507	0.456	
7		0.583	0.513	0.452	0.400	
8		0.540	0.467	0.404	0.351	
.						
.						
.						

Figure D.5

Partial table for present value of a dollar. This table is used to discount a dollar back to present value from the indicated years, using the indicated discount rates. More detailed versions of this table can be found in many accounting, finance, and economics books.

present value of this expense is \$4,500 × 0.797 or \$3,587. Fortunately, you don't have to calculate discount factors. There are tables similar to the partial one shown in Figure D.5 that show the present value of a dollar for different time periods and discount rates. Multiply this number by the anticipated cost or benefit to get the present value of that cost or benefit.

Returning to Figure D.4, we have brought all costs and benefits for our example back to present value. Notice that the discount rate for year 0 is 1.000. Why? The present value of a dollar in year 0 is exactly one dollar. It makes sense. If you hold a dollar today, it is worth exactly one dollar!

After discounting all costs and benefits, subtract the sum of the costs from the sum of the benefits. This is called the *net present value* of the solution. If it is positive, the investment is good. If negative, the investment is bad. When comparing multiple solutions or projects, the one with the highest positive net present value is the best investment. In our example, the solution being evaluated yields a net present value of $46,905. This means that if we invest $46,905 at 12 percent for 6 years, we will make the same profit that we'd make by implementing this information system solution. This is a good investment provided no other alternative has a net present value greater than $46,905.

SUMMARY

Feasibility is a measure of how beneficial the development of an information system would be to an organization. Feasibility analysis is the process by which we measure feasibility. It is an ongoing evaluation of feasibility at various checkpoints in the life cycle. At any of these checkpoints, the project may be canceled, revised, or continued. This is called the creeping commitment approach to feasibility. There are three feasibility tests: operational, technical, and economic.

Operational feasibility is a measure of problem urgency or solution acceptability. It includes a measure of how the users and managers feel about the problems or solutions. Technical feasibility is a measure of how practical solutions are and whether the technology is already available within the organization. If the technology is not available within the firm, technical feasibility also looks at whether it can be acquired. Economic feasibility is a measure of whether a solution will pay for itself or how profitable a solution will be. For management, economic feasibility is the most important of our three measures.

To analyze economic feasibility, you itemize benefits and costs. Benefits are either tangible (easy to measure) or intangible (hard to measure). To properly analyze economic feasibility, try to estimate the value of all benefits. Costs fall into two categories: development and operating. Development costs are one-time costs associated with analysis, design, and implementation of the system. Operating costs may be fixed over time or variable with respect to system usage. Given the costs and benefits, economic feasibility is evaluated by the techniques of cost/benefit analysis. Cost/benefit analysis determines if a project or solution will be cost-effective—if lifetime benefits will exceed lifetime costs. There are three popular ways to measure cost-effectiveness: payback analysis, return-on-investment analysis, and present value analysis. Payback analysis defines how long it will take for a system to pay for itself. Return-on-investment and present value analysis determine the profitability of a system. Present value analysis is preferred because it can compare alternatives that have different lifetimes.

PROBLEMS AND EXERCISES

1. What is the difference between feasibility and feasibility analysis?
2. Explain what is meant by the creeping commitment approach to feasibility. What feasibility checkpoints can be built into a systems development life cycle?
3. Visit a local data processing shop. Try to obtain documentation of their systems development life cycle standards or guidelines. What feasibility checkpoints have they installed? What feasibility checkpoints do you think they should install? (*Note:* Don't be misled into believing that only during phases labeled *feasibility* is feasibility analyzed. There may be other points in their life cycle where this also happens.)
4. What are the three tests for project feasibility? How is each test for feasibility measured?
5. What feasibility criteria does the data processing shop you visited for problem 3 use to evaluate projects? How do their criteria compare against the criteria in this book? Have we omitted any tests that they feel are important? Have they omitted any tests that we use?
6. Can you think of any technological trends or products that may be technically infeasible for the small-to-medium sized business at the current time? Defend your reasoning.
7. Whether or not you have data processing experience, you have experience with people who use computers (including friends, relatives, acquaintances, teachers, and fellow employees). Taking into consideration their biases for and against computers, identify issues that may make a proposed system operationally infeasible or unacceptable to those individuals.
8. What is the difference between a tangible and intangible benefit? Give several examples of each. How would you quantify each in terms of dollars and cents — a measure that manage-

ment can understand? Note that tangible benefits should be easy. Intangible benefits are harder, but pretend that management insists that you quantify the benefits.

9. What is the difference between fixed and variable operating costs? Give several examples of each.
10. What are some of the advantages and disadvantages of the payback analysis, return-on-investment analysis, and present value analysis cost/benefit techniques?
11. A new production scheduling information system for XYZ Corporation could be developed at a cost of $125,000. The estimated net operating costs and estimated net benefits over seven years of operation would be:

	ESTIMATED NET OPERATING COSTS	*ESTIMATED NET BENEFITS*
YEAR 0	$125,000	0
YEAR 1	3,500	$26,000
YEAR 2	4,700	34,000
YEAR 3	5,500	41,000
YEAR 4	6,300	55,000
YEAR 5	7,000	66,000
YEAR 6	7,700	75,000
YEAR 7	8,400	82,000

What would be the payback period for this investment? Would this be a good or bad investment? Why?

9. What is the ROI (return on investment) for the project in problem 8?
10. What is the net present value of the investment in problem 8 if the current discount rate is 10 percent?

ANNOTATED REFERENCES AND SUGGESTED READINGS

Gildersleeve, Thomas R. *Successful Data Processing Systems Analysis.* Englewood Cliffs, N.J.: Prentice-Hall, 1978. This book provides an excellent chapter on cost/benefit analysis techniques. We are indebted to Tom for the *creeping commitment* concept.

Gore, Marvin, and John Stubbe. *Elements of Systems Analysis.* 3d ed. Dubuque, Iowa: Brown, 1983. Chapter 13, "Feasibility Analysis" (equivalent to our use of the term *feasibility study*) suggests an interesting matrix approach to identifying, cataloging, and analyzing feasibility of alternative solutions for a system.

Wetherbe, James. *Systems Analysis and Design: Traditional, Structured, and Advanced Concepts and Techniques.* 2d ed. West, 1984. Wetherbe pioneered the PIECES framework for problem classification. In this module, we extended that framework to analyze operational feasibility of solutions.

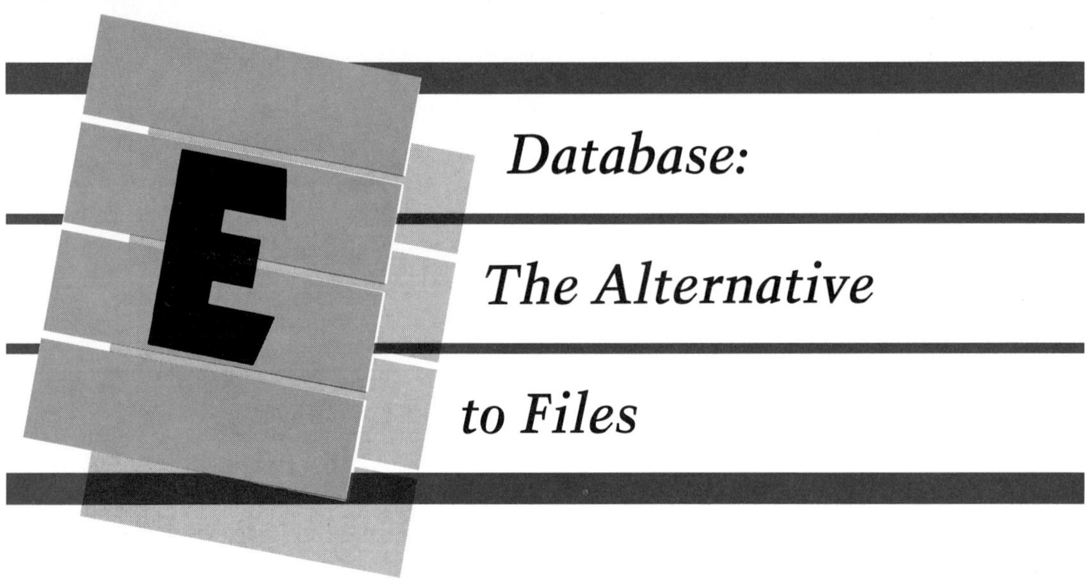

Database: The Alternative to Files

WHEN SHOULD YOU READ THIS MODULE?

This module should only be read after studying Chapter 12, "Designing Computer Files."

Database is often considered too advanced a subject to include in an introductory systems analysis and design course. But today, so many applications are being built around database technology that database design has become an important skill for the analyst. Indeed, database technology, once considered important only to the largest corporations with the largest computers, is now common for applications developed on minicomputers and even microcomputers. By placing the material in a module, we give you and your instructor the option of studying or omitting the material. This module won't make you a database systems analyst. However, it will make you database literate, an important first step.

DATABASE CONCEPTS FOR THE SYSTEMS ANALYST

The history of data processing has led to one inescapable conclusion: *data is a resource that must be managed.* Very few experienced data processing staffs have avoided the frustration of uncontrolled growth and duplication of data stored in their systems. As systems were developed, implemented, and maintained, the common data needed by the different systems werc duplicated in multiple files. This duplication carried with it a number of costs: extra storage space required, duplicated input to maintain the files, and data integrity problems (for example, the ADDRESS for Joe's Bar and Grill not matching in the various files that contain customer addresses).

Necessity, being the mother of invention, came to our rescue. Database technology was created so an organization could maintain and use its data as an integrated whole instead of separate data files. We can now develop a shared data resource that can be used by several information systems. This concept, illustrated in Figure E.1, was first introduced in Chapter 3. In this section, we'll survey the advantages and disadvantages of database versus conventional files. We'll also study the terminology and current state of practice in database environments.

Conventional Files Versus the Database

Before you conclude that the conventional file is the original sin of data processing, we should compare the file and database alternatives. Look at Figure E.2. It illustrates the fundamental difference between file and database environments. In the file environment, data storage is built around the applications. In the database environment, applications are built around the integrated database. The database structure is natural; that is to say, it is not dependent on the applications that will use it. Each environment has advantages and disadvantages.

Pros and Cons of Conventional Files Conventional files are relatively easy to design and implement because they are normally based on a single application or information system (such as accounts receivable or payroll). If you understand the user's output

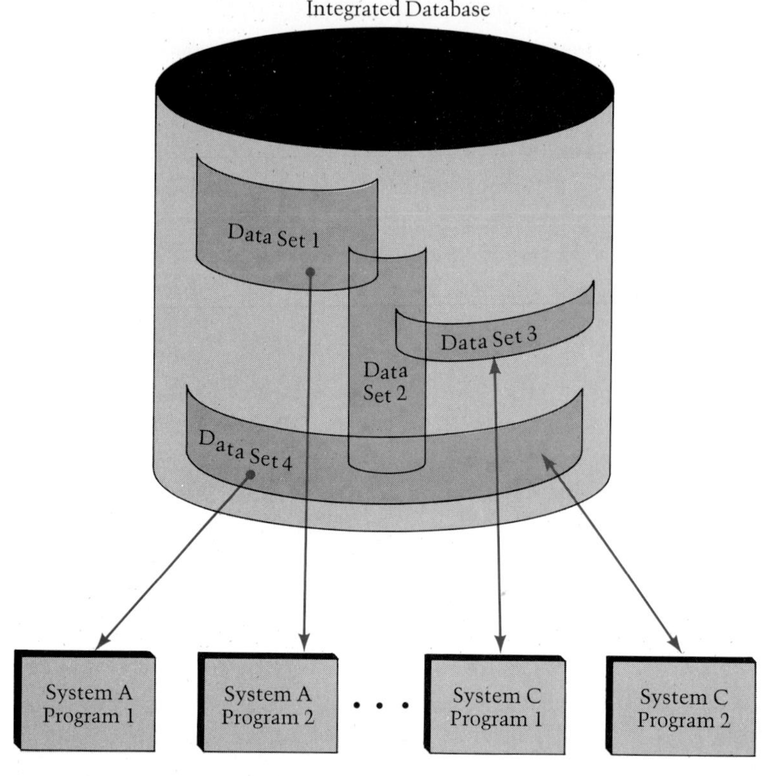

Figure E.1

The database concept. A database should be thought of as a shared data resource. Although each data record and item is stored only once on the disk, the data may be shared by multiple information systems. Most traditional information systems don't share their files with other systems.

needs for that system, you can both determine the data that will have to be captured and stored to fulfill those needs and define the best file organization for those requirements. That is the approach you learned in Chapter 12.

Another advantage of conventional files is processing speed. Database technology is complex and often too slow to handle large volumes of transactions with an adequate throughput. File organization techniques, as you will recall from Chapter 12, were selected to maximize file processing speed. Another advantage, often overlooked, is the fact that numerous file systems are already in place. Given the shortage of data processing personnel and the growth in

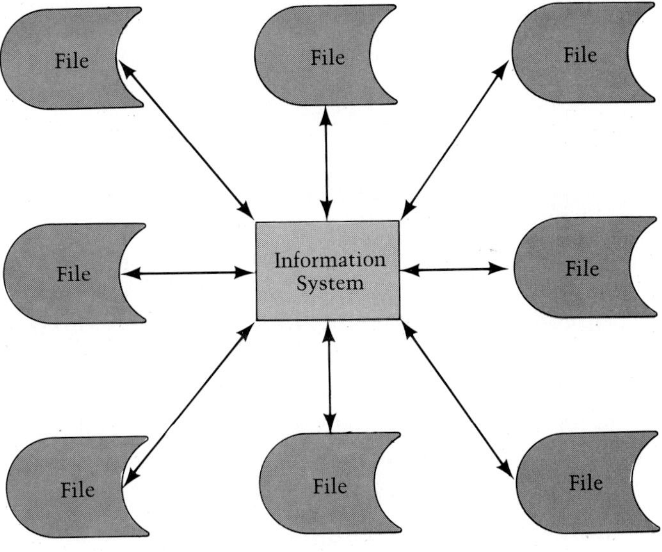

Conventional File Environment

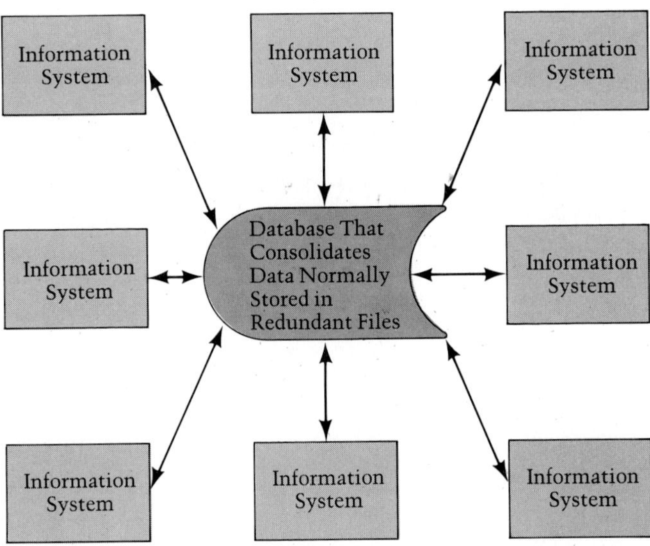

Database Environment

Figure E.2

File versus database approaches. File-based environments emphasize the application. As applications are developed, custom files are built around them. Database environments emphasize the database. The applications evolve around a central database. The database and applications are independent from one another.

demand for new information systems, many firms cannot afford the time or money required to redesign all of their current file-based systems as database systems.

The disadvantages of files have already been outlined, but a quick summary is in order. Duplication of data is normally cited as the principle disadvantage of files. Duplicate data results in duplicate input, duplicate maintenance, duplicate storage, and possible integrity errors. And what happens if the data format changes? Consider the problem faced by many firms if all systems must support a nine-digit zip code. Do you have any idea how many redundant files and synonyms would have to be located and changed in a typical organization? Add to this the enormous volume of programs that use the field, and you have one nightmare of a maintenance project.

Another disadvantage of files is inflexibility. Files are typically designed to support the user's *current* requirements. New information needs (such as reports and queries) often require files to be redesigned because existing files cannot support the new needs. If the existing files are restructured, all programs using those files may have to be rewritten; this would be quite impractical in most businesses. And if the files cannot be redesigned, then new, redundant files are often created to meet the new requirements!

Pros and Cons of Database Just as we were concerned that you unfairly condemned files, you should realize that database is no panacea. The principle advantage of database lies in the sharing of data. A common misconception about database is that you can build a single database that contains all data items of interest to an organization. This Heaven-on-Earth notion is doomed to failure. The complexity of such an environment is such that the database would take forever to build. Realistically, most organizations build several databases, each one sharing data with many information systems. Yes, there will be *some* redundancy between databases. However, this redundancy is both reduced and controlled (relative to the file environment).

Database technology also offers the advantage of storing data in more flexible formats. These formats allow us to use the data in ways not originally specified by the users. Different combinations of the same data can be easily accessed to fulfill new report and query needs. Database technology also offers the unique advantage of data independence. When fully realized, **data independence** permits data formats and structure to change (recall our zip code example) without having to change all the computer programs that currently use that data. Thus, new fields and record types can be added to the database without affecting current programs.

But there are no free lunches! Database technology is more complex than file technology. Special software, called a **database management system** (DBMS), is required. This flexibility provided by a DBMS usually makes it slower. Thus many organizations have to buy bigger computers. Also, the cost of developing databases is higher because analysts and programmers must learn how to use the DBMS. And the DBMS technology itself can be expensive to acquire and maintain. Still another problem is the increased vulnerability inherent in use of databases. Because you are using a shared data resource, you are placing all your eggs in one basket. Therefore, backup and recovery procedures and security issues become more complex and costly.

Despite the problems discussed, database usage is growing by leaps and bounds. The technology will get better, and performance limitations will likely disappear. But for the time being, we'll have to adjust to a world that uses both files and database systems.

Three Database Environments

Data becomes the central resource in a database environment. Information systems are built around this central resource to give both computer programmers and end users flexible access to the data. Let's examine this environment more closely by studying three different types of database situations.

Application-Oriented Databases Application databases are those that either were designed for or evolved around a specific information system. A single database consolidates the files that would have been needed for a single application (see Figure E.3). At first, this may seem like a slight variation on files. However, there are two significant differences. First, the single database is not as redundant as the multiple files. Second, the data is organized for more flexibility than is possible with files. Thus the information system will likely be more responsive to future requirements for that application. On the other hand, although there will be fewer databases than files, the number of databases can still be large — it will be equal to the number of information systems. Furthermore, the existence of

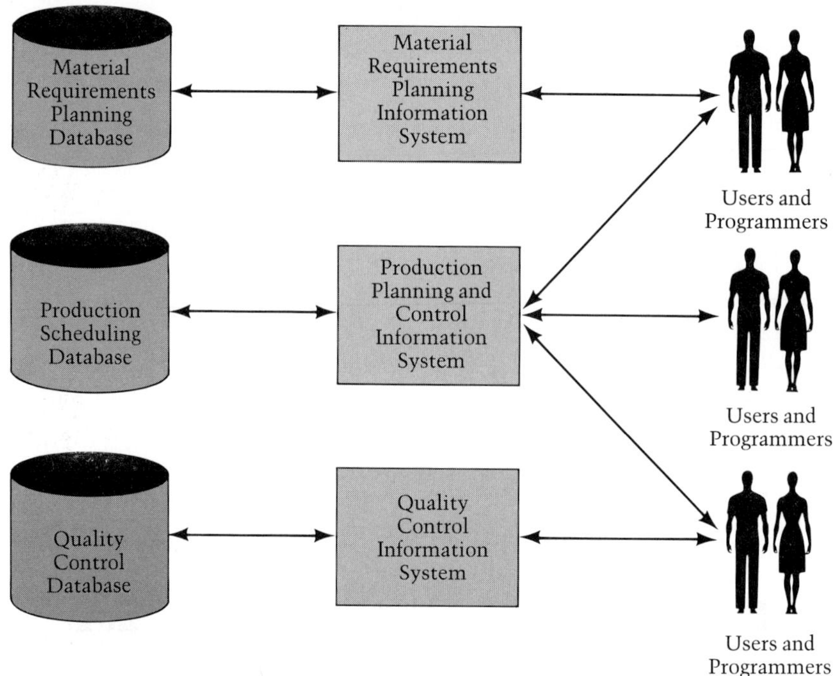

Figure E.3

Application databases. Application databases consolidate the multiple files normally used for a single information system into a single database for that system. This reduces redundancy within the system and increases flexibility. However, different application databases tend to be redundant against one another.

redundant data in separate databases developed for separate information systems is still a potential problem.

Subject-Oriented Databases Subject databases are designed around organizational subjects instead of specific information systems. Representative subject databases may include those built around data describing orders, customers, accounts, or products. Subsequently, multiple information systems may use a subject database. In addition, any information system may use more than one subject database. This is illustrated in Figure E.4. There will be fewer databases than in the application-oriented environment. Subject databases represent the most flexible environment because they are

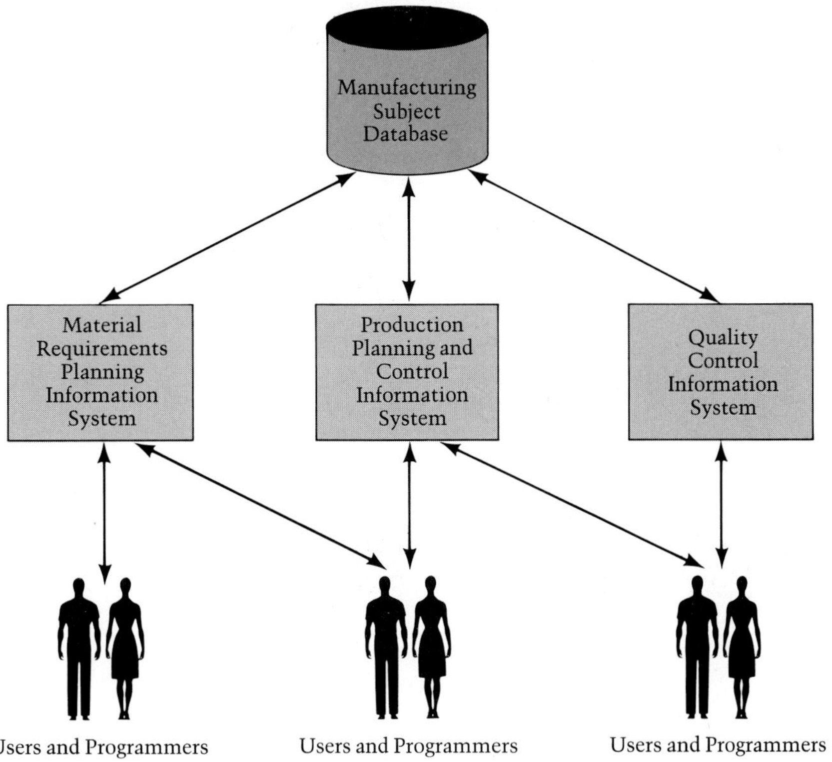

Figure E.4

Subject databases. Subject databases are defined and built independent of the information systems that use them (or will use them). Organizations that use subject databases tend to have fewer databases and less redundancy while maximizing flexibility. This is considered the ideal database situation; however, it is difficult to achieve.

designed around data, not around the use of that data. Data usage evolves in such an environment.

End-User Databases In Chapter 3, we discussed the current trend toward fourth-generation programming languages and their direct use by knowledge workers, called end-user computing. What we didn't tell you is that these end-user languages (such as *FOCUS* and *RAMIS*) are usually built around database technology. Data are extracted from other files and databases to create end-user databases.

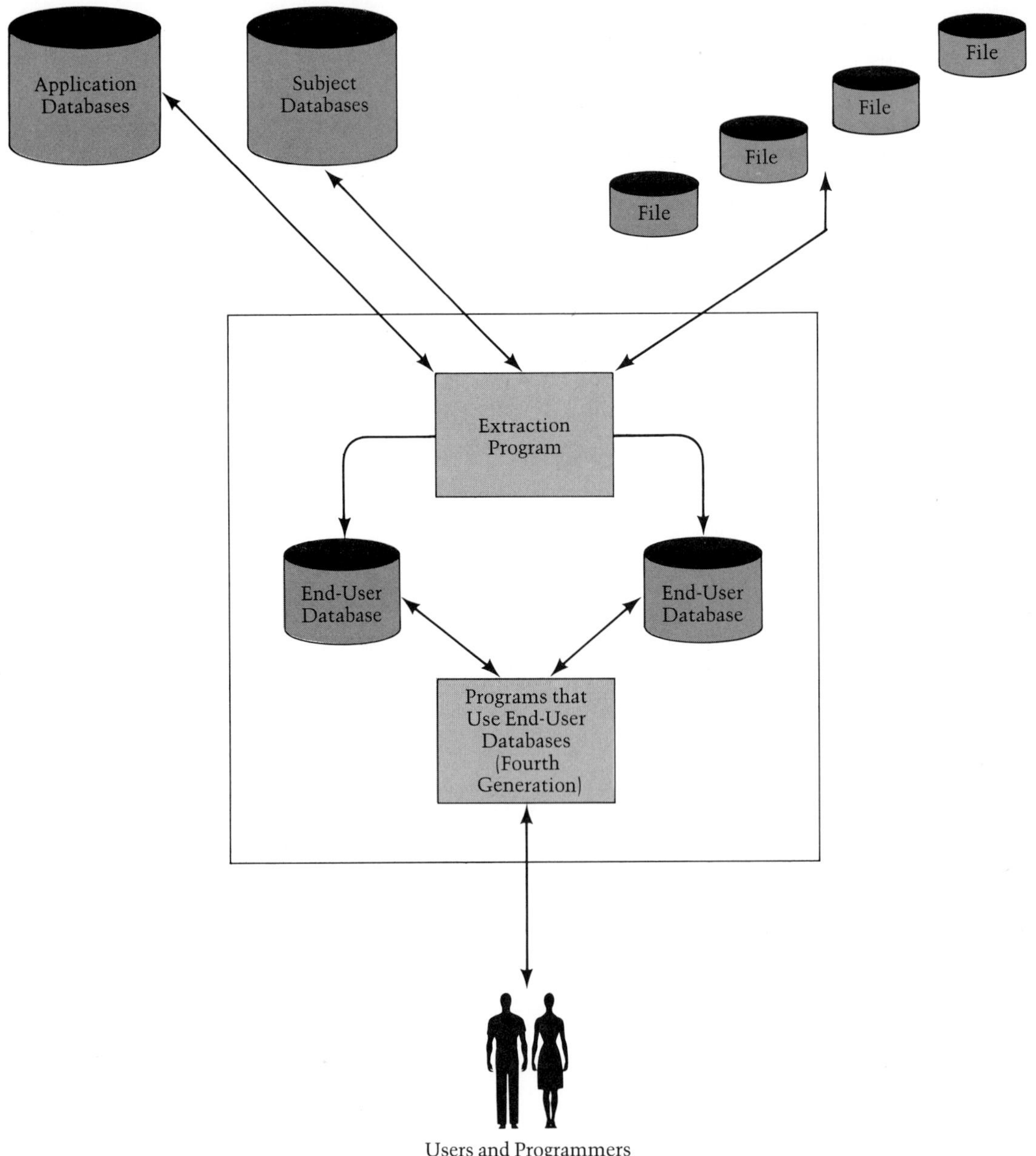

Figure E.5

End-user databases. End-user databases are built from the conventional files, application databases, and subject databases in one or more information systems. After they have been built, end-user databases are used to produce management reports and respond to decision support inquiries.

Using the end-user languages, analysts and users can quickly generate their own reports and inquiries against those databases (see Figure E.5).

Putting It All Together Figure E.6 illustrates the way many companies have been forced to ease into a database environment. Note that most companies have numerous conventional file-based information systems, most of which were developed prior to the popularity of databases. In many cases, the processing efficiency of files and the projected cost to redesign files prevent conversion of these systems to databases. Other information systems have been built around application and/or subject databases. Access to these databases is limited to computer programs that use the DBMS to process transactions, maintain the data, and generate regularly scheduled management reports. Some query access may also be provided. These databases are often referred to as production databases because they are heavily used to support the transactions for major information systems.

Many data processing shops hesitate to give end users access to production databases for queries and reports. The volume of unscheduled reports and queries could overload those databases. Instead, end-user databases are developed, possibly on separate computers (including micros). Data, extracted from the production databases and conventional files, are stored in these end-user databases. Both conventional and fourth-generation programming languages are used to generate reports and queries off these databases. Admittedly, this scenario is advanced, but many firms are currently using variations of it.

You might be disturbed by what appears in the scenario to be a lack of total commitment to subject and end-user databases. Just remember that economics, not theory, dictates how businesses are forced to operate. Existing file applications cannot be changed overnight. Application databases cannot be quickly converted to subject databases.

THE TECHNOLOGY OF DATABASE

Let's briefly examine how the database environment is implemented. The discussion is oversimplified but nonetheless adequate for introductory purposes.

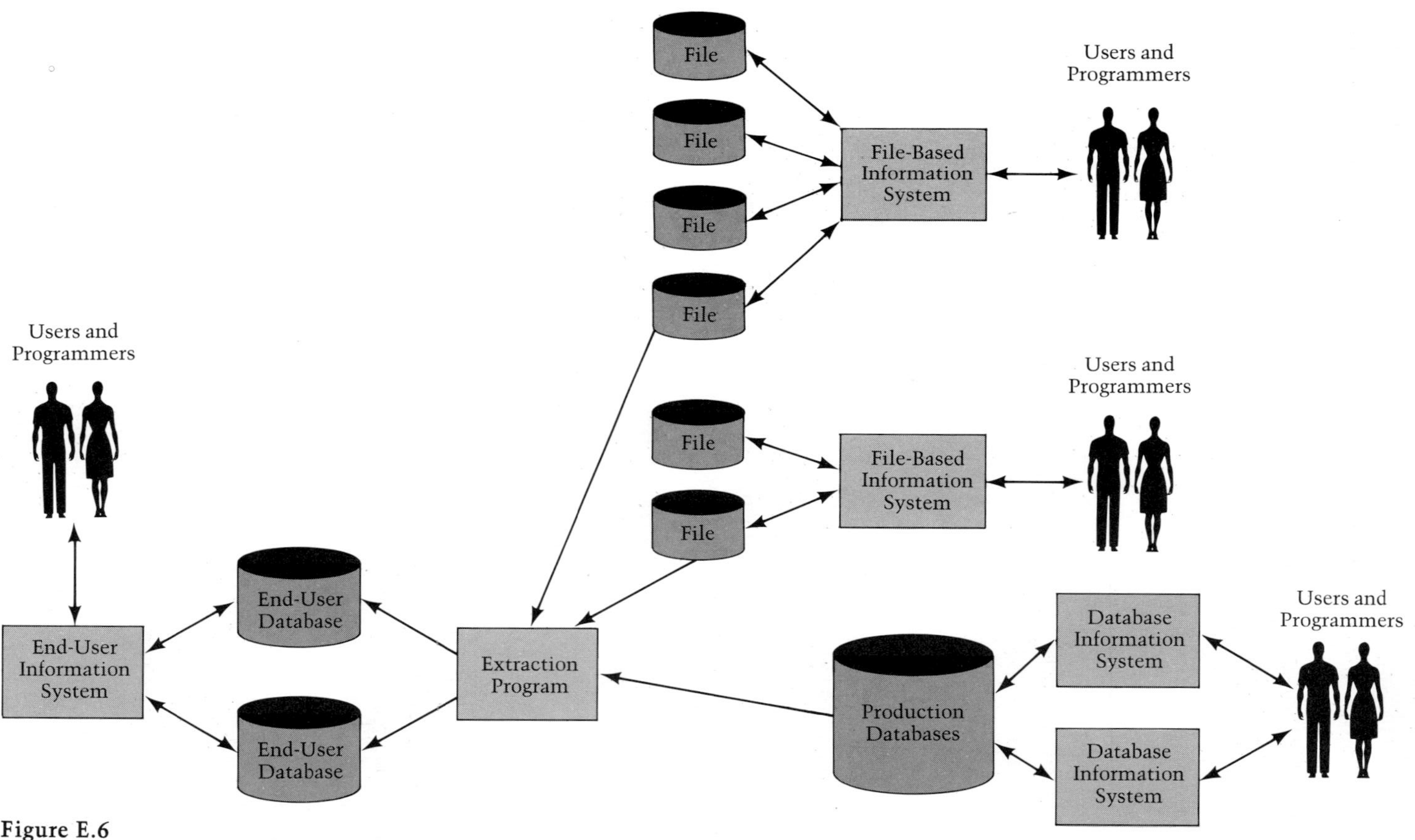

Figure E.6

A typical database environment. By today's standards, a typical database environment still includes numerous conventional files. Additionally, it may contain both production databases (of the application and subject variety) and end-user databases (also of the application and subject variety).

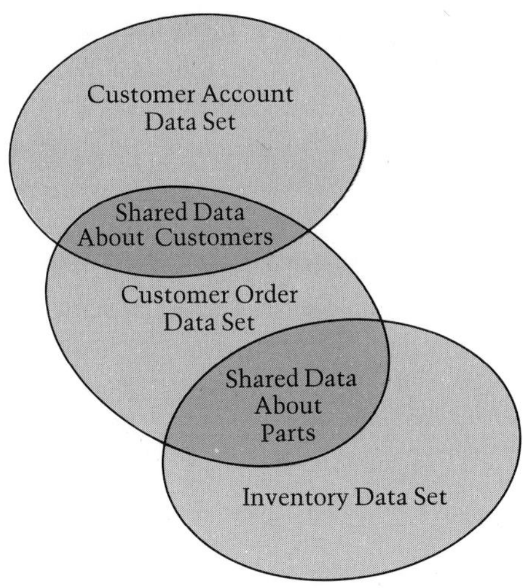

Figure E.7

Data sets in the database environment. A data set is a collection of different record types and their relationships to one another. A record may be contained in more than one data set. This allows the record to be shared by many programs and many information systems. Relationships are implemented by logical pointers that connect occurrences of different record types that are related.

Database Architecture

In a database environment, the notion of conventional files disappears. In its place, we have what we'll call data sets, which can overlap (see Figure E.7). Thus certain records and fields may be contained in (shared by) several data sets. For instance, PART data may be shared by the CUSTOMER ORDER and INVENTORY data sets, even though the part data is physically stored only one place on the disk.

Unlike a file, a data set can consist of many types of records. For instance, the ORDER data set could consist of CUSTOMER records, ORDER records, ORDERED PART detail records, and PART records. An INVENTORY data set may include PART records, MATERIAL records, and BILL OF MATERIAL records. Each record contains unique fields. Ideally, any given field, such as CUSTOMER NAME, should be stored in only one type of record. Different types of records are linked together by logical pointers to represent relationships between those records. For instance, each

CUSTOMER record may contain pointers to ORDER records placed by that customer (see Figure E.8). In turn, each ORDER record may contain pointers to ORDERED PARTs on that order. An ORDERED PART record will describe quantity ordered, price at time of order, discount given, and the like. Finally, each ORDERED PART points to exactly one PART record that contains such fields as part description, unit of measure, and quantity in the warehouse.

How does all this work? The database is created, accessed, and controlled through specialized computer software called database management systems (DBMS), which are available from numerous computer vendors. Let's examine what a DBMS is and what it does.

Database Management Systems

Figure E.9 depicts the database technical environment. A systems analyst, or a database analyst, designs the structure of the data sets, record types, fields, and relationships that were described earlier. This analyst then uses the DBMS's **data definition language** (DDL) to establish those data sets, records, fields, and relationships. DDLs record the definitions into a permanent data dictionary. Some data dictionaries include formal, elaborate software that helps database specialists keep track of everything stored in the database—including generation of data dictionary reports, analyses, and inquiry responses.

Computer programs are written to load, maintain, and use actual data. These programs may be written in a host programming language (such as COBOL, PL/I, or BASIC) that is supported by the DBMS. Using the host language, the programs call subroutines in the DBMS's **data manipulation language** (DML) to retrieve, create, delete, and modify records and navigate between record types (for example, from CUSTOMER to ORDERs for that customer). The programmers don't have to understand how the data is stored (file organization) or accessed. The DBMS takes care of such details. The DML refers to the data dictionary (DDL) during execution. The dictionary specifies valid data sets, records, fields, relationships, and constraints. The DBMS manages security and access to the database and audits and logs all database updates (for audit and backup purposes).

Alternatively, some DBMSs don't require a host language. They provide their own self-contained programming language that uses the DML but allows the user to avoid learning it. This is true of

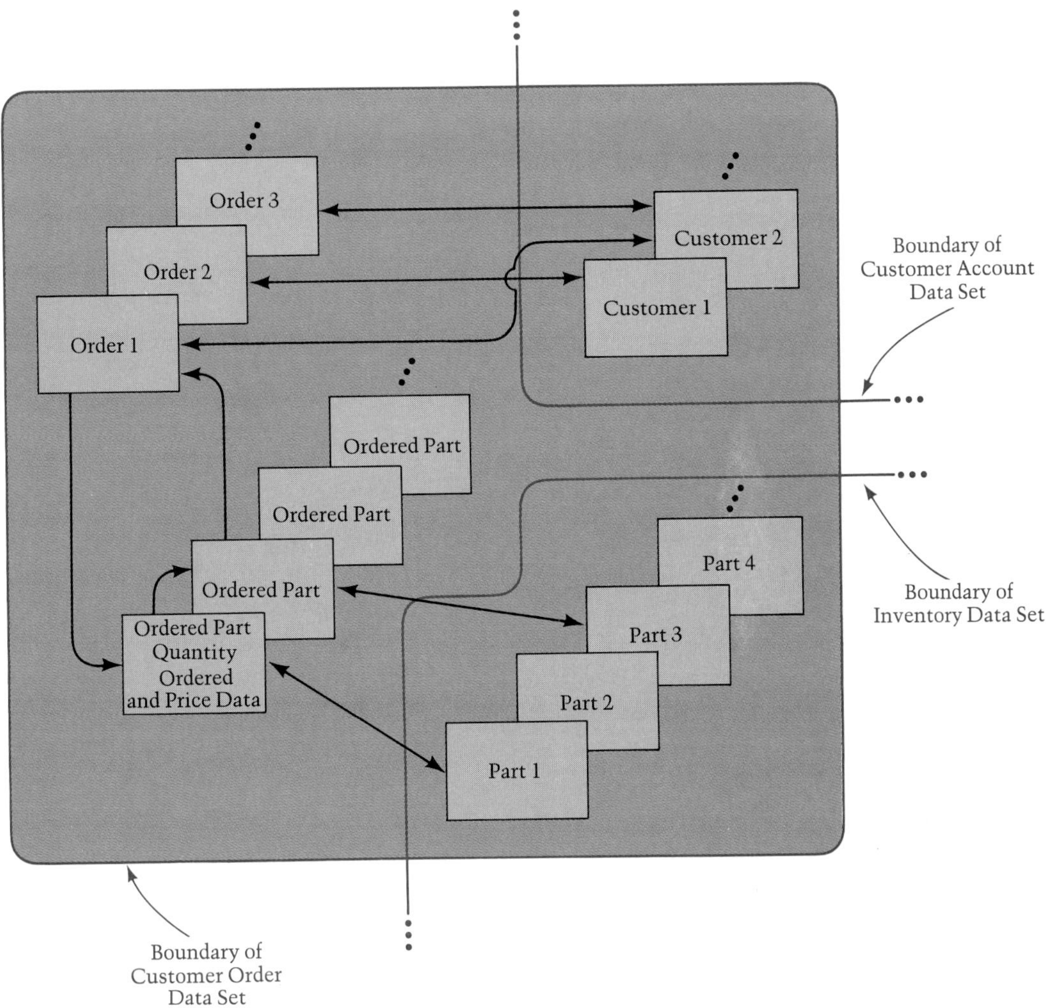

Figure E.8

Record occurrences in a database. This picture illustrates how a database works. Any given occurrence of one type of record is somehow linked to occurrences of another type of record. This allows fields to be stored in only one record type because those fields can be retrieved via the specified links.

fourth-generation languages, such as *FOCUS, RAMIS*, and *DBASE III*. Additionally, most DBMSs offer report writers and query languages for use with existing databases. These languages and features are generally designed to be simple to learn and use, so much

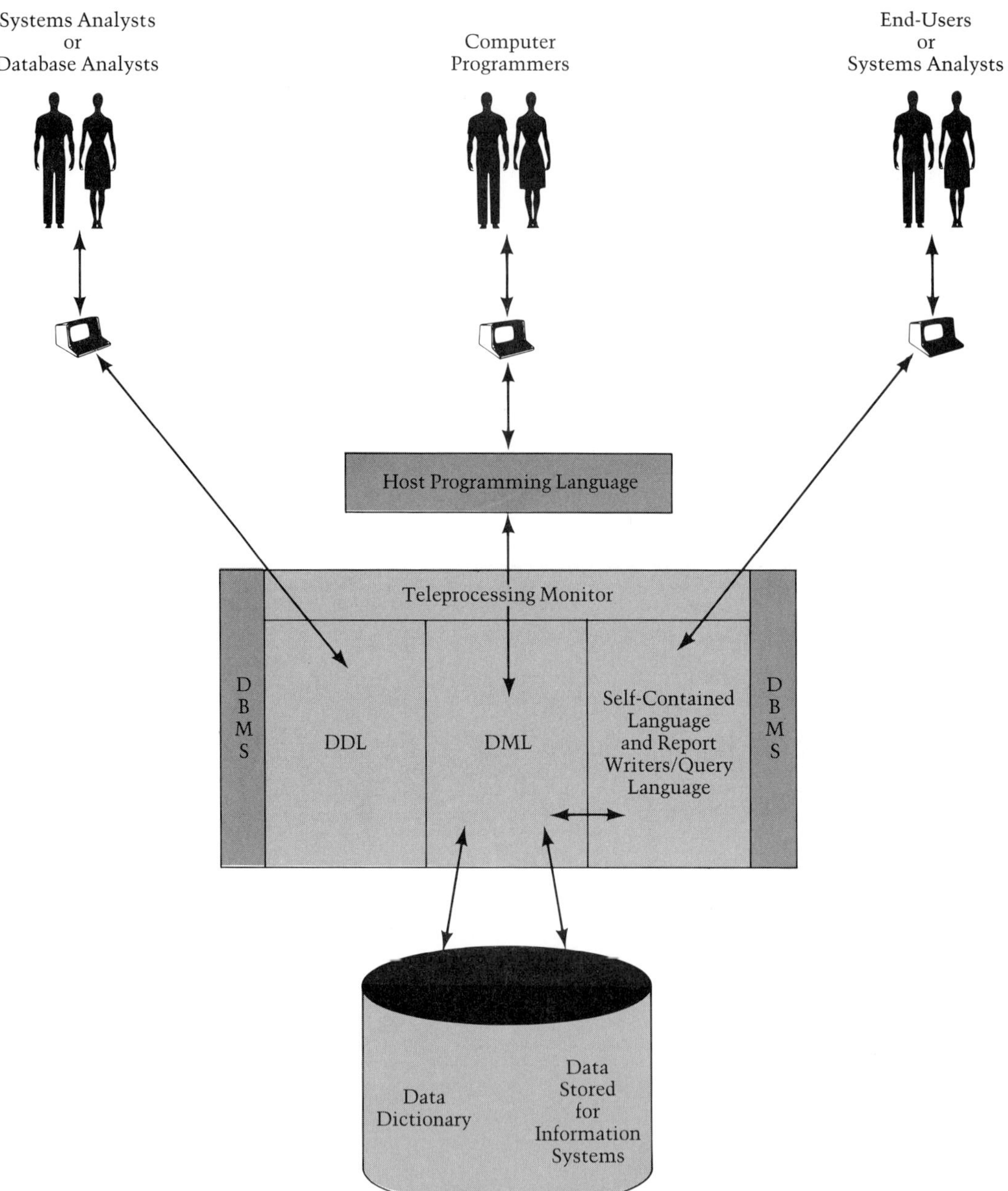
Systems Analysts
or
Database Analysts
Computer
Programmers
End-Users
or
Systems Analysts
Host Programming Language
Teleprocessing Monitor
DBMS
DDL
DML
Self-Contained
Language
and Report
Writers/Query
Language
DBMS
Data
Dictionary
Data
Stored
for
Information
Systems

◄ **Figure E.9**

Architecture of an ideal DBMS. Not all database management systems contain all the components shown in this ideal architecture; however, this diagram is representative of a typical DBMS. The key components are the data definition language (DDL—used to create and change the database structure) and the data manipulation language (DML—used to access and maintain the database).

so that experienced programmers can be replaced by analysts and users. This alternative is also depicted in Figure E.9.

Multiple-user DBMSs frequently include a teleprocessing or TP monitor. This is specialized software that supervises and controls access to the database via terminals in on-line environments. Most such systems can also interface with TP monitors other than their own (such as IBM's *CICS*).

Any given DBMS supports two views of the data, a physical and a logical structure. The physical structure defines how data is stored on the disk. That's right, database management systems don't replace file structures, organization, and access methods—they just hide them from the programmers and users. The physical view may include a variety of data and file structures including sequential, relative, or hashed records; linked lists; inverted lists; and indexes (these are all structures you learn in beginning and advanced programming courses).

The logical view defines the data sets, records, fields, and relationships that were discussed earlier. They differ primarily in how they implement relationships between different record types. There are three popular logical views supported by various DBMSs: hierarchical, network, and relational.

Hierarchical Database Management Systems Some DBMSs require that different record types be interrelated only via hierarchical relationships. For example, in Figure E.10, we see a schema for a hierarchical database. A **schema** is a picture that identifies the records and the interrecord relationships in a database. Hierarchical DBMS records are referred to as parents and children. A parent record can have several children, but a child can have only one parent. A record (such as ORDER) can be both parent and child as long as it doesn't violate the last rule.

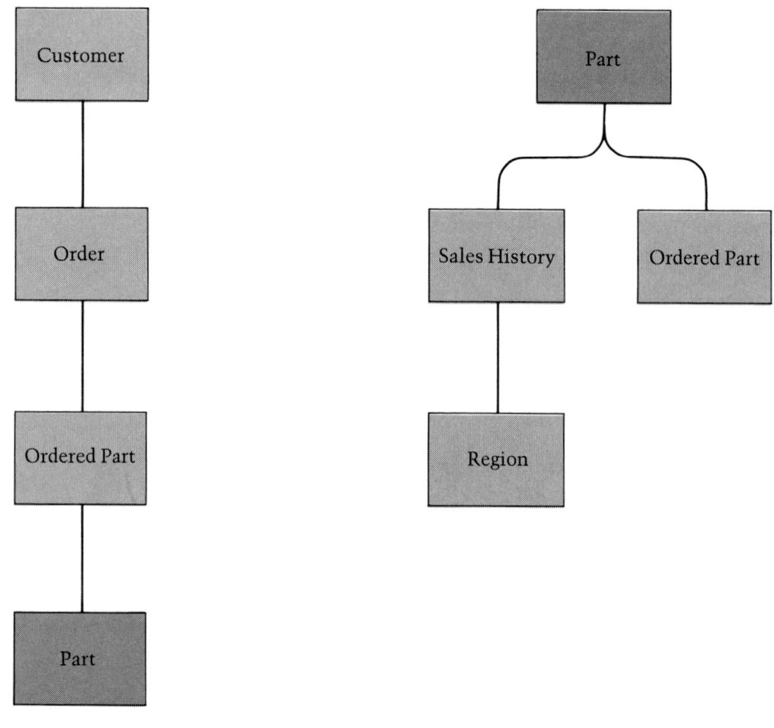

Figure E.10

The hierarchical logical data model. Hierarchical DBMSs require that related record types be linked hierarchically. No child record type can have more than one parent record type.

In our hierarchical schema, we see that we can retrieve all orders for a customer, all parts for an order, and specific part data for an ordered part (such as PART DESCRIPTION). As records are retrieved, we have access to their fields. In another hierarchy, we see that for a part, we can retrieve all occurrences of ordered part records as well as historical sales data. The identical records in the two hierarchies only look redundant. They are actually two separate data sets that happen to share the same record, which is stored only once on the disk.

Examples of commercial DBMSs that use the hierarchical data model include IBM's *Information Management System* (IMS) and

Intel's *System 2000*, and Information Builder's *FOCUS* (not exclusively hierarchical).

Network Database Management Systems Network database management systems provide a more flexible, albeit more complex, logical data model. The schema for a typical network DBMS is illustrated in Figure E.11. The key difference between the network database and the hierarchical database is that a record in a network database can be the child of more than one parent record. Notice in our example that we didn't need two data sets to depict the records in the hierarchical example.

Examples of network DBMSs include Cincom's TOTAL and Cullinet's IDMS. IDMS conforms to a network database modeling standard called CODASYL. TOTAL, on the other hand, is a network database that has some restrictions — for example, a TOTAL record cannot be both a parent and a child. You can learn more about CODASYL and TOTAL data structures in a typical database course or from a database textbook.

Relational Database Management Systems Relational databases use a model intended to greatly simplify database technology for programmers, analysts, and nontechnical users. Records are seen as simple tables (see Figure E.12). The rows are record occurrences, and the columns are fields (we are purposely avoiding relational terminology). Relationships are stored quite differently from the way they are stored in hierarchical and network models. Instead of relating records through logical pointers, records (tables) are related through intentionally redundant fields (usually keys) common to the different tables.

The DML for a relational DBMS doesn't navigate paths and pointers (which is what happens with hierarchical and network databases). Instead, the DML lets the programmer or user perform simple table operations to create temporary tables that can be used to write reports and answer inquiries. These operations include:

- Selecting specific occurrences from a table and creating a new table that contains only those occurrences. Criteria can be set to determine which records to select from the initial table.
- Projecting out specific fields from a table, thus creating a table that has fewer occurrences and fields.

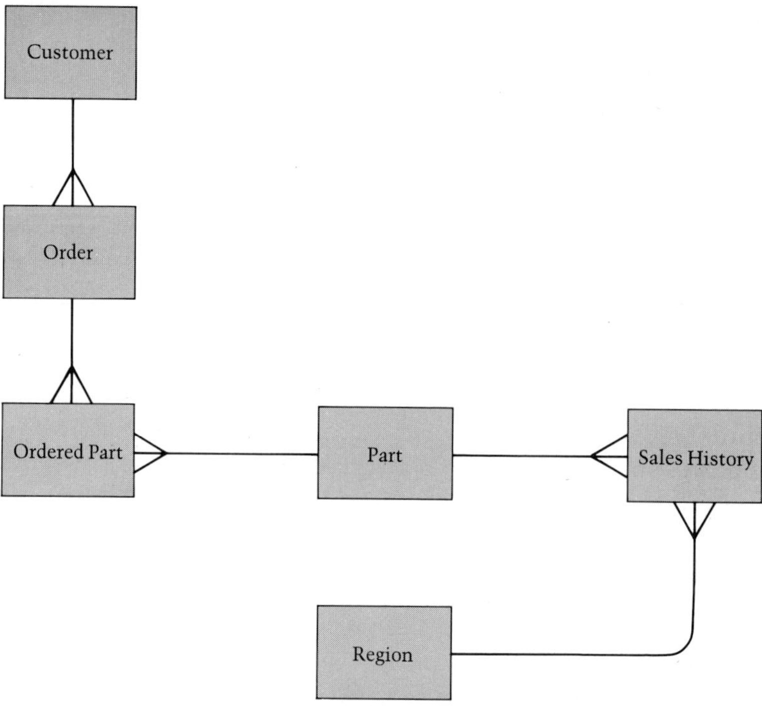

Figure E.11

Network logical data model. A network DBMS allows record types to have any number of logical relationships with any other record types. Notice that the line connecting CUSTOMER and ORDER indicates that there may be several occurrences of the record type ORDER for a single occurrence of CUSTOMER. And there may be only one occurrence of CUSTOMER for a single ORDER.

- Joining two or more tables across a common field (this is the same as navigating relationship paths in a hierarchical or network database). For instance, we can join the customer and order tables across the common field CUSTOMER NUMBER. This produces a temporary working table that has all the customer fields appended to each order record occurrence.

The data in the working tables can also be updated. When the program is finished with the working table, that working table disappears, but updates are stored in the original tables.

Examples of relational DBMS's include Information Builder's *FOCUS* (which is also hierarchical) and Ashton-Tate's *DBASE III. DBASE* is a remarkable success story because it brought the technology of database to microcomputers where it has been learned and applied, (because of the ease of use of the relational model) by many knowledge workers who possess limited computer experience and skills.

That's about all we want to say about the three common data models. Database textbooks and courses will offer entire chapters and units on each of the three data models.

The Database Administrator

Who manages the database environment? That depends on the size of the organization. In larger shops, a **database administrator** (DBA) oversees a staff of database specialists. These specialists design databases according to systems analysts' and users' requirements, load and maintain databases, establish security controls, perform backup and recovery, and maintain the DBMS software. They also plan and control database definition to minimize redundancy and keep track of where all data is stored and how various systems use that data. In smaller shops, a systems analyst may perform these duties.

DATABASE IMPLICATIONS FOR INFORMATION SYSTEMS DEVELOPMENT

What impact does database have on our systems development life cycle (SDLC)? Because database will force some changes on the entire life cycle, we should discuss database development in the context of both the systems analysis and systems design processes.

Ideally, databases should be independent of any one information system (recall Figure E.2). Along those lines, the ideal approach

Customer Table			
Cust. No.	Cust. Name	Cust. Address	...
	. . .		

Order Table		
Order No.	Order Date	...
	. . .	

Part Table		
Part No.	Part Desc.	Quant. on Hand
	. . .	

Part records describe data about parts in general. Ordered Part describes data about specific parts on specific orders.

Ordered Part Table			
Order No.	Part No.	Quant. Ordered	...
	. . .		

Figure E.12

Relational logical data model. A relational DBMS logical model depicts record types as tables. Tables are related to one another via redundant fields, usually keys. Relational DBMSs provide operators that build working tables from the tables that are physically stored.

would be to develop and implement a subject database before developing any applications that would use that database. Then you would build information systems using the SDLC. But as is the case with many ideals, this one often proves impractical. It assumes that you can easily define all records and fields for a subject database. This could consume considerable time and effort. Meanwhile, the user has nothing to show for all this work because information systems haven't been developed.

Consequently, databases tend to evolve as applications or information systems are built. You have to be careful because this approach can lead to development of application databases instead of the more flexible and less redundant subject databases. But it can be done! Let's study the database implications for the systems analysis and design phases of the life cycle for a new information system. (We are assuming that you are familiar with the general life cycle — Chapter 5 — and the detailed tasks of the analysis and design phases — Chapters 6 and 10.)

Systems Analysis in a Database Environment

Recall that systems analysis consists of three phases: study, definition, and evaluation. During the study phase, the systems analyst should be doing two things. First, you should identify the data that describes the application being studied. Second, you should look for opportunities to eliminate the redundant storage of data in the system. Although data flow diagrams are useful for documenting work and data flow in a current system, they can't, by themselves, support our needs in a database project. In the database environment, the data content of the data flows are important. The data that resides on current forms and files can be documented in a data dictionary.

During the definition phase, the systems analyst should define the requirements for the database. But we want the requirements to be specified independent from the requirements for the specific information system that we are currently developing — a *subject* database is our goal! In other words, the worst thing we can do is to begin by discussing the desired outputs with the user, which is precisely what you *would* do in a conventional file environment. Why would this strategy be wrong? Because it limits your thinking to the data and structure needed to support requirements that can be defined today and ignores future requirements! So what *should* you do?

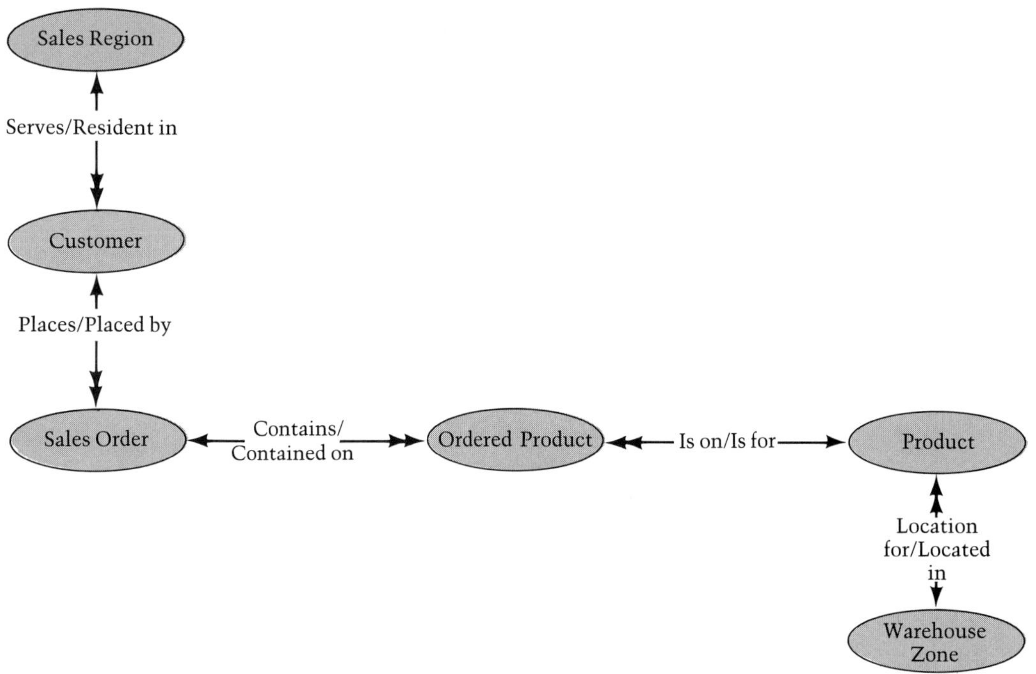

Figure E.13

Conceptual schema. A conceptual schema is a tool used by the analyst to define database requirements in terms of business entities and natural business relationships between those entities. The conceptual schema does not restrict itself with any of the logical data model capabilities or limitations.

Instead, identify those entities in the business about which we want to store data. Then define the natural relationships between those entities so we can implement the navigation capability that was introduced earlier in this module. Systems analysts often draw a special schema, called a **conceptual schema,** to describe the entities and relationships. The conceptual schema differs from the logical and physical schemas in that it presents only database requirements and does so independent of any DBMS's logical model and limitations.

A sample conceptual schema is shown in Figure E.13. There exist a number of conceptual schema symbologies. In this diagram, an oval is an entity about which we want to store data. A line between two or more entities indicates a natural relationship between those entities. A relationship defines a possible navigation path through the database. For instance, the relationship (places/placed by) between CUSTOMER and SALES ORDER suggests that we should be able to retrieve all ORDERs for a CUSTOMER, and vice versa. Relationships are named so that the names describe the relationship.

The number of arrows at the ends of the relationship lines describes how many occurrences of one entity may be connected to a single occurrence of the other entity. This complexity is always analyzed in *both* directions. For example, for one CUSTOMER, there can exist many ORDERs (two arrows). And for one ORDER, there can only exist one CUSTOMER (one arrow).

We would be remiss if we didn't introduce the concepts of conceptual data modeling and normalization. There are formal techniques for defining the conceptual schema. They are collectively called *conceptual data modeling.* An ideal conceptual data model or schema is one that structures the data independent from the way(s) the data will be used. Such a model is said to be stable—that is, future requirements are not likely to cause the conceptual model to be changed in such a way that, to implement new requirements, existing database applications would have to be reprogrammed or duplicate databases would have to be developed.

Normalization is a popular, formal technique for finding the ideal conceptual schema. A full discussion of normalization is beyond the scope of this introductory textbook (besides, it would take many pages and examples to cover it well enough for you to be able to duplicate the technique). However, you should absolutely learn this technique, either in database courses or advanced systems analysis courses. Suggested sources are listed in the readings for this module. The following is a very simplified explanation of the results of normalization:

- No record contains repeating groups of elements. In other words, all records are fixed length and all fields in the record occur once, and only once, for a single occurrence of the record.
- All fields in the record are dependent on the key of that record—that is, all fields describe the same business entity that the key describes.
- None of the fields in a record can be calculated from other fields in the record (calculatable fields can be eliminated from the database).

We cannot overstress that this summary is greatly simplified for this book. The important thing for you to realize is that normalization results in the smallest, most stable database possible. And the normalized database is flexible to meeting future requirements as they become known.

It is during the evaluation phase that the file versus database decision is actually made. It's not an either-or decision, and it's not an easy decision either. Initially, you need to find out whether any of the required data is currently stored in either conventional files or an existing database. If any are, you have to consider whether those files or databases can be used or changed (remember, changes to current files may cause existing programs to be modified).

Let's say that the data isn't stored in any current files or database. How are you going to store the data? You could implement data stores as conventional files. Or you could implement an integrated database. Or you could implement a combination of files and a database. The evaluation phase results in a decision based on the pros and cons of files and databases. In either case, you need to determine your data storage capacity requirements (bytes of storage) so you can learn whether you need additional capacity.

Systems Design in a Database Environment

Recall that systems design consists of two phases: selection and design. The selection phase is only applicable if additional storage capacity is required or if a DBMS is to be selected. Note that the selection of a DBMS is usually delegated to the database administrator's staff because the DBMS usually serves multiple information systems. However, the selection of a microcomputer DBMS is frequently the systems analyst's responsibility.

During the design phase, the logical and physical structures of the database are finalized. This structure is determined by constraints and features of the available DBMS. The task is not an easy one, particularly when the database is maintained on medium and large computer systems. First, the conceptual model of the database requirements may be merged into an overall subject database that has evolved through the development of other information systems. If your new system's requirements can be fulfilled by databases that already exist and if those databases can be supplemented to support your needs, why reinvent the wheel by building a redundant database?

Once the new system's conceptual data model has been merged and understood, it is translated into a logical data schema that can be supported within the restrictions of the DBMS and its logical data model (hierarchical, network, or relational). At this time, the DDL for the schema is generated. This schema must be made known to the systems analysts so they can easily complete the remainder of the design phase — output, input, terminal dialogue, and program design. Meanwhile, database specialists must design, redesign, or fine-tune the physical model of the database in order to achieve optimum performance (this is rarely done by the systems analyst).

In the last section, we suggested that the ideal conceptual data model is normalized. During the design of the logical database, the normalized structure is ideally preserved. In reality, the normalized data structure may have to be compromised when it is translated into a logical schema. Why? The designer is frequently forced to improve performance efficiency, and the normalized conceptual schema may not be the most efficient logical schema.

The design of a database is usually delegated to database specialists in large organizations. However, the systems analyst can expect to perform database design in smaller organizations. Also, because database specialists tend to focus on large, centralized databases, the analyst frequently designs those databases to be implemented on microcomputers.

SUMMARY

In this module, we changed our strategy somewhat. Our goal was not to teach you immediately applicable database design tools and techniques. That would have been impossible. Instead, we hope that we've enlightened you on one of the hottest topics in data processing — database. Database is an alternative to files where the data, normally stored in redundant files, is consolidated into nonredundant data sets. There are numerous advantages and disadvantages to both the file and database approaches; therefore, the two alternatives currently tend to coexist in many data processing shops. Ideally, databases should be built around business subjects rather than information systems applications. Subject databases are more flexible to future information systems requirements. End-user databases, which extract data from more active files and databases, are becoming popular.

Database technology revolves around special purpose software called database management systems (DBMS). Through a DBMS, programmers and users gain more flexible access to their data. Records are logically structured through the DBMS in one of three ways: hierarchies, networks, and tables (usually called relations). Records are physically stored on disk using traditional data and file structures that are transparent to the programmers and users.

Database technology has a significant impact on the analysis and design phases of the systems development life cycle. The analyst becomes responsible for understanding and structuring the data that describes a business problem. That data is then organized according to the capabilities and limitations of the available DBMS. More than anything, we've raised questions that point out (rather than providing answers to) the dilemma of database design. We hope you're now motivated to seek additional training on database design. You had better! Future systems analysts may be unable to function without a detailed understanding of database design!

PROBLEMS AND EXERCISES

1. Tammy, an Accounts Receivable manager, is considering a database management system for her microcomputer. She's not certain she really understands what a database is. In college, she took an introductory computer course and learned about files. She assumes *database* is the current buzzword for a collection of files. Write Tammy a memo explaining the difference between a file and a database environment. What are the advantages and disadvantages of each environment?
2. Briefly explain the differences between a data definition language, a data dictionary, a host programming language, and a data manipulation language.
3. What is the difference between a DBMS's physical structure and logical structure? What are three popular logical views supported by DBMSs? Prepare a simple schema for each type of logical view, and explain how they differ.
4. Visit your local computer store, and ask for a demonstration of

a microcomputer database management system (such as DBASE II or III, Knowledge Man, RBASE 4000, or a similar product). Get some literature on the product, and prepare a summary description (one or two pages) for the layperson (someone unfamiliar with computer technology and terminology).

5. Visit a local data processing shop that uses a database management system. Describe the existing database environment— Do they have application-oriented databases, subject-oriented databases, or end-user databases? What host programming language is used to load, maintain and use the data? Ask the systems analyst or database administrator to give you a brief orientation on the physical and logical structures supported by the DBMS. To what extent are conventional files used?

6. Discuss the impact a database would have on the following phases:
   (a) Study of the current system
   (b) Definition of user requirements
   (c) Evaluation of alternative solutions
   (d) Selection of computer equipment and software
   (e) Design of the new information system
   (f) Construction of the new information system
   (g) Delivery of the new information system

7. Visit a local data processing shop that operates only in a conventional file environment. Ask the systems analyst for information describing several of the master and transaction files. Do some of the files contain duplicate data? Is this data input several times? What impact has the duplicated data had on maintenance? Does the shop experience problems with data integrity? Have the analyst explain the impact of changing the format of one of the files.

8. If databases were created with the ability to solve many of the problems characteristic of conventional file-based systems, why aren't all data processing shops operating in a database environment?

9. For the database environment at a local business (problem 5), discuss the implications of the database for systems development. Does the analyst do anything differently from the way it would be done using conventional files? How do the analysts interact with the database administrator?

10. For the following simple systems, identify the basic business entities and relationships that would be stored in a database:
    (a) A course registration system
    (b) An order-processing system
    (c) An accounting system
    (d) A payroll system

    Try to identify at least four entities for each. Draw a data model diagram to depict the relationships.

ANNOTATED REFERENCES AND SUGGESTED READINGS

Flavin, Matt. *Fundamental Concepts of Information Modeling.* New York: Yourdan Press, 1981. This is a concise book on the subject of conceptual data modeling. The conceptual schema is similar, but not identical, to the sample conceptual schema in our book.

Gane, Chris, and Trish Sarson. *Structured Systems Analysis: Tools and Techniques.* Englewood Cliffs, N.J.: Prentice-Hall, 1979. Chapter 6, "Defining the Contents of Data Stores," presents a concise and relatively easy-to-understand treatment of normalization.

Koenke, David. *Database Processing.* 2d ed. Chicago: Science Research Associates, 1983. This is a popular introductory database textbook that surveys database concepts, technology, design, and implementation. If you don't have a database course available or can't fit one into your plan of study, this textbook would be one source of the fundamental knowledge of database.

Martin, James. *Managing the Data-Base Environment.* Englewood Cliffs, N.J.: Prentice-Hall, 1983. James Martin is one of the most noted authorities, writers, and lecturers in the database and data processing field — sort of a guru. No database reading list would be complete without at least one of his many titles. We chose this title because of its management orientation, which makes the book easy to read. The book introduces the database environment, its technology, normalization, applications, end-user databases, and database administration issues. This is a must reference book for the systems analyst's library.

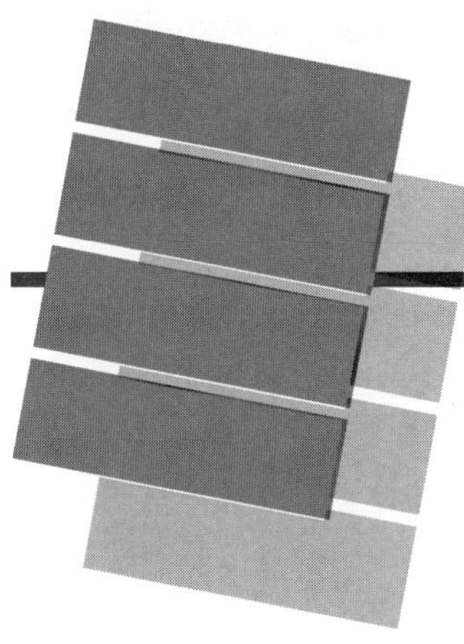

Index

NOTE: Italicized page numbers refer to illustrations.